INTEGRATED INTERDISCIPLINARY LEARNING BETWEEN THE HEALTH AND SOCIAL CARE PROFESSIONS: A FEASIBILITY STUDY

This book is dedicated to the memory of
my father David Derrick
(1924-1994)

Integrated Interdisciplinary Learning between the Health and Social Care Professions

A Feasibility Study

ROSEMARY TOPE
PhD (Wales), MEd (Wales), RGN, RCNT, RNT, Cert.Ed. (FE), DN (Lond)
Consultant in Interdisciplinary Health Studies and Advanced Nursing Education

Avebury
Aldershot · Brookfield USA · Hong Kong · Singapore · Sydney

Published by
Avebury
Ashgate Publishing Ltd
Gower House
Croft Road
Aldershot
Hants GU11 3HR
England

Ashgate Publishing Company
Old Post Road
Brookfield
Vermont 05036
USA

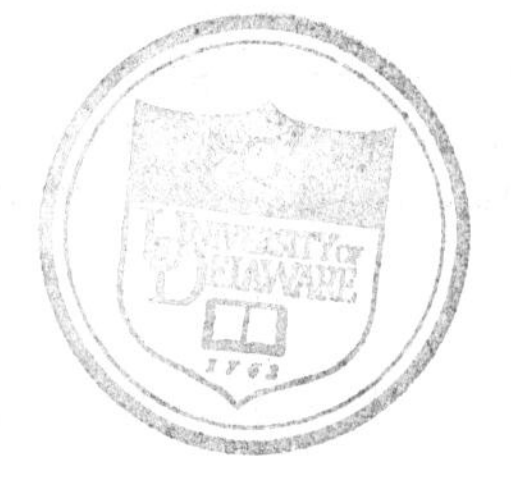

British Library Cataloguing in Publication Data

Tope, Rosemary
Integrated interdisciplinary learning between the health and social care professions : a feasibility study
1. Medical education 2. Interdisciplinary approach in education
I. Title
362.1 ' 07

ISBN 1 85972 357 8

Library of Congress Catalog Card Number: 96-84621

Printed in Great Britain by the Ipswich Book Company, Suffolk

Contents

Chapter 5 The results

Chapter 6 Interpretation and discussion of the results

Index to tables within the text

Chapter 2

Section 2.6: Interprofessional conflict

Section 2.7.3 Teamwork in primary health care

Chapter 5

Section 5.2 The fourteen curricula

Section 5.3 The reading lists

Section 5.4 The structured interviews

Section 5.4.1 The teaching staff

Chapter 6

Index to figures in the text

Section 5.5.1 The teachers

Section 5.5.2 The students

Section 5.5.3. The results by individual professions

5.5.3.1 The dentists

5.5.3.2 Dental surgery assistants and dental hygienists

5.5.3.3 The dental technologists

5.5.3.4 The medical practitioners

List of acronyms used in the text

ACTN	Advisory Committee on Training in Nursing
BIOSS	Brunel Institute of Organisation and Social Studies
BDA	British Dental Association
BMA	British Medical Association
BPS	British Psychological Society
CAIPE	Centre for the Advancement of Interprofessional Education in Primary Health and Community Care
CCETSW	Central Council for Education and Training in Social Work
CERI	Centre for Educational Research and Innovation
CHM	College of Human Medicine
CIHE	Cardiff Institute of Higher Education
CIPS	Centre for Interprofessional Studies (University of Nottingham)
COREPER	Committee of Permanent Representatives of the Member States
CONCAH	Continuing Care at Home
CPSM	Council for the Professions Supplementary to Medicine
CTI	Combined Training Institute
DHSA	District Health Authority
DHSS	Department of Health and Social Security
EC	European Community
EFPPA	European Federation of Professional Psychologists Association
EMPE	European Network for development of Multiprofessional Education in Health Sciences
FHSA	Family Health Services Authority
GDC	General Dental Council
GMC	General Medical Council
GNC	General Nursing Council
HCPEF	Health Care Professions Education Forum
HIU	Health Intelligence Unit
HMSO	His/Her Majesty's Stationery Office

HPAW	Health Promotion Authority (Wales)
ICN	International Council of Nurses
ICS	Institute of Community Studies
IFMSA	International Federation of Medical Students Associations
JTC	Joint Training Committee
LBTC	London Based Training Consortium
MBCT	Marylebone Centre Trust
MEP	Member of the European Parliament
MSC	Manpower Services Commission
MSG	Manpower Steering Group
NCVQ	National Council for Vocational Qualifications
NCOEIHS	Network of Community Oriented Educational Institutions for Health Sciences
NFER	National Foundation for Educational Research
NHS	National Health Service
NHSTA	National Health Service Training Authority
NHSTD	National Health Service Training Directorate
NVQ	National Vocational Qualifications
OWHS	Oliver Wendell Holmes Society
PMGI	Programa de Medicina General Integral
PSSC	Personal Social Services Council
RCN	Royal College of Nursing
SRHE	Society for Research into Higher Education (Ltd)
TCV	Team Care Valleys
TEHY	Union of Health Professionals (Finland)
TQM	Total Quality Management
UCH	United Cardiff Hospitals
UKCC	United Kingdom Central Council for Nursing Midwifery and Health Visiting
WFME	World Federation of Medical Education
WFPHA	World Forum Public Health Associations
WHA	World Health Assembly
WHPF	Welsh Health Planning Forum
WHO	World Health Organisation
WHO (SEARO)	WHO South East Asia Regional Office
WHPF	Welsh Health Planning Forum
YTS	Youth Training Scheme(s)

Glossary of terms

The following operational definitions have been adopted throughout the text unless specifically stated otherwise.

Accountability

"The test of accountability is that if a person did not do something, did it poorly or deviated from an established policy or procedure, the person could be considered negligent or to have breached their contract and sanctions could be applied as a result - an extreme sanction being that they could be sacked. Accountability cannot be delegated." (Ovretveit 1984)

Clinical autonomy

"The freedom to exercise discretion.........within available resources and other limits and without that discretion being overridden or scrutinised be a higher authority, unless negligence or infringement of limits is suspected." (Ovretveit 1984)

Community based education

"An educational programme, or curriculum, can be called community based if for its entire duration, it consists of an appropriate number of learning activities in a balanced variety of educational settings ie in both the community and a diversity of health care services at all levels." (WHO 1988b)

Competence

"The ability to carry out a certain professional function (eg a medical function, a nursing function) which is made up of a repertoire of professional practices. Competence requires knowledge, appropriate attitudes and observable mechanical or intellectual skills, which together account for the ability to deliver a specified professional service." (WHO 1988b)

Corporate responsibility
"Corporate responsibility is an ethical concept rather than a legal or managerial one i.e. it refers to team loyalties and responsibilities as perceived and felt by members." (BPS 1986)

Health care team
"A health care team is a group of three or more health care practitioners who working together, bring their skills to bear on a particular health problem or patient in order to achieve health care goals." (Feiger & Schmitt 1979)

"There can be no universally applicable composition of the health team." (WHO 1988b)

Health personnel
"All persons who carry out health care tasks (promotive, preventive, curative and rehabilitative) within the health system, whether they are community health workers, heart surgeons, dentists, nurses, chiropodists, sanitary engineers, social workers or any other manpower category." (WHO 1988b)

Integration
"Integration is a way of organising knowledge and skills to approximate to practice more closely than academic disciplines normally do." (WHO 1978c)

Professionalisation
"The process by which an occupational group secures a domain of activity against encroachment from other workers through the imposition of entrance criteria, special training programmes, codes of ethics to secure a domain of work which, in many instances, is eventually institutionalised when the state recognises it." (WHO 1981b)

Role
"Expectations enhance the probability that in a given social situation, individuals will act to a greater extent in a predetermined manner." (HMSO 1979d)

Strategy
"The broad lines of action required in all sectors to give effect to health policy." (WHO 1981)

Teamwork
"Teamwork implies that solutions to problems can be worked out as agroup rather than by individuals and that it is possible to arrive at a shared philosophy and to act as an organic entity. In this way teams can acknowledge and support the roles of its members." (Hannay 1980)

Acknowledgements

The author wishes to acknowledge and give sincere thanks for the invaluable assistance and support given in the conduct of this research from the following ;
The Smith and Nephew Foundation for awarding a 1992 Scholarship which enabled the visits to Sweden, Finland and France to take place.
Professor Hans Nils Areskog and all staff and students in the Faculty of Health Sciences, University of Linkoping, Sweden.
The Ministry of Education, Finland, and the staff and students in the Universities and Higher Education Institutes of Helsinki, Turku and Joensuu.
Professor Attali and all staff and students in the Faculty of Medicine and Health Sciences, Universite Paris XIII, Bobigny, France.
The Welsh Office for their participation in, and their financial support of the interdisciplinary workshop held in March 1993.
The Provost, the Deans of Faculties and the senior members of staff for their encouragement and their permission to access the teaching staff and students from the three participating institutions.
The twenty nine teachers and twenty two students representing the thirteen professions, who were willing to be interviewed.
The Principals of the Colleges in which the pilot studies took place and the ninety eight teaching staff and students who completed the questionnaires.
The three hundred teachers and one thousand three hundred and sixty three students who completed the main study questionnaires.
Mrs Vanda Fenn, Dr Glyn Johns, Dr Eleri Jones and Dr Alan Sutton for their constructive advice and criticism.
Last but by no means least, Dr Roy Nolan for giving me the confidence to believe in myself, for his being there at all times, and for his technical expertise and time that enabled my thesis to be converted into this book.

Foreword

I am delighted to have been asked to write an introduction to Dr Tope's book on interdisciplinary learning between the health and social care professions. It is not possible to have been involved in the clinical care of patients and the education of medical students (as I have been for many years) without being aware of our failure to promote effective teamwork between the various health care professionals by teaching them, both at undergraduate and postgraduate level, how they should go about it.

Increasingly, looking after patients, whether in the primary care setting or in hospitals depends on team-work between the individuals involved who will be members of different professional groups. There will be many examples of how this can be done well with consequent benefits for patients. Unfortunately, many of us are only too aware of how often interprofessional jealousy, conflict over roles and unhelpful stereotyping inhibit the provision of the best care.

Interdisciplinary learning, both at postgraduate and undergraduate stages, including the recognition of the roles, expectations, strengths (and yes, weaknesses) of other professions would seem to be the key to unlocking this problem.

Anyone who wants to set out to attempt this would be wise to read Dr Tope's book first. Based on her PhD thesis, this is a real "how to do it" manual. We can learn what has been done, where, by whom and did it work. Various models for interdisciplinary learning are described as well as the research which is still needed. I can only hope that anyone with an interest in health education will read this book and ask themselves why are we not doing this already? Once that question has been asked Dr Tope can show the way forward.

I R Cameron
Provost and Vice-Chancellor
University of Wales College of Medicine
Heath Park
Cardiff CF4 4XN

1 The need for the research

1.1 Introduction

The impetus for this research resulted from a growing awareness of the urgent necessity to address the problems of health professionals' education. The isolationalist approaches to curriculum development within each profession in particular, did not seem to reflect or complement the philosophy of holistic patient care. Whilst this tenet remains the crucial issue throughout, other factors have also contributed to the recognition of the need for innovation and change. These include an awareness of an increasing shortage of appropriately trained personnel, demographic changes and increasing financial constraints. The cultural shift in health care in which the patient has become the central focus, signifies an acknowledgement that the patient has a right to choose and normally direct decisions regarding his/her own life style and health behaviour. The emphasis on "health" rather than on "disease" has also influenced change. The evolution of the primary health team, in evidence throughout most of the world, has moved the emphasis away from the acute hospital sector and into the community. Maintaining healthy individuals within their own environment has become paramount in the quest for quality in health care.

Integrated interdisciplinary education in health care is a global issue (WHO 1948). Maintaining health, preventing disease and caring for the sick is now so complex a problem that it is impossible for any single health profession to deliver quality care in isolation (Schein 1972, Mazur et al., 1979, Ducanis and Golin 1979, Scott-Wright 1976, Mariano 1989). Light (1969) described health care as "an occupational jungle" in which new professional breeds were constantly proliferating and forming their own tribes. The mainstream professions in health care are usually controlled by statutory bodies. They include medical practitioners ("doctors"), dentists, nurses, physiotherapists occupational therapists, speech therapists, clinical psychologists, nutritionists and dietitians, podiatrists (formerly chiropodists), radiographers (both diagnostic and therapeutic), dental technologists, pharmacists, orthoptists, and ophthalmic opticians. A further profession inextricably linked with health and welfare is social work. Whilst this group is not directly classified as a health care profession, social workers make an essential contribution to the maintenance of a patient's biopsychosocial equilibrium.

Within the United Nations an agency with specific responsibility for international health matters was constituted in 1948. This agency is called the World Health Organisation (WHO). The constitution of the World Health Organisation states that one of its functions is to promote "improved standards of teaching and training in the health,medical and related professions" (WHO 1948).

In the same year a programme of education and training was adopted by the First World Health Assembly and guidelines for the implementation of the programme issued. Nearly three decades later Fulop (1976) assessed the progress to date. In a highly critical paper he identified many reasons why the integrated development of the health professions had become a "permanent problem". One of his major concerns was the lack of collaboration between the managers responsible for health care delivery and those providing education and training. He suggested that there was hostility and conflict between professional groups which was impeding the concept of a team approach to learning and in the delivery of care.

The WHO (1981a) set targets which need to be achieved in order to reach the elusive 'Health for All'. These include an increased focus on patients needs, an increased emphasis on the promotion of health through primary health care and a greater effort to develop the philosophy of effective teamwork. In order to meet these demands major innovations in the current educational programmes for health personnel will have to occur (Areskog 1988).

The problem of manpower shortage and the inadequate and irrelevant training that health carers received was addressed by the WHO in 1976. Appropriate education was perceived as *the* major factor in predicting the success of health care programmes throughout the world. The WHO recommended that all educational programmes should be developed in such a way that integrative teamwork resulted. The traditional medically orientated, curative care approach to curriculum development has been heavily criticised and is deemed to be largely irrelevant to changing health patterns (WHO 1973a, 1973b, 1976, 1981a, 1981b, 1987d). Kiereini (1985) adds to the debate of what constitutes changing health patterns by suggesting that the consumers of health care services, whether on a community or an individual basis, are more knowledgeable about changing needs and priorities than the professionals. Rigid and demanding educational programmes are commonplace. Passive learning and factual recall for examination purposes continue to take priority over problem solving and critical thinking skills (WHO 1973a, Steele 1987, Eron 1985).

By 1984 universities throughout the world were considering their contribution to health care. Approximately 350 delegates attended the 37th World Health Assembly. They were representative of most ministries of health, universities and national health services throughout the world. The focus of the assembly was to highlight the potential that universities have for influencing the outcomes of health care. A document was produced which recommended an increase in collaboration between all concerned. The document described this phenomena as "a partnership of opportunity" and clearly highlighted the *potential* role that universities could play as opposed to the *actual* role currently in vogue. It examined the philosophy of higher education and used the term 'university' generically throughout for all higher education establishments. (WHO 1984a, Resolution 37.31)

In 1984 it was perceived that universities were discipline rather than mission orientated. The trend towards greater specialisation and fragmentation of knowledge would reinforce academic disciplines rather than link higher education with the real world, "communities have problems , universities have departments" (WHO 1984a : p.13).

An interdisciplinary approach was suggested as being a more flexible, appropriate strategy for a new type of interaction with the consumer. As far as health care itself was concerned there was no suggestion that in most cases, highly qualified, competent practitioners were not produced. More time should be devoted, however, to the enhancement of communication skills. A problem solving rather than a discipline orientated approach was identified as being the best way forward. It was recognised that any attempt to restructure traditional curricula would be resisted by the academic traditionalists in the name of so called academic freedom. It was clearly acknowledged that, "a critical appraisal of the curricula of various health science programmes is a fundamental though daunting task" (WHO 1984a : p.15).

Adaptability and understanding were thought to be essential if an attempt to redirect curriculum development to implement interdisciplinary learning was to be made. The isolationist 'ivory tower' philosophy of universities was noted with regret. This was in view of the fact that universities were usually strategically placed regarding resources, delivery and promotion of health care in the communities which they purported to serve. They should play a far more fundamental role in helping to define health policies. Not all the criticism can be laid within the university sector. It was suggested that governments and most particularly ministries of health failed to capitalise on the academic's knowledge and experience in health related disciplines. If the recommendations set out above were adopted as a policy, wastage of resources, unnecessary duplication and general inefficiency would be diminished and possibly completely erased. The assembly called for a framework to be developed that would maximise each faculty's contribution to health care.

Whilst recognising that different models of management exist in different establishments it was deemed essential for a formally identified group of managers within higher education to coordinate increased collaboration. The deans of faculties were perceived to have a central role. The listing of programmes and courses important for national development regarding 'Health for All' was considered to be an initial step. Where possible these programmes should be extended from the 'ivory tower' into the society they serve. This, it was felt, would minimise the academic elitism fostered by most institutions. "Reform will come through enlightened leadership and the spirit of interdisciplinary collaboration." (WHO 1984a : p.17)

1.2 The nomenclature

Over one thousand references have been found which allude to interdisciplinary health care. It would appear however, that few authors have considered in depth the nomenclature which should be adopted when discussing integrated learning between the health professions. Various terms have been used interchangeably both between and within publications. Information has been collated for this study which has revealed the usage of the following terms:

interprofessional, intraprofessional, transprofessional, multiprofessional, multidisciplinary pluridisciplinary, transdisciplinary and interdisciplinary.

The Society for Research in Higher Education (SRHE 1977), Szasz (1969), McCally et al., (1977), Mazur et al., (1979), Owen (1982), Bair (1983), Ivey et al., (1988) Mariano (1989), Leathard (1990), have all addressed the problem of the correct terminology which should be used. The term 'interdisciplinary' appears to generate greater consensus than other alternatives when true integration and collaboration is evident, "common goals, cooperative relationships and coordinated activities are ideally the hallmarks" (Ivey et al., 1988: p.192)

Bair (1983) believed that only when the multidisciplinary team began to meet on a regular face-to-face basis did interdisciplinarity begin to emerge. Mariano (1989) was convinced that without a clear definition and an understanding of the concept of interdisciplinary care, the expectations and orientations of the different disciplines would continue to be diverse and divisive. Mariano suggested that a suitable definition would be "an entity that has a structure, a definition, a direction, an identification, a group energy or synergy." (Ibid : p.286)

The SRHE (1977) considered that when two or more disciplines have a close interaction on a regular basis that interdisciplinarity is occurring. Scott-Wright (1976), although incorrectly using the term 'multidisciplinary', concluded that it was therefore necessary for students of different disciplines to participate in some shared learning. This she argued would "avoid wasteful overlap of expertise" (p 77). She believed that the evidence was now "irrefutable". Owen (1982) supported Szasz (1969) in concluding that integrated learning was an extension of joint learning. Joint learning, they argued was the strategy most frequently adopted. Students from different disciplines might attend the same lectures or classes but interaction did not take place on a formal basis. This could justifiably be described as multidisciplinary joint teaching. When students from different disciplines work actively together on problem solving activities, or when they are dealing with common issues in small tutorial groups this can be described as integrated interdisciplinary learning. The question now arises of how many courses that are described as interdisciplinary should be reclassifed as multidisciplinary? For the purposes of this research it was decided that the words integrated and interdisciplinary would be used as the nomenclature and as such is a deliberate strategy.

Milio (1979) further supports the suitability of this decision when she described the development of a common curriculum for the education of the health professions. She stated categorically that it must be "integrative and interdisciplinary" (Ibid : 159). Perhaps Ivey et al (1988) have been the most succinct in their suggestion that true interdisciplinarity would result in, "a health care support system which is greater than the sum of its professionals" (Ibid : p.192).

1.3 Integrated learning

It is important to change or modify the beliefs of the more traditional managers as well as the academic staff directly involved with health care programmes. The formulation and evaluation of curricula will ultimately depend on the ability to identify the competencies required by the health care professions, which permit them to function in a way that enhances the total quality of patient care whilst retaining academic freedom (Hamburg 1984). A series of radical approaches have been advocated. One of these was to establish new training institutes in which shared learning could be implemented (WHO 1976 A29/15). A non orthodox approach to curriculum development was to be encouraged which reflected problem orientated programmes based "not only on biomedical but also on social and behavioural sciences (sic) including epidemiology , healthplanning and management." (WHO 1976 : p.26)

This would lead to the optimum utilisation of all health personnel, as the success of health care depends upon effective health manpower. The word effective is paramount as it implies that unhealthy competition, duplication of effort and conflict should be minimised in order to increase mutual cooperation and collaboration. The WHO had previously warned however, that such programmes should not replace those for individual health professions. They should be complementary to existing programmes. Adopting this approach they believed, would lead to an increased recognition of the unique skills deployed by each profession within the health team (WHO 1973b).

Steele (1987) suggested an alternative way to approach learning in health care. He considered optimal learning in health care as community orientated, individualised and flexible. Collier and Clarke (1986) paradoxically had found that most curricula were teacher centered, subject orientated, standardised, inflexible and in many cases obsolete. Steele (1987), heavily criticised "the lack of active participation" by students in the learning process and regretted that whilst there was a profusion of literature on the shortcomings of the present system, there was little available on what needs to be done and by whom. Steele berated the use of the lecture system and accused health educators of force feeding the student "an ill defined quantity of knowledge" (p3). As no student can retain the amount of knowledge to which he/she is exposed, Steele suggested that the prime responsibility for the teacher is to teach the student how to learn. Steele's philosophy would be strongly supported by Knowles (1984) who drew attention to the principles of adult learning and ensured that the term andragogy was absorbed into common usage in adult educational language. Goodlad and Hirst (1989) described student learning as making it possible to combine work with pleasure.

Debling cited in Burke (1990:80), argued however, that competence remained the central issue upon which vocational education and training should be based. He described a competent individual as being able to :

> perform a particular function or satisfy a particular role in a diversity of settings, over an extended period of time; and respond effectively to irregular occurences in environments having different characteristics.
>
> (Ibid 1990 : 80)

Each health care profession demands a measurable level of competence in students before they are recognised as autonomous practitioners. This indicates that the teachers function is to select *what* must be learned in order that students not only pass the statutory examinations, but also demonstrate safe practice.

In an ideal world, health professionals' education would be provided in a real life setting so that the knowledge and skills acquired could be applied immediately. The constraints however, in which professional education is currently delivered, mean that the best alternative would be a problem solving approach enacted in such a way that a real life situation could be simulated. If students interact with each other in the same way that qualified practising health professionals do in reality, then teachers will need to redefine their role in order to facilitate student learning. They should certainly do so before the student becomes a qualified, autonomous practitioner (Houle 1980, Knowles 1984, Guilbert 1984,Eron 1985, Steele 1987, Goodlad and Hirst 1989).

Smith and Bass (1982) linked health personnels' communication skills inextricably with the public image of health care. Good communication they argued, enhances the public's perceptions of the quality of health care whereas poor communication has a detrimental effect. They emphasised the diverse socio-economic, cultural and ethnic differences between health care workers themselves. Misunderstandings, prejudices, conflict and stereotyping were the inevitable concommitant of these differences. If an individual patient's own diversities were included in a given situation it could be a recipe for disaster. Many authors reinforce the individuality of patients but few consider the individuality of the professionals themselves. Professional elitism is not the answer to cooperative health care. Commitment to other people can only be established through collaboration. This includes the cooperation of the patients because the carers are dependent on their request for help.

One of the most frequent criticisms of the National Health Service in the United Kingdom is the lack of communication that exists at all levels, at all times (Smith and Bass 1982, Nelson 1989, Turrell 1989, Broome 1990). Jargon is frequently used in health care to the detriment of patient comprehension. Jargonistic terms are being assimilated increasingly into each profession with a further subgroup language evolving for specialisations within a single profession (Light 1969, Hockey 1977, Brooking 1991). Hockey (1977) during a one hour period of observation within a hospital ward, witnessed eleven different professionals in some form of verbal exchange with patients. The need for consistency and continuity of information must surely be exemplified by this example?

1.4 Recent developments

Over the past fifteen years, groups of professionals from different health disciplines have begun to address the problem of lack of interdisciplinarity. Several organisations have been founded on both an international and national basis. The European Network for Development of Multiprofessional Education in the Health Sciences (EMPE), founded in 1987 operates from Linkoping Sweden. The Network of Community Oriented Education Institution for Health Sciences (NCOEIHS) founded in 1979 is based in Maastricht Holland. The Centre for Advancement of Interprofessional Education (CAIPE) founded in London in 1985, and the Health Care Professionals Education Forum (HCPEF) founded in 1989 in the United Kingdom, are but a few examples.

Journals are also beginning to appear which concentrate entirely on the interdisciplinary approach to health care. In January 1992 the first specialist publication, "The Journal of Interprofessional Care" appeared. The contributors to the journal have all previously published extensively on integrated interdisciplinary teamwork with their names appearing on membership lists of several of the organisations identified above. The editorial preface of this journal is entitled "A New Beginning". It would appear that the philosophy of integrated interdisciplinary health care is becoming more widely accepted and that its implementation is growing rapidly. In order to realistically address the WHO 1981 directive, "Health for All by the Year 2000", all institutions which educate and train future health care professionals must urgently confront the issues.

1.5 Summary

In conclusion, universities, polytechnics, institutes of higher education and the national health services are currently facing acute financial problems (Turner 1990). Professional education and the delivery of health care by implication therefore, is constantly under review in order to maximise the available resources without reducing quality. The introduction of integrated interdisciplinary learning where appropriate and feasible, may be a solution which would address the problem in a tangible and altruistic way. Interdisciplinarity challenges the traditional curriculum because it portends academic fusion with the associated flexibility and adaptability that this would demand. For many educators in the health field a major re-orientation would be essential in order to reduce role conflict, professional boundaries and legitimate concerns regarding professional autonomy and accountability. Each profession is regulated in the United Kingdom by its own Statutory Body that controls its practitioners. Licence to practice must be sought by each newly qualified practitioner on the recommendation of the training institution. Within this structure it is very rare that an individual migrates from one profession to another mainly because legally he/she has to undertake additional training. All Statutory Bodies share the same aim of excellence in practice. Styles and Gottauk (1978), ruefully observed that the professions tended to talk as though they are interdisciplinary, whereas in reality, "they function as separate professional entities in a physical structure that houses different disciplines." (Ibid,1978 : 1979). The institutions in which this research took place epitomise the above statement. In 1993 three separate organisations existed which trained health professionals. They were all within a three mile radius. There were no less than fourteen academic schools providing specialist training in various forms. Turnbull (1982) recommended a major thrust towards shared learning and warned that there was no room for "tokenism". Manpower issues and financial constraints will most probably demand maximal utilisation of resources and whilst no one model of interdisciplinary learning can be projected as the optimum one, a critical analysis of the potential areas of shared learning between the health professionals should be undertaken with urgency. Perceived and identified change from within is always preferable to imposed change from external agencies (Broome 1990).

Mariano (1989) listed confusion, fragmentation and isolation as the inevitable outcome of a lack of theoretical understanding of true interdisciplinarity. Ducanis and Golin (1979) blamed a lack of empirical research which could underpin a theoretical framework on which a model could be built. They observed that the present system of rewarding individual accomplishment in academia de-emphasised and devalued collaborative endeavours. One of the first requisites for greater interdisciplinary collaboration would be institutional commitment in the form of time, space, legitimation, administrative support, motivation and reward (Mazur et al., 1979).

An increasing number of publications have appeared, citing examples of shared learning between two or more professions, most of which can be attributed to the behavioural sciences. Little evidence would appear to exist of shared learning in the biological sciences (see Appendix 1.1).

Many examples of integrated interdisciplinary learning would seem to have been subjected to anecdotal evaluation only. Spitzer (1975) argued that empirical data must be obtained on the effectiveness of such initiatives, only then could a conclusive and definitive statement be made. It was decided therefore, to explore the concept of integrated interdisciplinary learning and to empirically determine the feasibility of its introduction into practice, within the context of health care.

1.6 The aims of the study

From the foregoing considerations it became increasingly clear that a detailed analysis of all the various implications of implementing integrated interdisciplinary learning within health care was required. In consequence this study set out with the following aims:

1. To analyse the behavioural science content specified within current curricula for each profession in order to determine commonality.

2. To identify the behavioural science textbooks listed in the current curricula for each profession in order to determine replication.

3. To determine the opinions of a sample of both statutorily qualified and student representatives from each profession regarding :

   3.1 The concept of integrated interdisciplinary learning.
   3.2 The perceived advantages/disadvantages of integrated interdisciplinary learning.
   3.3. When integrated interdisciplinary learning should take place, if at all.
   3.4. The favoured learning methods which should be adopted.
   3.5. The level of interest in interdisciplinary learning.

3.6. Which professions would be acceptable to each other on an interdisciplinary learning basis.

4. To determine :-

    4.1. The operational strategies required to implement integrated interdisciplinary learning.
    4.2. The preparation needed by the teachers themselves prior to implementation.

5. To ascertain from the statutory and professional bodies :-

    5.1. Whether integrated interdisciplinary learning in the behavioural sciences would fulfil the statutory requirements of the individual professions.
    5.2. The level of support forany potential developments in interdisciplinary learning between the health and social care professions.

2 Review of the literature

2.1 Introduction

The review of the literature has revealed an extensive range of publications regarding interdisciplinary approaches to health care. More than a thousand such references have been reviewed to date and new papers seem to appear on a monthly basis. Many of these papers concentrate on the concept of teamwork and focus on teamwork in the community. Most publications referring to interdisciplinary learning describe initiatives which involve health professionals who have already qualified. These integrated learning programmes have therefore, been designed specifically as post graduate continuing education strategies. Far fewer have been found that describe under-graduate, pre-clinical integrated learning. This is in spite of the evidence, that will be subsequently discussed, which suggests that stereotyping and role conflict occur at the beginning of an individual's professional education.

Authors, on a global basis, have contributed to the debate of what constitutes integrated interdisciplinary learning, how and when it should be implemented, and which professions should be encouraged to participate. A few authors have developed their own theoretical frameworks upon which they recommend educational developments should be based. Despite an extensive search, most papers focus on the relationship between medicine and nursing. Whilst others concentrate on the dynamics between all the health professions, few examples have been found of authors from the paramedical professions publishing in their own professional journals on this subject. Inevitably the classification of this number of publications has proved extremely difficult, as many fit interchangeably into several categories. It has been decided, nevertheless, for convenience to divide the review of the pertinent literature into the following classifications :

2.2 A global overview

There are currently one hundred and sixty five countries contributing their knowledge and expertise to the World Health Organisation (WHO 1984a). The purpose of this collaboration is to achieve the WHO stated aim of 'achieving health for all by the year 2000' (WHO 1978). Although publications can be traced back to 1948 which refer to education and training in healthcare, it is only over the last twenty years that more attention has been paid to the problem of inappropriate and inadequate preparation for holistic patient care.

In 1973 a WHO Expert Committee (No 534) examined continuing educational opportunities for medical practitioners. They concluded that although most medical students were highly motivated at the beginning of their training, this was rapidly eroded because of the negative characteristics found in most medical schools towards learning. The expert committee believed that before innovative continuing education in medicine could be addressed, undergraduate training should be completely revised. They primarily blamed the educationalists themselves whom they suggested "must modify their curricula and teaching methods in a manner that will provide positive inducements to learning."(WHO 1973a : 10)

They explored the desirability of interdisciplinary programmes and advised that whilst such programmes could not and should not replace the traditional individual discipline programmes, they should be adopted as complementary ones. Adopting this approach, they believed, would lead to an increased recognition of the unique skills deployed by each profession working within a team, would increase role satisfaction, increase the general public's appreciation of the health care team and most importantly be a much more effective way of treating patients holistically. They emphasised the point that interdisciplinary learning must be an active process in which a common language is established and a common frame of reference adopted. They recommended that student members of each profession should be an integral part of curriculum development teams. It was deemed to be essential for students to contribute towards identifying the learning objectives, the teaching strategies and the evaluation process (WHO 1973a : 21). Co-ordination was seen as an essential criteria for the success of interdisciplinary learning. Significantly they concluded their report by commenting on the growing number of health care teams and recognised their importance in combating professional isolation. They warned however, that whilst these teams may create a climate which was more receptive to this kind of learning, any change would not occur automatically. Each member state of the WHO was charged to provide interdisciplinary programmes and the committee recommended that demonstration projects should begin immediately. In the same year the WHO published a Technical Report (WHO 1973b) which examined the training of teachers in the health professions. It stressed the importance of teachers grasping the principles of curriculum development. Examples were given of essential criteria which should be implicit in a successful curriculum. These included the educational philosophy, health care determinants, community issues, the sequencing of instruction and the assessment method devised to test professional competence. The sociology of the health professions was deemed to be an important part of a teacher's training, so that an understanding was gained of health care systems, the vocabulary of the health professions and the values used to judge acceptable and unacceptable performance.

Fulop (1976) suggested that problems in the health services were due, in part, to inappropriate preparation of personnel. These problems, he continued, were both qualitative and quantitative in nature. The qualitative ones Fulop believed were :

- the relatively low status accorded to health in plans for socio-economic development in some countries.
- an absence of well formulated health policies and plans.
- a lack of co-ordination both within the health sector and with other sectors in socio-economic development.
- no involvement by the community (i.e. the consumer) in the planning, management and evaluation of the health services available.

The quantitative ones were due entirely to a lack of empirical research. He accused health services generally of uneconomic utilisation of many categories of health personnel. Different values were placed on different disciplines with a consequent uneven distribution of resources. A geographical bias and prejudice in the allocation of resources was evident. Fulop appealed for a clearer definition of the functions of each discipline along with a "delineation of competence" (p 434). He postulated that many tasks carried out by highly qualified personnel could equally be undertaken by less highly trained individuals at a consequent lower cost.

The global effect of these problems was inadequate health care in developing countries and a deficiency in the quality of health coverage in developed countries. Fulop expressed concern that training institutions do not always belong to the same authority as the health manpower planning unit. This is an interesting statement in view of the fact that there is a rapid move for many more educational centres to become entirely independent of the health authorities in the United Kingdom this decade. Fulop maintained that as a result of this split "the production of health manpower develops quite independently from the real needs, both quantitative and qualitative, of the health services." (Fulop 1976 : 434 - 435)

Management of health personnel was also compromised by a lack of communication and coordination. The three main elements essential to the development of health services ; health manpower planning, health manpower production and health manpower management, Fulop believed were developing in an entirely uncoordinated manner. He introduced a model in which the inter-relationships between the three elements were clearly demonstrated (see Figure 2.1).

Fulop identified reasons for the difficulties in manpower planning. In many countries there were insufficient facilities available for training. Consequently this led to unmanageable and unwieldy numbers of students in other places. General shortages of teachers especially those competent to plan, implement and evaluate the teaching/learning process systematically compounded the difficulty. A wide chasm continues to exist between academic goals, service requirements and consumer expectations in a constantly changing socio-economic climate. As a result of the problems Fulop suggested, many of the present curricula are often unsuitable in that they do not meet the needs of the community. Health needs change rapidly and educational programmes that develop in isolation do not fulfil this need. The need to adapt existing educational programmes was evident, yet Fulop suggested a lot of talking was taking place but little action. Advances had been made, there was an increased emphasis on student centered learning and an
The Twenty Ninth World Health Assembly (WHO 1976 : WHA 29.72) considered that inadequate and irrelevant training impeded the health care available to populations. They affirmed theit commitment to interdisciplinary learning and referred to the need for a greater emphasis on the behavioural sciences (p6). Continuing education "should be developed in such a way as to favour the concept and practice of team work". (Ibid : p9)

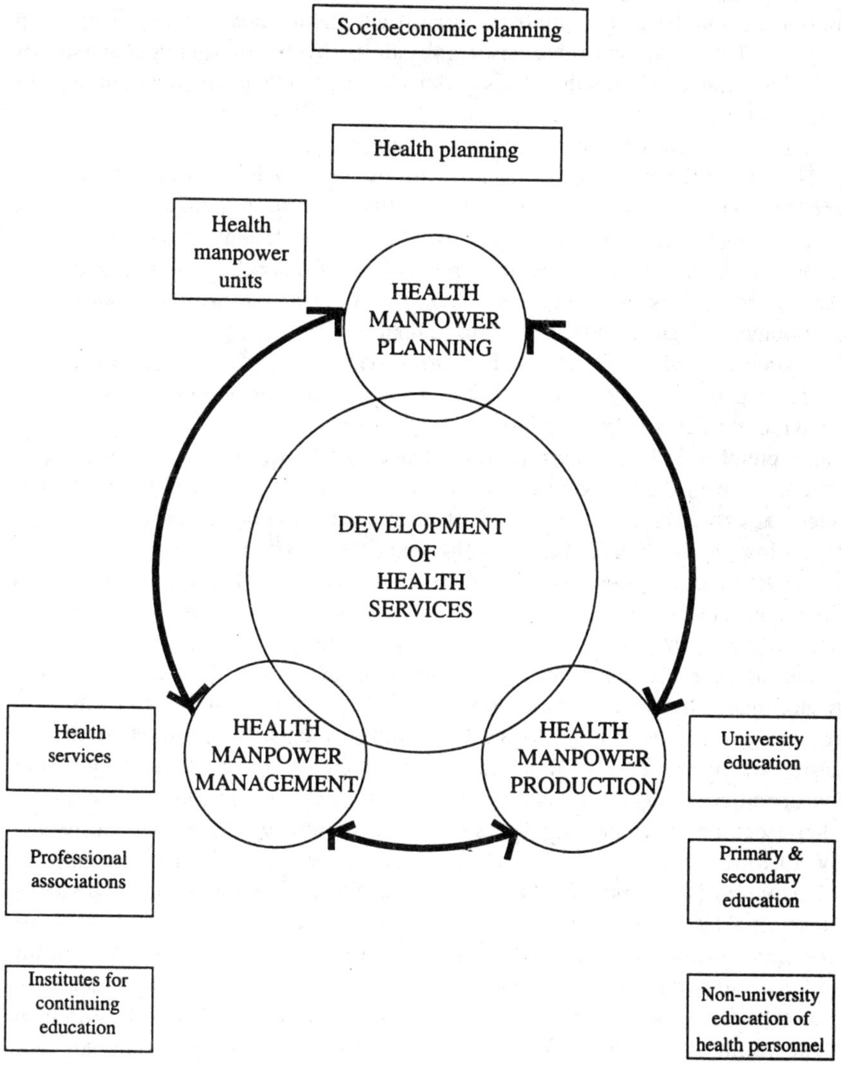

Socioeconomic planning

Health planning

Health manpower units

HEALTH MANPOWER PLANNING

DEVELOPMENT OF HEALTH SERVICES

HEALTH MANPOWER MANAGEMENT

HEALTH MANPOWER PRODUCTION

Health services

Professional associations

Institutes for continuing education

University education

Primary & secondary education

Non-university education of health personnel

National bodies involved: Ministry of Health (or equivalent); Ministry of Social Welfare (or equivalent); Ministry of Education (or equivalent); Ministry of Socioeconomic Development (or equivalent); Ministry of Planning (or equivalent); Ministry of Labour (or equivalent); National Research Institutes, etc.

Figure 2.1 Institutional interrelationships in health services and manpower development (HMSD) and some of the national bodies involved (Fulop 1976)

They noted 'the wide divergency' between theory and practice and the continuing emphasis on curative rather than preventative care. This, they believed, led to an ever increasing chasm between educationalists and the managers responsible for the delivery of care. This divide was not helped by "a hostile attitude on the part of certain influential professional groups to radical changes in health personnel education." (Ibid : 19)

They called for a radical change in the approach to health manpower development. They devolved the responsibility to a national level, thus enabling each country to define their own objectives. Unorthodox approaches were seen as the way forward. It was suggested that individual countries should reorientate themselves by establishing new training institutions with concommitant development of teaching staff and educational processes.

Integrated interdisciplinary, problem orientated educational programmes should be developed to enhance teamwork. These programmes should include the behavioural sciences, health planning and management.

In September 1978 a milestone was reached, when one hundred and thirty four nations convened at a conference in Alma Ata, in the former USSR. The delegates expressed an urgent need for all governments in the world to promote the philosophy of 'health for all by the year 2000'. The key to the solution was known to be prevention rather than cure and as such, a call was made for greater effort and more resources to be put towards primary health care. The delegates made a statement which has subsequently become known as 'The Alma Ata Declaration'. From this declaration health strategies throughout the world can be traced, indeed the all embracing term 'health for all by the year 2000' emanates from statement five (WHO 1978a : 3). Health strategies have been subsequently defined by the WHO as; "a broad line of action to be undertaken at policy and operational levels,nationally and internationally in the health sector and in other social and economic sectors to attain health for all by the year 2000." (WHO 1981a)

Kierini (1985) complained that not all governments had kept their pledge made within the Declaration, and of those who had, many had subsequently lost momentum. She believed that public expectations had been raised and health workers, supported by governments, should make every effort to meet these expectations. Kierini expressed particular concern about the third world countries, many of whom were adopting ideas from the developed world. This, she had found, was a mistake, as these adopted strategies took no account of local circumstances. Regretably, human resources and financial support were being wasted. Of even greater significance was the continued refusal to consult the local communities themselves.

The WHO (1986d Res.WHA 39.22) defended their position. They argued that whilst they had sought to develop more integrated health policies and programmes, the lack of national mechanisms for action and implementation of change coupled with inadequate resources, planning and commitment, militated against progress. They called for "major internal adjustments and reorientation" (p 15) within individual countries. The changing health profiles of nations in conjunction with changing socio-economic climates meant that the health policy makers had to take an overview of its peoples' health and plan accordingly using a flexible approach. The educationalists, both in health care and the university sectors, did not escape the attention of the WHO. They were charged with the task of "imparting a core of interdisciplinary knowledge" (p 91) and ensuring that the curriculum orientated health professionals towards "assuming greater responsibility as health educators" (p 124). Ineffective communication between the different disciplines was thought to be a major factor in the lack of collaboration.

Dr Halfdan Mahler (then Director General of the WHO) challenged educators' to produce programmes that maximised student's full potential and prepared them to work as a member of a health team (WHO 1978c : preface). Mahler complained of the irrelevant and inappropriate programmes which continued to place too much reliance on past experiences. The principle objective of the document itself, was to promote and develop health personnel of a calibre that would meet the needs of the community they served. In order to achieve this, both basic and continuing education programmes had to be made relevant and applicable to meet these needs.

In 1978 experiments in interdisciplinary, interprofessional, community orientated learning had commenced. The WHO was collating and publishing the results of these experiments. They required the anonymous institutions participating in the experiment to criticise their programmes constructively and disseminate the results. Of particular interest was any information which identified the factors that had facilitated or inhibited their programme development. Initial results suggested that with the shift towards primary care and the community, a greater emphasis on the behavioural sciences as a foundation study had evolved. An increased emphasis on team work was also evident. Many problems had been encountered with the introduction of interdisciplinary learning and with "some notable exceptions" the WHO detected frustration at the lack of progress. Although initiatives seemed reasonably successful in collaborative research projects, professional jealousies and insecurities were militating against the interdisciplinary programmes themselves. The WHO were convinced that in spite of these problems :

> Given that effective health care requires the services of personnel with different competencies, it is essential that trainees should appropriate experience of such cooperative endeavours and havethe ability to work towards a common goal, to communicate and share responsibility
> (WHO 1978c : 12)

The WHO emphasised that each case study was unique and that any institution considering interdisciplinary learning should develop its own strategy for introduction whilst remaining mindful of the problems reported by others.

Benor (1982) reinforced this point increasing recognition of the need for continuing education, although conceptual development had not progressed very far, emphatically "Interdisciplinary integration is required for educating a creative thinker; but there is not and cannot be one proper method of integration." (Ibid : 36)

In 1979, as a result of a meeting held in Geneva in 1977, the WHO published a document concerning "the training and utilisation of health care workers in the third world". There was increasing concern regarding the limited impact the recent increase in health expenditure and advances in medical care had made on the third world. Without addressing this problem 'health for all by the year 2000' would remain entirely elusive. Training programmes for these health care workers were identified. A detailed examination was undertaken of the health care structures within rural areas on an international basis. There was general agreement that the correct strategy would be the introduction of a three tier system:

1. *Primary health care*, within each village or community, where health personnel would provide basic preventative, curative and rehabilitative services.
2. *Secondary care*, where preventative, curative and rehabilitation services would be offered, and where health care workers had the responsibility of maintaining and improving health by using more specialised skills.
3. *Tertiary level*, provided by professionals who would treat disease and solve health problems.

They indicated that each tier "should function in a working relationship with the others" (WHO 1979b : 11). By involving everyone from within the community and the health care team, problems could be identified, analysed and priorities set for a plan of action to be drawn up and implemented.

Guilbert on behalf of the WHO (1984b) was still challenging educators to address the issues concerning the appropriate preparation for future health care workers. He accused the curriculum developers of "indiscriminate borrowing" from other sources which led to curricula that did not meet the needs of the community; "It must be obvious that the preparation of any health practitioner for his/her role in a given society or culture must be based on the health problems of that society or culture." (WHO 1984b : 6)

Part of the problem Guilbert believed, was due to territoriality of specific disciplines which preclude innovation and change. Tradition he continued, appeared to be the dominant factor in curriculum development. This entrenchment led to "education by ritual" (p 9) and "learning by rote" (p 6).

Miller (1977) had previously argued that institutions would not reach their potential in health care preparation if they continued to "guard jealously individual and departmental autonomy" (p 12).

Guilbert (WHO 1984b) further highlighted the inevitable waste of institutional, faculty and student resources whilst the curriculum content continued to fail to prepare the students for what they needed to know in order to become competent practitioners. The WHO (1984b) requested the International Council of Nurses (ICN) and the World Federation of Medical Education (WFME) to participate in a study which examined the preparation of nurses and physicians for their future role. Guilbert and his colleagues were the project leaders. The ICN approached 337 schools of nursing and the WFME 614 medical schools on a global basis, asking for their cooperation in the study. In the first phase all were asked to send a copy of their institutional objectives. One hundred and forty two (42%) of the schools of nursing and 164 (27%) of the medical schools complied. Of these, 84 schools of nursing and 58 medical schools fulfilled the (unspecified) criteria for inclusion in the study. These schools were then included in the second phase. A detailed questionnaire (not reproduced in the publication) was sent requesting information on curriculum development, student involvement, teaching and learning strategies, aims and objectives. Forty two schools of nursing (N = 84) and 21 medical schools (N = 58) responded.

The methodology, as the researchers admitted themselves, was badly flawed. Lack of clarity and language problems led to misinterpretation of terms in those schools which had responded and therefore led to unreliable results. In addition the final response rate itself was very low in comparison to the original number of schools approached (N = 337 and 614 respectively) so cannot be deemed representative. There were however, some generalised observations of relevance to this present study. In both the medical and nursing schools, students were rarely consulted and patient's views were almost universally not included in developing the appropriate curriculum to meet their needs. Another point of interest was that the nursing curricula included more on health issues and patient needs than those of the medical schools. Guilbert et al., wryly noted that too many educational establishments had devised a curriculum which ensured that students passed the examinations rather than enabling them to develop as competent practitioners. They suggested that "policy makers need to give attention to this" (WHO 1984b : 46). Harnack cited by Guilbert et al., succinctly summarised the issue "a curriculum that is unchanging is an educational programme in trouble. Times change, needs change, goals must then change." (WHO 1984b : 49)

Whilst reminding readers of the difficulties of drawing any valid conclusions from their study, Guilbert et al., pleaded for an increased sensitivity by educators to the damage that narrow and exclusive disciplinary interests could bring.

In 1984 worldwide economic recession was causing a crisis in higher education funding. The WHO (1984a) convened a conference in which representatives on an international basis considered the role of universities in health for all. Whilst the impetus for this conference was the identification of a more efficient utilization of resources, many interesting and pertinent points were raised which reflected the increasing need for integrated interdisciplinary learning. Dr Al-Refaie, a Kuwaiti physician, observed that whilst the emphasis remained on academic targets there was a general failure to develop in the student "those qualities in social and behavioural sciences that form an indispensable complement to the medical sciences." (WHO 1984a : 36)

Al -Refaie maintained that a doctor bereft of knowledge of the social health of the society in which he/she worked had no chance of comprehending the "economic and legislative framework" (p 36) on which medical care is based. The Russian representative Professor Vartanian, challenged the tradition of medical schools being based within universities and espoused the value of Institutes of Medicine. In the USSR all health related training is housed within these institutes which are an integral part of the health system. Professor Vartanian suggested that by adopting this approach medical education would adapt more easily to curricula changes in the future.

Professor Thoeun representing Kampuchea, had already attempted to adapt the curriculum in order to help students grasp their social responsibilities. The universities in his country had resisted the change by demanding the traditional disease orientated training. He pleaded for the WHO to act as a catalyst which would encourage all the United Nations countries to progress towards a greater emphasis on interdisciplinary learning, most particularly in the behavioural sciences. Dr Greep of the Netherlands charged all universities with assimilating the global concept of health by making a fundamental change in their health programmes. This included the "adoption of teaching methods based on teamwork in the field" (p 44). He continually emphasised the need for an integrated approach to health care which, in turn, concentrated on primary health care with its constituent health promotion and education programmes. Dr Guzman from the Phillippines, fully endorsed Dr Greeps comments. However as he rather wryly observed "It is easier to move a mountain than to change a university curricullum" (WHO 1984a : 46).

He recognised the increasing importance of the behavioural sciences in equipping all health personnel to practice effectively. He suggested that this could best be achieved by the immediate introduction of interdisciplinary workshops.

Sir Kenneth Stuart, on behalf of The Commonwealth Secretariat, seemed to rather miss the point ! Whilst eschewing the reluctance of universities to adapt their curriculum to meet the needs of students in their preparation towards professional practice, he referred constantly to the medical student in isolation from others in the health care team. He justifiably warned that all the emphasis on the team approach "should not make one lose sight of the need for training appropriate specialists" (p 51). The WHO was challenged with establishing a direct link with universities in order that the changes in emphasis could be accelerated. The WHO it was suggested, could most effectively achieve this by agreeing to become the coordinating body for the dissemination of research, information and the evaluation of innovative curriculum changes.

Dr Acevedo described some of the changes that had occurred in Mexico and reported the difficulties encountered if a curriculum had bits tacked on. He advocated, at the very least, a modification of the existing curriculum and wherever possible the development of an entirely new one in which integrated interdisciplinary learning was incorporated. He emphasised that each curriculum should be discrete in most areas of preparation for individual professions, but in areas that could be identified as common to all, shared learning should be encouraged. Dr Ghai from Ghana, pleaded for the establishment of much broader based concepts. He argued eloquently on behalf of the third world countries, that the philosophy of primary health care could never be truly addressed, by any establishment, without first studying in depth the structure and function of the society that the establishment purported to serve. This, he continued, was fundamental to all health care and could be addressed only by shared learning. Dr Prywes from Israel reinforced Dr Sai's remarks and suggested that each country should examine all the different models of integrated interdisciplinary learning that were available and then adapt the different approaches in order to develop a model appropriate to their own needs. In this way, he believed, a sense of ownership would evolve.

Dr Hamburg, as chairman of the conference, closed the proceedings by posing the question; "How can the WHO facilitate the changes in perceptions that will be necessary, the awareness of mutual benefit, in other words, an enlightened self-interest view on both sides?" (sic) (WHO 1984a : 66)

The solutions, he suggested, were for the WHO to use its coordinating power more effectively and more diversely. It should foster networks, encourage international research and act as the link between institutions which were involved in educational and/or service innovations. Most importantly it should provide leadership and commitment to integrated interdisciplinary learning.

In 1987 no fewer than eight documents pertinent to integrated interdisciplinary learning were published by the WHO (WHO 1987 a, b, c, d, e, f, g, and h). The chronological sequencing is difficult to determine as most are discussion papers and have no references to each other. Nevertheless, several seem to be inextricably linked (WHO 1987b, c, d, and e). The authors of these papers, Richards and Fulop (WHO 1987b), Kantrowitz et al, (WHO 1987c), and two unnamed working groups (WHO 1987d and WHO 1987e) studied experimental programmes in health professionals' preparation and training. Kantrowitz et al, (WHO 1987c) concentrated on interdisciplinary initiatives *within* medical education only whilst the working groups examined a broader remit and used the generic term 'health worker'. Examination of these papers has revealed the extent to which Dr Tamas Fulop, Director of the Division of Health Manpower Development (WHO) has been involved with all these initiatives.

In 1979 the Network of Community Oriented Educational Institutions for Health Sciences (NCOEIHS) was founded with the specific purpose of assisting institutions who had made a decision to introduce innovation in the training of their health personnel. Richards and Fulop (WHO 1987b) studied ten of these institutions in depth. The focus of their study was to determine what progress had been made and to what extent any progress made had effected the delivery of health care, most particularly in the primary health care field. The stated aim was to identify what constituted a successful curriculum and paradoxically what indicated an unsuccessful one. At least one institution was included from each of the six regions in the WHO. Richards and Fulop justified this by stating that "it helped obtain a global perspective on the issues involved" (Ibid : 3)

The ten included in the study had all been established since the nineteen sixties and were known to include either a problem based learning approach or a community orientated approach in their curricula. A brief description of the institutes was included and it was of interest to note that all ten had previously been described by Katz and Fulop in the previous decade (WHO 1978c). A fuller description of these ten will be included at the end of this section of the review (2.2). Richards and Fulop (WHO 1987c) singled out principles that underpin curricula development in health professionals' education. The prime concern should be the imparting of the information that is considered essential for a student to know if he/she is to become a competent practitioner. The competencies themselves need to be clearly defined as students undertaking any innovative programmes must still meet the statutory requirements of their profession and must therefore still acquire a defined body of knowledge, attitudes and skills.

A working party commissioned by the WHO added to the debate of competency and practice (WHO 1987e). They argued that a competent practitioner in any health discipline should be able to respond to the health needs and demands of the community. In order to achieve this the competent practitioner should be able to provide preventative care, provide curative care, educate the population in health matters, manage services, participate in health team work, train other members of the team, participate in research activities, problem solve and take responsibility for his/her own continuing professional development (p 45, 46). A subsequent document published by the WHO clarified the position regarding what precisely was meant by 'competence' :

> The ability to carry out a certain professional function (eg a medical function, a nursing function) which is made up of a repertoire of professional practice Competence requires knowledge, appropriate attitudes an observable mechanical or intellectual skills, which together account for the ability to deliver a specified professional service . (WHO 1988b : 680)

The WHO (1987e) group also emphasised the importance of understanding ethical values and demonstrating social skills. This was necessary they believed, so that the professions were conscious of their "moral responsibility" and therefore protected the community from "unethical and incompetent actions" (p 46). They specifically included in 'social skills' awareness, perception, judgement, empathy and the ability to communicate effectively. The working group argued that health care students should undertake much more learning in the community itself. They identified six reasons why this approach should be adopted:

1. It gives students much greater insight into sociological concepts and the needs of society. Health is inextricably linked to these concepts.
2. It encourages the integration of theory and practice.
3. It builds bridges between the professions, the general public and allows students to become actively involved with the community.
4. It constantly updates the curriculum itself by absorbing change as it occurs.
5. The competency levels of students will increase by utilising the resources available.
6. The quality of the community health services will improve.

(WHO 1987e : 12,13)

The working group noted the reluctance of teachers involved in parts of the curriculum to allow an infringement into their time. That there is a risk of the quality of patient care diminishing with more time spent in the community has not been confirmed in practice or theory. Buttery and Moser (1980), Phillips et al.,(1982). Prwyes (1983) found that community based education was a powerful means of upgrading the quality of health services. Prwyes suggested that this may be because of the comparative youth of the students. Their youth allowed them to remain open minded towards philosophies of care, thus placing them at an advantage when meeting clients in the community.

The group (WHO 1987e) recommended that as each course was redesigned, community orientation should take a much higher priority. Evidence of this change can be witnessed in the Project 2000 programmes devised as an innovative curriculum for nurses in the United Kingdom. Evidence collated by the National Foundation for Educational Research (NFER) shows a much greater emphasis on community care in twelve demonstration colleges of nursing (NFER 1992). A major problem envisaged by the WHO (1987e) working group was that this type of approach would not be viewed as 'academic'. The potential involvement of students in community activities was seen by some academics as placing in jeopardy "the intellectual qualities of the student" (p 16). More alarmingly still there was the implication that understanding human problems should be left until a student was qualified and thus more mature and able to cope.

Medical students evaluate community based education highly. Friedman et al, (1980) Boren (1982) and Richardson (1983) all found that students reported that they had learned aspects of medical care not available elsewhere. Bass and Paulman (1983) demonstrated that there was a correlation between the students who ranked this experience 'very highly' and those who subsequently chose to specialise in primary care. Richards and Fulop (WHO 1987c) also reported similar findings. Arlton (1984) in her American study reported that seventy five per cent of the student nurses who had undertaken community based education, had subsequently sought employment in the community sector. Arlton's cohort unfortunately was very small (N=30) and so no conclusions can be drawn. In addition, in her introduction, she described them as nurses who had expressed an interest in this type of experience, so the probability of a biased sample is raised.

The WHO (1987e) working group attempted to measure the effectiveness of interdisciplinary community based education in relation to the rest of the curriculum in fifteen medical schools (ten of which have been described by Richards and Fulop (WHO 1987c). Their findings however were inconclusive as they found that quantity did not reflect the effectiveness or quality of each programme. It also did not correlate with the students evaluation of the programmes effectiveness. The group suggested that there was an urgent need for further research to be undertaken.

Great emphasis was made of the fact that health problems were so complex that no one single profession could manage them alone. Through working together, each health team member could assess and compare his/her own role and responsibilities in relation to others in the team. They acknowledged that "There is no universally acceptable composition of the health team as the requirements will vary with the public health problem in question." (WHO 1987e : 40)

Throughout the entire paper there was no attempt to separate or identify any discrete profession. Each reference is attributed to the generic term 'health worker' . This implies that *all* personnel involved in health care should be exposed to these aspects of 'moral responsibility'. In order to achieve interdisciplinarity in health care they recommended that teachers of different disciplines should be involved. They warned however, that these teachers must be adequately prepared for such a role so that they could cope with the additional demands (p 34).

A list of recommendations was made (see Appendix 2.1). Nevertheless the authors were keen to emphasise that each stage should be modified in order to adapt to the individual institutions resources and the specific needs of the communities they served.

Kantrowitz et al., (WHO 1987c) at the outset of their study examining changes in medical education, wondered why institutions providing professional health care programmes had failed to respond to the challenge of innovation and change. They concluded that the main reason was because they were "steeped in tradition, jealously guarding departmental power bases and the status quo against newer 'alien' ideas." (Ibid : 19)

In their opening chapter, Kantrowitz et al., described the 'brick wall' of resistance that individuals faced when trying to innovate change. They highlighted the value of NCOEIHS membership by institutions for its support in helping to initiate change. When implementing major changes in educational programmes they suggested some precautionary ground rules. These included the identification of teachers who perceived the need for change and were willing to participate in any experiment. Teachers should be, wherever possible, from different disciplines. This would help overcome professional jealousies and traditional training boundaries, as an integrated curriculum implicitly implies an interdisciplinary approach. The WHO subsequently developed this theme of appropriate teachers and even produced a suggested profile of a good teacher (1988b : 71,72). Time and space should be allowed for innovators to plan, develop and modify the new approach. Wherever possible or practical, an integrated common core curriculum should be developed rather than relying on negotiating small periods of time within the traditional programmes (often at the cost of resentment and hostility of colleagues). Mahler (WHO 1988a), Nelson (1989), Broome (1990) would support these guidelines, as their texts on the management of change advise a similar approach.

Kantrowitz et al., (WHO 1987c) did not anticipate any major ethical problems providing that a group volunteered rather than being coerced into any trial. They suggested that any experiment should be directly controlled by staging a comparison between a traditional group (ie the control group) and the volunteer group (ie the experimental group). Eight innovative schools were studied. Each school sent representatives to a conference held in Alberquerque. The representatives were asked to come prepared to discuss, amongst other issues, their successes and perhaps more importantly their failures, so that other educators could learn from their mistakes. The organisers recognised this was a difficult request. Indeed they stated :

> This was not only a difficult and complex assignment but also an uncomfortable one for many of the participants. We are more comfortable presenting a favourable face to the world - describing our achievements. Describing our failures can be embarassing, yet it is of inestimable value to other educators, since they can more easily identify with and learn from, an open account of the problems they themselves face. This is the basis for a road map to change.
>
> (WHO 1987c : 23)

The eight schools had previously completed a detailed questionnaire. One of the questions asked was what had motivated them to change. All eight responded in a similar manner that an "excess of passive learning and a lack of curricula integration of basic and clinical science" had been the motivating factor (Ibid :

49, 61). The eight stated that the overall aim was to produce a more active learner and a more scientific thinker. Kantrowitz et al., concluded that "integrated student centered problem based learning finds a broad supportive audience among medical educators." (Ibid : 49)

The validity of this statement must however be questioned. Only eight schools participated and as already described by the authors, were innovative and keen to change. This suggests that they were in the forefront of medical education and that the vanguard traditionalists were not represented in this statement. This highlights an ethical dilemma. Kantrowitz et al., advocated "volunteer participants" in any experiment, but volunteers who are likely to perceive the need for change will not be a representative sample of the student population as a whole and could therefore, introduce the distinct possibility of bias.

Interestingly it was reported that all eight schools used small interdisciplinary planning groups to develop their programmes (p 51). The results of the questionnaire do not support this as only six reported using these strategies and the other two did not ! One of the most important points to emerge in this paper was the need to maintain traditional faculty work alongside any innovative programmes. All eight schools insisted that this was vital. The students ranked their preferred learning methods as small group teaching followed closely by peer teaching and lectures. If an innovative track could be developed that encompassed all three strategies, then an analysis could be undertaken to test its efficacy.

Mager (1961) studied student learning situations in which the teacher only answered questions. He found that each student used a different approach when learning about a topic. During the learning process individuals continually made sure that they fully understood what they had previously learned. Mager also found that the sequence of learning not only differed but was contrary to what had been previously thought was appropriate. Steele (1987) implied that students would feel that their individual learning needs would be only marginally met through lectures and that the resulting frustration would actively deter them from participating in the learning process. He referred to the profile of a health professional and suggested that as well as the traditional skills of diagnosis, treatment and cure, skills should also be evident in "interpersonal communication, fact gathering, problem solving, teaching and collaboration with colleagues within and outside the healthcare team." (Steele 1987 : 4)

Steele suspected that in most traditional programmes, these skills were not an integral part of the curriculum and had tended to be addressed on an 'ad hoc' basis. Eron (1985) suggested that the current emphasis on academic skills had psychological implications for the students which fostered such attitudes as cynicism and indifference in them once they had qualified. Steele (1987) warned that failure to accept the need for the assimilation of these new skills would be a serious error and argued that peer learning through close personal contact develops effective interpersonal skills in a way that a lecture could not and would not. Steele stressed that it was not a question of forcing a dichotomy between tradition and innovation, but more a question of effectively integrating the two in such a way that they complemented each other.

In 1988 a technical report was produced on behalf of the WHO by an expert group (WHO 1988b). The report was entitled "Learning Together To Work Together For Health". The report restated the position of the WHO regarding the concepts of interdisciplinarity, teamwork and holistic patient care. The authors went to great lengths to reinforce the need for a continuation of specifically designed curricula for each individual health profession. Nevertheless they advocated the introduction of shared learning strategies that would complement the existing programmes and enhance the quality of care. This declaration reinforces the work of Kantrowitz et al., (WHO 1987c). The expert group (WHO 1988b) recognised that reliable evidence for advocating the introduction of integrated interdisciplinary learning was lacking, but were convinced that "community oriented, multiprofessional education of health personnel has an important place in strategies for achieving health for all" (Ibid : 11)

The technical report was a clear attempt to clarify the advantages of interdisciplinary education (p 16,17) the educational principles behind such an innovation (p 25) the conditions necessary for its successful implementation (p 39-49), and the difficulties and constraints in introducing this approach. The suggested strategies for successful implementation are very similar to those suggested by the WHO working party in 1987 (WHO 1987c) and these are compared in Appendix 2.1. As such this report has emerged as a core document and will be referenced throughout this current study. It has particular relevance to and implications for the design of the research and consequently will be considered in detail in Chapter Three - Design of the Research.

In 1986 at a conference in Tokyo, nurses were being challenged to take the lead. Approximately fifty per cent of health personnel were nurses yet they still failed to take the initiative or build up the confidence to influence the changes needed:

> The nursing culture is heavy with insubordination without influence.
> It is burdened with obligation without power even in directing, heading
> and controlling its own education, practice, research and management.
> Such an ethos militates against the emergence of positive initiative.
>
> (WHO 1986a : 5)

Consumer views were also perceived to be influential on the reluctance to change. Culturally, many societies hold conservative attitudes towards health professions' education and prefer a medically orientated, curative approach rather than one based on health promotion (WHO 1986a : 19). The conference called for a quantum shift in health professionals' education with a fundamental restructuring of the curriculum content. With the emphatic change in emphasis envisaged from acute hospital care to community care it was recommended that common foundation courses should be identified which would enhance teamwork and interdisciplinary interactions. It was suggested that because nurses were predominantly female they had been traditionally assigned a passive subordinate role. Untapped potential far exceeded the present performance it was believed. In order for this potential to be realised opportunities had to be made available which would develop the professional confidence needed for effective interdisciplinary collaboration and integration.

Nurses are in the ideal position to influence change because of the very nature of their work. They provide care at all levels, in all situations, to all people at all times. The need for committed and dedicated leaders of nursing, both in education and management is paramount. Potential leaders, ones who are value driven, motivated, who 'think as well as do' should be helped to channel their intellectual energies into improving the breadth and depth of the education available for health professionals (Houle 1980, WHO 1986a, Steele 1987).

In 1988 the Director General of the WHO (Dr Mahler) reported on the progress of member states in developing a comprehensive nursing/midwifery component in the "health for all" strategy. He stressed the need for action if nursing's full potential was to be realised. He referred to the lost opportunities in all aspects of planning for the future (WHO 1988a : 10). He criticised the entrenched attitudes of all health professionals as far as the continuing emphasis on the acute sector was concerned. He regretted that, on the whole, interdisciplinary learning opportunities were not available which thus prevented students from gaining a "knowledge and appreciation of each others roles" (p11). Mahler referred at length to the difficulty of changing attitudes and regulations. He recognised that resistance to change was common, but insisted that change was fundamental if the goal for health for all was to be achieved. He praised the nursing professions for the educational developments which were beginning to emerge but reminded them that still more effort was required in order to meet the consumers' needs. He talked of "collaboration within and among schools" (p 13) and was convinced of the need for interdisciplinarity (p 14).

In March (1988) the WHO and the ICN met in Riga. The purpose of the meeting was to review the progress to date since the Alma Ata conference in 1978 in which the declaration "health for all by the year 2000" had been made. The report of this meeting was published the following year (WHO 1989a). The consensus was that at the half way point, progress had been made , but that much remained to be done. As a result, a meeting was subsequently held in Ferney-Voltaire in order to assess the nursing profession's position. The major problem impeding progress was "little or no precedent for multisectoral cooperation in the management and control of health problems" (WHO 1989a : 4) .

Great emphasis was placed on nurses being part of a team whilst remaining autonomous practitioners. Such abilities, it was argued, were acquired by practice and not by theory alone. In other words 'the knowing came with the doing'. In order that nurses embraced the concept of health for all several pre-requisites were identified. One of these was in the realm of continuing education where nurses were exhorted to develop programmes that were "problem based, practice orientated, multiprofessional and team focussed" (WHO 1989a : 8)

Reference was made to Richards and Fulop's work (WHO 1987c) and whilst the delegates at the meeting acknowledged that each institution faced different problems and constraints, common strategies could be identified and should be used as a framework for the implementation of change. They postulated that many obstacles which impede change could be removed and that any innovations should be "encouraged, implemented and evaluated" (p 10). Any research proposals which addressed the problem should receive immediate attention. They continued this theme by suggesting that, "If nurses are to undertake such studies, appropriate training including the award of fellowships from the WHO and other organisations, should be made available and encouraged." (WHO 1989a : 11)

In order to encourage nurses to undertake this synergistic action, it was deemed essential that a fundamental change of attitude within the profession itself occurred. One of the inhibiting factors was that tradition discriminated against the emergence of a predominantly female group. This was particularly evident in the third world countries where the women were poorly educated, academic entry criteria for training were low, the salary meagre and schools of nursing lacked material resources. A continuing emphasis on the medical model in health care was also thought to be a contributing factor in the failure to progress. The elitism and isolation of individual disciplines led to a lack of integration and collaboration which in turn led to "interprofessional tensions and difficulties" (p 15).

2.2.1 Innovations in specific countries

From the review of the literature pertaining to innovative changes in health professionals education on a global basis, it has been possible to gather a large amount of information from different countries. In order to present a reasonably representative picture, a summary of each country's progress on an individual basis is presented.

2.2.2 China

In China the structure of medical education is highly traditional and derived from both European and North American models (Xue-Min and Yi-Fei 1987 cited by WHO 1987c, Nutter 1983) Students are taught didactically with little application of integrated theory to practice. Few opportunities exist for community health experiences or primary health care. In Shanghai four hundred and twenty students are admitted to medical school each year. From 1987 thirty of these per year would undertake a new problem orientated curriculum. The proposed innovative curriculum appeared to be biologically science orientated with no mention being made of the behavioural sciences at all. The teaching methods adopted were lectures, laboratory work and case study material. It is difficult to criticise this 'innovation' in the absence of further information into what was described as 'traditional training'. It would seem however, that China is many years behind other countries in its approach to medical training. Xue-Min andYi-Fei described in detail the political ideology in China and the constraints it made upon all educational developments. Education is prescribed by the Central Committe of the Communist Party. A glimmer of hope was expressed by the authors in that the Ministry of Public Health had undertaken to improve standards of health care by encouraging scientifically based medical education. The existing problems that needed to be overcome, before any major change occurred, were identified by the authors as:

1. The passive learning role adopted by students. There was no encouragement of student initiative, participation or creativity.
2. The students were saturated with endless facts. They therefore had no time to undertake self directed learning and lacked the skills needed.
3. There was no integration in medical education at all. What was learned in the pre-clinical years was forgotten or could not be applied in practice.
4. Clinical courses did not challenge the students to solve patient's problems clearly.
5. Moral guidance was neglected by the teachers.
6. There were no comprehensive evaluation methods used to assess the quality of the students learning. The only measurement being the grades obtained in examinations.

No other information was found on health professional's education in China.

2.2.3 The Phillippines

This country was experiencing major problems in manpower distribution with many of the rural communities being without health care at all. Seiga-Sur and Varona cited by the WHO (1987c) had commenced an experiment using a step ladder curriculum. The philosophy behind the change was described as the need to train health professionals for the underserved regions of the country. The curriculum consists of five steps that eventually produces a multi-skilled worker. A student may progress from level one 'health worker', to level five 'doctor of medicine'. Registered nurses reflect level three but do not have the equivalent recognition in other countries. The step ladder curriculum inevitably means that true integrated learning is taking place as each individual progresses through each stage. Fifty percent of their time is spent in the community, 'learning on the job'. Seiga-Sur and Varona indicated that the training is based on the Fillippino cultural value 'utang na loob'. This value consists of a depth of loyalty and commitment which is perceived as never fully repaid. It would appear to relate to sponsorship offered by the community from which the student hails. This the authors recognised was a novel selection process but a powerful one. There was no mention of schooling, literacy or ability influencing the selection process. The major problem to date was the unrealistic expectations of the students themselves. They all wanted to be doctors. Of the one hundred and ninety students who had completed the programme, ten had fulfilled the criteria for level five. All ten had failed to return to the community that had sponsored them. This then was a self perpetuating problem as the communities that so desperately needed health care could only rely on less highly qualified workers and they had lost their investment. In 1992 the problem appears to have worsened. In the 'Nursing Standard' world news section a short report commented that almost ninety per cent of nurses and sixty per cent of doctors who have qualified in the last ten years have left the Phillippines (1992 Vol 6. No 19 : 11).

2.2.4 Thailand

Thailand experiences similar problems to the Phillippines. In Bankok the doctor/ patient ratio is 1-1000. In rural areas it is 1-50000 (Suwanwela et al cited by WHO 1987c). A programme was designed in 1976 to try to redress the balance. Great emphasis has been made on creating good working relationships within the health care team and the curriculum uses a biopsychosocial approach to care. Health education features strongly and there is a commitment to continuing professional education. The learning strategies include creativity, rational thinking and problem solving skills. The use of the term interdisciplinary was somewhat misleading however, as it seemed to embrace the notion of physicians, surgeons and pathologists working more closely together. There was no mention of any other professions besides medicine. A follow up of the programme ten years after its inception found that 'many' of the students were indeed working in the rural areas. This, the authors suggested was proof that programmes could be designed that would solve the problem of manpower shortages in specific areas. Further evidence of the successof this strategy was provided by Arlton (1984) in North America. Interestingly in 1978 Buri and Katz described a programme in Thailand in which teaching responsibility for the programmes was undertaken on an interdisciplinary basis (WHO 1978c). The course was health problem orientated and so specific topics such as epidemiology, health economics and the behavioural sciences were integrated extensively "when opportunities arise during the course of instruction and wherever problems are encountered." (Ibid : 162)

2.2.5. Algeria

In Algeria emphasis is made on health team training and in helping to improve communication and cooperation amongst all the agencies contributing to the health of the nation. All basic sciences are taught in an integrative way which was adopted as a direct result of an acute shortage of manpower ("Comite Pedagogique" cited by WHO 1978c). The aim of the training institute was to train the health professionals to "implement the health policy of the country" (p

22). There were three basic concepts, the health team, the application of theory to practice and the interdisciplinary approach. The whole ethos of the programme was to promote the ability of students to function effectively as team members. This meant helping them acquire a respect for others "while still maintaining confidence in their own professional identities" (p 23). Salary differentials had been reduced, teaching staff taught on an interdisciplinary basis, there were shared facilities and resources and an increased collaboration with the social services.

2.2.6 Turkey

Turkey has tried to address the problem of manpower distribution, overspecialisation and poor quality of training. A department of community medicine was established, the aim being to, "promote a philosophical commitment to community medicine as a holistic approach to all promotive, preventive, curative and rehabilitative activities acting on individuals, environment and community." (Fisek cited by WHO 1978c : 170)

In 1967 this was indeed a radical forward thinking approach for a medical school. The teaching of the behavioural sciences, epidemiology and preventive medicine were seen as essential components of the curriculum in order to enhance the overall aim. Training for health personnel is well established in Turkey. A six to seven year medical training is undertaken after eleven years compulsory schooling is completed. A four year college or university based training is undertaken by nursing students after a minimum of eight years compulsory schooling. The philosophy for community medicine was clearly and precisely stated and could be used as a model for many medical schools. The staff displayed great courage in breaking away from the traditional constraints of curriculum development and designed a programme which was innovative and exciting.

Preliminary experiments in behavioural science teaching by staff from the social sciences department was not perceived as valuable by the students. This Fisek (1978) suggested was due to the failure of the students to make the link between social science and medicine. The students therefore did not acquire a satisfactory basic knowledge in the social sciences. The problem was solved by an integrated and specific course entitled 'social sciences for medicine'. It may be that the original teaching failed to apply theory to practice thus adding weight to the argument that students must perceive the relevance of what they are taught.

2.2.7 The Cameroons

Nchinda (1974) described the farce of a physician being the first point of contact for the sick patient in underdeveloped countries. Physicians in rural communities he maintained, should only be used as a consultant with the first point of contact for a sick person being a voluntary health care worker. He suggested that most of the population in the Cameroons would be extremely lucky to have access to any health care at all. In order to address this crisis the University Centre for Health Sciences in Yaounde was created. The goal of the centre is to educate members of health teams in meeting the severe shortages of health manpower. Monekosso and Quenum (1978) cited by the WHO (1978c) described the increasing emphasis on developing and implementing a curriculum which would enhance the creation of effective health teams. The genesis of this project was the acute shortage of all categories of health personnel. It was deemed that students from any of the related disciplines should be able to adapt to working in any rural area. There had to be therefore, an appropriate mix of personnel in terms of levels and nature of training. Co-ordinated team work and not isolated individual effort was seen as essential for the enhancement of patient care. Individual students whilst pursuing specific courses for individual health professions share common core programmes with all the other students. The emphasis is on participation by all students in practical team training exercises "students thus get a chance to practice their future role and to appreciate the roles of other team members." (Ibid p 196)

A preliminary review of these courses revealed that whilst the students are still learning and thus qualifying in different professions, shared learning has taken place and motivation to integrate was clearly evident. The tutorial staff from all disciplines were highly commited to shared teaching and learning in spite of the additional difficulties of bilingualism, ie French and English. The personal observations by Monekosso and Quenum included the difficulties and pitfalls experienced in the introduction of this challenging programme. The students had problems in accepting the role of 'guinea pigs', although this anxiety soon lessened as they recognised the benefits. Large student numbers were difficult to manage with the existing resources available and new staff tended to be very disorientated. Recognition was also made of the need to select staff carefully who were committed to the concept of integrated teaching as there was no place for staff who inherently believed in traditional methods. The attributes required of staff involved with the project included good organisation and management skills, flexibility, problem solving abilities and a high level of competence within their own field. A virtual paragon of a professional ! All members of the faculty needed to develop a sense of ownership with no inferiority or superiority complexes. The success of the project was attributed to the staff within the university, the Cameroonian Government who gave 'unflinching support' and the WHO. The opinion of the authors was that the programme should continue to be supported and expanded and that the experience could be whole heartedly recommended to both developed and developing countries.

2.2.8 Sudan

Hamad (1982) described a programme that was designed to blend medical education with rural developments. It had been introduced by the University of Gezira and involved medical, economics, agricultural and science students learning together. Increased problem solving, research skills, community orientation and teamwork were the desired behavioural changes. Groups of students were made responsible for the development of their 'chosen' village. Their remit was to identify problems, plan, implement changes to eliminate or minimise these problems and then evaluate the success of their strategies. Hamad did not publish an evaluation of the programme so it is impossible to comment on its effectiveness. What his paper clearly demonstrated however, is the breadth of interdisciplinary learning that students in third world countries now share. The philosophy behind these developments would appear to be sound and it could be argued that primary health care should encompass all the disciplines that contribute to a healthy lifestyle.

2.2.9 Fiji

Medical training in Fiji is not recognised in the Western World. Pathik and Goon (1978) argued however that Fijian students who trained abroad were not equipped to practice medicine in Fiji as the emphasis in training was entirely different. Students qualifying in their motherland were more realistic about the resources available and consequently were more flexible. The objectives however were remarkably far sighted:-

> Promote the physical, mental and social wellbeing of the nation.
> Protect Fijis young and old from illness and disease.
> Provide adequate clinical facilities and staff to satisfy the medical and dental needs of both urban and rural populations.
> Promote a better standard of living through a lower birth rate.
>
> (Ibid : 81)

Emphasis was made on the role of health assistants who undertook a three year training and became deputy doctors. These students along with physiotherapists, dietitians and pharmacists shared basic science teaching programmes. No mention was made of the nursing profession. The attrition rate for medical students was extraordinarily high, up to sixty five per cent. The authors identified inadequate pre-entry preparation and disciplinary problems as being the main causal factors. Major problems were obviously being encountered in Fiji and it would appear that they had to be addressed urgently. Ironically, if the programme were to be discontinued it would mean that in most instances there would be no supervised health care at all in most of the country. Continuation of this training therefore can be justified.

2.2.10 Hungary

In 1972 'social medicine' was introduced in a substantial way into the traditional medical training. Students were admitted to medical school after spending one to three years in health care as nurses, ambulance workers or health technicians. Other entry criteria are equally firm, good school performance in biology and physics, along with an appropriate social background. Preference was given to those individuals whose parents were employed as industrial workers, farm labourers most particularly in areas which were currently poorly supplied with medical services. An intensive interview was also conducted with the potential students to try and ascertain aptitude for health care. Whilst it may be thought that students who come from the lower social classes and districts bereft of medical care have not had the opportunity to obtain a good academic record in biology and physics, this did not appear to be the case. The number of suitable applications outweigh the number of places available by three to one. The social medicine aspect of the course sought to give the student the historical background, political ideology and an understanding of the sociological and physiological aspects of medicine. Tigyi (1978) and his fellow teachers had adopted the sound philosophy that diagnosis and therapeutic management change so fast that the student and then graduate will always meet new challenges and problems. They firmly believed that it was "necessary to instil a spirit of inquiry rather than a passive reliance on memory" (Ibid : 103).

Whilst major strides have been made towards the concept of holistic care with the erosion of disciplinary boundaries, health care remains entirely medically orientated with no apparent evidence of any shared learning.

2.2.11 Israel

The University Centre for Health Sciences was established in 1974 and is based within the Ben Gurion University of the Negev, Beersheva. Three major goals were identified:

1. The delivery of preventative, curative and rehabilitative care in an integrative way.
2. The merging of the health care system into one authority.
3. To produce a graduate who could work in both the hospital and the community sectors.

This called for a radical review of the traditional curriculum offered in other Israeli universities where the content was both disease and specialty orientated with little or no mention of community care or health promotion. There was an additional problem in that preventative and curative medicine was controlled by different authorities. A consortium was established with the aim of integrating these two authorities. A spiral curriculum was adopted in Beersheva with core competencies identified. Students were expected to reach a specified level of proficiency in each of the core competencies. Further competencies were then identified by the individual students in consultation with their tutors in the form of electives. The tutors were held accountable for the outcomes. Although in the paper it is not made clear, there is the implication that the degree was of a modular format.

Segall et al., (1978) cited by the WHO (1978c) placed great emphasis on the development of optimal problem solving skills. They stated categorically that this could only be achieved through "considerable interdisciplinary learning" (p 120). This was achieved by a short introductory block in each medical discipline followed by problem centred interdisciplinary teaching. It was not made clear which teaching methods were used. Unless some interaction had taken place between the students themselves then interdisciplinary learning could not be said to be taking place. Segall et al., issued a word of warning regarding the need for competency as well as enthusiasm on the part of the tutorial staff involved in developing innovative curriculum. Competency could not be replaced by enthusiasm and the teachers who were not competent should not be involved. Generalisations regarding innovation in programmes could not be made they believed, as innovation "often develops out of circumstances which are specific to individual institutions" (WHO 1978c : 122).

2.2.12 Mexico

In the WHO (1987c) publication, Valle et al. contributed a chapter on the innovative changes which were occurring in Mexico. There had been a major shift in emphasis towards community care and away from the traditional specialisation in the acute hospital sector. This had been a direct result of a recognition that students were being prepared to pass examinations rather than act as effective practitioners in the community they served. The overiding concern of the curriculum developers was to:

> develop professionals not only with a sound scientific and technical knowledge, but also with a deep and realistic appreciation of Mexicos social, economic and health problems. Graduates had to possess a clear concept of man as a biological, psychological and social being.
>
> (Ibid : 74)

The curriculum at Programa de Medicina General Integral (PMGI) aimed to avoid fragmentation into separate disciplines. It introduced students to the concept of scientific, humanistic patient care with the additional philosophy of service to patients, their families and the community. The PMGI programme was initiated in 1974 as a viable alternative to the traditional route. Final examinations were however to be shared. The hidden agenda was that a direct comparison of 'fitness to practice' would be available through the examination results. Theory applied to practice was the framework upon which the whole PMGI programme was built and a Piagetian approach was chosen. Piagetian theory postulates that knowledge is arrived at by an inductive process of building and synthesising experience and information. Diagnostic and problem solving skills were high on the agenda using a biopsychosocial approach. This approach Valle et al. believed, would help the facilitation of integrated knowledge. Each academic year was divided into a series of modules. Students were assessed at the end of each module in three core areas, knowledge, clinical skills and attitudes. The programme itself met with much resistance from the traditionalists who accused the innovators of producing second rate practitioners. The problem the staff involved with the PMGI programme faced was that they could not refute the allegations until the first student cohort graduated (and presumably not for a few years until their competence had been proved). Valle et al., reported that the results showed a slightly improved overall achievement in the PMGI students than those on the traditional route. No data was produced to support their claim. It may be possible however to accept the reported success of the programme as in 1985 the traditional programme was eventually discontinued entirely in favour of the PMGI one. As the authors pointed out this programme was not only daring but also risky particularly as the Alma Ata Declaration was not made until 1978, four years after the inception of the PMGI programme. Their foresight however has enabled them to be one of the world leaders in innovative changes in medical education.

2.2.13 Brazil

Medical training began at the University of Brasilia in 1966 and is an integral part of the Faculty of Health Sciences. The Faculty also trains allied professions including nursing and dietetics. An additional discipline, not normally associated with such a Faculty, is physical education. Sobrel and Mejia cited by WHO (1978c) did not indicate whether any integrated learning took place or whether it was just a case of the different disciplines being housed in the same building and sharing the same resources. It seemed that the educational programme discussed referred only to medical training but this was not clear. The curriculum however seemed innovative and exciting for 1966. It was based on several concepts:

1. Health as a multilevel state with organic and psychosocial dimensions.
2. Disease is a state based on several causal factors.
3. Medicine is an endeavour directed towards holistic patient care.
4. Medical education is an integrative learning process.

The curriculum was developed as a direct result of qualified physicians dissatisfaction with the training they had received, which they evaluated as being too biologically orientated. This had consequently left them ill prepared to cope with patients psychosocial problems. This paradigm acted as the blueprint for further developments which allowed for greater community orientation and greater flexibility towards individual learning needs. This it was hoped would help produce a physician "more adapted to the delivery of primary health care under conditions of restricted resources in rural settings or impoverished areas" (WHO 1978c : 56).

No evidence was found that indicated that any shared learning took place with other health related courses. The medical students were isolated within the Faculty in a similar manner to so many other establishments which pay lip service only to interdisciplinary learning.

2.2.14 Africa

Little written evidence has been found of interdisciplinary learning in health care in spite of a rigorous search. It is possible that local initiatives have been undertaken but have failed to be reported in international journals published in English. All WHO reports have an English language version and constitute an important reference source, but have yielded little information regarding Africa.
In Zimbabwe reorientation from the acute hospital sector to the community has been taking place since 1980. Eighty eight per cent of the twenty two thousand health workers are nurses. Nurses have therefore taken a predominant role in changing educational practice. Following a review of the curriculum for medical and nursing students a programme was devised that enabled them to learn together. Thus the concept of teamwork becomes a natural approach at the beginning of their training (WHO 1986b, Mehlomakhulu 1991). In Kenya it would seem that nurses again take the lead by organising regular interdisciplinary meetings and seminars (Kierini 1985).

2.2.15 Canada

In 1969 a pioneering school of medicine was founded at McMaster University Ontario. The programme was unique and described by Walsh (1978) as 'risky'. It encompassed a problem solving approach using integrated subject matter rather than a discipline based course. The aims of the course were described as :-

1. The identification and definition of health problems and the searching for information to resolve or manage these problems.
2. Given a problem to examine the underlying biopsychosocial mechanisms.

Other significant aims included self development, self appraisal, functioning with a small group appropriately and the ability to work in a variety of health care settings. The admissions staff selected students who demonstrated self esteem, an inquiring mind, an ability to communicate and an ability to solve problems. The successful students whilst having academic qualifications did not necessarily have a scientific background. More than two thousand applied each year and one hundred were admitted.

The whole ethos of the course was based on problem solving which is developed and enhanced by the extensive use of small group tutorials. In the initial stages of training, Walsh (1978) reported, students tended to experience anxiety as there were no defined limits to the requisite amount of knowledge. This of course is very different to the traditional approach where parameters are set according to the amount and depth of knowledge that is needed in order to pass an assessment. Although Walsh stated that after six months this problem was minimised he did not offer any data to support his claim. In the first year the students spent a large amount of time attached to a physician practising in the community. This was a deliberate decision on the part of the curriculum developers who wished to discourage specialism and elitism by encouraging students to view medicine as primary care and prevention rather than disease orientated. The students gained experience in both urban and rural practice. A longitudinal comparative study is being undertaken between the McMaster students and those from other Canadian medical schools. Results from the first four groups of graduates revealed a 'better' pass rate by the McMaster students than the rest and the students themselves were functioning 'very effectively' within the health care system.

2.2.16 The United States of America

In the USA two main groups of health workers are described, doctors and nurses. These professions collaborate with twenty six allied health professions. It was in the early nineteen seventies that the concept of health personnel working collaboratively as a team first received attention. Predictably, many examples of innovation and interdisciplinary approaches to health professionals education have been culled from the American literature and will be referenced throughout this study. Nevertheless there are a few which have been described as 'innovative tracks' and therefore merit inclusion in this section. In 1964 the College of Human Medicine (CHM) in Michigan State began planning a curriculum based on the premise that the behavioural sciences should receive as much attention as the biological sciences. The CHM ran two programmes simultaneously. Track 1 was the traditional model with discipline based lectures and laboratory work being the most commonly used teaching strategies and Track 2 was the innovative approach which placed great emphasis on problem solving. Medical students chose which Track they wished to follow. Brazeau et al., (1987) stated that approximately one third of the one hundred students that registered each year opted for Track 2. No other data was given although the authors implied that more females than males chose this Track. Developing problem solving skills was a high priority and the authors commented on the inevitable resistance to the change by many of the traditionalists. They regretted that this resistance had inevitably led to compromises which had a detrimental effect on the programme. In 1982 a study had commenced that will compare the performance of Track 1 with Track 2 students over a ten year period. Interim results reveal more Track 1 students opting for specialist training such as surgery after qualification whilst the Track 2 students tend to opt for family practice and psychiatry. There was no raw data to support these claims and the authors themselves pointed out that as students are able to choose which Track they enter it may indicate that those who opted for Track 2 already had a specific interest and commitment to the integration of the behavioural sciences into health care.

Brazeau et al., considered that Track 2 students had learned 'at least' as much as those undertaking the traditional programme and that the stability in numbers rendered it a viable programme. The student satisfaction ratings, the authors indicated were "very good" and the resistance by the traditionalists was diminishing. No evidence in the form of data was included in the publication so most of the statements cannot be substantiated.

Eight students only commenced an alternative preclinical curriculum at the Rush Medical College in Illinois. Small group problem solving using a holistic approach was adopted. Specialist facilitators were utilised where appropriate. Gotterer et al., cited in WHO 1987c identified the reservations expressed by the staff about the new curriculum. These included an excessive demand on faculty time and a concern that there would be a lack of academic rigour. Students complaints on the traditional programme however included, too great an emphasis on rote learning, too little attention paid to the application of knowledge and problem solving abilities, little or no opportunity to think creatively, little opportunity to develop sensitivity to individual needs and no opportunity to attain the skills necessary for life long learning or critical inquiry. Gotterer et al., summarised these complaints by stating that students "see themselves as sponges required to soak up as much information as possible" (p 187). It was disappointing to find no evidence which demonstrated that health promotion and primary care were seen as essential pre-requisites prior to studying disease processes. The Rush experiment is however, still in the formative stage with the first cohort due to graduate in 1992. It may be that this omission will be corrected.

There are three pathways at Harvard medical school through which students can graduate. The latest was introduced in 1985 and is known as the Oliver Wendell Holmes Society (OWHS). Important changes include a greater emphasis on small group learning, a greater application of theory to practice using a holistic approach and a greater emphasis on health promotion and education. Clinical experience includes visits to health centres and community health initiatives. Data is being kept of the students progress and is due to be published in 1994. A problem that had been encountered by Ramos and Moore (WHO 1987c) was that students who were not included in the innovative programme felt rejected and insignificant. The authors reported both subversive and openly hostile behaviour by these students towards the students on the OWHS programme. An important lesson can be learnt here for anyone contemplating introducing new and innovative programmes. The perceived value and continuing esteem of both students and staff on established programmes must be maintained and upheld otherwise their negativity will inevitably sour the success of the new innovation.
The University of New Mexico, Alberquerque changed their approach to medical education as a result of the realisation that the training was not equipping students to work in primary health care. In addition, by adopting a passive role in learning they were not subsequently able to assume responsibility for their own

continuing learning. The students complained that they were treated like children (Mennin et al.,WHO 1987c). Confrontation eventually took place between the faculty staff and the students themselves and as a result the urgent need for change was accepted. A similar programme to the one described by Brazeau et al., has been implemented but its efficacy has not yet been tested.

Boyer et al (1977) described a rather different interdisciplinary course in that it was conceived, planned, implemented and evaluated entirely by the students themselves. Boyer and her colleagues unfortunately did not make clear their own role in the project and their profession and status was not given. The origin of the course was attributed to the predominantly female nursing students who challenged the sexual stereotyping they were encountering. An impromptu meeting was held with medical students which ended with the medical students accusing the nurses of taking themselves too seriously. Both groups did meet again and jointly proposed the introduction of an interdisciplinary course which would help foster mutual respect and improve communication. Two members from the nursing, medical, occupational therapy and physiotherapy professions volunteered to plan the course. Social workers and dental students declined the invitation to join in. The planning team devised a set of objectives which included learning about each others professional backgrounds by identifying the role of each within the health team. The planning team decided that facilitators in the form of qualified professionals should be appointed. Two members of the medical profession declined as they doubted that a team approach was more desirable than the traditional model with a physician in charge. Eventually one doctor (from another medical school), two nurse lecturers and a medical sociologist were enlisted. Boyer et al observed that at the beginning of the course the medical students seemed to display less commitment than the others. While this is obviously an entirely subjective comment Boyer et al would appear to be justified if these medical students were modelling themselves on the two members of the medical school described previously.

The other groups appeared totally commited to the concept of teamwork. Many sessions were undertaken and not surprisingly at the end of the course the student evaluations revealed that more time was desirable. They felt that they were just beginning to make progress and increase understanding and collaboration. The students unanimously voted for a repeat of the course providing some alterations were made. One of the most interesting suggestions was the inclusion of hypothetical situations which required problem solving skills. This recommendation provides the first real evidence of the value that students themselves perceive in practicing problem solving. Although no raw data was given this paper was a useful one to review as it gave the student perspective of the value of interdisciplinary learning when student led and when the autonomy of the course also remained with the student body.

McPherson and Sachs (1982) reviewed progress in interdisciplinary learning initiatives in the USA and Canada and noted that a change in philosophy seemed to be taking place. They attributed this to three causal factors, medicine had adopted the concept of holistic care, secondly the US Government had made available large sums of money for interdisciplinary projects (although as McPherson and Sachs rather cynically suggested economic recession was the main reason for seeking cheaper ways of training) and finally the growing recognition that certain client groups had multiple problems that required an interdisciplinary approach to address them. These reasons had previously been outlined by amongst others Siegel (1974) and Mazur et al (1979). McPherson and Sachs circulated a questionnaire to all medical schools asking whether any part of the curriculum addressed the teamwork issue. Of the 141 medical schools 105 responded and 30 (N=105) included formal teaching on teamwork, 11 in the clinical years, 10 in the pre clinical years and 9 throughout training. Interestingly they found that the teaching in the pre clinical years only indirectly related to team building such as the concept of primary health care whereas in the clinical years role negotiation and conflict management were identified topics in the syllabus. The most important finding was the total lack of any interdisciplinary learning. The multidisciplinary team concept was addressed by one discipline in isolation from all the others which constitute a team.

2.2.17 Australia and New Zealand

Despite an intensive search, very little literature was found that described interdisciplinary activities in either Australia or New Zealand. The most prolific author would seem to be Owen, a lecturer based in Adelaide, South Australia. In conjunction with some colleagues named Furler, Moss and Pigott, Owen presented papers at conferences in Perth and Sydney in 1977 and 1981. Owen himself, subsequently referenced these in a paper published in Medical Teacher in 1982. Conference Proceedings were available then but an attempt to obtain these was unsuccessful. A further attempt was made to communicate directly with Owen himself, but no response was received. Owen (1982) was one of the few authors identifed who attempted to address the problem of how to deliver an interdisciplinary programme. He explored the concept of joint and integrated teaching on multidisciplinary community health programmes in Adelaide. He differentiated between joint teaching which he described as "the type of situation where students of different disciplines are in the same lecture.........dealing with the same academic or clinical material"; and integrated teaching which he described as "students additionally working together on solving problems or reaching agreement on practical solutions to case material, or dealing with common ethical issues and programmes for health problems" (Owen 1982 : 47)

He concluded that there was a clear continuum between the two types of teaching. He did not attempt to differentiate between multidisciplinary, multiprofessional, interprofessional and interdisciplinary learning and indeed used them all interchangeably and randomly throughout his paper.

Since 1976, Adelaide has provided a:

> multiprofessional programme for students of nursing, occupational therapy, pharmacy, medicine, physiotherapy, psychology, social work, speech pathology, nutrition and dietetics, health education, health administration and health surveying
>
> (Owen 1982)

The aim of the course was to increase the students awareness of teamwork, health promotion and communication. The course was an integral part of the profession specific training programmes and students attended on a weekly basis for two hours. Owen advised that students should not commence too early in their training as they "may not have developed sufficiently different personal identities ....to achieve the objectives" (Ibid : 48).

This was a mistake because this is precisely why students should be integrated from the beginning of training, so that professional territories have not been found, entrenchment has not begun and negative stereotyping about the other professions does not exist. These concepts will be further explored and the evidence given to substantiate this statement in Section 2.6 Interprofessional Conflicts and Section 2.7 Teamwork in Health and Social Care. The multiprofessional programme described by Owen will be discussed in detail in Section 2.9 Integrated Interdisciplinary Learning Frameworks. No further evidence of interdisciplinary programmes was found.

2.2.18 Summary of global overview

Evidence has been found of many 'integrated interdisciplinary' programmes. Few appear however, to reflect the true ethos of this concept. Much attention has been paid to innovations in medical education and there are numerous publications concentrating on this aspect alone. Little reliable empirical data exists on the efficacy of these programmes and many of the authors have exhibited subjectivity in the evaluation of their innovation's success. Important factors have emerged nevertheless. Shortage of skilled personnel and inappropriate training commensurate with each individual country's needs have been the most influential factors in accepting the need for change. This is particularly evident in the Third World countries where the socio- economic climate militates against a replication of the Western models. For this reason the Third World, in many ways appears to be in advance of the more developed countries. The importance of primary health care in the community has received far greater attention in the developed countries in the last decade and thus curriculum developers have turned to their Third World colleagues for inspiration and guidance.

2.3 A European overview

Despite an extensive search for pertinent literature, few relevant publications have been found. The two major contributing sources have been the European Community, Brussels and The World Health Organisation European Regional Office in Geneva. Many of the documents are not available in the United Kingdom and could only be obtained directly from Geneva or Brussels. Consequently it may be that many of the educators responsible for curriculum development are not aware of their existence. As the EC and the WHO documents are published independently they are reviewed separately.

2.3.1 The European Community

On January 1, 1958 the Treaty of Rome was signed by six countries in Europe and this signalled the beginning of the European Community (EC). The six countries were Belgium, France, West Germany, Italy, Luxembourg and the Netherlands. The key aims of the Treaty were to establish the foundations of an ever closer union among the European peoples and to ensure economic and social progress by common action in eliminating the barriers which divide Europe (Lawson 1962, Quinn 1978, Collins 1983). In 1992 the EC consists of twelve member countries with several other countries applications for membership currently being considered. The recent events in Eastern Europe have enabled Poland, Hungary and Czechoslovakia to express a keen interest and they may well join in the next five years. The European Community structural organisation is clearly delineated (see Appendix 2.2). Within this structure there are four divisions which influence or even dictate the decisions made regarding health policies in Europe.

1. *The European Commission* is the 'Think Tank' of the Community and consists of seventeen Commissioners. These individuals must swear an affidavit that they will act independently of their own national interests. The Commission is responsible for drafting, adopting and implementing legislation and relies on information supplied by Advisory Committees.
2. *The European Parliament* consists of five hundred and eighteen individuals (1994) (Members of the European Parliament, MEP) who are directly elected by the population from the twelve member states. It has less power than a national parliament and does not adopt legislation although it debates and gives its opinion on legislative proposals.
3. *The Committee of Permanent Representatives* of the Member States (COREPER) consists of civil servents from the fifteen countries. It is in this Committee that any initial discussions take place.
4. *The Council of Ministers* are enabled to take final decisions and this is where legislation is adopted. Some of the proposed laws can be adopted through a majority vote while others require unanimity.

In the field of health care Advisory Committees on nursing, medicine and dentistry are in existence. They all fulfil a similar function in that they help ensure standards of health care training across the Community (CEC 1990b). The Committees were set up as a result of a decision made by the Council of Ministers in 1977. Each member country has representatives on these committees who are either experts in clinical practice or in education. Each committee meets individually on a twice yearly basis in order to exchange information on the type, level and structure of the training in each country with the overall aim of developing a comprehensive approach to the standard obtained and to review current developments in each member country. The importance of these committees, which report the results of their deliberations directly to the European Commission, cannot be over emphasised in the light of the Single European Act (1986) which came into force in July 1987. The Act concentrates on the necessity for a single internal market within the European Community. While much of the Act focuses on trade and finance, education and training has also received attention and the "free movement of goods, persons, services and capital" had to be in evidence by the target date of 31 December 1992 (EC 1991a). Consequently the Advisory Committee on Training in Nursing (ACTN) for example, had the unenviable task of trying to ensure that the standard, kind and content of nurse training within each country not only continued to satisfy the Statutory Regulating Body (in the United Kingdom it is the UKCC) but also that it satisfied each other member countries' requirements. Achievement of this means that Registered General Nurses, in the first instance, are able to practice anywhere within the European Community. Obviously other considerations such as an ability to speak the language of the host country are imperative. The implications for the nursing profession in the United Kingdom are therefore enormous as so many other Europeans speak excellent English and may well apply to work here. Because of the insularity of the British, far fewer individuals speak an European language to an acceptable standard and there is little likelihood of many British nurses working in other European Countries for the foreseeable furture. In 1991 the ACTN published guidelines for the training of general nurses in primary health care (EC 1991, Doc 111/F/5370/2/90). One of the many pertinent recommendations made in this document was:

> primary health care requires the acquisition of knowledge over a wide area and demands a team approach. For this reason there must be a multi-disciplinary approach to teaching. To this end it is important that other disciplines and professionals should contribute to nurse training to achieve greater understanding of the respective roles.
>
> (Ibid:1)

This unequivocal statement demonstrates an acknowledgement of the necessity to encourage ever increasing collaboration between the health care professions. Further evidence of the European Community interest in the future of the nursing profession was evident in 1989 when a symposium was held which addressed the issue of "Health Care and Nursing Education in the Twenty First Century" (CEC 1989: EUR 12040: EN). Chaired by Lord Cockfield, Vice President of the Commission of European Community. This symposium provided nurse experts from many countries with the opportunity to share their vision of future developments. One speaker believed that the only way forward was, "to train nurses with other members of the health professions, in some subjects which they both (sic) have to study, and this applies to both theoretical and practical training." (Diniz de Sousa : 80) Using this approach, Diniz de Sousa was convinced, would prevent conflict between the professions at a later stage.

2.3.2 The World Health Organisation : The European region

The regional office for the WHO is based in Geneva and consists of thirty five member states. It is characterised by the many different languages spoken in the region and it publishes papers in English, French, German and Russian. Following the acceptance of the strategy of health for all, regional targets have been adopted and reflect the view of all participating members. There are thirty eight targets in total many of which indirectly refer to the education of the health professions. One however specified the approach which should be adopted (Target 36) and considers in detail the problems and solutions which are inherent in the Target statement; "Before 1990, in all Member States, the planning, training and use of health personnel should be in accordance with health for all policies with emphasis on the primary health care approach." (WHO 1986d: 141)

The statement which followed this target suggested that one of the main problems was that planning did not always reflect the real needs as far as education and training was concerned. The theory and practice gap was well described and the need to make training more relevant to primary health care was emphasised. The Target solution included :

> .... a systematic review of undergraduate and postgraduate syllabuses for different categories of health personnel in order to discuss any changes that might be needed in curricula, training methods and the ways in which the numbers trained are matched with anticipated needs.

(WHO 1986d : 145)

To achieve this, the paper continued, self directed learning should be encouraged and the opportunity given for students to learn together in order that they can solve problems of concern to all disciplines working in health care.

Continuing education for health professionals was considered in 1979 by the WHO European Region. A meeting was convened in Helsinki in order to identify the way forward and while discussions centred on continuing education, inevitably initial training was reviewed. The delegates viewed interdisciplinary education as 'complementary to' rather than 'instead of' individual professional training. They believed that it was essential that the concept of teamwork was emphasised right at the beginning of all training programmes and that a common language and frame of reference was adopted. They acknowledged that while self motivation was fundamental to learning, all educationalists involved in health care training should foster the idea that the most effective way of improving health care was to ensure that all disciplines learned together (WHO 1979a).

In 1984 the WHO European Region was assessing the impact of training in the delivery of primary health care (WHO 1985a). The discussion centred on two key questions; what were the training needs of doctors and nurses in order to prepare them adequately for primary health care and how these identified needs could be met? Primary health care itself was thought to be disadvantaged as it was perceived to be low in professional esteem. It was seen as imperative that a move away from the medical model of care occurred with a concommitant move towards the adoption of a biopsychosocial model. A framework was suggested which would help achieve this aim. This summarised the proposed change in emphasis under four main headings; focus, content, organisation and responsibility (see Appendix 2.3), Apart from the change in emphasis from illness to health, there were several references to interdisciplinary teamwork and collaboration. It was suggested that many of the problems could be solved through a change in the educational approach. The involvement of 'lay members' such as environmental health workers should be included in this shared learning. This suggestion is an illustration of the shift towards the third world models previously described in section 2.2 of the literature review. The Alma Ata Declaration (1978) had stressed the need for teamwork yet it was noted with regret in Helsinki that most medical schools in Europe had not heard of the Declaration let alone incorporated the recommendations into their curriculum (WHO 1985a: 7). The working group denounced medical education in that it remained isolated and in many ways inappropriate for the future medical practitioner. They were not much more impressed with nurse education and its preparation for working in primary health care. They warned that basic nurse training, however good, was not adequate preparation for the job. This was undoubtedly true in 1984 but it could justifiably be argued that in the United Kingdom at least, the introduction of Project 2000 has ameliorated the criticism. Nursing is the first profession radically to alter the curriculum in order to meet the needs of the population it serves. The recommendations made in Helsinki included the introduction of interdisciplinary education through the foundation of health science faculties and more theoretical and practical experience in primary health care for all health professionals. The nursing profession as a whole adopted many of the proposed changes and between 1984 and 1988 many debates took place at a local, national and European level which culminated in a Conference held in Vienna in 1988 (WHO 1988c and WHO 1988d). The focus of the conference was on nurses' potential in ensuring equity in health, community participation, primary health care and international collaboration. The delegates at the conference were representing more than four million nurses' views which had been collated as the result of six hundred and forty five meetings being held in four hundred and seven locations in thirty European countries. In total 77,500 nurses attended these meetings. Amongst the topics discussed at length was the issue of team and multisectoral collaboration. Many called for "models of excellence in curriculum development" (WHO 1986d:8). A definite trend was identified in the move away from the medical model towards one that placed greater emphasis on interpersonal relationships, decision making and the ability to work as a team. The following year the Chief Nursing Officers of each European country met to consider the impact of the findings of the Vienna Conference and concluded that progress, although slow, was being made. The WHO Regional Office in conjunction with the Chief Nursing Officers devised a five year plan which included a commitment by the WHO to assist member states in the development of interdisciplinary educational programmes (WHO 1988a).

The most comprehensive document of any pertaining to interdisciplinary education in Europe was an unpublished one obtained directly from the WHO in Geneva. This paper (WHO 1986c) reported the proceedings of a conference, held in the regional office, which was attended by twelve temporary advisers and five staff members. The purpose of the meeting was to analyse progress and trends in interdisciplinary education, devise strategies for the implementation of interdisciplinary programmes and identify any co-operative activities currently underway in Europe. This paper was one of the few found that gave an operational definition of its terminology and was emphatic in its assertion that multi professional education should not be confused with multi disciplinary training. The latter the group believed "consists in exposing the same group of students to the teaching of different disciplines." (WHO 1986c : 2)

Multi-professional education indicated the grouping of students from the different disciplines who then shared common learning themes within the health team concept. This, the delegates believed, constituted the whole philosophical framework. The purpose of such an education was described as enabling students to solve problems, share care, undertake collaborative research, and plan, implement and evaluate the care given. Delegates from nine European countries reported their experiences in multi-professional education, Belgium, Finland, France, Greece, Portugal, Sweden, the United Kingdom, the USSR and Yugoslavia. The reports from France, Greece and Sweden concerned initiatives taken at an undergraduate level whilst the others reported initiatives at the continuing education stage.

Collectively, the institutions reported shared learning experiments in the following topics; teamwork, communication, behaviour, interpersonal relationships, biopsychosocial aspects of health care, management, environmental health, information technology, research methods and statistics. The topics appear to have a bias towards the behavioural sciences but the reasons for this were not explored. It may be that there is a tacit acceptance that the breadth and depth in teaching the biological sciences is decided on a 'need to know' basis. Medical students, for example, without doubt require a greater depth of knowledge in the biological sciences than nursing students. The topics described above are essential knowledge for all personnel involved in health and social care and should therefore be evident in each professions curriculum. The report is one of the most comprehensive discovered pertaining to the rationale for introduction of interdisciplinary learning and as such will be discussed in greater detail in sections 2.8 and 2.9 of the literature review. It will also contribute to the description of the methodology employed in this study. Two international interdisciplinary organisations have been traced, the first of which was founded in 1979 in Kingston Jamaica. Dr. Tamas Fulop and Dr. Fred Katz were the individuals behind the idea and at the inaugural meeting, twenty schools for health professions education enrolled. One of these was the University of Limburg in Maastricht, Holland which is now the headquarters of the organisation. This organisation was named the Network of Community Orientated Educational Institutions for Health Sciences (NCOEIHS). One of its principal objectives is to assist institutions who aim to introduce innovations in health personnel training. The overall aim is to improve health and thus contribute in a significant way to the WHO Strategy of 'Health for all by the year 2000'. In 1989 the principal objectives of the NCOEIHS were reviewed and updated. They can be summarised as follows :

1. A strengthened emphasis on instititutional support and capacity through increased exchange and dissemination of information, improved communication and an encouragement of relevant publications.
2. A new emphasis on partnerhsip between universities, governments and communities in order to reach the aim of health for all by the year 2000.
3. A focus on research and development, particularly towards education of the health care professions.
4. Management of growth

(NCOEIHS1991:14)

The NCOEIHS holds annual meetings but it is noted with regret that in 1987 only three representatives from the United Kingdom were present. All three were already involved in community based education and interdisciplinary learning within university departments, Dr. Godfrey from Southampton, Professor Seager from Sheffield and Dr. Walton from Edinburgh. At the conference it was agreed that because of the widely varied health problems encountered on an international basis one of the stated goals should be to increase the health status of a given population by ensuring that the education the professionals received was appropriate. The delegates examined the feasibility of analysing existing data, prioritizing it and changing the curriculum content of medical schools to accommodate this. They concluded that it would be feasible and recommended that this idea should be extended into other health professions educational programmes (NCOEIHS 1987).

The second organisation of note is the European Network for the Development of Multi-Professional Education in Health Sciences (EMPE). The inaugural meeting of the EMPE was held in Paris in 1987. The stated aim of the network is to foster a change in attitude among health care professionals by enhancing the concept of teamwork through multiprofessional learning. The promotion of information exchange, collaborative research, the development and evaluation of models of learning and the dissemination of research results was seen as the main function of the EMPE. The network itself operates from the Faculty of Health Sciences, Linkoping, Sweden with Professor Nils Holger Areskog being the General Secretary. Areskog has been a prolific author, speaker and advocate of interdisciplinary education and his signature can be found on many of the WHO publications. Newsletters are published on a regular basis with information regarding forthcoming conferences and abstracts of pertinent interdisciplinary research. What has become increasingly clear from the information gathered and the literature reviewed is that credible academic organisations with political influence and most importantly enthusiasm and commitment to innovatory interdisciplinary learning have emerged. Although operating independently and based in different countries, an interdependent network has developed in which each organisation mutually recognises and supports each other. It is interesting to note that institutions which have joined this interdependent network tend to belong to both NCOEIHS and EMPE. In addition they then belong to national networks. The support for the concept of interdisciplinary education would appear to be growing rapidly with more institutions joining these organisations each year. Individuals from all health disciplines are also encouraged to join at a very reasonable subscription and both organisations are most willing to provide any information, help and advice to anyone interested in developing an interdisciplinary educational programme (EMPE 1990a, 1990b).

2.3.3 Innovations in specific European countries

2.3.3.1 The Netherlands

Interdisciplinary learning in the Netherlands was first described in 1978 by Bouhuijs, Schmidt, Snow and Wijnen (cited in WHO 1978c). A programme had been introduced in 1974 at the University of Limburg, Maastricht. A particular emphasis was placed on primary health care with students being given considerable responsibility for their own learning and self assessment. Maastricht was one of eight universities in the Netherlands offering medical training. It differed however from the others because it chose to concentrate on community care. The curriculum aimed at problem orientation rather than discipline orientations and specifically identified co-ordination and collaboration between the professions, the acquisition of social skills and a commitment to continuing education. No lectures were given and the course was based entirely on shared learning between the students and tutorials with a member of staff. The curriculum was divided into a six week modular system described by Bouhuijs et al as 'instruction units'. The units were planned by multidisciplinary groups with each unit forming part of an overall matrix. Successful completion of each unit was necessary in order to complete the matrix and qualify. The programme was described as being very successful but no evidence was offered to support this statement and consequently the claim should be treated with caution.

2.3.3.2 Finland

In 1990 there were 22,200 students undertaking training in the health professions (Ministry of Education, Helsinki 1990). All health care courses are taught at one or other of the seven H.E.institutions in Finland. The Union of Health Professionals (TEHY) represents every health profession in Finland thereby immediately inviting cohesion and collaboration between the professional groups as there is common ground (TEHY 1991a). Medical staff have in addition their own professional organisation. In common with other countries, the majority of health care students in Finland begin their training straight from secondary school. A one year core curriculum of health care education is mandatory for all students where more than eight hundred hours are devoted to such subjects as communication, ethics, sociology, psychology, epidemiology, environmental health issues, research methods, statistics and teamwork. Having completed the common core curriculum the students then begin to concentrate on their chosen speciality. Shared learning to a lesser extent continues throughout their training (TEHY 1991b). Although most students have decided on the profession which they wish to join before they commence the common core, there is the opportunity for students to make a final decision during this first year. Isokoski (cited in WHO 1986c) described multiprofessional training at the University of Tampere. The course itself was limited by the fact that it trained qualified health personnel for health care administration. Nevertheless, there are some important observations to be made. A total of 1217 people had completed the course at the time of publication. The participating professions were physicians, dentists, nurses, managers, veterinary surgeons and 'others' (WHO 1986c : 35). The diversity of the personnel would not be of importance because the principles of good administration would be the same. The overall aim was described by Isokoski as enabling the students to become 'competent administrators'. Interdisciplinary small group tutorials constituted the main learning method and the reader was informed that the demand for places on the course far exceeded the number of places available. Again no empirical data was included which substantiated the claim of success. On this occasion it could be argued that the number of applicants for the course supported its efficacy. A course which does not meet the needs of the students will eventually fail as the number of applications received diminishes. This report also highlights the need for a fundamental shift in thinking towards subject orientation rather than professional orientation. If knowledge of a topic is essential in order for an individual to perform his/her job competently then the professional category becomes irrelevant. Through the assimilation of this knowledge the individual should then be able to apply this into professional practice.

2.3.3.3 Belgium

The need for a multiprofessional training programme in health education was identified by the then Minister of Health in 1984. As a result several universities entered into a collaborative partnership in order to address health education training on a large scale. The proposed student cohort comprised school teachers, nurses, social workers and army officers, an innovative multidisciplinary mix indeed. Piette (cited in WHO 1986c) described the problems that the tutorial staff had encountered in identifying the most appropriate level at which to teach, not least the problem of differing expectations from the students and the range of prior knowledge identified in those students. Piette emphasised that it was not a matter of different levels of academic achievement but a different orientation towards health education. This had led to a lack of tolerance and a lack of acknowledgement between the students of each others' expertise . The first programme was currently underway in 1986 and a self administered questionnaire was planned for the students at the end of the course which would be repeated twelve months following completion. Piette commented that "no one had as yet thought of training them in working as a team" (WHO 1986c : 18). This was a most illuminative statement as Piette obviously had identified this need but had either not been allowed to do so or she did not view this as a priority. Requests for further information have proved unsuccessful and consequently the student evaluations were not available. The criticism could be levelled that this innovation was too much, too soon. No evidence of any other interdisciplinary courses relating to health care has been found. It may be that Belgium would be well advised to introduce a programme which offers common themes for health professions in the first instance, in order to enhance co-operation between those groups. An early introduction to the concept of teamwork would also seem to be imperative.

2.3.3.4 France

The University of Paris-Nord, Bobigny belongs to the network EMPE (previously described in section 2.3.2). D'Ivernois, Cornillot and Zomer (cited in WHO 1986c) were convinced that along with the University of Linkoping in Sweden, Bobigny had been the most committed to introducing interdisciplinary programmes at both undergraduate and postgraduate levels. The programme was first introduced in 1977 with a common core of health sciences. Interestingly the subjects were described as anatomy, physiology, histology and biochemistry. No attempt was made to introduce the behavioural sciences. It appeared to be an introductory course to medical school and the choice of topics would seem to reflect the emphasis on biological sciences common in medicine. The authors reported that any student who failed the summative examination at the end of the one year programmme was given the opportunity to transfer to another discipline in health care. By 1984 the programme was far more complex. The two year course was designed with the specific intention of a common core for all students who then subsequently chose which professional training they wished to enter. The principle aim was that "everybody who is interested in health sciences may find his proper way" (WHO 1986c : 51). The students usually enrol straight from secondary school although according to the authors, the number of mature students was increasing rapidly. There was a fundamental shift in orientation in this new curriculum. The introductory module consisted of psychology, sociology, economics and experimental sciences. On successful completion of the module, which was assessed by a 'diagnostic test' the students commenced the next module entitled 'Option Sante' (Option Health). The contents of the module were described as epidemiology, community health, psycho-sociology, economics, biology, ecology, decision methodology and health education'. The rationale for this was described as "the concepts of community health consitute the real common core of the health sciences and are much more relevant than the basic sciences." (Ibid : 52)

The students as a result of interviews with their personal tutors then make a decision about their professional career choice. Subsequent modules are discipline orientated although, where possible, shared learning continues. The professional training offered in Bobigny consists of medicine, dentistry, seven (un-identified) paramedical professions, nursing, midwifery and health management. Several interdisciplinary degrees at Masters level are also in existence along with specified courses which address such issues as 'health and sport', 'mental health' and 'natural medicine'. The authors of this most informative paper continually referred to the concepts of a 'corporate mentality' and the 'genesis of teamwork'. They concluded that the courses should be based on methodology rather than content and that the core issues were communication, behaviour, relationships with patients and assessment of their quality of care. Along with other related subjects, they believed that this approach seemed "to offer more opportunities of exchange and mutual enrichment" (p.54). They also insisted that the only way that interdisciplinary education would truly be achieved was through a modular programme with the aims of each module being very clearly specified. Bobigny were also confronting the problems of "the granting of exemptions based on the recognition of professional experience" (p 55). They were convinced that the present system of repeating previous theory and practice would have to change if effective learning was to take place. The Bobigny programmes seemed to have all the hallmarks of true interdisciplinarity and as such could be adopted as a model upon which other institutions develop their own modular programmes in health care.

2.3.3.5 Greece

In the University of Athens there is a School of Health Sciences where medicine, dentistry, nursing and pharmacology are taught. Lanara (cited in WHO 1986c) described the co-operation that currently existed between the disciplines although this seemed to be based almost entirely on an administrative and shared resources basis. Some cross disciplinary teaching was evident with students from all disciplines attending common lectures. This could only be described as multi-disciplinary learning as there was no evidence of any interaction taking place between the disciplines and the use of lectures as a teaching method militates against interaction. It should of course be pointed out that Lanara presented this paper in English and consequently her choice of terminology was limited on occasions. Her description of the 'lecture' may not therefore have been absolutely correct although her call for closer collaboration indicates that there was little interaction in existence. Lanara requested more commitment from the WHO and the EC towards interdisciplinary learning and commented that these two organisations were in an ideal position to encourage international research into the subject. A multi-professional committee had been established in Greece in 1986 which had been given the remit to act as an advisory body to the Minister of Health in all educational matters. Lanara was very hopeful that rapid progress would now be made. She did not make it clear whether she was a member of this committee but it seems quite likely in view of the fact that her name appears as the nursing representative for Greece on the Advisory Committe on Training in Nursing to the EC. Lanara is therefore according to the EC an expert in the field of nurse education (EC 1991, Doc 111/F/5370/2/90).

2.3.3.6 Portugal

The University of Lisbon contains a Centre for Educational Studies for Health Development. According to Rendas (cited in WHO 1986c) the centre acts as a catalyst in bringing the different health professions together. Since 1982 student teachers of the professions have trained together, collaborative research has been undertaken and a consultation service has been offered to the whole of Portugal. The concept of teamwork has been adopted as the central tenet of the Centre with the belief that a holistic approach to health problems is essential. Rendas reported the commencement of a large empirical study which involved the task analysis of the different professions with the aim of establishing an integrated curriculum. The Portugese were questioning the inflexible stance that many of the professions were taking towards shared clinical skills. They believed that it was essential for core skills to be adopted by health care workers in order to maximise efficiency in rural areas. While no evidence was forthcoming about shared learning this paper was suggestive of an embryonic development in closer collaboration. Rendas did not identify which professions were involved in the scheme but Portugal in common with many other countries has a very limited number of health care disciplines.

2.3.3.7 Sweden

Evidence was found of two interdisciplinary initiatives in Sweden. The first described by Engstrom (1986) will be analysed in detail in section 2.7 of the literature review, teamwork in health care. Engstrom conducted an empirical study in communication and decision making in multi-disciplinary teams. It can never the less be stated that interdisciplinary case conferences were in existence in Sweden before 1982 (Engstrom 1986). The other initiative has been described by Areskog in several publications (Areskog 1988, also cited in WHO 1984c, WHO 1986d and WHO 1988b). This took place in Linkoping under the direction of Areskog himself and has already been described as the centre from which the EMPE operates. Although small interdisciplinary projects had been in evidence for some time in Linkoping a new regional health university was opened in 1986. Former colleges of medicine, nursing, occupational therapy, physiotherapy, laboratory assistants and social workers amalgamated into this new venture. The aim was described by Areskog as ensuring "the students acquire a basic knowledge using scientific methods, develop a common reference frame and prepare themselves for teamwork" (WHO 1986c : 64).

A core curriculum is in operation for the first ten weeks of training and Areskog included an example of the scheme in operation which was based on an educational objectives approach. Knowledge, skills and attitudes were categorised separately with lists of lower order objectives moving through to higher order objectives. A great deal of emphasis was placed on the use of problem solving, assimilation and synthesis although such terms were not actually used by Areskog himself. In addition to this initial course further periods of shared learning took place between two or more disciplines when appropriate. For some reason these periods were termed 'streaks' although, as has previously been discussed, this may be the result of a word in the Swedish language being translated literally into English. An example of a 'streak' was given as a situation in which medical students and physiotherapy students jointly studied the subject of trauma of the upper extremities. Over a one week period the students were given a free choice of tutors and other resources within the orthopaedic department. The aim was to diagnose, treat and plan the rehabilitation of patients with arm injuries. Several of these courses had been completed and Areskog reported that the student evaluations had been very positive. No evidence of these evaluations was given and so Areskog's assertions cannot be substantiated. He briefly referred to a similar initiative taking place in Tromso, Norway but no other references to this could be found. The rest of the paper concentrated on other interdisciplinary programmes on a global basis and as such have already been reviewed.

2.3.3.8. Summary of interdisciplinary initiatives in Europe

No evidence was found of any other programmes in operation in European countries. There are several possible explanations for this. The journals reviewed have been predominantly in the English language and it may be that countries such as Germany do not contribute to these publications. It is surprising that the WHO publications do not refer to any such programmes in Germany along with Italy, Spain, Luxembourg, Switzerland, Denmark and Ireland who all have representatives based in the WHO European Regional Office in Geneva and therefore obviously contribute significantly to the development of health strategies and the setting of targets.

These countries are all very active and committed members of the EC but any information from the EEC has not been forthcoming. It would appear that no such information exists as both the WHO and the EC have been instrumental in providing papers, references and the names of individuals who have contributed to the quality and quantity of this literature review. There have been numerous reports of developments in interdisciplinary learning throughout Europe yet they are mostly descriptive, anecdotal and lacking in persuasive data. Many of the reports refer to several disciplines but it has become evident that few countries train or employ many of the paramedical professions. Most appear to concentrate on medicine, nursing and dentistry. There would appear that less interdisciplinary learning is taking place within the European region than there is in the Third World. This may indicate that one of the prime reasons for its introduction is to utilise resources both in manpower and finance to the maximum effect. The funding of health care is now of major political importance in most countries. With the spiralling costs of health care, accountability and a sensible rationalisation of resources has become paramount.

Whilst the educational rationale for a greater thrust towards shared learning may be ignored from an altruistic basis the argument for the rationalisation of resources may well persuade the policy makers to turn their attention to its potential. Interestingly in October 1990 a Council of Europe Conference of Health Ministers was held in Nicosia, Cyprus. These Ministers decided to create a group to co-ordinate an ongoing research study commencing in 1991. The focus of the study would be interdisciplinary learning approaches in the training of health care staff. Both undergraduate and postgraduate programmes are to be monitored in a number of countries.

Representatives from primary health care and the acute hospital sector are co-opted and the group is of an interdisciplinary nature. The study is in its early stages and no indication has been given of when any published results might be expected. Although the rationale for the study has not been revealed it is suggestive of a move towards the better utilisation of financial resources and manpower.

2.4 The United Kingdom perspective (excluding Wales)

Since as early as 1920 various reports have been published which refer to the need for increased interdisciplinary collaboration in health and social care in the United Kingdom. Many of these reports have been commissioned by the Government and have therefore appeared under the umbrella of HMSO. Inevitably, because of the difficulty in separating the references many have been adopted under the name of the person who chaired the working party (HMSO 1920 - The Dawson Report, HMSO 1951 - The Cope Report, HMSO 1959 - The Younghusband Report, HMSO 1968a - The Todd Report, HMSO 1968b - The Seebohm Report, HMSO 1969 - The Cohen Report, HMSO 1972 - The Briggs Report, HMSO 1973 - The McMillan Report, HMSO 1974a - The Otton Report, HMSO 1974b - The Halsbury Report, HMSO 1975 - The Merrison Report, number one, HMSO 1976a - The Court Report, HMSO 1979a - The Merrison Report, number two, HMSO 1979b - The Jay Report, HMSO 1980 - The Nodder Report, HMSO 1981 - The Harding Report, HMSO 1986 - The Cumberledge Report, HMSO 1989 - The Griffiths Report.) In addition to these reports HMSO has also published others which do not appear to have acquired nomenclature (HMSO 1968, 1971, 1976, 1977, 1978, 1979, 1985, 1986b, 1988, 1989a and 1989b). To further complicate the issue not all reports have been assigned a command number and some refer to previous reports by their adopted name only. Other reports have also been commissioned by organisations such as the Royal College of Nursing over the years and these too have adopted the names of the chairperson. Two reports in particular that have emerged through the RCN made specific recommendations regarding interdisciplinary education (RCN 1964 ,The Platt Report, RCN 1985 - The Judge Report). The sheer number and extent of these reports militates against individual written analyses and consequently common themes have been identified and the reports considered collectively. Many reports have also been published in Wales, most particularly by the Welsh Office. It has been decided to review publications pertaining solely to Wales in a separate section of the literature review (section 2.5) as many of these have direct implications for the feasibility of introducing interdisciplinary learning described in this current study.

2.4.1 Collaboration between the Health and Social Services

For many years great concern has been expressed about the divisions which exist between the National Health Service and The Social Services. Several reports have emphasised the inextricable links which occur between the two and have insisted that this should not only continue to be the case but that these links should be strengthened. The Younghusband Report (HMSO 1959) commented that it had found considerable resistance to this concept from both the NHS and the Social Services. It highlighted the fact that the resistance was due to different professional groups jealously guarding their own territory by rejecting any suggestions which were believed to threaten the expertise and autonomy of each profession. Numerous authors have studied this phenomenon and interprofessional conflict appears to have a major constraining influence on interdisciplinary developments. (Evidence of interprofessional conflict is analysed in depth in section 2.6 of this literature review). In 1959 primary health care in the community had not assumed such a high profiile as it has in the last two decades. Nevertheless Younghusband (HMSO 1959) referred to health centres and stressed the need for social workers to be employed within them as part of the health team. Forty years earlier The Dawson Report had considered the future provision of medical and allied services (HMSO 1920). Oblique references were made to primary health care in that the working party foresaw a shift away from the emphasis on caring for the patient in hospital towards maintaining health and caring for the individual in his/her own environment wherever possible. The Report on Local Authority and Allied Personal Social Services (HMSO 1968) and The Otton Report (HMSO 1974a) made similar observations and considered in depth the implications of such a strategy. The Otton Report, whilst acknowledging the difficulties of increased collaboration between the Social Services and the NHS, insisted that the only way the needs of the patient would truly be met was through "a genuine interprofessional partnership with each member of the team making his appropriate contribution to the pattern of care" (HMSO 1974a : 16, 17). Otton and his colleagues were particularly concerned with the problem of how to ensure continuity of care and asserted that teamwork was imperative if this was ever to be achieved. They believed that continuity of care "demands a system which will ensure that there is a team responsibility to co-ordinate any action and prevent either overlap or gaps in the help offered" (HMSO 1974a : 51).

Further evidence concerning the lack of collaborative care has been traced through the last two decades. Many working parties have been commissioned by the British Government with the remit of identifying good working practice and paradoxically exposing what was considered to be bad practice. The Personal Social Services Council (PSSC) published their findings in 1978 (HMSO : 1978). They had found situations in which a large number of agencies contributed collaboratively to the care of an individual in the community. On occasions these agencies dealt with acute problems which were ameliorated by prompt co-operation and action between several different professions and the PSSC noted that mutual support and counselling was readily available in these cases. These situations were praised by the PSSC as examples of 'good practice'. Where 'bad practice' was identified the working party noted that there was a noticeable absence of joint planning, not only at an operational level but frequently at a strategic level as well. Inadequate resources and services were also contributory factors. In some instances the main reason for the bad practice was the inappropriate action taken by the professionals themselves. The causal factor included "failures in communication which led to inadequate information and ignorance of roles, skills and outlooks of other professional groups". (HMSO 1978: 12). Blame for this was attributed equally to the Health Service and the Social Services. Ominously the working party reported that while ignorance of each others roles contributed to the failure to work as a team the single most important factor was "due to professional perceptions of the world and the balance of power between different professional groups and between professionals and clients". (HMSO 1978: 19).

In 1981 the Harding Report pursued a similar theme and suggested that a "respect for the different orientations" (HMSO 1981: 9) was essential if these problems were to be overcome. The need for integration was stressed, which would be achieved only through the adoption of common objectives, a clear understanding of the role of each team member, and a flexible approach to care. Educators were charged with ensuring the "proper preparation of all those taking part" (p 48) and they continued, the obvious way was through training. They concluded with the following statement; "We are convinced that conscious efforts towards preparation for teamwork need to be made during formative professional training, preferably on a multi-disciplinary basis. (HMSO 1981: 50)

The Royal Commission on the NHS (HMSO 1979) commonly refered to as the Merrison Report, had reached similar conclusions. The Commission was charged with the task of identifying how to best use the financial and manpower resources available within the NHS. They collected 2460 written submissions for evidence, 2800 informal interviews were conducted and 58 individuals gave formal oral evidence. As a result of the mass of information Merrison and his colleagues collected, they reached the following conclusions; teamwork was at a very early stage in its development therefore more joint training activities were of considerable importance (p 71 para 7.4); within the existing multidisciplinary clinical teams questions of leadership, corporate responsibility, legal responsibility and confidentiality seemed to cause the most conflict and uncertainty and these issues should be resolved as rapidly as possible (p 171 para 12.38) ; a skill mix analysis of staff in difference contexts should be undertaken urgently (p 181 para 12.65). Medical training was particularly criticised as not being appropriate as it concentrated on acute hospital medicine and that it; "produced a doctor whose skills, attitudes and expectations were sometimes poorly related to the health problems and needs of the community." (HMSO 1979: 277)

Several attempts have been made to respond to this criticism, the latest being a report published by the Kings Fund (Towle 1991) which is analysed elsewhere in this review. An important development however was a seminar held at the University of Exeter chaired by Dr. Pereira-Grey. The seminar was arranged in the context of the WHO Regional Strategy for Health for All. The remit was to consider how undergraduate medical education could be altered in order to increase doctors' competencies in primary health care (WHO 1983). The group stressed that while many countries continued to emphasise the biological sciences to the detriment of the behavioural sciences in medical training, progress would be slow. A multi-disciplinary approach was suggested as this the delegates believed, most accurately reflected primary health care. The development of Regional Health Universities was considered as being one possible model for integrating health care and the education of health professionals as they would facilitate interdisciplinary education and training. It could be argued however that this structure already nominally exists as all medical schools are within the University sector as are most other allied professions. Teaching hospitals are also linked directly to the university sector with many of the professionals holding joint appointments between a health authority and a university. The contribution of psychologists and sociologists from their own university departments might also be at risk if there was to be a splintering away from mainstream higher education. It was suggested that the concept of health should be taken as a starting point in medical training with an insistence on epidemiological awareness and an increasing trend towards preventive measures. The authors of this report advocated a greater concern with core objectives, for by incorporating these, core competencies could be developed. The emphasis on core objectives and learning together also continued as a central tenet of the Merrison Report (1979) with one of its conclusions being "there are few things more important for the NHS than that its health professionals should work well together". (Ibid : 278).

Merrison and his colleagues came to no firm conclusions about the relationship between the NHS and the Social Services. They noted that many of the individuals who sent evidence proposed that the two services should be integrated in some way (p 37). Willcocks cited in Cypher (1979) also commented on the great divide between the two. Again while reaching no firm conclusions he suggested that this was a deliberate ploy by both services in order to maintain professional competition. Hargreaves also cited in Cypher (1979), thought that it really did not matter as the end result of any re-organisation would mean that nurses and social workers in particular were going to have to be prepared to work more closely together. Both the Jay Report (HMSO 1979b) and the Nodder Report (HMSO 1980) considered the need for an integration of the NHS and the Social Services in order to improve the quality of care for the mentally handicapped and the mentally ill. The reports highlighted the major problem of differing authorities being responsible for two services each with totally different methods of allocating resources. In reality this meant that many of the potential recipients of care failed to receive help from either service. This anomaly continues in 1992 for both the mentally ill and the elderly. Delays caused by arguments over which service should take prime responsibility for an individual frequently mean that individuals fail to receive the care they need. It is interesting to speculate whether professional conflict and the attempt to expand responsibilities in fact diminishes considerably when it comes to deciding which service should pay the bill for an individuals care. It is suspected that in such cases each service would readily hand over responsibility to the other! Nodder and his colleagues nevertheless recommended that joint training initiatives between the Health Service and the Social Services should be implemented as a matter of urgency. Lord Cohen (cited by Kogan and Pope 1972) observed that the need for cooperation was "now generally, if not quite universally accepted" (p 8). The British Government however in 1986 was still expressing concern about the inefficiency in the delivery of care due entirely it believed to the "lack of adequate understanding between team members at present" (HMSO 1986b: 47). This would suggest that there is not a general acceptance of the need for cooperation nor much evidence of an attempt to address the problems. Evidence has been found however which refutes this. The UKCC (1992) in the Code of Professional Conduct (see Appendix 2.4) charged all nurses, midwives and health visitors to; work in a collaborative and co-operative manner with health care professionals and others involved in providing care and recognise and respect their particular contribution within the care team. (Ibid : 2 : Clause 6)

The UKCC also recognised that the issue of confidentiality caused a problem in so much that sharing information with other team members may undermine a patient's confidence. Clause 10 of the Code of Professional Conduct addressed the issue and previously in 1987, the UKCC published a pamphlet entitled "Confidentiality". It emphasises that "confidentiality is a rule with certain exceptions" and recognises that in some circumstances particularly where certain vulnerable groups are concerned "practitioners should always take the opportunity to discuss the matter fully with other practitioners." Significantly they pointed out that this did not necessarily mean just other nurses. Several of the professions allied to medicine are currently developing similar codes and it seems a pity that the medical profession does not do likewise. The statements within the Code are ideal for teaching and learning purposes as each constitutes a position statement which reflect attitudes, values, legal implications, ethical issues and professional competency.

Paradoxically in 1985 The Royal College of Nursing published the Judge Report. It was commissioned because of increasing concern about nurse education and its inappropriateness to the real world. The Report acknowledged that the general public, providing it received a 'good service' may not perceive the need for change. The Report overall made a significant number of recommendations and made the observation that "at the core of the education of the general nurse still lies the teaching which bears most directly upon the practice of nursing". (RCN 1985 : 9)

This is unarguably the case and should remain so. However, the Commission then expressed the opinion that this core could not be isolated from a body of knowledge which contained anatomy, physiology, biology, pharmacology and mathematics. The Report did however justify the infusion of psychology and sociology in to the curriculum. In 1964 the RCN had also considered the reform of nurse education (The Platt Report). A fleeting reference to joint education of health care professionals was made and the report mentioned the desirability of a degree in social and human biology which would act as a preparatory course for those entering the professions (RCN 1964: 26: para 105). It was recommended that an individual's social, emotional and physical factors should be the core topics with a concommitant involvement of the family and the community. Environmental factors, cultural differences, social policy and the promotion of health and welfare should all be included. The Briggs Report (HMSO 1972) reviewed the role of nurses, midwives and health visitors. In this Report the function of the extended team was considered and such words as 'dove-tailing', 'overlapping', 'collaboration' and 'colloboration' were used liberally. The Briggs committee envisaged that the role of doctors and nurses would become complementary and interchangeable on occasions as in many instances it was difficult to decide which profession should take the lead. Communication between the two professions was seen to be the key to integrated patient care (p 45). The Report also identified an overlap in some duties between physiotherapists and nurses, radiographers and nurses. This was found to be particularly the case in intensive care and accident and emergency units. The relationship between social workers and nurses was examined. The Report concluded :

> There is a lack of awareness among many nurses or social workers and this highlights the need for nurses in training, particularly those with a special interest in preventive health, to be given an understanding of the role of the social worker and vice versa.
>
> (HMSO 1972 : 50)

A further point of interest in this Report was the survey in which 3000 nurses were asked to comment on the suggestion that the theory of nursing should be taught in technical colleges. Some 75% thought that "the only place to learn nursing is in hospital" and 78% "prefer to learn only with other nurses" (p 69). These findings do not seem to have had any influence on the move to affiliate nurse education with higher education or indeed the trend towards integrated inter-disciplinary learning. Twenty years ago however, little experience was available of either concept and it may well be that attitudes have changed. For 1972 the Briggs Report was remarkably futuristic in relation to both the education and practice of nursing. Many of the proposals and recommendations are finally coming to fruition twenty years later with the advent of Project 2000. Briggs also envisaged a 'common' induction course for nurses and the professions allied to medicine. In direct contrast to the preferred isolated learning described by the nurses in the Briggs Report, the Jay Report (HMSO 1979b) received written evidence (N = 613) that the concept of a common core training was highly supported along with a strong preference for an interdisciplinary approach to health care for the mentally handicapped. This Report also recommended that the professional group most suited to adopting the role of team leader was social work. Even more contentiously they envisaged that ultimately mental handicap nurses would no longer be under the aegis of the General Nursing Council (GNC), which has now become the UKCC. Fourteen years later this controversy has still not been resolved, mental handicap nurses remain under the statutory control of the UKCC although their job has altered considerably. Caring for the mentally handicapped has moved very firmly away from the biological model to the psychosocial model and without doubt nurses and social workers employed in this specialty would benefit from far more integrated interdisciplinary learning.

Analysis of the literature has revealed numerous 'common' educational programmes, but usually in the form of post-graduate multidisciplinary study days, which have stated their aims as increasing cooperation between the professions. In 1985 a multi professional group of doctors, nurses and social workers founded the Centre for the Advancement of Interprofessional Education in Primary Health and Community Care (CAIPE). The purpose was to :

> promote development, practice and research in interprofessional education for practitioners and managers involved in primary health and community care, in order to foster and improve inter-professional co-operation.
>
> (Horder 1991 : 18)

Its first task was to commission a national survey which identified interprofessional initiatives in England, Scotland and Wales. The Institute of Community Studies (ICS) completed the survey and published the results in 1989. The report is the most comprehensive analysis of development in interdisciplinary learning to date although as the authors observed, by the date of publication further initiatives had commenced. The terms of reference were; "to establish the extent and nature of recent initiatives in interprofessional education involving primary health care professionals in mainland UK." (ICS 1989: 1)

The information was gathered through a nationwide postal survey which although having too many variables to make it scientifically valid gave an indication of the developments taking place. The inclusion criteria for the study was that the reported initiative must have education as the primary aim and that any two groups of general practitioners, social workers, district nurses, health visitors and community midwives were learning together on an interdisiplinary basis. Reports of student interdisciplinary groups were also accepted as valid. The authors (Shakespeare, Tucker and Northover) recognised that the inclusion of these five groups excluded other professions who equally contributed to health and social care in the community but apparently resource limitations necessarily dictated this. It should be noted that all five professions included in this study were qualified practitioners and therefore most reports would inevitably involve interdisciplinary learning at a continuing education stage. Stereotyping, cloistering and interprofessional conflict (subsequently described in section 2.6 of the literature review) would be already in evidence. Attention should also be drawn to the fact that three of the five groups were all registered nurses in the first instance and therefore collectively constituted the largest group in the survey. The information requested consisted only of those initiatives that had taken place within a specified time scale of one year and concentrated on factual non evaluative data. Of the 1518 questionnaires sent, 1105 responses (75%) were received. Of these 470 (43%) indicated that they had not participated in any interdisciplinary learning, 156 (14%) indicated that they had, but the details given failed to meet the original inclusion criteria and 479 (43%) confirmed their participation and gave valid examples which were included in the results. Some of the 479 positive responses described more than one initiative. In total 695 (excluding duplicate) responses were received. The number of notifications from each professional group varied considerably, 474 from nurses, midwives and health visitors, 90 from social workers, 202 from doctors and 78 from 'others' (N = 844). Health visitors reported 612, district nurses 504, social workers 318, general practitioners 256 and community midwives 224 initiatives (N = 695). Health visitors and district nurses therefore participated in many more initiatives than the other groups. Regretfully the total number of shared learning experiences undertaken by medical students and student nurses totalled 20 (N = 695) thus re-inforcing the suggestion that most undergraduate students learn in professional isolation. Of the total number of initiatives (N = 695) only 43 (6%) involved the five groups collectively whereas 315 (43%) involved only two groups. Predictably the most common combination of professional groups was that of district nurses and health visitors sharing learning opportunities (136 occasions where N = 695). The authors concluded that the reason for this was due to the UKCC being the Statutory Body which controls the training of both groups and also the fact that it is usual to find health visitor and district nurse training in the same building thus allowing greater opportunity for shared learning.

Other professions participating in shared learning reported in this study included nurses from many different disciplines; teachers, voluntary agencies, the police, physiotherapists and occupational therapists. Hospital nurses participated in 168 (N = 695) initiatives. The authors suggested that this may well be due to the relevance of certain topics to both the hospital sector and the community. Another observation they made was that conferences and study days on child abuse was the main reason for the participation of the police force (55 occasions) and teachers (60 occasions). The Court Report (HMSO 1976a) which examined child health services had recognised the importance of collaboration between the health professions, the police and teachers in child care and welfare and had called for opportunities to be made available for these groups to learn together and share their expertise. It is difficult to judge whether any of the initiatives reported in the ICS (1989) study were developed as a direct result of the Court Report recommendations but it can be assumed nevertheless that Court and his colleagues would have approved of these developments. The Court Report however in its deliberations on training strategies recommended an even more collaborative approach to child care :

> Because .....children will require a multi-professional approach, so communication assumes a new importance. One way to foster this would be through common core training and multi-professional inservice training schemes.
>
> (HMSO 1976a : 336)

The ICS (1989) survey revealed some interesting findings in the types of agencies that offered opportunities for interdisciplinary learning. Schools of nursing organised 102 (22%), higher education establishments 73 (16%), health authorities 64 (14%), social services 37 (8%) and the general practitioner vocational training scheme 40 (11%). The remaining opportunities were offered by a variety of agencies. The authors highlighted however that the health authorities having a broader remit than the schools of nursing tended to offer courses for the greatest number of disciplines whereas the schools of nursing "were almost invariably for the nursing professions only" (p 18).

The respondents in this survey were asked to decide amongst a list of other objectives, whether the interdisciplinary programmes were primarily organised for convenience or for promoting teamwork and collaboration between the professions. 367 (53%) indicated that it was to promote teamwork and enhance understanding, the schools of nursing however arranged these courses "for reasons other than the promoting of teamwork and interprofessional understanding" (p 20). In total one in ten continuing education programmes centred on teamwork whereas one in four undergraduate programmes did. It should not be forgotten however that only 20 initiatives at an undergraduate stage were described and so according to these results only five undergraduate courses centred on teamwork.

The number of particpants on each course varied considerably. There were less than 10 on 35 initiatives, less than 20 on 222 initiatives, less than 50 on 249 and more than 50 on 142 occasions. The educational methods varied from group work and discussions (597 occasions), lectures (505 occasions), experiential methods (97 occasions) to exhibitions, tutorials and demonstrations. Amazingly the courses with the greatest number of participants (> 50) indicated only a slightly higher tendency in using lectures. These large courses however tended to last for only a short duration, frequently one day or less. Many initiatives (201) were also 'one off' with others held on a once yearly basis (60). However, 125 were instigated several times a year. The most encouraging finding was the 128 incidences of one or more sessions that were incorporated into an established course. This may indicate the adoption of integrated interdisciplinary learning as a philosophical approach into these established courses which is a most encouraging development. The final point of interest in this report was the finding that only five per cent of the continuing education initiatives were compulsory whereas more than 40% of the undergraduate interdisciplinary initiatives were mandatory. This raises the question of interested volunteers choosing to attend interdisciplinary courses. Any evaluative studies may tend to be biased in the results because it could be postulated that the respondents have a positive attitude towards those of shared learning anyway. It would seem that the only way to overcome this possibility is to randomly sample individuals from each professional group giving each person the opportunity to refuse to participate if he/she wished. Whilst this ICS survey had acknowledged flaws it did represent a reasonable picture of the current position in 1987/8.

One of the courses surveyed which lasted more than twelve weeks was the MSc at the University of Exeter which commenced in 1988 and has been subsequently described by Goble (1991). Further Bachelor and Masters degrees have since been validated around the United Kingdom (Leathard 1992). The approved titles of these usually reflect the interdisciplinary nature of these courses with the most favoured word seeming to be 'interprofessional'. The adoption of the prefix 'inter' supports the decision made in chapter one of this study to use the term interdisciplinary rather than multidisciplinary as it implies meaningful interaction between the professional groups.

In 1986 Cumberledge was appointed by the Government to review community nursing (HMSO 1986a). In the forwarding letter to the Secretary of State, Cumberledge stated very clearly the need for primary health care teams. Cumberledge and her team identified several areas of weakness in the overall excellence observed. One of the weaknesses was that duplication occurred between several of the health care disciplines which meant that as many as four or five different people assessed a client. If interprofessional protocols were developed an assessment could be undertaken by one individual only. Cumberledge suggested that community nurses were trapped within their own discrete roles and bound by tradition. The working party found little evidence of a clear understanding of the roles of primary health team members and even more alarmingly little evidence of mutual respect. The report rather ruefully observed that many 'teams' existed in name only. It recommended that community nurses should become more generic although practice nurses and occupational health nurses seemed to be excluded from this suggestion which rather negates the idea of cohesiveness. It could indeed be argued that the adoption of this strategy may be rather divisive. The Report also recommended that community nurses should be managed by a community nurse who has credible clinical experience but equally importantly has been "fully trained in management skills" (p 24). This emphasis is pleasing as too often individuals in professions such as medicine or nursing are promoted into senior management positions without adequate preparation to take on this role. While it is recognised that the working party was given only six months to investigate the problem, collect the data and produce the report, it must be noted that the overall impression that the recommendations give would be one of chaos if fully implemented. Re-organisation of community nursing was long overdue and this was obviously the intention of the Government. Perhaps all that can be concluded is that the recommendations implied re-arrangement rather than an improvement in the organisation of the service. Section 8 of the report considered improving teamwork and urged that the proposed neighbourhood nursing service should complement rather than compete with the primary health care team. The recommendations included the negotiation of a written contract between the two parties with the veiled threat that if general practitioners did not enter into this contract then they would not be consulted about future nursing apppointments in the community (p 36). A coherent argument could be made however that an interview panel should always consist of different professional representation if the applicant is going to work in an interdisciplinary team. (This point is further developed in section 2.7.3. of the literature review). One of the recommendations made in this report was the introduction of a generic training for all those nurses wishing to work in primary health care. It was suggested that a Diploma in Community Nursing or similar should be adopted. This recommendation has indeed been addressed and there are now several centres which specialise in primary health care nursing that offer a generic diploma level qualification. The Cumberledge Report was full of pertinent observations about the current weaknesses of the system, the wasted resources in manpower and the urgent need to re-organise. Cumberledge and her colleagues regretted the poor response from the questionnaires that had been distributed (no raw score was given for the numbers distributed or returned). Many protests were made by the community nurses to the working party about the impossible time schedule. Cumberledge, judging by her introductory remarks obviously agreed with the protests and was well aware that six months was far too short a time to do justice to the complexity of the problems in the community. The most glaring omission in this hasty report was the lack of a reference section, in spite of quotes being included in the main text. This meant that tracing the original sources was sometimes an impossible task.

The final document relating to the collaboration of health and social services was the Government White Paper "Working for Patients" (HMSO 1989). The White Paper emphasises caring for people wherever possible in their own homes. The Government recognised that failing to clarify the responsibilities "had led to confusion and had contributed to poor overall performance" (p 5). One of the key changes was that local authorities should collaborate with the health professionals in organising appropriate care in the community for individuals. The relevant professions were charged with the task of recognising; "particularly at the working interface there is frequently much common purpose; to cross refer cases when appropriate and to seek and share advice and information when relevant." (HMSO 1989: 13)

In order to enhance this idea, the White Paper suggested that; "Training authorities may wish to adapt existing training programmes and consider providing such training in a multi-disciplinary setting in order to enhance understanding between health and social service professionals." (Ibid : 36)

The National Health Service Training Authority (NHSTA) in 1990 produced the first of what will doubtless be many modules as part of the PICKUP programme for members of the NHS involved in teamwork in community care. It is a module of high quality which explains in detail team dynamics, team values and the problems which team members can encounter. It mentions democratic decision making, leadership styles, effective communication strategies, mutual support, respect and trust and the importance of flexibility. What a pity that the NHSTA did not work with the Social Workers training body (CCETSW) and develop a collaborative module. Although the module is ideally suited for social workers the fact that the NHS has sole ownership as far as the development is concerned, further contributes to emphasising the divide between the NHS and Social Services. Until far more truly collaborative programmes are developed in which both sides have collective ownership, progress will continue to be slow.

2.4.2. The professions allied to medicine

In 1949 a series of eight committees were set up to consider the supply and demand, the training and qualifications of almoners (now called social workers), chiropodists (now called podiatrists), dietitians, medical laboratory technicians, occupational therapists, physiotherapists, radiographers and speech therapists. The chairman and two other members were common to all committees. As the individual committees were considering their terms of reference, it became increasingly apparent that there were many common problems. For this reason it was decided to publish the findings of the committees collectively under the auspices of the HMSO and it is now known as The Cope Report (HMSO 1951). Although part of the terms of reference included the examination of current training it appears that apart from recommending greater autonomy and control by the professions themselves, thereby implying that the medical profession should relinquish some of its control, the issue of the curriculum was not examined. The Cope Report recommendations did however contribute significantly to the Professions Supplementary to Medicines Act (HMSO 1960).

In 1972 a working party chaired by McMillan was convened by the then Secretary of State, Sir Keith Joseph (HMSO 1973). The remit of the working party was to make recommendations on the future role of the remedial professions in relation to the other health care professions and to the patient. The remedial professions were described as physiotherapy, occupational therapy and remedial gymnastics. One of the major problems identified was that of overlapping responsibilities between the professions. Many similarities between occupational therapy and physiotherapy were identified and it was believed that the difference between the latter and remedial gymnasts was barely distinguishable. All three remedial professions suffered from a lack of autonomy in that medical practitioners prescribed treatment for patients and dictated the way in which the treatment was to be implemented. The working party concluded that this state of affairs was unacceptable as the remedial professions themselves had a superior knowledge of treatment strategies than did the medical profession. They observed that ideally the medical and remedial professions should work together collaboratively in a situation in which the doctor would decide the desired outcome and the therapist decide the best way of achieving this outcome. The relationship between nurses and therapists was also examined. It was acknowledged that nurses were "involved in rehabilitation in the broadest sense" (p 13) and that the patient received the best care when there was close collaboration between the two groups. A team approach was recommended which utilised the skills of all professions along with a formalised interdisciplinary teaching commitment.

A major and controversial recommendation was the convergence of the three remedial professions in order to make "one comprehensive and unified remedial profession" (p 18). To achieve this, integration of training was seen as both urgent and essential. It was recommended that a basic course of less than three years duration should be commenced with a second phase in which specialisation took place. A degree level qualification was seen as desirable but not essential. Nearly twenty years later the effects of this report could be described as minimal. Although remedial gymnastic training has been discontinued, an all graduate status has been approved in most of the professions allied to medicine. No evidence has been found that implies the total integration of physiotherapy and occupational therapy. Interdisciplinary learning appears to be minimal or absent.

The Council for the Professions Supplementary to Medicine (CPSM) was particularly concerned with the effectiveness and efficiency of the basic education and training of eight professions (CPSM 1979). They reviewed "the opportunities for and the constraints upon the collaboration between" (p 2) chiropody, dietetics, medical laboratory sciences, occupational therapy, orthoptics, physiotherapy, radiography and remedial gymnastics. No rationale was offered for the exclusion of speech therapy. The aim was to make more effective and efficient use of the resources available. The Council argued that over the next decade degree level studies should be introduced to stimulate "genuine scientific enquiry in order to foster a climate in which provenly ineffective methods whether new or old can be abandoned...." (CPSM 1979 : 4) They also concluded that the introduction of degree courses would increase the quality of interaction with other professions. They warned however, that the acceptance of this idea by the more traditional professionals would ultimately depend on a measurable improvement in the quality of patient care. They emphasised the necessity of each profession demonstrating observable skills and the mastery of a complex body of knowledge. They urged caution regarding the implementation of change for changes sake but continued; "Yet everything about present methods is ripe for review and evaluation jointly by those responsible at every level and in every sector......most of all the supplementary professions need to learn from each other." (CPSM 1979: 28)

They recommended the introduction of joint contracts, course collaboration and common lectures and concluded that all staff and students should be "intermingled and in no way artificially divided" (p 28). They also addressed the issue of 'competence' and decided that in all professions it meant that an individual possessed the knowledge, skills and attitudes to perform efficiently at the basic level needed to fulfil their professional role. The Report described the opportunities that were missed for integrated interdisciplinary learning, mainly because of a failure to grasp the initiative. A common core was perceived as being an appropriate area for limited experimentation as the authors believed it implied a logical progression in curriculum development.

The introduction of a common core for health care assistants in the early part of this decade may just be the embryogenesis of such a programme. Indeed a feasibility study undertaken by Price Waterhouse in 1987, (commissioned by the Department of Health and Social Security, Manpower Services Commission, the UKCC and the NHSTA) concluded that a Youth Training Scheme (YTS) should be introduced as soon as possible. A model syllabus was suggested within the final report which included core competencies such as the philosophy and practice of caring, the individual and society, health, illness and disability, human development and body function, health and social services and communication skills. The implication of this Report was therefore that a curriculum undertaken by school leavers, considering a career in one of the health professions, should contain elements common to all the professions. Integrated interdisciplinary learning would then have been introduced prior to any undergraduate training whatsoever.

Increasingly numerous advertisements are appearing announcing interdisciplinary conferences, more resources are being allocated to such initiatives and more staff are indicating their willingness to attend such gatherings. Some conferences are oversubscribed and apparently could be repeated several times in the same venue, an example of this being the CAIPE conference held in June 1992 entitled "Working Together or Pulling Apart". All these developments are most encouraging for those health and social care professionals who are convinced of the need for closer collaboration in order to produce quality care.

2.5 The Welsh perspective

In 1988 the Welsh Office published a document which outlined "The Corporate Management Programme for the Health Service in Wales". It primarily constituted an agenda for action, described the projected timescale for implementation and listed key objectives with accompanying classification of the importance of each objective. The stated aim of the Programme was :

> to detail the management action that must be undertaken, on an all Wales basis, to maximise the effectiveness of the NHS in the Principality to the benefit of patient care and to help authorities deal positively with the problems they face in common.
>
> (Welsh Office 1988: 6)

Evidence of the shift towards an integrated interdisciplinary approach to health care can be traced throughout the above document with frequent references being made to collaboration, joint planning, integration, teamwork, effective communication, co-operation, skill mix, defined accountability and joint research initiatives (p 8, 9, 11, 17, 22, 25, 37, 41, 44, 46).

Since 1989 the Welsh Office has published several documents which state the Welsh position in response to the Government White Papers, "Working for Patients" (HMSO 1989 : Cmnd 555) and "Caring for People" (HMSO 1989 : Cmnd 849). The Welsh Office outlined the future strategies for health care in Wales, (Welsh Office 1989a, 1989b, 1989c) with it's NHS Directorate responding directly to the challenge by describing the overall strategic intent as "To take the people of Wales into the 21st Century with a level of health on course to compare with the best in Europe". (Welsh Office 1989d : 3).

The strategic direction adopted to meet this intention identifies three key "strands" i.e. the NHS in Wales should be "Health Gain Focused, People Centred and Resource Effective". These three factors are interdependent and are the central tenet of all subsequent publications issued by the NHS Directorate (Welsh Office 1990a, 1990b, 1990c, 1991). Fundamental to these developments in Wales is the emphasis on Total Quality Management (TQM) at both a national (The Welsh Office) and a local level (District Health Authority and Family Health Services Authority). Management of the proposals has been devolved to the local level but direct accountability to the Welsh Office remains.
This change "is intended to achieve a better fit between national priorities and local needs" (Welsh Office 1989d : 11)

Ten key areas of proposed health gain have been identified most of which this review of the literature suggests would be most effectively addressed fron an interdisciplinary perspective (maternal and child health, mental handicap, mental illness and cancer care being examples). The NHS Directorate in Wales recognises that resources will always be limited and that priorities will need to be identified. Value for money has become a major issue in health care and ways in which this can be achieved whilst maintaining a quality service are constantly being reviewed. The motivation and commitment of all NHS employees is seen as being central in achieving the Strategic Intent and a stated aim is "to provide a satisfying, rewarding and supportive environment for all NHS staff and to enable each of them to maximise their potential." (Welsh Office 1989d : 23).

High quality training, the Welsh Office suggested is one of the ways of fulfilling this. A companion paper to the Strategic Intent was published simultaneously which prescribed a fresh approach to local strategic planning (Welsh Office 1989e). The Welsh Health Planning Forum (WHPF), established in 1988 by The Secretary of State for Wales, offers "expert advice on the planning of health services" (p 2) in distinguishing between the purchaser/provider roles. The DHAs' were requested to submit their procurement plans based on local needs which would "spell out how the response strategy could be implemented within the available resources and who the providers would be." (Welsh Office 1989e : 10)

A collaborative response was required from the Directors of Public Health Medicine, the DHA's, the FHSA's, the Health Intelligence Unit (HIU) and the Health Promotion Authority for Wales (HPAW) working with the WHPF to produce local profiles. The three central strands, health gain, resource effective and people centred were to remain the central focus for all strategic planning. Although the training of health personnel was not explicitly mentioned in this document, potential staff shortages (p21), links between the acute and community sectors (p 20) and rising client expectations (p 21) were. Retaining staff, maintaining and increasing links between the acute and community sectors and meeting client needs have all been described as positive outcomes of undergraduate, integrated, interdisciplinary education.

An example of a District Health Authority response to the Welsh Office directive can be seen in the South Glamorgan Health Authority Mission Statement (1990) which states that in order to achieve total quality management it intended to "develop a team approach in securing the delivery of a friendly and helpful service offering people time, commitment and privacy."(Ibid : 1990).

Evidence has been found of previous attempts in Wales to rationalise some of the numerous training programmes for the health professions. In 1964 the Joint Training Committee of the United Cardiff Hospitals was given the remit of considering and advising; "on matters of common policy concerning training schools for medical auxilliaries and other allied trainings and to make recommendations where appropriate." (JTC of UCH : 1964)

An unsigned, undated memorandum by this committee outlined the concept of integration in order to "economise in space, lecturers time and to foster better relationships and communicationsbetween the disciplines." (JTC of UCH : undated)

The previous year Crighton and Crawford (1963) presented a report to the Welsh Staff Advisory Committee entitled "Disappointed Expectations". In the report Crighton and Crawford remarked upon the expectations of health personnel regarding interdisciplinary health care. Achieving this had eluded them to date which had resulted in frustration and disappointment for all concerned.

In 1973 Collins investigated the possibility of rationalising some of the courses at the Combined Training Institute (CTI), University Hospital of Wales, Cardiff. The CTI had somehow acquired an international reputation as a multidisciplinary training school, which it patently was not. In 1996 this sadly remains the case. Collins found that within the CTI a number of courses were separately administered, taught and managed with the only interdisciplinary contact being the student common room. No shared learning occurred at all. Collins wrote despairingly, "The Institute would appear to have reached the make or break stage". (Collins 1973 : 75) Over twenty years later the status quo still exists and Collins' words are still applicable.

Collins interviewed the principals of the paramedical schools based within the CTI, attempting to ascertain whether there was a common core of material relevant to all training programmes and also to assess the value placed by each profession on independence of action. Optimistically Collins hoped that shared learning may be perceived as an increased opportunity to improve patient care. She discovered that shared learning was perceived to be a threat to professional competence and status and consequently any adaptation of existing curriculum was going to be strongly resisted. In 1973 some of the principals believed that the courses trained the student rather than educated the student. As a direct result "the development of treatment skills must take priority in the allocation of time available" (p 74). There was the suggestion of one enlightened principal who thought that the answer was to recruit the calibre of student who would take responsibility for continuing their own education in order to addresss other concepts in health care. A major limiting factor, identified by Collins was the prescribed length and content of training regulated by each statutory training body which ultimately had the power to register an individual as a practitioner. Collins, during her interviews, managed to identify topics which appeared to be acceptable to more than one profession. These included learning to understand people, learning to understand themselves, learning to appreciate other workers skills and the management and organisation of the NHS. In 1992 no evidence was found that any of these subjects were taught on an interdisciplinary basis. The principals in 1973 were quite firm that linking background knowledge to specialist knowledge could not be shared. Collins did not interview any students to find out whether they agreed with this conclusion.

The Faculty of Health and Community Studies, Cardiff Institute of Higher Education also undertakes the education of some of the professions allied to medicine and social work. These complement rather than duplicate those offered in the CTI and collectively the two centres train most of the health and social care professions other than medicine, dentistry and pharmacology which are based in the University of Wales College of Medicine and the University of Wales Cardiff. No evidence has been found that shows any previous attempt to encourage interdisciplinary learning at CIHE at an undergraduate stage. In May 1992, however a Masters degree in Interprofessional Health Studies was validated by the University of Wales and commenced within the Faculty of Health and Community Studies in October 1992. A firm commitment to the philosophy of interdisciplinary learning therefore has been adopted by this Faculty.

The current education of health personnel in Wales has been examined in depth in another key document (Welsh Office 1989f). In the introduction the NHS Directorate emphasised that the "key to success" for the NHS in Wales was the staff and "in having the right people in the right place at the right time" (p 1). The remit of the Manpower Steering Group (MSG), founded in 1986, was to "develop and promote a comprehensive manpower strategy for the NHS in Wales" (Welsh Office 1989f : 3).

It was the MSG that was instrumental in producing this document. Section 3 reported the findings of a working group who had reviewed the Combined Training Institute. Chaired by Mr Alwyn Roberts, the group was commissioned by the MSG and South Glamorgan Health Authority and given the following specific terms of reference :

1. The manpower strategy for the NHS in Wales.
2. The relationship between the CTI and other relevant training institutions within and outside the NHS in Wales.
3. The place of the CTI in the broader UK training framework for the professions supplementary to medicine and others.
4. The present and potential contribution of the CTI to training both within Wales and more widely.
5. The appropriateness of current arrangements for the management and funding of the Institute with particular regard to its' capacity to meet future developments as may be identified as necessary by the review.

(MSG 1989 : 1)

All schools with the exception of the School of Nursing were included in the review. Thus the schools of physiotherapy, occupational therapy, orthoptics, diagnostic radiography, medical photography and operating department practitioners were included. Other training schools were also taken into account, clinical psychology in-service schemes in both North and South Wales, occupational therapy in Mid Glamorgan, dental hygiene and dental surgery assistants at the UHW Dental Hospital, all those within CIHE, therapeutic radiography at Velindre Hospital and the schools of diagnostic radiography in Mid Glamorgan, West Glamorgan, Gwent and Clwyd. The overall majority of training schools are therefore still based within a small geographical radius in South Wales. This reinforces the report produced by Crighton and Crawford (1963) in which they commented on the training schools close proximity. There has been no major change in this arrangement for the last thirty years apart from an increase in the number of professional disciplines. The Working Party emphasised that the review was not a "retrospective examination and assessment of the standards of training" but to plan for the future manpower requirements within Wales into the next millenium (MSG 1989 : 3). One of the most significant recommendations made by the Working Group was "*A Common Core Syllabus* drawing together the areas of knowledge and skill common to several professions should be developed." (Welsh Office 1989f : 8).

A further recommendation of relevance to this present study was the introduction of degree level training *along with* a common core. By 1992 most of the professions allied to medicine had commenced degree level studies but there is still no real evidence of integrated interdisciplinary learning at an undergraduate level.

In 1987 The Welsh Office published a document which considered the position of the nursing profession in the community. A team approach was advocated and several references were made to the necessity for all members of the primary health care teams to share experiences during training (Welsh Office 1987 : 14, 28, 29, 53, 54, 66). The report noted that while there were undoubtly problems with interprofessional jealousy, accountability and duplication of effort there was also evidence of primary health care teams working most successfully together (p 28). The mark of success, the report continued, seemed to be each profession taking responsibility for their own clinical decisions but doing this in a collaborative way through discussion and negotiation with the other professions (p 53). The authors hoped to see an increase in interdisciplinary initiatives although they recognised that this "may have to be a long term rather than a short term aim given the different vocational training regulations that would have to be reconciled." (Welsh Office 1987 : 66).

MacDonald (1988) discussed the work of the health and social professionals in the care of people with mental handicaps in the valleys of South Wales. He paid tribute to the All Wales Strategy (Welsh Office 1983) which aimed to solve the problems of an uncoordinated service delivery. Social workers, nurses, teachers and general practitioners all interacted with the patients and their families "without any real shared awareness of the plans and purposes of each one" (Welsh Office 1983 : 65). MacDonald (1988) had previously remarked that the consumer does not usually associate a social problem with a particular discipline and with the increased contribution of physiotherapy, clinical psychology, occupational therapy, speech therapy and other disciplines the problem would be exacerbated. MacDonald (1988) believed that whilst specialist work should continue to be based on a specific training, "communicating work" should be interdiscplinary. Communicating work was often devalued and MacDonald identified stress and overwork as contributing factors as he believed that stressed professionals "hang onto their core identity". In a further undated document MacDonald reported on a series of workshops held at the Brunel Institute of Organisation and Social Studies (BIOSS), entitled Working Together: Professional Expectations and Understanding. The emphasis was on the needs of people with a mental handicap and the problems encountered between health service and social service objectives. He argued that if the patient has a need, the patient has a right and therefore there is a demand to provide the service required. MacDonald postulated that in the mental handicap field nurses were the core group of carers as they had a twenty four hour responsibility for meeting the clients needs. However, he continued, other disciplines also had responsibilities and accountability for meeting the needs and successful collaboration depended on successful communication between the different professional groups. While doctors and nurses complement each others' roles in mental handicap other disciplines complain that the afore mentioned groups "do not understand their potential value" (p 6). In view of the implied interdisciplinary nature of caring for people with a mental handicap, an attempt has been made to set up multidisciplinary teams (MDT). MacDonald emphasised the need for a shared language and the adoption of a shared theoretical framework as "recording, predicting and communicating can lead to a test and refinement of therapeutic practice" (p 8). The same point was made previously by Osborne and Wakeling (1985).

The Team Care Valleys initiative was a pilot project which focused on post-graduate multidisciplinary training in the South Wales Valleys. Developed through a series of discussions with the UWCOM and the Welsh Office and taking into account the Government White Papers, "Promoting Better Health" (HMSO 1987), "Working for Patients" (HMSO 1989a) and "Nursing in the Community" (Welsh Office 1987) amongst other publications of importance, the purpose of the initiative was described as supporting "extended vocational training for health professionals working in the area" (Team Care Valleys 1990 : 3). References to teamwork, mutidisciplinary activities in learning, auditing and management featured frequently throughout the document and as such could be seen as a central tenet of the initiative. Team Care Valleys presented a high profile as an innovative and dynamic approach to primary health care. Unfortunately the project was discontinued in 1994 as a result of cost benefit analysis findings. The developments in health care in Wales over the past eleven years have been phenomenal, mainly due to the number of Strategic Documents issued by the Welsh Office. While the unprecedented pace of change has undoubtedly caused great anxiety and uncertainty for both the organisations and the individuals who work in the health care field, there have been some positive changes towards achieving quality health care. One of the most exciting developments has been the change in emphasis towards the necessity for integrated teamwork. It would seem opportune to grasp the initiative by introducing the professions to each other at the earliest possible stage in training.

2.6 Interprofessional conflicts

Efforts have been made for many years to address the conflict, jealousy, negative stereotyping and stress that professionals experience when working together in health care. Territorial issues affect the quality of health care. Whilst the individual professions defend their institutions, their roles, and their operational areas, logical development of quality health care will continue to be impeded. Professional qualifications and license to practice are designed to protect the general public from incompetence, but they also serve to protect the territory of one professional group from another (Berkowitz and Malone 1968, Dana and Sheps 1968, Johnston et al 1968, Martin 1969, Kenneth 1969, Pluckhan 1970, Banta and Fox 1972, Rosenaur and Fuller 1973, Lloyd 1973, Bendall 1973, Beckhard 1974, Ratoff et al 1974, Kendall 1977, Alaszewski 1977, Parkes 1977, Westbrook 1978, Challela 1979, Kuenssberg 1980, Lonsdale et al 1980, Beales 1980, Pritchard 1981, Turnbull 1981, Lishman 1983, Williams and Williams 1982,Webster 1985, Osborne and Wakeling 1985, Wright 1985, Linsk et al 1986, Guy 1986, Webster 1988, Iles and Auluck 1990, Brooking 1991, Fawcett-Henesy 1991, Mocellin 1992).

Williams and Williams (1982) defined stereotyping as an "attempt by an individual to understand his or her social environment" (p 17). They postulated that people within certain groups are not perceived as individuals but are held by the observer as behaving in a certain manner pertaining to that group. Snodgrass (1966) and Mullaney et al (1974) suggested that stereotyping may be a coping mechanism adopted by individuals who do not have a well defined boundary within which to operate. If this statement is accepted then it seems reasonable to conclude that the ill defined boundaries, which exist within health care teams, will lend themselves to stereotypical attitudes from one profession to another, and will often be of a negative nature (Church 1956, Discher 1974, Bracht et al 1975, Pritchard 1981). Williams and Williams (1982) believed that in order to maximise positive stereotyping, groups of professionals had to act as "functional equals on a common task" (p 18). This declaration would have been much approved by Swift and MacDougall (1964) who had written of the need for functional equality between doctors and nurses in primary health care. Evidence has been found of residential courses being held on an interdisciplinary basis with the specific purpose of dissipating prejudices, clarifying roles, and establishing common ground (Bennett et al 1972, Mond 1972, Hasler and Klinger 1976, Brunning and Huffington 1985). Bennett et al (1972) were convinced that the identification of common ground was essential in order to manage the "diverse patterns of request for help which are not tidily assembled" (p 605) into discrete professional roles. The current state of affairs, they continued, meant that far too frequently patients were referred to other professionals as a bureaucratic manoevre which not only inconvenienced the patient, but was a source of irritation to all concerned. For this reason alone it could be argued that interdisciplinary learning should be introduced as early as possible for, as Bennett et al observed, most health care professionals had to admit to an embarassing deficiency in their knowledge and understanding of each others roles.

Dana and Sheps (1968) considered the problem in depth and concluded that :

> Interprofessional behaviour does not require members of related professions to think alike but rather to act together. .... It asks that the professional person puts problem ahead of profession and/or institutional auspices......and necessitate that he respect both himself and others as having knowledge, understanding, skills and most importantly, equal rights to participate in the problem solving process.
>
> (Ibid : 37)

Martin (1969) expressed the opinion that there appeared to be a lack of clarity concerning the role of the professions supplementary to medicine, whilst Osborne and Wakeling (1985) queried the posssibility of influencing the quality of care through education and training. They were particularly interested in improving the quality of care available to the mentally handicapped. They introduced an educational programme for nurses and social workers at both a pre and post qualifying stage. They justified their early intervention in training by declaring their intention to change attitudes for, they believed "Unless students have sufficient evidence of the value of collaboration during their training, they may lack the will to make it a reality." (Osborne and Wakeling 1985 : 23)

They argued that whilst there were many situations that divided the professions there was one that inextricably bound them together.... the patients and the services they required. Competence in care would only develop through interdisciplinarity, and interdisciplinarity would only develop through a diminution of conflict, stereotyping and professional jealousy. Gomes (1985) believed that interdisciplinary learning would remove the competitive rivalry existing between the health care professions as it would encourage each individual participant to focus all his/her attention on the patient. Ling et al (1990) questioned however, some of the assumptions being made about interdisciplinary learning. They were concerned about the serious role conflict that may occur as a result of losing professional 'uniqueness' for the common good. They suggested that a critical examination should be undertaken which assessed the contribution of interdisciplinary learning in diminishing role conflict. If, they asserted, it was shown to be of value, then it should be adopted wholeheartedly.

Alaszewski (1977), a sociologist, examined the changing relationships between the health care professions and the emerging independence that the paramedical professions had claimed. He considered that the term 'paramedical' was unfortunate and inappropriate as it implied subordination and a dependence on approval by the medical profession. He explored the concept of professionalisation and concluded that the; "key differentiating characteristic between professional and non professional occupations is the control and application of a body of knowledge to solve certain problems for society." (Ibid : B1)

This, he described as the functionalist perspective as it emphasised the characteristic traits of practitioners within each discrete profession. Alaszewski was particularly interested in the impact of organisational changes on professional relationships and the effects that those changes had upon the autonomy of each profession. He referred to the Council for the Professions Supplementary to Medicine (CPSM) and wryly noted that although each profession had a majority on their own Statutory Boards the CPSM itself consisted mainly of medical staff and thus the medical profession retained overall control. He noted with satisfaction, the increasing number of graduate practitioners within the professions allied to medicine, along with the concommitant increase in research and the subsequent inclusion of non medical subjects in each curriculum. This he believed, broke away from the traditional model which had dominated all health professions training for such a length of time. Nevertheless he warned that without careful planning the curriculum would be overloaded and lack integration. He then turned his attention to the NHS itself and suggested that practitioners within the health professions either gave direct patient care or else they contributed indirectly. In direct patient care the "the practitioner is the producer and the patient is the consumer" (p B2) whereas in indirect care specialities, such as radiology, pathology and bacteriology, it is the clinical practitioners giving direct care who are the consumers as it is this group which request the services of the indirect practitioners. Alaszewski argued that the same principle applied to the paramedical professions. He suggested that whilst medical colleagues in indirect care specialities would always be described as equals by the direct care practitioners, there was a distinct air of patronage when considering the paramedical professions services. This was in spite of the fact that they were mainly involved in direct patient care. Alaszewski foresaw "contractor status" becoming more common where the paramedical professions became independent of the physicians management control. Their specialist expertise would then be bought in on a contractual basis. He was alarmed by the thought that management, whilst attempting to resolve these problems, could become the focus of interprofessional conflict itself. Within remarkable and uncanny accuracy he prophesised in his concluding statement; "The NHS could fragment into a series of independent and uncoordinated medical and paramedical services. The victim of such a process would be the patient." (Alaszewski 1977 : B4)

Hancock (1990), a nurse and General Secretary of the Royal College of Nursing (RCN) gave a keynote speech at the Physiotherapy Congress. She addressed the issue of partnership in health care in the twenty first century. She re-iterated Alaszewski's warnings by drawing the delegates attention to the need for putting patients first. This meant the lowering of the "barriers of professional exclusivity" with the consequent development of an "interlocking, mutually supportive multidisciplinary team" (p 670). Interdisciplinary education was the key, she believed, to achieving a true partnership.

Shortell (1974) asked three hundred and one subjects to complete a questionnaire which evaluated their perceptions of the occupational prestige of forty one categories of medical and allied health professionals. The respondents consisted of physicians, hospitalised patients and business school students. Of the forty one categories, twenty three were specialities within medicine itself and the other eighteen were nurses and the professions allied to medicine. All three groups of respondents similarly rank ordered the categories with the overall results revealing that the 'specialists' or 'consultants' in medicine were the most highly rated with general practitioners appearing half way down the list. Social workers, occupational therapists, nurses and technicians were all placed near the bottom of the list. Shortell had used Szasz and Hollanders (1956) list of propositions to analyse his data. In summary these consisted of three types of doctor/ patient interaction:

1. *Activity - passivity.* The doctor is active and the patient passive.
2. *Guidance - cooperation.* The doctor tells and the patient complies.
3. *Mutual cooperation.* The patient acts as an active and equal partner.

Shortells findings' indicated that where the doctor was active and the patient passive (in cardio-thoracic surgery for example), these doctors were accorded the highest occupational prestige. In general practice or in the dental surgery where the professional tells and the patient complies, the professional was accorded a middle ranking. Where mutual cooperation is the adopted model (in nursing, social work and occupational therapy) the professionals are perceived to be at the bottom of the occupational prestige league. Shortell (1974) concluded that; "the basic nature between the specialist and his patient in terms the degree of control over outcomes is much more related to a speciality's prestige than it's ability to carve out a separate domain over it's work." (Ibid : 6)

This finding has potentially important implications for the emerging professions. It would appear that identifying specialist knowledge and skills in order to fulfill the criteria for becoming a recognised profession will not in itself raise the occupational prestige of any group. Szasz and Hollanders model cited by Shortell (1974) would seem to indicate more accurately the perceptions of an occupations value. Nunally and Kittross (1958) reached a similar conclusion. They did not refer to the work of Szasz and Hollander but they undertook a similar study of the lay person's perceptions of the medical and allied professions. The medical profession was ranked the most highly of all the professions. Within the medical profession 'consultants' were ranked the highest with general practitioners accorded middle ranking and those doctors involved in mental health the lowest.

Furnham et al (1981) designed a study which explored the hypothesis that; "health care professionals might be expected negatively to evaluate professionals who seek to appropriate a field of knowledge, style of operation or particular client group that is under their control and jurisdiction." (Ibid : 292)

They aimed to systematically examine this concept of health care as they believed that there were potentially serious consequences for teamwork and ultimately for patient care. This study was one of the very few found in which empirical methods had been adopted and an extensive parametric analysis undertaken. As such the work of Furnham et al has been quoted extensively by numerous authors addressing the problems of stereotyping and role conflict. One hundred and twenty five professionals participated in the study in total. All subjects had been working as qualified practitioners for at least eighteen months prior to the commencement of the study. The professional groups and the numbers involved were as follows :- 25 female nurses, 25 female occupational therapists, 25 female health visitors, 25 doctors (18 male, 7 female), and 25 social workers (13 male, 12 female). Each individual completed a questionnaire in which they rated twelve occupations, 'consultant' doctors, clinical psychologists, dentists, general practitioners, health visitors, medical laboratory personnel, nursing assistants, nurses, occupational therapists, medical specialists, speech therapists and social workers. The inclusion of nursing assistants seems rather questionable as whilst the argument continues over what constitutes a professional occupation, this group most certainly do not meet the criteria on any of the scales. In addition ninety four of the total cohort were female (N=125). If Webster's (1985) paper holds any credence then the effect of gender loyalty may well outweigh professional loyalty and this would then bias the results. Furnham et al (1981) devised a research tool which consisted of ten seven point bi-polar scales. Ten attributes were generated from information gained in a pilot study in which twenty subjects participated. The subjects were asked to complete a free response form in which they listed the attributes of health care professionals. Validity of the scale was ensured although reliability was not tested apart from a subjective judgement of similarity. The ten scales were listed as :

Approachable......................................Non Approachable
Highly Trained....................................Little Trained
Skilful..Non Skilful
Radical...Conservative
Powerful...Non Powerful
Accessible..Non Accessible
Essential...Non Essential
Highly paid...Badly Paid
Sympathetic..Non Sympathetic
High Status...Low Status

The respondents in the main study completed the questionnaire within their own professional groups and in the presence of a researcher. Furnham et al obviously wanted to prevent communication between and within the groups to ensure individual responses. This increased the reliability of the data collected. A multivariate analysis of variance was completed across the five professional groups for all ten scales. The Scheffe test was applied in order to test for significant differences between any two groups on a specific scale. Within the publication itself only results that achieved a significance of at least $p<0.05$ were reported. Each of the five groups indicated "substantial differences in their perceptions of themselves and others" (p 293). The results were presented both in tabular and descriptive form which enabled clear visual and literal interpretation. Each professional groups results were presented individually and consequently will be discussed in the same manner.

General Practitioners These respondents perceived themselves more negatively than the other four groups perceptions of them. They saw themselves as approachable, sympathetic, accessible, highly trained, powerful and essential. On the whole, the other groups agreed with them although the social workers perceived the general practitioners less favourably than the other groups regarding approachability and sympathy. Occupational therapists and nurses perceptions were very similar to those of the general practitioners themselves. All four other groups indicated that the general practitioner was 'very' powerful and 'very' highly trained. The doctors themselves did not perceive the same level of power or training.

Nurses This group perceived themselves mainly positively in that they were highly trained, skilful, approachable, essential and sympathetic. They also saw themselves as non powerful and poorly paid. General practitioners and health visitors tended to agree with the nurses. The occupational therapists and the social workers however, found nurses significantly less approachable, less highly trained, less skilful and of lower status.

Health Visitors This group also tended to perceive themselves positively with characteristics similar to those of the nurses. The other professions however, did not perceive them in so positive a manner. Occupational therapists and social workers in particular, believed that the health visitors were non skilful and non powerful, whereas nurses saw them as more powerful and better paid. On the whole the health visitors were perceived positively. Surprisingly, the closest result to their own was that of the general practitioners perceptions.

Social Workers Perceived themselves as approachable, accessible, sympathetic, of low status and poorly paid. All the other groups agreed that the social workers were not highly trained and no other group valued social workers as highly as they did themselves.

Occupational Therapists Self perceptions by this group revealed themselves as being approachable,accessible, sympathetic, highly trained but badly paid. All other groups saw occupational therapists as being non powerful and less highly trained with the nurses and health visitors seeing them most negatively.

Furnham et al did not present the results of the other seven professional groups previously mentioned for two reasons, the first being the rationale that the other professions were not usually included in the primary health care team and the second that the authors were subject to word limitation in the publication itself. An overall table of the ten scales within the twelve 'professions' was nevertheless displayed. A detailed format was given of the top three and the bottom three 'professions' in the rank orderings. 'Consultants' were perceived as the most highly trained, skilful, highly paid and with the highest status. Dentists and general practitioners were ranked second and third respectively for the same attributes. Nursing assistants were the least skilful, lowest trained and of the lowest status. Social workers and psychologists were the most radical. Nurses were perceived as the most accessible, essential and sympathetic, whereas social workers were perceived as unessential with the psychologists the least essential of all. Consultants were unapproachable, unsympathetic and inaccessible. Interestingly, health visitors (who are qualified nurses) were perceived as moderately unskilful and unessential. Medical laboratory personnel scored badly on most of the scales. Remembering that only five groups participated in the completion of the questionnaire itself it is interesting to note that the two professional groups who do not by definition participate in clinical skills (social workers and health visitors) and are the least involved in the 'medical model' of care concentrating instead on the 'psychosocial model' were perceived the most negatively of all. Role conflict and professional jealousy between these two groups caused by the problems in their blurred roles (Ratoff et al 1974, and Kendall 1977), can only serve to further isolate these two groups from the other professions and indeed between themselves. Furnham et al (1981) concluded that adverse stereotyping based on prejudice decreased the likelihood of teams working effectively in health care. In summary, the hypothesis that "health care professionals might be expected to negatively evaluate" (p 292) other professionals who threatened to encroach on their territory was quite clearly demonstrated in this study. It would appear that this negativity has a detrimental effect on collaborative holistic patient care. Furnham et al recommended that the problem be addressed by increasing interdisciplinary contact early in each individual's professional training. The same recommendations have been made by Tanner et al (1972), Owen (1982), Dickens et al (1985), Knox and Thompson (1989).

Paradoxically Mazur et al (1979) advocated the introduction of interdisciplinary team training at a later stage as they believed that students would be unable to participate as team members until they were familiar with the demands of their own discipline. They recommended that shared learning just prior to qualification would be the "most practical and productive time" (p 712). Mazur et al introduced a programme for students from six health disciplines with the aim of improving students abilities in problem solving, conflict resolution, decision making, the delivery of holistic care, teamwork and leadership styles. Mazur et al admitted that most of the learning experiences were observational rather than participatory and that many of the students resented the artificiality of the programme. The forty two students who volunteered to participate in the programme were paid one hundred US dollars a week over a period of nine weeks. A criticism could therefore be levelled that the students were motivated by financial reward rather than any altruistic desire to improve the quality of learning. In order to evaluate the success of their programme Mazur et al used the Traits Questionnaire which had previously been described by Snodgrass (1966). This questionnnaire assesses the perceptions held by individual disciplines about others and Snodgrass's results revealed stereotyping similar to those later described by Furnham et al (1981). Mazur et al (1979) produced similar positive and negative stereotyping but at the end of the nine weeks they demonstrated an increase in positive stereo typing and a subsequent reduction in negative stereotyping. Mazur et al regretted that there were no valid and reliable instruments which measured the quality of team effectiveness. In 1992 a search for such a research tool has proved equally unsuccessful. There is without doubt a paucity of reliable methods for evaluating teamwork. Those which have been identified tend to be subjective and badly flawed.

In an American study, Challela (1979) focused on a theoretical framework for an interdisciplinary health care team and discussed the role of the nurse within this model. Areas of potential conflict were identified and possible resolutions explored. Challela suggested that with the emphasis moving away from hospital care and disease orientation towards community care and health orientation the fundamental philosophy of all health professions was going to have to change. How the resolution of conflict was to be achieved depended a great deal on how the professions understood "their own roles within an interdisciplinary milieu" (p 10). The Interdisciplinary Model (IDM) developed by Challela hinged on the ethos of unitary programming defined by Challela as; "A maximum utilisation of the different resources of the individuals who comprise the group or team which in turn requires effective communication between the team members." (Challela 1979 : 10)

Challela also stated the necessity to establish priorities of client needs in order to establish the responsibility of each discipline. By establishing these it would be possible to achieve true commitment to the client rather than maintaining professional egos. In other words Challela was challenging the professions to stop thinking about themselves and put the patient first. She further explored the conflicts and jealousies theme by suggesting that if autonomy was the distinguishing criterion of a profession then any outsider that challenged this would meet a closing of the ranks and would effectively be shut out. Challela implied that the outsider was in fact the patient who was supposed to take priority. The IDM would allow a developing influence and shared power between the disciplines which would allow for negotiation in the choice of team leader depending on the presenting situation. Aradine and Hansen (1970), Beloff and Korper (1972), Bloch (1975), The British Psychological Society (1986) and Brandt and Magyary (1989) all reiterate Challela's philosophy of the team leader being flexible and suggested similar models or frameworks which would facilitate this philosophy. As Challela succinctly concluded; "interprofessional behaviour.......is an entity of its own that does not require members of related professions to think alike but rather to act together .... It requires knowledge, values, skills that transcends the professions." (Challela 1979 : 15)

Brunning and Huffington (1985), two clinical psychologists, designed workshops on an interdisciplinary basis in order that 'interprofessional jealousies' could be identified and aired. Doctors, nurses, social workers, occupational therapists and psychologists were the workshop participants. This was a small scale social experiment using role play. The impetus for these workshops was the evidence of the negative perceptions and stereotyping that each profession was expressing about the other. Brunning and Huffington also believed that "each professional group tends to perceive itself more positively than it perceives any others." (Ibid : 24)

This belief has previously been described by Shortell 1974, Merrison 1979, Furnham et al 1981 and Nitsun et al 1981. One of the most important aspects of Brunning and Huffington's workshop was to help the participants explore their perceptions of what it may be like to work in the other disciplines. Each participant was labelled 'doctor, nurse, social worker' etcetera regardless of their true occupation. They were then grouped according to their labels and asked to discuss their feelings about their 'roles'. A list of statements was then drawn up and revealed to the other groups. The 'real' professionals were then asked to agree or disagree with the statements. Many positive correlations were found. The role play doctors made the statement that they felt vulnerable and that they were only human yet society expected infallibility all the time. Eight of the nine 'real' doctors strongly agreed with this statement. The number of statements collected in total from five groups equalled eighty four. Most of the statements were categorised as negative ones and in most instances the 'real' professionals agreed with them. Occasionally there was strong disagreement but analysis suggested that this was because the statement was a direct criticism of a particular group and the profession naturally refuted it. A good illustration of this was the statement "my desire for authority and control conflicts with the stress of being a God like figure". This statement was made by the role play doctors. All nine 'real' doctors categorically denied that they desired authority and power. Bennett (1987) a consultant psychiatrist, obviously was not one of these doctors! He warned that with the increasing advent of the other professions adopting therapeutic interventions "doctors can well feel that their unique status is under threat" (p 72). He did however continue that this would not necessarily be a disadvantage from the patients' point of view, merely from the doctors. Brunning and Huffington (1985) identified three main themes which were common to all the participants. There was lack of clarity in roles, an uncertainty in all disciplines about their roles within an interdisciplinary team and dissatisfaction about the roles of the other disciplines. Brunning and Huffington reported the following findings. Both the doctors themselves and the other professional groups seemed to have a rather ambivalent attitude about the role of the doctor in the interdisciplinary team. Whilst the doctor remains on a pedestal the other professions will continue to let the doctor take all the responsibility and in addition take any blame that may be apportioned. Two of the more junior doctors in the group complained that the results did not emphasise the great problems they encountered in the divide between senior and junior doctors. It is perhaps not surprising that the senior doctors did not see this as a problem or even acknowledge that a divide existed. The statements regarding the nurses portrayed a passive complaining group who were 'used' by the other disciplines. Statements such as the complaint that no notice was taken of their opinions, were confirmed by fourteen of the sixteen 'real' nurses. Inner conflicts were again revealed within the hierarchy. The social work statements tended to identify the conflict between the differing demands of society and particularly whether they should be accommodated within the NHS or within the Social Services. The 'real' social workers all agreed with the statement that society had unrealistic expectations of them. Doubt was expressed by the social workers themselves and by the other professions about how social workers could integrate into a health care team in view of the fact that they were accountable to the Social Services and not the NHS. Younghusband (1959), Seebohm (1968) and Abramson (1984) all concluded that social workers should remain in the direct control of the Social Services in spite of the difficulty this presented for teamwork in health care. Occupational therapists were perceived by the role players and the 'real' ones as being misunderstood in their 'basket weaving' reputation. An outcome of this workshop was that occupational therapists were challenged into attempting to better define what they actually did and then to share this information with the other professions. Both the role playing psychologists and the 'real' ones seemed uncertain whether they should be training the interdisciplinary team from the outside or whether they should be working within it. This was an interesting finding as all the workshop participants were working in the field of mental health. In this field psychologists are an integral part of the team and it would seem reasonable to assume that their sense of cohesiveness would have been evident. The end of the workshop elicited many plans that would increase interdisciplinary collaboration. The authors however were disappointed to report retrospectively that no dramatic changes had taken place. They recognised that a regular forum should have been arranged in order to keep the momentum going.

Thorne cited in Hughes et al (1973) would have fully endorsed these sentiments and is a most persuasive advocate of interdisciplinary learning and teamwork. He described the phenomena of isolation, conflict, negative stereotyping and professional jealousy as the result of 'cloistering' and noted with regret that if members of the different health professions did learn to relate to each other it was more by luck than judgement. This, he was sure, compromised the efficacy of effective teamwork. Kirkland (1970) a medical student, complained bitterly of his isolation from other health care professionals. He asked how the physicians of tomorrow could "justify sharing ever increasing responsibility with other health professionals about whose training he has little but hearsay knowledge." (Ibid : 278)

He strongly advocated the concept of shared learning at the undergraduate stage through a common curriculum. This he postulated, would benefit the patient as a common knowledge would increase collaboration in solving clinical problems. Two years later Parker (1972) blamed the system of training for medical students isolation. MacDougall and Elahi (1974) believed that the medical students would inevitably have great difficulty in working within an interdisciplinary team as they were not given the opportunity to understand the capabilities of the other team members. It would be both unrealistic and unreasonable to even expect them to work effectively in a team without adequate preparation or having been exposed to a problem solving approach to patient care. Pascascio (1970) in a complementary paper to Kirkland (1970) recognised that medical students were isolated but so, she believed were all the other professions. She acknowledged however that physicians were key members of a team and insisted that the only way to overcome the problem was to learn to work together by actually working together.

In other words nothing can replace or better real experience. This experience should be complementary to and not instead of individual professional training. Schreckenberger (1970) found it difficult to address the problems of teamwork because he did not feel part of a team even though he was supposed to be working within one. He wrote that no team action was evident at all. His profession was not disclosed but it would be reasonable to suppose that he was a physician as he rallied his co-professionals to take up the challenge as the health team leaders by encouraging a "spirit of comradeship". He concluded his paper by calling for urgent changes in the curriculum that would allow everyone to learn together. Hockey (1977) reviewed the situation from the nurses point of view. She believed that collaborative care is based on mutual trust and respect. Consistency and continuity were essential if quality of care was to be achieved. For this reason "nursing cannot be practised in a vacuum" (p 148) and would always be "tangential to other disciplines" (p 149). Hockey was a firm believer that all health disciplines depended in part on knowledge gained from other disciplines and looked forward to the time when there would be a much greater pooling of knowledge. Her dream was to witness; "a significant upsurge in interdisciplinary education and research which would prepare the ground for the kind of team activity that the complexity of modern patient care demands." (Hockey 1977 : 152)

Larkin (1984) was particularly interested in the occupational imperialism and monopoly that the health care professions displayed. He suggested that a strategy was adopted for the specific purpose of moulding the division of labour to each profession's maximum advantage. He accused each profession of "poaching desirable skills" (p14) and delegating other less desirable ones with the intention of securing status and control. It all hinged he suggested, on establishing advantageous relationships with allied groups. This destructive situation was further complicated by the conflict evident within each professional sub-group. Smith cited in Duncan and McLachlan (1984) was convinced that health professionals would be less likely to regard each other as adversaries if they were given the opportunity to understand each other through shared learning at an early stage. Margaret Clark, the Chief Nursing Officer for Scotland in 1984, viewed the problem from the opposite end of the spectrum. She emphasised that each profession had areas of competence superior to others but that there were areas of shared and equal competence. She warned that until this idea was accepted, the effective utilisation of skills by each member of the health team would not be evident. The patient was the person who had the most to lose. Houle (1980) warned of the consequences if individual professions continued to claim exclusivity in learning. Thorne (1973) observed that training in all professions tended to be isolated and self contained. The claim to an esoteric and unique body of knowledge encouraged exclusivity, isolation and inevitable conflict. Paradoxically, professions also claimed that their existence hinged on a universal body of knowledge. Thorne was convinced that this led to "A chronic strain between the exclusive and the general, between intellectual isolation and ties with others" (p 71). Medical students in particular were criticised by Thorne in that they expected to dominate situations which had an "equalitarian ideology" (p 80) and that in medicine there was frequently a "condescension towards occupations lower in the hierarchy" (p 80). Stanfield (1990) stated categorically that respect and understanding would be crucial for all future health care workers. Fragmentation and complexity posed a constant threat to comprehensive, continuous care in which quality and cost efficiency would be the key indicators. She predicted that in the next decade in the United States of America service coordination and integration would have the highest priority. She foresaw the situation in which social workers and nurses working in primary health care would develop common skills in many areas. The increasing number of elderly people and the care they would require, would necessitate this as a matter of urgency as the appropriate utilisation of the professions would be critical to maintaining a large elderly population at their optimum potential.

Turnbull (1982) concentrated on the nursing profession and challenged the nurse educators to take a long hard look at the monodisciplinary training which was offered. Whilst she knew that some educators would respond positively to the challenge, others would remain ingrained and more traditional in their approach. The latter group were likely to be perceived by many as the ones who were remaining loyal to their profession. Turnbull defended these attitudes in that the nursing profession's struggle for autonomy did not seem to reflect interdisciplinarianism which implicitly indicated the need to compromise, negotiate and change. Lenz (1985) also examined the deliberate maintenance of boundaries in the field of nursing. She reinforced Turnbull's paper by discussing the insularity evident in nurse education and drew attention to the fact that an almost total reliance was placed on nurse authorship and nursing journals. This, she argued, was the complete antithesis of encouraging increased interdisciplinary collaboration. Campbell (1969) remarked that nursing could not afford to become insulated, parochial or egocentric and should make every effort to become more cosmopolitan. Other authors nevertheless have stated categorically that nursing is a distinct entity with its own science base (Bloch 1981, Norris 1982). Lenz (1985) found that an increasing number of nurse educators were gaining an increasing number of qualifications in both the biological and behavioural sciences in order to teach those subjects. This she observed, was not a desirable trend as it would increase nursing's insularity. Whilst survival in academia may depend on nurses controlling nurse education and thus claim this unique 'knowledge', the demands of the patient dictates a more open and receptive approach to shared learning. Furthermore, disciplinary gate keeping discourages students of nursing from enriching their knowledge by reading the literature from the other disciplines. The same criticism could of course be levelled at other disciplines and their recommended reading.

Lenz (1985) described a small study in which she had sent twenty five top nursing administrators (deans or directors of nursing) a questionnaire. The study group were a random sample from the directory of nursing establishments in the USA. Sixteen responded. The questionnaire contained five sections in which the characteristics of the school, the numbers of nurse educators and non nurse educators, where the non nurse educators were employed within the organisation and how their role was perceived, how the non nursing content was taught and how it was evaluated were all elicited. Lenz also requested information on any proposed changes. This request was couched in the terms of if there were unlimited resources which changes would be desirable. Of the sixteen respondents eight reported that nurse educators only were employed. The remaining eight reported between one and fourteen non nurse educators in each faculty. Many of these were employed on a part time basis, in the larger schools where masters and doctoral programmes were offered. Lenz found to her dismay that the numbers of non nurse faculty members had actually declined over a five year period. Interestingly Lenz also discovered that where non nurse faculty members were employed there was a marked increase in student / teacher contact (p 238). The most favoured strategy for teaching the behavioural sciences was to employ a nurse teacher who had specialist knowledge in that subject, most usually a degree.

Whilst it is laudatory that nurse educators seem to be so versatile the question does arise of whether nurses would be so magnanimous if a psychology lecturer undertook the minimum training to register as a nurse and then presumed to teach nursing to psychology undergraduates. It also adds credence to the claim that nursing is not a discipline in its' own right and consequently encourages the 'isolationists' to continue to promote nursing as a distinct entity. The acceptance that each discipline has its' own specific body of knowledge that each profession can share by introducing theoretical concepts applied into clinical practice by knowledgeable practitioners, would seem to be the best option for both the individual disciplines and for interdisciplinary learning. Lenz (reporting in the same article 1985) confirmed her suspicions that all was not well by undertaking a second study. She sent a questionnaire to fifty four named non nurse lecturers who were employed in faculties other than those which Lenz had used in the first study. Forty four (81%) completed and returned the questionnaire.

Their responses confirmed the earlier findings. They were being used less frequently than previously and any specific non nursing books and journals they recommended were not generally accepted or promoted within the faculty itself. Lenz was unable to undertake any correlational analyses as the sample sizes were too small. She admitted that the mean figures gave a somewhat biased presentation. An obvious example of this could be seen in the results. The total number of non specific nursing articles identified in the second study by the forty four respondents were presented as a mean of 11.3, ten respondents however indicated that no articles of a non nursing nature were included in their faculty whereas one respondent returned eighty two named articles. This respondent appeared to be given complete autonomy within the faculty of nursing and was therefore able to introduce a wide range of non nursing materials. Lenz herself acknowledged that exclusive reliance on nursing publications was common practice. Lenz concluded that not only was there evidence that nursing was isolationist as a discipline but that a "continuation even intensification" seemed likely (p 331). This would appear to be against the general trend expressed by other authors in their observations of the increased demand for interdisciplinary collaboration (Crane 1972, De Leon 1979, Sarason 1981). Lenz forecast that the inevitable outcome for nurse education would be a diminution of both quantity and quality of health care knowledge in which the ultimate loser would be not only the patient but the nursing profession as well.

2.6.1 The physician / nurse conflict

Many authors have published their concerns about the conflict that exists between the medical and nursing professions and the detrimental effect that this has on holistic patient care. Much of their attention has inevitably concentrated on teamwork on an interdisciplinary basis. A number nevertheless have examined the reasons for conflict, jealousy and stereotyping between these two groups alone (MacGregor 1960, Akester and McPhail 1964, Schlotfeldt 1965, Rosinski 1965, Pelligrino 1966, Peoples and Francis 1968, Bates 1965, 1966, 1970, Berkowitz and Malone 1968, Hoekleman 1975, Kalisch and Kalisch 1977, Burkett et al 1978, Steele 1981, Singleton 1981, Mechanic and Aiken 1982, Ahmedazai 1982, Goodwin 1982, Coluccio and Maguire 1983, Ferguson-Johnston 1983, McClure 1984, Kurtzman et al 1985, Webster 1985, Whitehouse 1986, Keddy et al 1986, Copp 1987, Garvin and Kennedy 1988, Brooking 1991).

Pelligrino (1966) described the communication crisis between the two professions and blamed the sub language barrier and the professional blueprinting that existed. He challenged both groups to resolve their differences in order to achieve optimum patient care. Pelligrino advocated the introduction of shared learning at an early stage in training although he did not believe that biological sciences were suitable for inclusion owing to the different levels of knowledge required in the students professional lives. He recommended that the behavioural sciences however were suitable for shared learning purposes. Pelligrino was himself a physician in 1966 and it could be argued that he was claiming exclusive knowledge and superiority for the medical profession in the biological sciences but that the behavioural sciences were of less importance to this group and they were therefore willing to share. Peeples and Francis (1968) examined the values, attitudes, beliefs and sociocultural structures which influence the work relationships of physicians and nurses. They explored the concept that conflict occurs not because of individual behaviour but as a result of social and cultural structures which inevitably occur in groups. A major problem was thought to be the fact that even when in the midst of conflict health professionals may not perceive it as such. They subdivided problems of social structure into the following :

1. *The Occupational Gap*

Not only is there a gap in social prestige between doctors and nurses but there is the additional problem of sub groups within each profession. Psychiatrists do not have the same prestige as surgeons. In nursing the same occupational snobbery exists with mental health nurses being perceived as less prestigious than general nurses (MacGregor 1960).

2. *Social Class Orientation*

Doctors tend to belong to higher social classes than nurses.

3. *Income Breach*

In 1968 nurses' income reflected only one fifth of a physicians' even though nurses spend a minimum of three years qualifying and doctors a minimum of five.

4. *General Status Disparity*
Physicians enjoy the most esteemed position in society. The nurse is way down the social scale, below the level that her educational achievements and clinical responsibility indicates. Peeples and Francis described this phenomena as a "social anaemia" (p 30) and suggested that this may be one of the causal factors of low esteem and morale in the nursing profession.
5. *The Technology Factor*
Because of the rapid technological advances within each profession, sub groups are emerging which separate those who can use technology and those who cannot.
6. *The Occupational Identity Struggle*
Ideological ambivalence must be minimised so that each profession presents a clear picture of what it is to the other and also to the general public.

Peeples and Francis also subdivided problems of attitudes and beliefs :

1. *Florence Nightingale Stereotypes*
The lady of the lamp and the well educated autonomous nurse are disparate in the minds of the general public.
2. *Nursing - The Work of Females*
The public perceives men as physicians and women as nurses. This enhances segregation and discrimination.
3. *Nursing - Work for the Soft Hearted*
Linked with the female image nurses are seen as 'tender and sympathetic'.
4. *Task Status Differential*
Nursing tasks are seen as routine and less demanding. Peeples and Francis highlighted the paradox in that manual dexterity has low prestige yet a surgeon who relies entirely on this enjoys such a high prestige.
5. *The Fantasy of Medicine*
Hospitals are seen as high drama institutions by the general public. Physicians and nurses have the highest profile in this but the nurses role involves obeying the physician's orders. (Kalisch and Kalisch :1977) have perhaps been the most prolific researchers into this area of controversy).
6. *The Perfection of Scientific Medicine*
The physicians knowledge is perceived as absolute whilst nursing is not believed to be scientifically based.
7. *Baccalaureate Nurses = Technical Incompetence*
Degree nurses are seen as clinically inexperienced as they spend more time in college than in gaining clinical expertise. In 1992 this argument was still being used by the traditionalists who maintained that the advent of Project 2000 in the United Kingdom will produce the same result. No evidence has been found to

support this hypothesis and it could be argued that this is the result of defensive stereotyping.

8. *The Physician - The Natural Leader of the Health Team*
   This belief is strongly held by the medical fraternity, even though they are infrequently at the patients bedside. A physician does not have the opportunity to know the patient as well as the nurse primarily caring for that patient. The debate concerning who should be the team leader will be subsequently discussed in the section of the literature review which addresses 'teamwork' (Chapter 2 Section 7).
9. *Therapeutic and Somatic Medicine*
   Many physicians resist the concept of holistic care by negating the contributions of psychologists, social workers and nutritionists by dismissing it as 'fringe medicine'.

(All headings have been described by Peeples and Francis)

Bates (1969) a physician herself, undertook a fascinating study in Kentucky USA in which she attempted to define the critical requirements in nurse physician teamwork. The focus of the study was to gather specific data which demonstrated physician behaviour that helped or hindered nurses in giving good patient care. The methodology was then used inversely and nurses behaviour that helped or hindered physicians was likewise identified. The two part study took place in a teaching hospital with two hundred and fifty beds. All patient care areas were involved. One hundred and fifteen nurses and ninety physicians participated in the study. In part one of the study nurses were asked to report specific incidences of physician behaviours which affected patient care. No attempt was made to influence the proportion of positive or negative incidents.

Eight hundred and fifty eight incidents were collected. Of these twenty two were discarded as being non specific. Of the remaining eight hundred and thirty six, three hundred and sixty three (43.4%) were described as helping actions and four hundred and seventy three (56.6%) were described as hindering actions. The results are presented in the seven categories as Table 2.1

The critical factor in the interpretation of these results however was whether the incidents were seen as positive or negative ones. In category one the total is somewhat misleading. Analysis of the minutiae revealed that when a physician explained a medical condition, a diagnostic technique or gave a demonstration the communication was perceived as helping (32 helpful incidents and 2 hindering ones). Communicating with the nurse in a calm courteous manner was viewed mainly negatively as was the giving of adequate orders on which the nurse could act (28 helpful incidents, 60 hindering ones). The coordination of physician/ nurse activities was seen in a positive way with 32 helpful and 18 hindering incidents. Cooperation with the nurse yielded a near equal number of incidents (18 helpful, 20 hindering). The startling result was that of category five in which the nurses perceptions of whether physicians performed their own role effectively. In a total of 392 incidents, 246 were seen as being hindering

Table 2.1
Critical incidences in nurse/physician teamwork (Bates 1969)

Critical Incidences	N= 836	%
Communication with the nurse	258	31.00
Co-ordinates physician/nurse activities in implementing care	50	0.60
Co-operates with the nurse. Responds positively to suggestions by nurse	38	0.50
Recognises & conserves limited nursing resources	57	0.70
Performs effectively within own role	392	47.00
Works effectively with other physicians & medical students	28	0.30
Honours the policies & codes of his service, institution or society	10	0.10

particularly those of being available to the patient when needed. Other hindering factors in this category included the maintenance of patient safety and attention to patient comfort. Communication with the patient was also included within this category. The other unexpected result was that of category seven. No helpful incidents were noted but 10 hindering ones were. What can be surmised from these results? The physicians in the study appeared to be confident and competent in communicating with the patient when they were able to demonstrate a superior knowledge of diagnosis, disease or surgical technique. They did not however, appear to be able or willing to communicate in a helpful or positive manner with the nurses. The results did not allow for analysis of individual physician responses because they were presented as a numerical mean. Some physicians could therefore have scored highly on helpful interactions whilst others were given mainly hindering incident scores. These results must therefore be treated with caution. Nevertheless it can be assumed that the lack of helpful communication between these two groups overall would not enhance the concept of collaborative teamwork.

In the second part of the study physicians were asked to categorise helpful and hindering incidents that they perceived in the nurses interactions with them. A total of five hundred and twenty incidents were recorded. Fourteen were discarded as unsuitable, two hundred and thirty three (45.3%) described helpful interactions and two hundred and eighty one (54.7%) described hindering ones. They were grouped into five main categories and are presented as Table 2.2 :

Table 2.2
Helpful and hindering incidences (Bates 1969)

Incidences	N = 504	%
Provides the physician with assistance	101	20.00
Follows the physicians orders	140	27.00
Communicates effectively with the physician	133	26.00
Performs effectively within own role	130	25.00
Willing to deviate from institutional policies	10	0.20

Again analysis of the data revealed that it was not the total number of incidents that were so interesting but the weighting of the helpful versus the hindering incidents. In category one no significant difference was seen between helpful (N=55) and hindering (N=46) actions. In the category describing 'following physicians orders' however a startling finding emerged. Only 10 helpful incidents were recorded against 130 hindering ones. It would not seem to be a problem in communication as the category 'communicates effectively with the physician' identified 101 helpful and only 32 hindering ones. Could it be that whilst physicians believe that nurses communicate well with them the nurses do not appreciate the way in which the physician speaks to them? (See category one part one of the study). If this was the case it may be that the nurses gave negative non verbal cues that signalled the displeasure that they were experiencing in the way that the physician was speaking and gave the impression therefore that they had no intention of following the physician's orders. Another major difference emerged in the category that described nurse's effectiveness in performing their own role. Unlike the physicians the nurses conveyed the impression that half the time they were performing well , particularly when communicating with the patient or family (20 helpful, 9 hindering incidences).

In the final category, nurses showed less willingness to deviate from institutional policies with 3 helpful and 7 hindering incidences. This finding is not surprising. Insitutional policies are written to protect and safeguard both the patient and the employee from harm. Lack of adherence to policy is usually a disciplinary matter, one in which if the deviation is serious enough the withdrawal of licence to practice may result. What is surprising is that so many physicians were prepared to deviate from their own codes of practice and policies thereby leaving themselves subject to possible disciplinary procedures. One factor that should be considered when discussing the limitations of this study was that these helpful/hindering incidences were perceived in relation to good patient care. Bates pointed out that no definition had been offered or sought by the respondents as to what constituted 'good patient care'. With this in mind it means that every individual in this study would have an element of subjectivity and a philosophy of 'good and bad' patient care. In her conclusion Bates remarked :

> As the interdependence of the physician and nurse continues to grow it becomes increasingly important that each member of the team should have some understanding of the viewpoint of the other and of the factors in his/her own behaviour which influence the ability of the other to function effectively. Lack of understanding leads to frustration, antagonisms and ultimately to poor if not hazardous patient care
>
> (Bates 1969 : 80)

Her study has highlighted the need to improve communication between these two groups of health professionals. Introducing communication skills, teamwork and conflict avoidance at an early stage in training would help to minimise these problems.

In a further article Bates (1970) comprehensively reviewed the literature pertaining to the roles and relationships between physicians and nurses. She asserted that both medicine and nursing had the common goal of preserving and restoring health. She suggested nevertheless, that the role of each profession differed, the role of the physician being primarily that of diagnosis and treatment, and that of the nurse being primarily one of caring, helping, comforting and guiding (p 129). She emphasised however, that neither role was an exclusive domain. Lewis and Resnick (1966) found that medical students identified mainly disease orientated objectives and physiologically based treatments whereas nursing students identified patient orientated objectives and social factors thus proving, they felt, the different viewpoints and emphasis the two professions held on patient care. Bates (1970) described physicians as the; "last of the autocrats who consign other allied health personnel to a non professional limbo regarding those persons as working for him rather than working for the patient." (Bates 1970 : 130)

Bates acknowledged that socio-cultural factors contributed to this position. In 1970 physicians were predominantly men, nurses were predominantly women and male dominance usually prevailed. Physicians also tended to be older and come from a higher socio-economic class, they had a stronger knowledge base, a greater prestige and a greater financial reward bestowed on them by society. Tanner and Soulary (1972) reported similar divisions. Bates (1970) defended medical students' attitudes by firmly blaming the traditionalist medical curriculum which did not provide the student with any opportunity to recognise the contribution that the other disciplines made to patient care. Bates described the evolution of the clinical nurse specialist, the extended role of the nurse as bridging the gap between the two professions. Disappointingly in this article Bates for the first time demonstrates her lack of conceptual understanding of what nursing really is. Her solution to the problem was to allow nurses to become more like physicians. Twenty years later in 1992, experience has shown that the extended role of the nurse has had the marked effect of reducing the workload of physicians in such tasks as administering drugs through an intravenous cannula or an epidural infusion. Lengthy debates are currently being conducted and position papers regularly published which refute many of the extended roles as not being the job of a nurse (UKCC 1989, 1990, WNB 1989, 1990, 1991).

Steel (1981) described the successful collaboration she enjoyed with a physician. They were equal partners in a joint practice. She warned that true collaborative practice does not happen automatically and that it is something that is achieved through a number of stages of development. The philosophy of Steel (a nurse) and her partner Waltman (a physician) was that through explicit determination of mutual goals and the negotiation of each individuals contribution to meeting those goals, each could be "independent in his own area but interdependent in the delivery of health care" (p 964). Steel's first stage of development was the 'contract' where each partner agreed to examine his own role and responsibilities and agreed to recognise the role, responsibility and the contribution that the other could make. Steel reported that considerable time had been spent in "flexing professional muscles" and in identifying professional boundaries. The second stage involved the execution of this contract where formal guidelines were developed. Steel noted that at this stage they appeared to be collaborating. The third and final stage was refining the contract. Steel and Waltman discovered that they had become mutually supportive, had developed greater
insight into each others roles and contribution and that their mutual goals were now consonant. Steel made the important observation that not only did they recognise each others competence but also the not so competent areas. Mutual trust appeared to be the main issue on which the success of the joint practice hinged. Steel's observations reinforce the work of earlier authors all of whom had blamed the deterioration in the quality of patient care as a result of poor communication skills and a lack of collaboration between physicians and nurses (Christman 1965, Kalisch and Kalisch 1977 and Hoekleman 1978).

Mechanic and Aiken (1982) concerned themselves with the interface between medicine and nursing and examined the competitive strains that had developed between them. They believed that much of this could be alleviated if the two groups would only recognise that they had differing but complementary skills which if used collaboratively would enhance the quality of patient care. They were convinced that much of the dissatisfaction would disappear if the groups learned to collaborate at the beginning of their training. Closer academic ties were of paramount importance.

Ahmedzai (1982), a medical registrar, devised a questionnaire for junior hospital doctors working in Glasgow. The purpose of this was to ascertain their views on caring for the dying. Of the one hundred and fifteen questionnaires sent out seventy eight (66%) were returned. Only thirteen per cent felt that they had coped with the situation well with only four per cent feeling that their preparation for this role had been adequate. Whilst many of the responses related to physical symptom control, the rank ordering of the problems that these junior doctors had identified revealed that the psychological problems experienced by the terminally ill were the most difficult of all for the doctors. Ninety six percent believed that their own stress and anxiety levels would have been considerably reduced if the opportunity to discuss patients behavioural symptoms had been addressed. In other words there was a clear demand for the behavioural sciences to be introduced into death education. The respondents were also asked to rank the relative contributions of health care professionals in terminal care. In the wider aspects of care seventy five per cent ranked nurses as the major contributing group. Of even more significance was that in the 'medical management' of terminal care, fifty one per cent still ranked nurses as the major contributors. Additional comments included "we are thrown in at the deep end" and "we need to acquire counselling skills". Many indicated their respect and envy of the nurses abilities to address the psychosocial aspects of care. Most respondents offered spontaneous comments including their pessimism about medical schools ability to teach communication skills. The comments revealed vulnerability, anxiety and pleas for help. These doctors would have undoubtedly benefited from learning with the nurses whose skills they so envied when they were being introduced to the concepts of caring for the dying.

In an anecdotal paper Coluccio and Maguire (1983) discussed the effect that the introduction of primary nursing had on collaboration between nurses and physicians in a Seattle hospital. They suggested that collaborative practice was the natural evolution of primary nursing. A desirable consequence of primary nursing has been the increase of communication between the patient and his/her nurse and the physician. Previously all communication had tended to be conducted from the patient to a nurse who reported to the ward sister who told the doctor. Frequently this tortuous route would then be repeated in a reverse pattern. As a result of the improvement in communication in Seattle a collaborative practice committee had been formed. According to Coluccio and Maguire the physicians were very keen to become involved declaring that they had been calling for such an innovation for years. The nurses were equally enthusiastic. The inaugural meeting defined the terms of reference and goals. Communication was felt to be the key issue in the need to plan, implement and evaluate patient care. Integrated teaching rounds were introduced on both a formal and informal basis and were conducted primarily at the patients bedside thus involving them as active participants. In a purely subjective conclusion the authors stated that the positve outcomes included "more comprehensive patient care resulting in higher levels of satisfaction for patients, nurses and physicians" (p 63). They also claimed earlier detection of patient problems and complications. There was no evidence however of an audit tool being used to accurately measure these findings and the question must be asked whether because the authors were the instigators of these innovations, ownership had the effect of biasing their subjectivity towards a favourable outcome.

Ferguson-Johnston (1983) described what appeared to be the total breakdown in relationships between the medical and nursing staff in Greater South East Community Hospital, Washington and how efforts had been made to heal this rift. This paper classically described the situation which is known in the vernacular as 'if it wasn't so serious it would be funny'! In 1978 the nursing staff turnover and wastage rate was unacceptably high. Ferguson-Johnston identified some of the reasons as the nurses feeling and indeed being undervalued, performing patient care only on physicians orders and lacking information. Nurse expertise was not used or even welcomed by the physicians. Where the nurse tried to make an appropriate intervention the physician would often ignore it. As a result no communication took place at all except through written orders. The situation deteriorated to the point where both groups were constantly "dumping daily disputes on the doorstep of the medical director and the director of nursing" (p 67). At this point, not surprisingly, the administrators took over and identified the common goal of enhancing patient care by both doctors and nurses through increased collaboration. Devereaux (1981a) identified five essential components for building a collaborative relationship, communication, competence, accountability, trust and support systems. Greater South East used these concepts by starting out with "straight talk" (p 67). This was hardly surprising as somebody obviously had to do something rapidly. An action plan was designed to improve the nurses' credibility, establishing joint planning committees, improving joint management skills and increasing nurse participation on various hospital committees.

Both the nurses and physicians were told in no uncertain terms that they were to be held accountable for communication with each other on behalf of the patients. Performance indicators were introduced and those that could not or would not meet the prescribed standards left. The effect on the staff was an increase in self esteem, the quality of documentation improved and the number of complaints diminished. The medical and nursing directors refused to see complainants before they had been considered by the line management structure. Rather incidentally, one feels, Ferguson-Johnston commented "Obviously emergency situations are handled expeditiously" (p 69). The joint practice committees initially focussed on problems, however latterly they became a form of information sharing and mutual learning and appeared to be generating respect and cooperation. The physicians were candidly sharing their problems and nurses had explained their need to know the physicians goals for specific patients. The hospital's slogan has become "Why argue?, collaborative practice works", Ferguson-Johnston informed the reader in her concluding paragraph. The question must be asked whether any of these so called professionals were fit to practice? This paper has a universal message for all health professionals. It is vital to learn and share together so that mutual self respect is fostered otherwise professional jealousies may reduce staff to behaving like kindergarten children.

Webster (1985) examined the problems of interprofessional relationships between medical students and nurses from the medical students perspective. She considered individual, interpersonal and institutional factors which might be detrimental to interdisciplinary relationships. The methodology used to collect data from the sixty medical students involved participant observation and intensive interviewing. The medical students were stratified on the basis of the year in medical school and gender and then were randomly selected. Ten males and five females from each of the four years comprised the sample (N=60). Webster described this sample as comprising five per cent of the total number of medical students. Webster described the participant observation period as varied. She accompanied the students on teaching rounds, attended lectures, observed seating patterns in refrectories, visited operating theatres, intensive care units, emergency admissions and the wards. Additional information was gleaned from the directors of medical education and nursing education which related to policies and procedures, patient populations and professional relationships between medicine and nursing.

A number of questions arise from the participant observation period. Webster did not clarify whether the students she observed were the same as those included in the interviews. It would appear that they were not. The information that she obtained from the above sources was not included in the paper and so the possibility of observer bias cannot be excluded. There was no mention of the number of independent variables which would seem inherent in this type of study. Furthermore the reader was told that Webster visited three large urban hospitals and six affiliated private ones which yielded patients of various ages, ethnic backgrounds and differing medical conditions.

In phase two of the project, the intensive interview, demographic data was collected from the respondents in order to identify thirty two factors presumed to have a potential influence on relationships. A further forty items using open ended questions and probing to clarify the subjects meaning was adopted. Webster used three of her colleagues to determine face validity of the interview guide and a reliability of ninety six per cent was obtained. The data obtained from the interviews was coded to allow retrieval of information in any given category. Cross classification tables were also included which stratified gender and year in school thus making it possible to quantify trends. The results themselves were not displayed so a critical analysis could not be undertaken.
Webster's own interpretation appeared to yield some interesting results. First year medical students of either gender described the health team using broad concepts with some listing as many as nineteen different categories of staff. In distinct contrast the fourth year students organised the health team around an individual patient's needs. Definitions of professionalism varied widely but seventy per cent of male students (N=28) stated that the physician should be the

team leader. Of the female students only forty five per cent (N=9) thought this should be the case. The numbers however are so small that no conclusions can be drawn. The data also revealed that the female students were far more likely to demonstrate a knowledge about nurse education and the role of the nurse in health care, most particularly those in the first two years of medical school. Male medical students used far more disparaging terms concerning the nursing profession than their female counterparts.

Webster acknowledged that the implications for nursing from the data were merely suggestive. She had previously mentioned that female medical students shared halls of residence with the nurses and that they therefore personally knew many of them. Stereotyping was evident in these results but Webster did not draw attention to the gender factor which would appear to be significant in this small study. It could be argued that the results hinged entirely on the male/ female equality issue. The male medical students displayed a superior chauvinistic attitude towards female nurses, whereas the female medical students tended to support their female nurse colleagues. Initial impressions obtained from the abstract of this paper appeared to be promising but critical reading has exposed the study as inherently flawed and therefore invalid.

In 1988 Webster published a further discussion paper on the same issues. Whilst her review of the literature seemed to demonstrate her grasp of the subject, her presentation of the same project that she had undertaken in 1985 showed no further insight into the weaknesses of the study.

Keddy et al (1986) examined the evolution of the doctor nurse relationship. They used a grounded theory approach in order to analyse the data they gathered in recorded interviews with thirty four retired nurses who had worked in Nova Scotia in the nineteen twenties and nineteen thirties. Semi-structured interviews were used, with a non random selection of respondents. The non random selection was hardly surprising in view of the age these retired nurses must have been. Keddy et al described the snowball technique by which the sample was gathered. As the possible respondents were traced they were asked to suggest names of their former colleagues who were still alive and who may be prepared to participate in the study. It should be pointed out that Keddy and her colleagues were all nurses who, judging by their comments, were aggrieved by their subordinate role with physicians. As the respondents were also all nurses it could justifiably be suggested that an element of bias crept in as no physicians of a similar era were asked their opinions and memories.

Stern (1980) described grounded theory as a useful method for generating fresh ideas from stale experiences. As the empirical data is collected it is placed into codes which are then clustered into broader categories. These categories are then reviewed in order to generate new concepts. These concepts are then broken down into general categories. This method was described as 'reduction' by Stern (1980) and 'core variables' by Glaser and Strauss (1967). With this stage completed, selective literature sampling follows which further supports the theory. Using this approach Keddy et al (1986), through the data obtained from the semi structured interviews with the retired nurses, identified the key concept as the detrimental effect that the physician nurse relationship had on health care in the past. Their literature review supported this concept. They found that a physician's approval was the power behind the success, or otherwise, of both an individual nurse and of the nursing profession itself. There was a marked power differential between the two groups which related to the sexual divisions of labour within society. This finding reinforced the view of Navarro (1977) who was convinced that many of the problems had evolved from the power which had been invested in physicians thus allowing them to decide what should be learned by nurses and then to educate them accordingly. Keddy et al (1986) cited Rushmore (1940) who had written " it is the doctors duty to educate nurses and say what level is acceptable".

Nearly forty years later Kalisch and Kalisch (1977) were debating what made a 'good' nurse. They decided as a result of a content analysis of a number of films, made by the media for the general public which portrayed doctor/ nurse relationships, that good nursing care (in the eyes of the media) was equated with the fulfilment of the doctor's orders. In terms of quality of care, no evidence was found that led Kalisch and Kalisch to suspect that this had any influence on the outcome. Raisler (1974) wryly commented that a physician would perceive the nurse as 'good' as long as she continued to 'help' him, regardless of the patient outcome. According to Raisler any show of intelligence by the nurse was most definitely not welcomed by the physician. Canham (1982) blamed nurse education and was convinced that the root cause was the history of humility and passivity that was instilled in nurses in the traditional training methods adopted.

Keddy et al (1986) would have agreed with this as they discussed role behaviours and stereotyping. They believed that role behaviour was learned at an early stage in training, that role models within each profession were emulated by the students themselves and that the problem was therefore self perpetuating. Hoekleman (1975), a physician, recognised this role modelling phenomena and called for interdisciplinary educational efforts which would diminish the problem. It was obvious that this enlightened physician had not worked with the nurses' interviewed by Keddy et al (1986) as he was very forcibly making the case for an equal status. He challenged nurses to push for recognition as he maintained that the existing conflict would continue until society recognised the true value of the nursing profession and equated it with the medical profession. Smoyak (1987) believed that the two professions' worked best together when there was mutual agreement, equality in status, and a shared knowledge base. Trust and respect would then be the natural concommitant of such a development.

Copp (1987) suggested 'primary health care' in the form of prevention and early intervention for the professions themselves. Without the conflict being urgently confronted the situation was likely to deteriorate beyond redemption. Goodwin

(1982) wrote in a similar vein when she wrote bitterly of her attachment, as a health visitor, to a general practitioner. Territorial conflicts had caused a complete breakdown in the working relationship between the two. The (unnamed) general practitioner attempted to justify why he banned "health visitors from visiting my patients" (p 14). Goodwin pointed out the use of the possessive pronoun and suggested that this may be the result of the general practitioner viewing patients as actually or potentially ill and therefore in need of medical treatment. Goodwin's personal perspective was rather different "as a health visitor.......I focus my concern on the healthy and spend my time assisting them in learning how to stay that way" (p 14).

Brown et al (1979) studied joint practice between nurse practitioners and physicians and found that there was no reason for this territorial conflict. The patients in this study were described as fit and well and wanting to remain that way for as long as possible. Brown et al demonstrated that if and when these patients were ill they preferred to consult the physician. Nevertheless, for minor complaints, advice and counselling the patients evaluated the nurses in a more positive way than the physicians. Areas in which the nurses were awarded the highest score included examination skills, allowing more time, the completeness of the health history taken, the amount of health information given and the total overall satisfaction (p 97-98). These findings confirm the work of Beloff and Korper (1972) who had undertaken a very similar study.

Brooking (1992) called for a blurring of the roles which would allow a true partnership to develop between the two groups. Brooking was convinced that medical dominance was diminishing. This is contrary to Ovretveit (1985d) who was sure that medical dominance was as powerful as ever. Brooking (1992) firmly believed that in spite of the increasing numbers of shared research projects and shared learning initiatives "relationships between nurses and doctors have deteriorated to the point where patient care suffers" (Ibid : 24).

Brooking reviewed the reasons for the continuing medical hegemony, but she also recognised and clearly empathised with her medical colleagues who were complaining of increasing isolation and alienation from their nursing counterparts. Brooking called for a truce. The accepted nursing domain of 'caring' and that in medicine of 'curing' was no longer true. With the greater emphasis on holistic care using a biopsychosocial model these discrete domains no longer existed. Brooking advocated that, all things being equal, tasks which could be competently performed by an individual lower in the professional strata should be delegated. She was not in any way suggesting that incompetent, inadequately trained individuals should perform skilled work normally undertaken by experienced practitioners. She regretted the bureaucratic constraints of the separate statutory bodies', registration systems and funding bodies and suggested that these were the main contributing factors to the lack of interdisciplinary education. She "found it impossible to see" why shared learning could not and did not take place. She described as a "modest proposal" the introduction of shared learning in twenty five per cent of the curriculum and pondered whether monodisciplinary conferences would still be appropriate by the next century.

Brooking's attitude was particularly refreshing for a professor of nursing in the United Kingdom as she warned of the dangers of the "pseudo-philosophical mumbo jumbo" of the language that had been assimilated into nursing's sub culture. Nursing had come of age, she concluded, and as a profession it could therefore afford to collaborate with medicine more closely. Sadly not all Brooking's fellow professionals are so assertive, confident and challenging. It is interesting to note that in a publication only six weeks prior to that of Brooking, a staff nurse discussing patient advocacy wrote; " As doctors' are the most powerful members of the team, it is likely to be their attitudes which determine whether nurse advocates receive the support and understanding they need." (Marshall 1991: 29) At the 'shop floor' level it would appear that many nurses still play and indeed accept the subservient role.

2.6.2. Social workers and other professional groups

Hooper (1970), a clinical psychologist, described social workers as "bona fide members of the treatment staff" (p 90). Both Buttrym (1967) and Hooper (1970) considered the role of social workers in health care. They alerted the profession to the dangers of presenting themselves as the only experts in the use of relationships. Buttrym, in particular, thought that this would inevitably lead to confrontation and conflict with the other professions. Hooper predicted that conflict would occur as a result of the markedly different educational aims of social work when compared with, for example, those of medicine and nursing. Hooper suggested several reasons for this conflict, the first of which would undoubtedly be refuted by the medical and nursing professions; " the social worker may wish to enhance the individual autonomy of a patient in the interests of recovery whereas the nurse and doctor may well wish to diminish this, again in the interests of recovery." (Hooper 1970 : 91)

Patient autonomy is highly valued as a philosophy by the caring professions (Hockey 1977 and Horder 1991) and Hooper's inflammatory comment would undoubtedly increase the confrontational situation. Hooper suggested that a further problem was one of control. He made the point that whereas a radiographer, occupational therapist or a physiotherapist could all accept a fragmented view of the patient a social worker could not do so. The above named professions were not given the opportunity to defend their position. Hooper made some very contentious assumptions in his paper which whilst perhaps appeasing social workers' sensibilities, would have precisely the opposite effect on the professions he mentioned. Perhaps he hoped that a publication in a social work journal would not be reviewed by members of any other profession!

Hawker (1977), a senior manager in a social work department, warned of professional disaster if closer cooperation between the professions was encouraged. Whilst he continued, he was not against cooperation or coordination *per se* "There comes a time when the level of those activities is such that it threatens our ability to do the particular job we are trained to do" (Ibid : 18). He eloquently continued his argument by describing cooperation as "falling into masterly inactivity as we go about confirming our work ability" (Ibid : 18).

Hawker's fears are voiced by many individuals in the caring professions that the inevitable dilution of skills and knowledge will occur. The literature has not revealed the desire for a trend towards a generalist health carer, but rather the need to enhance a greater understanding of each profession's role so that a comprehensive holistic approach to client care can be achieved. Hawker demonstrated throughout his discussion paper, a vulnerability and a desire for professional elitism so criticised by other authors (Berkowitz and Malone 1968, Dana and Sheps 1968, Kendall 1977, Pritchard 1981, Ferguson- Johnston 1983,Webster 1985, Osborne and Wakeling 1985, Copp 1987, Horder 1991 and Brooking 1992). Bywaters (1986) also argued that any collaboration should not be unconditional as it would inevitably lead to a decreasing emphasis on the sociological welfare of the client.

Kendall (1977) described the basic philosophy of social work as enabling clients "to attain their full potential for quality of life and to prevent the perpetuation of the cycle of deprivation" (Ibid : 262).

Writing in the journal "The Health Visitor", Kendall, a director of social services discussed the role relationship dilemma between health visitors and social workers. He seemed to endorse the Seebohm Committee Report (1974) which had concluded that the notion of health visitors becoming all purpose social workers was misconceived. He described social work training as covering aspects of psychology, sociology, human growth, law and administration and an understanding of group dynamics. Whilst this may indeed be true, examination of a health visitor syllabus reveals a mirror approach. Social workers, Kendall argued, must be part of the primary health care team, where their expertise could be utilised fully. Health visitors should concentrate on health promotion and illness prevention. It was paramount that health visitors and social workers collaborated but Kendall was certain that the role of the health visitor was being diluted owing to the fact that they were continually becoming involved in problems which should be addressed by the social workers. He recognised that because of the current numbers of unqualified social workers this was inevitable as they were realistically unable to provide an adequate service through lack of training and knowledge. He quoted alarming figures which highlighted the extent of the problem. In 1974 of 11,800 full time social workers in the United Kingdom only 4,500 were qualified. In the last few years this problem has been addressed and the number of places on social work courses has increased dramatically. The role dilemma between health visitors and social workers may also diminish as a result of the move towards a more generic community nurse recommended in the Cumberledge Report (1986). If this generic nurse is to become more clinically orientated then the social interventions will have to be referred to and dealt with by social workers.

Other authors have also recognised the possible advantages that interdisciplinary learning may hold for nurses, health visitors and social workers. In spite of a few reservations, most seem to conclude that such an initiative should be encouraged (Hirschon 1976, Quataro and Hutchinson 1976, Williams et al 1978, Brooks 1987, Nursing Standard Editorial 1987, Henk 1989, Allen 1991, Peryer 1991).

Williams and Williams (1982) examined interprofessional perceptions and experiences between hospital social workers and nurses. Their study demonstrated that the greater the contact between the two groups, the less the stereotyping occurred. Their small scale project was methodologically sound and the data collected subjected to statistical analysis. Two hundred and thirty seven nurses and sixty social workers were used as a retrospective comparison group. They completed a self administered questionnaire which was presented in three sections. Part 1 requested demographic information, part 2 assessed the kind and amount of contact each profession had with the other, part 3 consisted of twenty statements which were presented on a semantic differential scale consisting of strongly positive characteristics through to strongly negative ones. Parts 1 and 2, whilst revealing interesting data, had no real relevance to this current study apart from the fact that whilst both groups reported regular contact in practice, neither group had experienced any contact during their training. Part 3 however, revealed negative characteristics about each other on an almost equal basis. The negative statements included 'over-extended, meddling, domineering and emotionally unstable'. There was no statistically significant difference between the two groups perceptions of each other using the T-Test ($p < 0.1$). Positive characteristics (such as committed, dedicated, non prejudiced, interested in people) yielded similar results in that there was no significant difference between the two groups ($p < 0.1$). An interesting and encouraging finding was that the fewest number of negative stereotypes were reported by those social workers and nurses who reported the largest number of contacts with each other in their daily professional lives.

Several authors have considered the relationships between social workers and general practitioners (Lambert and Muras 1967, Bennett et al 1972, Goldberg and Neill 1972, Ratoff et al 1974, Schenk 1979, Samuel and Dodge 1981, Pritchard 1981 and Butrym and Horder 1983). Ratoff et al (1974) described the relationship between general practitioners and social workers as 'poor'. In a discussion paper they identified the important issues that divided the two groups. One important factor was the number of social workers who could not be called 'professionals' as they were untrained and held no statutory qualifications. This meant that they could not be held legally accountable for their actions. General practitioners were justifiably concerned about their patients revealing confidential information to an individual who was not bound by a code of conduct to maintain confidentiality. Bennett et al (1972) had previously expressed the same concerns. Ratoff et al (1974) commented on the different nomenclature used by both groups, with the general practitioners referring to 'patients' whereas social workers referred to 'clients'. This they believed caused a fundamental division at the grass roots level. Even in situations where social workers were qualified, the two groups had entirely different orientations towards the patient/client. Social workers laid emphasis on family relationships and the community whilst general practitioners concentrated on individual human functioning particularly from a biological stance. An illuminative thought by Ratoff et al described the social workers' perceptions as consumers of health care. All social workers will at some time experience the role of a patient and the nature of that experience will colour their attitude towards health care. Most general practitioners will not personally require the services of a social worker and do not therefore have consumer insight into their contribution.

Goldberg and Neill (1972) believed that the language barrier was the biggest stumbling block. They suggested that words such as 'chronic' and 'urgent' had entirely different meanings for the two groups. To doctors 'urgent' meant dealing with the problem immediately or at the very least within the next few hours, whereas for social workers it may mean within the next few days. They illustrated this point by outlining the (then) current procedure for compulsory admission to a psychiatric hospital in which on rare occasions it was desirable that an individual was immediately admitted in order to protect either him/herself or other members of the general public. Through delay in the social services department tragic consequences had been recorded. Ratoff and his colleagues defended social workers however by explaining the legal statutes under which they were constrained. In addition whilst general practitioners were mostly autonomous, social workers had to contend with a complex hierarchical structure. Their paper concluded with the suggestion that a period of joint training prior to qualification would help diminish the conflicts experienced at a later stage.

Pritchard (1981) also considered stereotyping between the two groups. He found that very negative perceptions were held by each group about the other. Amongst those held by general practitioners about social workers were a lack of confidentiality regarding patients records, a lack of professional identity, lack of training, part of a bureaucratic organisation in which nobody takes responsibility or makes decisions and that social workers gave mainly material benefit rather than emotional support. Social workers perceptions about general practitioners included the observations that they were egocentric, enjoyed an unjustifiably high salary and social status, they were too disease orientated, they did not attempt to address a clients problems but prescribed drugs instead, and they could not be trusted with confidential information.

In 1983 Butrym (a senior lecturer in social work) and Horder (a general practitioner) co-authored a book in which they hoped to uncover; " some of the causes of misunderstandings which still exist between two vitally important helping professions, whose objectives and tasks are closely related." (Butrym and Horder 1983 : 1)

They made some very challenging statements asking the reader to consider whether it would not be better for doctors and nurses to concentrate on medical problems and leave personal and social problems to the remit of the social workers. They were convinced that this was neither possible nor desirable because medical and psychosocial problems were inextricably linked. Attention paid to one aspect only of an individual's personna was bound to be of limited value. Separate expertise should not indicate an ignorance of each other's roles.

Ignorance led to "narrow mindedness and a restriction of the opportunities of providing the most appropriate forms of help to patients/clients." (Ibid : 1-2) They subscribed to a holistic conception of health care and regretted that the medical model of training continued to concentrate on physical needs at the expense of psychosocial needs. They suspected that interprofessional rivalry militates against successful collaboration between the two groups. Both groups should learn to be more flexible and positive in order to build up trust, respect and a sharing of expertise. Opportunities for learning on a shared basis was an important strategy which should be adopted in order to achieve this. They challenged educators to try and make a convincing case for not introducing shared learning. They maintained that it was not possible.

2.6.3 Nurses and dietitians

Bersky et al (1987) issued a stern warning that anybody who was under the impression that different disciplines automatically adjusted and worked together harmoniously was naive. Wessell (1981) pointed out that part of a nurse's readiness to begin practice was his/her understanding of the nature of other health care professions. Bersky et al (1987) described an experiment in shared learning between nursing and dietetics students at the University of Illinois. The aim of the sessions was to enable them to clarify their roles in relation to each other and to build a foundation upon which conflict, interprofessional jealousy and rivalry would be non existent. The total number of participating students was very small (N=38). The programme commenced with an exploration of the concepts of teamwork and professional identity. The students formed pairs, one from each profession and were asked to conduct an interview with a 'simulated patient'. The interviews were videotaped and reviewed by the two students, the 'patient', a nurse lecturer, a dietetics lecturer and a psychologist.

The students evaluated their own performance and also received feedback from the others. As a result the students then formulated a joint care plan. The application of each profession's theory to practice was deemed as essential by Bersky et al and evidence of this was looked for in the completed plan. Students evaluated the experience as unique and positive. They observed that the experience had enabled them to decide that their own contributions enhanced rather than conflicted with each other and that the end result was a much better understanding of each others contribution to health care. Several students expressed the opinion that this experience should be mandatory for all the health care professions.

As a result of this positive feedback Bersky et al (1987) repeated and extended the programme. The number of participating students was not given neither was any evidence offered of the inclusion of any other disciplines. No conclusions can be drawn from this study as the numbers involved were so small and the quality of the report was not rigorous. It seems however to point the way to the introduction of shared learning on a small scale and would not be difficult, all things being equal, to introduce into faculties in which more than one discipline exists.

Dickens et al (1985) described a course for nursing and dietetics students which aimed to clarify role functions and increase collaborative planning. In total 38 students (19 nurses and 19 dietitians) enrolled. Introductory sessions addressed the issues of interprofessional communication, teamwork and role definitions. Simulated interviews with a 'client' were undertaken by two students (one from each discipline) simultaneously. The objective was to compare the similarities and differences in the kind of information needed by each discipline, to discuss suitable communication strategies and to develop a collaborative care plan. Vignettes of suitable clients were given to the students prior to the interview in which information on the disease status was included. The 'clients' were asked to retrospectively evaluate the session in terms of the relationship established, the clarity of the information provided and the sensitivity of the students interviewing skills. The students were also asked to evaluate their own performance and 88% of them stated that they had improved as a result and that the programme was 'extremely successful'. This reinforces Rosenaur and Fuller (1973) and Ballassone's (1981) findings in which mutual trust was described as essential for critically appraising another professional's strengths and weaknesses in interviewing techniques. The students in Dickens et al (1985) were able to establish collaboratively one priority diagnosis and collectively set treatment goals. These were then recorded on the care plan. In Rosenaur and Fuller's study (1973) 50% of the joint care plans submitted by medical students and nurses identified the need to consult with other professions, the most frequently mentioned being the social worker.

Caliendo and Pulaski (1979) also described the level of interaction between dietetics and nursing students in simulated case conferences. They concluded that such learning strategies "clearly facilitates role clarification between the two health professional groups" (Ibid : 574).

2.6.4 Summary of interprofessional conflicts

The review of the literature has revealed many publications which address the problems encountered by the different health care professions regarding their role in holistic care. Much descriptive and anecdotal evidence has been identified but little empirical work would appear to have been completed. Role conflict, interprofessional jealousy and elitism, medical hegemony, the struggle of the emerging professions, the fight for autonomy within practice and the desire by the professions to develop their clinical practice based on a sound theoretical framework has led in many instances to an ever deepening entrenchment. Tradition, fear, vulnerability and cloistering has reinforced this position. Most of the attention with regard to interprofessional conflict seems to have concentrated most particularly on three of the caring professions, physicians, nurses and social workers. References to the other allied professions have been sparse and when found have tended to focus on the overall concept of teamwork in health care. It was decided therefore to consider any such publications in the section of the literature review which considers teamwork. None of the authors reviewed have suggested that any one individual profession is exempt from the problem of conflict and isolation. Students from the different disciplines are beginning to demand interdisciplinary contact at an early stage in their training.

2.7 Teamwork in health and social care

The team concept in health care has developed slowly over the last four decades although the earliest evidence found of formal collaboration between two professions was that of a biologist and a physician working together in 1926 in London (Pearce and Crocker 1943 cited by Reedy 1981a). The need for closer collaboration began with the firm conviction that an interdisciplinary approach to health care was essential. The earliest evidence found of an embryonic multidisciplinary team was in 1949 at the Montefiore Hospital, New York where Cherkasky (1949) described the initial success of a home care programme instituted collaboratively by a physician, a nurse and a social worker. Kindig (1975) suggested that the concept of team work evolved at this time as a direct result of poverty following the second world war and was therefore due to financial constraints imposed by the US Government. Kindig developed his discussion on the historical development by stating that the causal factors, whilst crucial to the argument, should not detract from the idealism behind it. He was in no doubt that if one individual health profession could perform all the tasks needed to care efficiently then a team approach would not be necessary. This however, was not the case and invaluable contributions could be made by each profession whose unique skills could be identified clearly.

It would seem that communication is central to the concept of effective teamwork and is implicit in both cooperation and coordination. Simon (1961) argued that no matter how committed to the concept of cooperation a team was, teamwork would always be ineffective in the absence of coordination. He recommended that a corporate set of behaviours should be identified and adopted rather than individual ones. Furthermore he advised that all prospective team members should indicate their willingness to adopt these behaviours. Shaw

(1970) believed that; " Communication lies at the heart of the group interaction process.......the free flow of information......among various members of the group determine to a large extent the efficiency of a group and the satisfaction of its members." (Ibid : 75)

Batchelor and McFarlane (1980) were the co-authors of a King Edward's Hospital Fund project paper which was submitted to the Royal Commission on the NHS in 1979. This core document considered multi-disciplinary clinical teams and identified a number of problems relating to this concept. These included, leadership and who should take this role, the nature of corporate responsibility and it's effect on individual members, confidentiality, communication, legal responsibilities and finally the specific problems of primary health care teams. The following year (1981) the Harding Report was published. Harding and his colleagues considered that there were four basic requisites for true team collaboration, an accepted common objective, a clear understanding by each team member of his/her own role and area of responsibility, a clear understanding by each team member of the roles and responsibilities of other team members and a flexible approach to teamwork by each team member with a constituent mutual respect for each others' contributions. The last requirement was described by Harding et al as a "fundamental pre-requisite" in order that each team member could "exploit their professional skills to the full" (p 63). The choice of the word 'exploit' is perhaps unfortunate in the light of previous findings as it implies that each profession would be indulging in undesirable overlap (Milne 1980a).

Harding et al (1981) were quite justified in calling for clear team objectives and a corporate identity. This they suggested, could be achieved through proper preparation before the team worked together, an objective evaluation of existing teams already working together in order that their objectives could be reviewed and a recognition and acceptance of the need for more interdisciplinary training. Nevertheless they were encouraged by the increase in interest in this topic although they regretted that most shared learning appeared to take place at a post graduate level. They urged initial preparation at the undergraduate stage, although they recognised the inherent difficulties. These were described as the differing lengths and levels of training, the different teaching methods adopted and the differing expectations of the professional groups themselves. The authors gave the impression that they had collected evidence from some of the personnel with experience in interdisciplinary post graduate education although this was not absolutely clear. They commended the use of role playing and case studies as learning strategies and placed great emphasis on the merits of undergraduates visiting established teams who functioned well in practice.

They offered a solution to the problem of interpersonal conflicts within a team. A trial period should be available for a new team member to allow the individual and the existing team to assess cohesiveness and compatability. This sounds ideal but within the present contractual arrangements of district health authorities and the family health service authorities it would be logistically extremely difficult to move after a few months. It also does not take into account limited geographical mobility. An additional problem would be the possible interpretation of failure if an individual did not meet the team's expectations or vice versa. Loss of confidence and self esteem may be the end result in this situation. Management and organisational factors were considered widely but of particular relevance were the deliberations by the working party of management within the team itself. Leadership was frequently mentioned as a source of conflict with some members of the working party opting for the physician because of his "ultimate responsibility" (p 32) whilst others believed that it should be flexible and depend on the patient's presenting problems. They continually referred to lack of communication as being the fundamental problem in teamwork and called for more purpose built premises which would ensure more formal and informal contact.

This statement was subsequently reinforced by Bond et al (1987) in their empirical study which indicated an increased level of communication when premises were shared. Hamel-Cooke and Cope (1983) and Harding and Taylor (1990) also produced similar results. Iles and Auluck (1990) examined the problems encountered in developing effective interdisciplinary teams. They were convinced that organisational development with its emphasis on process rather than task was paramount for successful development of teamwork. Beckhard (1974) identified the problems of team organisation as being due in part to the professional rather than managerial orientation, the hierarchical multiple power level, the differing goals and priorities of individual professionals, the role conflict and the negative stereotyping between the professions. Iles and Auluck (1990) concluded that these constraints led ultimately to decision making within teams which is "often authoritarian rather than collaborative" (p 51).

Kinston (1983) considered interprofessional behaviour and its effect on patient care in relation to hospital organisation. He described the hierarchical structure and the negotiated order in existence in the NHS. He argued that organisational structure was imperative in order to constrain the boundaries of negotiation. While sub divisions within professions had created highly skilled care for patients it had also increased demands for integration and co-ordination. Numerous reports have been published on behalf of the British Government which have examined the role of health care professionals and the organisation within which they work but few have formulated concrete plans as they are usually dominated by professional values (Dawson Report 1920, Cope Report 1951, Younghusband Report 1959, Briggs Report 1972, McMillan Report 1973, Otton Report 1974, Halsbury Report 1974, Merrison Report 1979, Jay Report 1979, Harding Report 1981, Cumberledge Report 1986). Boundaries and professional constraints have inevitably caused strain and conflict between the professions and the question has already been asked whether an agreement when reached will be negotiated or imposed (Goldie 1977, Eaton and Webb 1979).

Forces exist within the existing organisational structure which are detrimental to patient care. Wilson (1982) identified three main factors, resources and budgeting, pressure because of accountability, and the need for long term planning. Kinston (1983) identified other constraints, primarily expediency and staff self interests. He admitted however that the loss of patient focus was accidental but he charged the health professions to maintain the vision of patient centred care. Kinston suggested that all staff should accept the need for collaboration in their work.

Abramson (1984), a professor of social work, posed several questions about ethical decision making and whose responsibility those decisions were in interdisciplinary teamwork in health care. She argued that ultimately a decision could be the responsibility of an individual or collectively within a group. In group decision making she continued; " the opinion of any one member of the group is invariably modified by the others. Each team members decisions and actions is both enhanced and restrained by the rest of the team." (Ibid : 39)

This realisation may cause a real dilemma for an individual as in order to maintain unity within the team, compromises may be necessary. This may mean that an individual's own internalised code of ethics and values may directly conflict with the team decision. Abramson listed several words which she believed reflected the real definition of collaboration. These included consensus, cohesion, negotiation, common understanding about team goals, roles and procedures. She asserted that as a profession social workers value mediation, co-operation, mutual respect, participation and co-ordination. No evidence was offered to substantiate this claim so it may have been an entirely subjective view. Nevertheless there was no doubt of Abramson's commitment to the concept of teamwork. She offered guidelines which would help enhance collective responsibility in teams when making 'ethical' decisions. She advocated the adoption of a common moral language. While medical terminology was reasonably common place in health care and used by most of the professions, moral and ethical terms were not. Concepts such as autonomy, paternalism, confidentiality or quality of life were not usually considered on an interdisciplinary basis. Individuals within a team needed to learn to articulate their thoughts so that ambiguity was reduced but confidence was gained, thereby allowing healthy disagreements to be discussed at length. The group needed to spend time clarifying both individual and collective values and principles in order that critical objective analysis could be made of more complex ethical dilemmas. Abramson concluded her paper with the powerful statement :

> The ultimate goal of interprofessional co-operation is good care of the patient.. To this end, professionals with different bodies of knowledge and skills are brought together in various types of collaborative groups to pool their resources in attaining the ultimate objective of the best care
>
> (Abramson 1984 : 42)

Ovretveit has been a prolific author on the subject of multidisciplinary teams. He expressed a particular interest in their organisation and management (1984a, 1985a, b, d and 1986a, b, d). He observed (1985b) that rhetoric frequently obscures the problems experienced in teamworking and regretted that so many teams develop without well defined objectives. He advocated developing a sense of ownership amongst the individual team members in order that decision making can become collective. Team members could not pretend to be a closely knit group if autonomous, hierarchical decisions were made by managerial superiors external to the team. Ovretveit suggested that the team itself should formulate an operational policy which addressed such issues as key working and the aims and objectives of the team. Ovretveit's papers are unfortunately similarly titled as well as similar in content. This similarity on occasions leads to direct repetition and therefore makes it extremely difficult for the reader to differentiate between them. Nevertheless there are specific points which can be gleaned from each publication. He examined case responsibility within health care teams and noted that consultants had traditionally been viewed as in overall charge of patients' clinical needs (1986a). He had previously written that in his opinion, medical dominance was not in significant decline (1985d). (This reference is variously described with two titles both used interchangeably by even Ovretveit himself ...... see reference section). In his 1986a publication he made an extremely important point "Every professional owes a duty of care to clients and may be held to account in a court of law for their actions and may be liable for negligence" (Ibid :2)

He referenced the Zangwill Report (1980) to substantiate his comments. It would appear that this potential liability depends upon working within agreed policies and if any individuals work is proved to be substandard, disciplinary action then becomes a probability. Ovretveit advocated the use of a 'prime' or 'key' worker who coordinated the work of the team. He did not venture an opinion as to which profession, if any, should undertake this role although he did make clear that this person should not scrutinise or over ride a team member's professional decision (1986a : 3). He did not believe that there was an ideal model for teamwork (1986d). The circumstances and purpose of setting up a team should vary depending on the locality and resources available. Exactly the same rationale had previously been expressed by Owen (1982). It is interesting to note that Ovretveit in all his publications refers to the 'multidisciplinary' team and never the 'interdisciplinary' team. He categorises the multidisciplinary team into subgroups :

1. *Formal teams* The regular meeting of members of the different professions. Information and tasks are shared and it is possible to state who belongs to the team and who does not. Other authors would disagree with this interpretation and would reclassify this as an interdisciplinary team (Szasz 1969 and Owen 1982).

2. *Managed teams* Those which consist of a single discipline. An example of this being the team of nurses working on one hospital ward.
3. *Joint accountability teams* Ovreveit (1986d) also described this as the democratic team where shared accountability is the accepted norm, but where each team member emphasises their independence and autonomy. Szasz (1969) and Owen (1982) would argue that this constitutes a multidisciplinary team.
4. *Coordinated teams* Managers within the hierarchy identify key workers and bring them together to form a team of experts in a given situation. This would seem to reflect the ethos of 'working parties' or 'advisory bodies'.
5. *Core and extended teams* A nucleus of individuals from one or two professions constitute the core. Other professionals form the extended team and are coopted in when appropriate. This is of physicians and nurses as the key workers with the most interaction with hospital patients. When necessary the patient is referred to other disciplines such as physiotherapists, podiatrists or dietitians.

Ovretveit (1986d) recognised the limitations that can be placed on individual professions by Codes of Practice. Competence and license to practice permits some members of a team to fulfil certain duties that other members cannot. The UKCC Code of Conduct for Nurses, Midwives and Health Visitors (1992) exemplifies this. Nevertheless there are common competencies which allow several disciplines to undertake the same procedures.

Many authors have identified the necessity of all team members having a working knowledge of the behavioural sciences in order to increase a team's effectiveness. Goal setting, role clarification, communication skills, leadership patterns, problem solving and management of conflict have all been identified as essential behaviours within an effective team (Lewis and Resnick 1964, Duncan and Kempe 1968, Szasz 1969, Beloff et al 1970, Howard and Byl 1971, Parker 1972, Mason and Parascandola 1972, Carlaw and Callan 1973, Wise et al 1974, Siegal 1974, Kindig 1975, Boyer 1977, Lowe and Herranen 1978, Mailick and Ashley 1981,Nason 1983, Kane 1983, Margolis and Fiorelli 1984, Germain 1984, Irwin and Bamber 1984, Knox and Bouchier 1985, Newman 1987, Archer 1987, Marcer and Deighton 1988, Sands 1990, Gregson et al 1991, Opoku 1992, Kingdon 1992, Trowell 1992).

Kindig (1975) succinctly summarised the rationale of the need for any health team's understanding of the behavioural sciences. He forecast that over the following decades consideration of the environment would play an increasingly important part in health care which would require the professionals to address the psychosocial needs of patients/clients. Kindig did not prescribe which professions should constitute a health team. Indeed he always referred to 'any' health professional thus emphasising the flexibility of the situation. This stance supports the work of Siegal (1974) which described eight different structures which he had identified existed and even then Siegal admitted that there was likely to be infinite variation. Kindig (1975) made an amusing but pertinent analogy between health care teams and football teams. He highlighted the importance of practice before playing the game of football and suggested that health teams "require a similar investment in practising their play in order to work together effectively in patient care" (Ibid : 102).

He supported the idea of learning together before experiencing the reality of teamwork in clinical practice. He had noted previously that additional training in learning to work together was necessary. This he concluded was the result of isolated educational experiences for each professional group and posed the question of whether this additional training would be necessary if interdisciplinary learning had taken place at an undergraduate level ; he suspected not. He believed that the impetus for shared learning had been generated by student demand and referred to the Student Health Organisation which had been founded in the USA by the students themselves. The organisation had set up its own interdisciplinary projects entirely independently of qualified practitioners. Further evidence of this innovation was found in McGarvey et al (1968). McGarvey and his colleagues were the actual students involved and their paper described the positive side of student anarchy and revolt. A further example of student initiative was described by Boyer et al (1977). The independent stance taken by both these groups was the direct result of the failure by medical educators to listen to the students demands for more appropriate preparation for their professional careers. According to both papers there was no shortage of interested and committed student volunteers prepared to take the matter into their own hands. In 1992 The Student Health Organisation still exists and remains a powerful influence in identifying student needs. It is encouraging to report that the medical educators now work collaboratively with this organisation in order to enhance student training.

This literature review has revealed that conflict is a natural and inevitable development of interdisciplinary teamwork. From the perspective of problem solving, conflict is desirable and therefore provides a catalyst for growth (Nason 1983, Kane 1983 and Margolis and Fiorelli 1984). Germain (1984) described conflict resolution as a stage in developing interdisciplinary collaboration. Team members from the different disciplines will progress from; "fragmented thinking about the patient and context based on disciplinary specialisation to a holistic or systemic view of patient/environment relationships bearing on health and illness." (Ibid : 203)

Von Schilling (1982) postulated that whilst each profession continued to approach the client unilaterally "enormous problems of duplication and other inequities are created for the client" (Ibid : 73).

The philosophy of team care therefore should be driven by client need rather than by interprofessional rivalry. Lowe and Herranen (1978) discussed the possibility of two major competing philosophies, one of which was that of the professional groups who saw themselves as patient advocates (nurses and social workers for example) and those who were primarily concerned with collecting factual evidence on the existence of clinical syndromes (physicians, dentists and speech therapists being examples of these). The difference in professional values, socialisation and thereoretical perspectives will lead to conflict (Mailick and Ashley 1981). Coser (1956) attributed this to a rigid social system, where the expression of conflict is suppressed. If however the social system was flexibly organised, he reasoned, so that the conflict was not central to the existence of the group, it would revitalise social norms, release tensions and maintain relationships within a team. Coser described this as the "Social Conflict Theory". Sands et al (1990) further expanded this idea when they blamed different values and theoretical perspectives for causing divergent opinions within a team. They identified the need for a common language, common values and a shared conceptual framework. Indeed they were convinced that "the most salient issue of conflict centres on terminology" (p 60).

There has been much debate regarding interdisciplinary teamwork in health care. Whilst most authors accept and support the concept, arguments continue to rage over who should belong to the core team and what is more who should be the acknowledged leader of this team. Fulop (1976) described a health team as :

> a group of persons who in their work share a common health goal common objectives, determined by community needs, towards the achievement of which each member contributes in a coordinated manner, in accordance with his or her competence and skills and respecting the competence of others. The manner and degree of such cooperation will of course vary and has to be solved by each society according to its' own needs and resources. There can of course be no universally acceptable composition for a health team.
>
> (Ibid : 436)

Lewis (1986) issued a list of observable behaviours which he believed should be identifiable in an effective team - equal clinical authority within own particular areas of competence, direct personal and legal responsibilities for their own omissions and actions, a consensus decision about care and treatment, no individual able to over ride the others except those of an exclusive professional domain and a mutual respect for the roles and skills of each team member. Lewis would appear to support equality but as with so many of the papers published on this subject there remains room for doubt as there are so many grey areas. The exclusive professional domain, as has been previously discussed is one of the greatest causes of insecurity and interprofessional rivalry. Many of the professions would claim exclusive rights to the same skill or expertise and until this problem is resolved Lewis' list is unworkable. The British Psychological Society (BPS) (1986) were sensibly less pedantic in their considerations. They produced an excellent pamphlet in which the unnamed authors tackled the problem in two parts. The first part was devoted to the consideration of professional responsibilities in which they clarified the terminology in common usage and the key issues and in the second part they considered the specific responsibilities of a clinical psychologist in multidisciplinary teams. They implied that a multidisciplinary team consisted of some or all of the following elements : different professionals who meet regularly with each member allocating a significant period of time pursuing the agreed and explicit objectives of the team, these objectives should determine the structure and function of the team rather than vice versa and should be clearly identified in policy documents. The work of the team should be both administratively and clinically coordinated but not necessarily by the same person on all occasions and the team should share a defined geographical basis. They concluded with the statement that in order to be effective the team needs to clearly differentiate those skills and roles which are specific or unique to individual members and those which are common or shared. In this document the authors made the important distinction between 'medical' and 'clinical' responsibility :

> Medical responsibilities arise from formal training, qualification and experience in training. The term 'clinical' has come to cover a variety of skills, professions and settings and is ....too general to identify clearly areas of professional responsibility
>
> (BPS 1986 : 2)

They challenged the right of physicians to assume prime responsibility in each case as they suggested that medical intervention was not always the first and most important action that should be taken when a client seeks help. Examples of this would be the urgent need for social intervention when it may be appropriate for the social worker to be the key worker, in cases of acute psychological distress it may be appropriate for a clinical psychologist to be identified as the key worker. The important point, the authors stressed, was that the key worker should be able to recognise a problem outside his/her own remit and thus refer the case to colleagues in the relevant discipline for further action.

As the pamphlet emphasised, no single discipline has an all encompassing knowledge. The key worker may, or may not, be the team leader. The key worker is usually designated the contact worker for a family, in times of acute illness of a family member it would be appropriate for the general practitioner to take responsibility. The authors suggested that a team could and should still function democratically in spite of the person with prime responsibility. Any outcome of decision making should reflect a general consensus of opinion. They rejected the term 'ultimate responsibility' as being unworkable and untenable and urged other health workers to do the same. Usually no one member of an interdisciplinary team has formal managerial authority. Informal authority frequently occurs as a result of convention, status or experience. One problem which may be experienced by those working in an interdisciplinary team may be that of divided loyalties. This, the writers felt, may become even more prevalent as dual accountability becomes more common. This may be the direct result of being accountable to a manager who does not belong to the same profession as the practitioner, but the practitioner will be also be accountable to a senior member of their own profession. The Government Report "Implementation of the NHS Management Inquiry" (HMSO : 1988) did not take account of this. A professional cannot be professionally accountable to a manager who is not of the same profession.

Brill (1976) discussed the important contribution that each individual's own personal and professional values can bring to a team. He suggested that it was a major factor in developing team cohesiveness in that it "promotes a critical attitude and examination of the principles involved" (p 64) which underpin the whole philosophy of health care. Rowbottom and Hey (1978b) commented that different professions must be able to work flexibly and modify or exchange their roles to a significant degree. The BPS (1986) pamphlet also emphasised the importance of flexibility. Regular team meetings were seen as essential even though members often work closely together anyway. They recommended that a skills audit be undertaken of each team member so that the team can collectively decide who has the most to offer in a given situation. Their proposed skills audit consisted of five main areas, which are self explanatory :

1. *Required clinical practices or procedures* An example of this would be the Mental Health Act where it is legally prescribed who does what when a patient is detained under section.
2. *Restricted practice* This relates to professional qualifications. A medical practitioner is the only professional who is allowed to prescribe controlled drugs.
3. *Core skills* An area of expertise normally expected of one particular group. Behaviour therapy is usually undertaken by clinical psychologists but in the field of mental handicap, qualified nurses are also taught to use this approach.
4. *Basic skills* These are shared by all professions, for example interviewing, assessing and planning care.
5. *Specialist skills* Usually acquired through personal interest, for example counselling, or complementary health therapies.

The authors made some interesting comments concerning the maintenance of confidentiality. They deemed it essential for some information to be shared. The parameters of confidentiality nevertheless must be defined and strictly observed within the team. As they pointed out, it is the responsibility of the person disclosing the confidential information to the rest of the team to disclose only what is deemed essential. They also emphasised the need to obtain consent from the clients themselves or, in the case of children, from the parent or guardian. If explicit consent is not obtained then this must be respected although this would inevitably limit the effectiveness of the team in dealing with the clients' problems. Jacques (1978) did not seem to be able to accept the possibility of maintaining confidentiality within a team. He warned that team decisions implied responsibility of the whole group for the care of an individual patient. Such an arrangement he thought, impaired the right of the patient to a personal and confidential relationship with one person in connection with his/her health care and undermined the ultimate sense of responsibility that an individual professional should experience. He suggested that if the whole question of accountablity and autonomy could be sorted out for once and for all then most of the problems encountered with interdisciplinary teamwork would disappear. He was convinced that if this problem was resolved then the need for teams may even diminish because collateral working relationships would be established with equal status. It would seem that the crucial issue in achieving true collaboration in interdisciplinary teamwork is based on where the responsibility for individual cases lies. It is an easy assumption that teams can undertake collective responsibility, however this does not address the question of what happens when things go wrong. Generally it may be agreed that there is a fundamental obligation for any individual licensed to practice by virtue of his professional membership, to act in certain ways in certain situations. Interdisciplinary teamwork can only effectively work provided there is freedom within the various professional and legal requirements. Rowbottom and Hey (1978) claimed that the most important change needed in order to achieve this freedom was in the personal attitudes of the staff concerned. This they maintained would achieve better continuity, a greater cross fertilisation of ideas and more opportunities for demonstrating and explaining the contributions of the various disciplines.

2.7.1 The leader of the team

One of the most critical factors which seems to affect collaborative interdisciplinary teamwork in health care is the continuing, often bitter, debate of who should lead the team. Medical organisations have argued consistently that a physician should be the team leader as in their opinion only a medical practitioner is adequately trained to take on this role (British Medical Association 1974, Hodkinson 1975, Mitchell 1984 and Webster 1985). Indeed some physicians do not support the idea of a team at all. Appleyard and Madden (1979) launched a vitriolic attack on the concept of teamwork by declaring "....as we see it the multidisciplinary team completely undermines the concept of the registered medical practitioner." (Ibid : 1306) They cited numerous examples of bad practice which had led them to come to this conclusion. Perhaps predictably none of the fault was attributed to medical practitioners ! They may have had a genuine cause for concern as only two years previously the General Medical Council (GMC) had declared that legally the medical practitioner retained ultimate responsibility for the management of patients and if the responsibilities normally undertaken by the doctor were delegated to a person who was not medically qualified then the doctor was liable to disciplinary proceedings (GMC 1977). Appleyard and Madden (1979) eloquently described the problems that they envisaged would arise if there was a conflict of professional interests and suggested that any one individual could sabotage the whole team. Social workers, clinical psychologists and educational psychologists were targetted for particularly harsh criticism. They were accused of causing a dichotomy by their inaction in cases of children with special needs "sometimes when they are asked to do something with which they do not agree, they do not bother to do it or delay taking action for so long that it is ineffective". (Appleyard and Madden 1979 : 1305)

It does not seem to have occurred to Appleyard and Madden that perhaps sometimes the doctor is at fault by failing to take account of the psychosocial reasons that may be the causal factors in causing a child to have problems. Some social workers and all psychologists are, after all, qualified to make these judgements as this is precisely what their training prepares them to do. Traditional medical training which concentrates on the biological disease orientated approach most patently does not. The authors had no doubt that teamwork had "eroded clinical care in geriatric medicine, in psychiatry and in paediatrics" (p 1307). Whatever the rationale behind their discomfiture, it would seem that lack of knowledge, lack of respect for others' expertise and to put it charitably their own insecurity and vulnerability had led to a total breakdown in perception by Appleyard and Madden. This surely strengthens the argument that increased interdisciplinary learning would help alleviate this type of entrenchment. Examination of the letters page in the British Medical Journal (published weekly) for the six months following Appleyard and Madden's publication revealed no response from other medical practitioners at all. It is therefore impossible to state whether others agreed with the authors or not.

Hodkinson (1975) thought that it was essential for the doctor to assume the coordinating role as he was the best person to ensure effective communication within the team. The BMA (1974) put the case more emphatically. Whilst they were sure that all doctors would cooperate with the nursing profession and with other 'medical workers' it did not mean in any way that doctors should "hand over his control concerning the treatment of his patients to anyone else". It is no wonder that there is so much conflict within the caring professions when directives like the above are published. The term 'medical worker' implies assistant to the doctor and the emphasis on 'his' patient does not lead one to believe that the patient has any control over his/her own destiny whatsoever. Webster (1985) found that more than two thirds of the male medical students she questioned believed that physicians were the only appropriate team leaders. They supported this response by highlighting the legal responsibilities that doctors had and the fact that they had the best education and experience. In the same study however, less than half of the female medical students thought that the physician should automatically assume responsibility.

Ferguson and Carney (1970) asked the patients their opinions. Whilst focussing on the relationships between doctor/patient, nurse/patient and social worker/patient they found that the nurse had the most valued relationship with the patient as perceived by the patients themselves. Ferguson and Carney (both consultant psychiatrists) used a psychiatric day hospital for their study. Their hypothesis was that social skills were more necessary than intellectual or diagnostic skills in health professionals when assessing patients' relative values of the above relationships. The main therapeutic emphasis in the day hospital was based on group discussion and patient participation. The quality of the relationships was measured by using simple direct questions in the form of a consumer schedule. Ferguson and Carney collected data for one year from 115 patients. The patients were asked to evaluate their relationships with the staff on a rating scale of one to four with one equating "very valuable" and four indicating "no value at all". Five doctors, three nurses and one social worker were evaluated.

The results demonstrated that in this instance the patients highly valued the relationships they had with the nurses. Of the total number of patients (N=115), 99 (85.8%) ranked the nurses in the top two categories on the rating scale, 69 (60.9%) ranked the doctors in a similar way whilst only 22 (19.2%) valued the social worker as highly. Ferguson and Carney suspected that this result could have been biased by the patients' overall experience at the day hospital. Analysis of different data showed that this was not the case as patients who had recorded their experience as unfavourable were concordant with the enthusiastic group (N=32) in their opinions of the staff. The researchers were also interested in whether a favourable clinical outcome had influenced the patient's choice. 'Favourable clinical outcomes' were classified by the physicians and the social workers as follows :

1. *Category A*. The patient was symptom free and socially fully functioning.
2. *Category B*. The patient had persisting symptoms but was socially fully functioning
3. *Category C*. Persisting symptoms interfering with social functioning.
4. *Category D*. Severe persisting symptoms causing great interference with social functioning.

Ferguson and Carney acknowledged that many independent variables would influence these results, however as they pointed out it was not the causal factors they were examining. Of the patients who were classified in Category A (N=22), ten ranked the nurse first and three the doctor first. The remaining nine patients did not express a preference. Of the patients in Category D (N=20), ten ranked the nurse first, one the doctor, the remaining patients (N=9) expressed no preference. The numbers were too small for statistical analysis, but the two groups yielded similar results.

Ferguson and Carney suggested that a possible explanation for the patient's high evaluation of the nurses was the amount of time that nurses spend with the patients in comparison with both doctors and social workers. A valid point was also made in that there was a mutually shared geographical background between the nurses and the patients that was not evident in the two other groups. This resulted in concommitant "language idiosyncracies and semantic nuances" (p 402) between the patients and nurses. The doctor/ patient relationship they felt was still bound by differential respect and awe and although the social worker was present in the unit for many more hours than any one of the doctors, she was largely ignored. This, Ferguson and Carney suggested, may have been because of a perceived stigma of receiving help from the social services. This small study was of interest and relevance as it was one of the few that measured quantitively patients' attitudes towards the professionals caring for them. The results add credence to the argument that nurses would be the most appropriate people to act as team leaders as they have the greatest number of interactions with the patients and are the most highly valued by the patients themselves.

Parker (1982) believed that leadership should alter depending on the demands being made upon the team at the time. In assuming patient management and co-ordination it could, in her opinion, only be provided by the physician. On the other hand, management of the team itself should be undertaken by a trained manager. From the patient's point of view it would be the person to whom the patient most closely relates (according to Ferguson and Carney (1970) this would be the nurse). In clinical decision making the physician would normally take the lead but sometimes, according to Parker (1972), this could equally be done by a nurse. For charismatic leadership she continued,the team should indirectly elect an individual by allowing, or even encouraging, them to emerge in that role. Kindig (1975) advised a team to determine its individual resources and based on their conclusions select the most appropriate individual to lead the team regardless of their profession. Nodder (1980) advocated a similar approach. Von Schilling (1982) was even less prescriptive. She suggested appointing an external consultant advisor. In her case she was the external adviser to a health team in another European country. It appeared however that she was consulted in circumstances which required some form of mediation. This is therefore suggestive of the need in some situations for a team to go for arbitration, which is not encouraging if the concept of collaboration is to work.

George 1971, Kinston (1983) and Newman (1987) all questioned the traditional hierarchical team structure where the physician was in charge. Kinston (1983) was convinced that team cohesiveness was most evident when it was not accepted as inevitable that the doctor was in charge. Newman (1987) was not sure that doctors were the most appropriate people to "judge the patients' best interests" (p 192). McFarlane (1980) blamed the problems of medical dominance within a team on the traditional disease orientation associated with health care. She suggested that a radical rethink was necessary wherein the patient was always included as part of the team as nothing could be done anyway without his/her consent. She did not wish to imply that the doctor should not be the main decision maker where there was a medical problem, but she reasoned that in many instances patients seek help for psychosocial reasons rather than with ill health requiring a medical diagnosis and that in this instance it was more appropriate for other professions to take the lead.

Abercrombie (1966) further complicated the issue by contending that it was not really necessary for a group to have a leader but he did concede that when a group had a task to perform that it would be accomplished more effectively if a leader was elected. Abercrombie's comments are not helpful, as it is implicit in teamwork in health care that the task to be performed is that of ensuring the highest standards of care for all patients/clients and consequently the task is never completed. For this reason Abercrombie's contentions must be discarded.

Salkind and Norrell (1980) did agree in part with Abercrombie (1966) as they reported that by regularly changing the leadership within their team they were continually revitalised. Ward (1979), a plastic surgeon, believed that providing each team member was regarded as an equal partner then there was no need even to discuss the issue of leadership because as he pointed out, each and every individual was essential for the welfare of the patient. Nevertheless Mitchell (1984) found that doctors had great reservations about nurses acting independently in an autonomous role, whilst Hamric and Spross (1984) warned that if a nurse was to assume either a leadership role or an autonomous role he/she must also be seen as a credible practitioner. Wright (1985) believed that "in theory......the most appropriate leader emerges according to the patients needs" (p 36). Campbell- Heider and Pollock (1987) argued that whilst doctors exercise the most authority, nurses possessed the greater informal power (p 423). They suggested that a collegial arrangement should be agreed in which interdependent practice should be encouraged. Ritter (1989) also referred to collegial teams but wrote that in order for such a team to evolve there must not be a hierarchical leader.

It would seem that there are several differing points of view regarding the leadership of health care teams, some of the arguments are persuasive in that a key worker should be identified according to a patient's specific need (British Geriatric Society and the Royal College of Nursing 1975, Nodder 1980, Parker 1982, Ward 1979, Wright 1985, Ovretveit 1986a, Newman 1987, Campbell-Heider and Pollock 1987, Ritter 1989) whilst others regard stability within the team as being dependent on an identified team leader, frequently the doctor (BMA 1974, Hodkinson 1975, Mitchell 1984). The emphasis on a changing leadership within the team depending on the needs of the patient is the most attractive option, but if this was adopted on a general basis it would still require a co-ordinator who could ensure that each team member was fully informed of any developments. This ethos has in some way been reflected in primary health centres where the 'practice manager' has emerged as a new occupation. Whilst having no clinical knowledge or responsibilities these managers do exactly what they were intended to do, manage and co-ordinate.

There appears to be no dispute concerning the statutory right of the doctor to make a final decision regarding a patient's medical problem, there does however appear to be divergent opinions in other areas of health care. Batchelor and McFarlane (1980) cited the example of patients being cared for in a nursing home. It was obvious to them that the nurse in charge should be the one to make the decisions regarding care unless the patient developed a further medical problem. In these circumstances then it was only right and proper that a medical practitioner should be consulted and then take charge of the case for as long as it was deemed necessary. A further example of the need only to consult a medical practitioner if medical complications occur has been the decision that in normal circumstances a pregnant woman will be cared for and delivered by qualified midwives rather than by obstetricians. The new emphasis will therefore be on the fact of pregnancy being a normal and healthy part of life for a woman. If however, potential or actual complications occur to either the mother or the foetus then she will be immediately referred to an obstetrician (Winterton 1992).

Jacques (1978) described the shift in emphasis for prime responsibility as a default. He identified areas such as care of the elderly, mental health and mental handicap where this change was readily apparent. Tolliday cited in Jacques (1978) expressed a particular interest in autonomy and it's concommitant responsibility. He described autonomy as "............it's possession allows the practitioner to use his judgement without it being subject to scrutiny and modification by anybody else." (Ibid : 43-44). This appears to clarify the issue for all professions who are licensed to practice. Tolliday unfortunately, immediately complicated his statement by then adding: "it entails the right of the client or patient to choose his practitioner and the right of the practitioner to refuse an individual as his client or patient." (Ibid : 44).

In 1996 only physicians and dental surgeons have this right, all other professions unless self employed must accept all patients into their care. It is also questionnable whether patients when dependent on public health services can refuse to accept care from an individual. Nevertheless Tolliday recognised that prime responsibility was a difficult concept as health care was (and still remains) very rarely within the competence of one profession. Batchelor and McFarlane (1980) were quite emphatic that the answer to this problem was that an interdisciplinary team should not have the power of veto over one of it's members when it came to a professional judgement, the individual had to remain responsible for his/her own actions. Rowbottom and Bromley (1978) were also sure that each individual had to be held responsible for his/her own actions otherwise nobody would take responsibility for things going wrong which inevitably from time to time occurred. It was however vitally important that agreement through negotiation was reached even though a regular review of that decision may well need to be taken.

Tolliday (1978) described this situation as one of 'primacy'. He added an interesting footnote to his paper by suggesting that the concept of primacy remained true only while one profession had a greater body of knowledge in a given circumstance than any other profession. He suspected that in certain areas of health care such as mental health, mental handicap and care of the elderly the body of knowledge was becoming increasingly established on an interdisciplinary basis. He believed that the end result may well be an individual who was qualified and practiced "*de facto* as fully fledged practitioners of the discipline" (Ibid : 47) Tolliday seemed to be implying that eventually in some areas of health care the professions would merge and new ones would evolve. An interesting proposition which it is suspected would be rigorously resisted by the members of the established professions. Rowbottom and Jacques cited in Jacques (1978) questioned whether multi-disciplinary team work was what was required in child guidance. They also discussed the merging of the professions as an option because, they continued, of the considerable amount of overlap, both potential and actual, that existed in this field.

They concluded that individuals are bound by the team approach because they have to agree to conform to certain established values, norms and procedures. They raised the subject of 'networks' where practitioners may or may not be known to each other, do not have to consider mutual personal acceptability and do not necessarily work face to face over an extended period of time. The only individual who was not mentioned in their deliberations was the patient.

The issue of confidentiality has already been discussed in this section of the literature review but it should be considered again in this context. One of the most difficult problems to resolve is that of safely maintaining a patient's confidential information. It is a subject of endless debate and rightly the general consensus of opinion amongst the professions is that only when necessary should confidential information be shared with other members of the team (an example of this would be a case conference). When an individual practitioner shares this information with another colleague it is done on an understanding of mutual trust and confidence in each other that this information will go no further. All professions who need access to a patient's notes are bound by law to maintain confidentiality (Batchelor and McFarlane 1980, Dimond 1989). If a 'network' emerged in place of these multi-disciplinary teams, where health care professionals frequently did not know each other, the mutual trust and confidence would inevitably be eroded. This may then result in vital information being withheld or paradoxically highly confidential information being publicised.

Pritchard (1984) suggested a solution to these potential problems when he advocated the introduction of three categories of teams. The first he described as an 'intrinsic team', one which responds to a given situation and changes in composition as a patient's needs change. The team then devolves as the problem resolves. This team needs clearly defined aims and quick reliable communication networks. This team would be ideal for critically ill patients who need a variety of experts to attend to their needs. The second type of team identified by Pritchard was the 'functional team', a team within a team, nurses or social workers work within their own professional teams but they also constitute part of a full team and contribute to strategic planning and policy making. The third team identified by Pritchard was the 'full team' which consisted of all the people working together in any context. Meetings would then consist of functional teams presenting certain agenda items for full team debate. Pritchard's suggestion does in reality exist to a certain extent in 1996. It certainly minimises the problem of maintaining confidentiality as much of the personal information pertaining to a patient can be kept at the intrinsic team level. Sharing of information at the other levels is then possible as the anonymity of an individual can be kept absolutely.

Temkin- Greener (1983) reviewed the existing literature looking for evidence of empirical work which would clarify many of the issues surrounding the controversy of teamwork but she found very little. In 1996 the situation remains much the same although some evidence has been found relating to primary health care. These papers will be discussed in section 2.7.4. which considers teamwork in primary health care.

2.7.2 Teamwork in a hospital setting

As early as 1964 teamwork in caring for the mentally ill was being advocated. Barker (1964) described the success of psychiatric teams in Shropshire U.K. Patients were allocated to health care teams who then became totally responsible for their patients welfare. Barker (a consultant psychiatrist) described the team as consisting of the patient, a consultant psychiatrist, a trainee psychiatrist, a psychiatric nurse, a psychiatric social worker, a mental welfare officer and the general practitioner. Barker described as a constant feature "frequent discussions and communications between all members of the team........ in which patients are encouraged to participate" (p 286). Unusually for 1964 the team was involved in both the care of the patient when in hospital and then the continuation of care in the community. The overall aim was to maintain wherever possible the patients in their own homes. The success of this strategy Barker claimed was that the number of readmissions to hospital was much lower. No data was given to support this claim and so the report must be treated with caution. Nevertheless it would appear that the team concept worked and certainly nearly thirty years ago it was both innovative and futuristic.

Court (1972) a paediatrician, considered the health team's contribution to child health. For 1972 this was a remarkable paper in that Court put parents firmly in the leadership role. He also included in his team school teachers, general practitioners, health visitors, nurses, paediatricians, social workers and speech therapists. The order in which these professions were presented is interesting in that the description of the team starts with the concept of the healthy child and then moves through the continuum to the sick child involving the other professions when necessary. It was assumed far too often, according to Court, that mutually defined and acceptable working relationships existed in childrens health care. He regretted that this was not the case. His suggested solutions for improving matters included the adoption of interdisciplinary case notes, joint development of ward policies and shared learning in the professions. He accused the medical and nursing professions in particular, of developing in "parallel rather than partnership" and rather cynically continued "we must hope that both professions are still teachable" (p 52). Court believed that tensions between the professions would lead to a destructive and disabling pathology. He advocated primary prevention or at the very least early diagnosis and treatment as a way to achieve collaboration.

In a paper presented to the American Society of Pediatrics (sic), Wise challenged paediatricians to become less blinkered in their approach to child health (Wise et al 1974). Wise insisted that the only way to ensure quality care was to take a collaborative care approach allowing each discipline to make its own unique contribution. This kind of approach he asserted "has far greater potential........than the piecemeal approach that is common today" (Ibid : 538)

There were, in his opinion, two major barriers to making this concept a reality. Inappropriate training leading to role conflict and the traditional organisation structures. It was naive to bring together a group of highly diverse people and expect that by calling them a team they would behave as one. Because of the traditional hospital structure the staff actually delivering care were frequently passive recipients of decisions made at the top of the hierarchy. Wise cryptically remarked that "the last kind of nurse wanted on a hospital ward is a problem solver" (p 538). Nurses must take charge instead of receiving orders, as nursing, according to Wise, was the profession which could ensure continuity of care. Role ambiguity, role conflict and role overload are the critical factors which affect team working. Wise described the problems faced by the Dr Martin Luther King Medical Center in the Bronx and identified the greatest barrier to effective teamwork and decision making as "the diverse cultural backgrounds of team members" (p 540). High status members Wise observed, tended to speak first and most convincingly on all issues. This meant that other members of the team tended to keep silent and not challenge or confront the speaker. The result of this strategy was that conflict was buried and any positive feelings which may have surfaced were effectively ignored. Wise admitted that their interdisciplinary team was not working and was a problem that he and his colleagues had needed to address urgently. The question was posed of how the team could become autotherapeutic. Wise decided to use an action research approach in which he collected relevant data, summarised the findings and disclosed them to the team, planned action to be taken and then collated the evaluations of the action taken and discussed the results with the team.

At the beginning of the project each individual team member was interviewed in order to ascertain his/her personal perception of team goals, own contribution and preferred decision making styles. Marked similarities and differences were identified. The most positive outcome at this stage was the expression of relief that the problems had been exposed for all to see. Wise noted that from this time the team members seemed to share ownership of the problems. The action planning stage involved collectively developing priorities, suggesting alternative solutions, developing a clear set of objectives, allocating individual and sub-group responsibilities and identifying a mechanism which would accurately monitor progress. Wise saw his role, as leader of the project, as helping the team to develop positive attitudes towards change. One observation made by Wise of relevence to this current study, was the plea for a greater knowledge of the behavioural sciences made by several members of the team. Wise justified this plea by explaining that without a knowledge of cultural norms and values, group dynamics, interpersonal skills and self esteem an interdisciplinary health team's "internal processes are inappropriate, it is likely to be no more than a collection of single entities treating sub-parts of single patients." (Wise 1974 : 542) No data was presented in this paper and Wise did not disclose the number of staff interviewed or the professions represented. The action research model did however seem to be an appropriate methodology to adopt should a more rigorous study be undertaken.

In the only article found on teamwork in dentistry, Craig (1970) concentrated on the problems of delivering effective dental care in England. It was an anecdotal, superficial paper which did not evaluate the effectiveness of teamwork. The team described by Craig was understandably very specialised and small. It consisted of a dental surgeon, a dental nurse, a dental hygienist and a dental technician. The team goal was to provide comprehensive dental care with the dental surgeon as the team leader who developed the treatment plan. It could be argued that the team concept was not described here at all and the same would be true in most dental practices in 1996. It would be more accurate to describe a group of individuals with specialist expertise who are employed by the dental surgeon who prescribes the treatment that the others then undertake. Effective communication between all the staff would be paramount but mutual decision making would appear to be less evident in dental practice.

Evers, (1977, 1981) a psychologist, focussed on the existing patterns of work organisation in hospital wards. She posed the question of whether these patterns enhanced total patient care as she considered that patient care was not exclusive to any one profession. Nevertheless she recognised that with the relative autonomy of the different professions it was unlikely that exact agreement on priorities could be achieved. She believed however that it should be possible to work towards the common goal of quality total patient care by ensuring that "specific problems be quickly resolved by smooth negotiation" (p 590). In order to achieve this integrative approach, mutual understanding of the different professions must be reached. In this small piece of empirical research Evers was particularly interested in the views of the nursing profession. She justified this by explaining that nurses without doubt were the only group that had continuous contact with the patient over a twenty four hour period. Evers described the work of the nurse as being pivotal in any hospital organisation and in informal communication channels. Evers (1977) interviewed nurses (N = 46) from three different wards in the same hospital. Five ward sisters, ten staff nurses and thirty one student nurses comprised the sample. Each were asked to try and ascertain their perceptions of working relationships with medical staff, physiotherapists and social workers. The ward sisters saw themselves as having regular working links with the other professions. Nine staff nurses held the same views. The significant finding was that only three student nurses (N=31) perceived themselves as regularly working with the other professions. It was on this result that Evers concentrated her discussion. She concluded that the students who spent more time at the bedside than the trained staff appeared to be working in isolation from the other professions. Nevertheless their motivation towards establishing stronger interdisciplinary relationships was extremely high.

Evers recognised that student nurses were the least stable members of the team as they tended to change wards every few weeks but she still believed that they had much to contribute to interdisciplinary discussion. She also considered the question of when the apparent transition of perceptions took place. As the trained staff saw themselves as having links with the other disciplines and the students did not, at some stage they must change their minds. Evers recommended that shared learning should take place at an early stage in training in order to minimise the perceived isolation of students. This small study, although inconclusive was worthy of inclusion as Evers was one of the few authors found who considered the contribution that student nurses make towards total patient care. The results of her study provided the information which could have been extended into a much larger project in which nurses from different specialities could have been interviewed. This may have highlighted differences between mental health nurses and surgical nurses for example. It would have been valuable for Evers to have interviewed the doctors, physiotherapists and social workers who worked on the three wards she used in her study. This may have revealed a very different perspective of the perceived working links on the ward.

Four years later Evers (1981) was still studying work organisation and its effect on the concept of teamwork. She focused her attention this time on the process of how elderly patients were managed in the light of any strategies and goals identified. Patient outcomes were measured in terms of ‘well being’ or ‘ill being’ as Evers wryly commented. This project was largely descriptive and was grounded in observational methods. Eight wards, each in different hospitals, were studied and ten to twelve patients were selected from each ward. Evers spent three weeks on each ward collecting data which she obtained through informal conversations with both staff and patients and by analysing the content of written records. A measure of patient/nurse dependency was used and staffing levels were monitored on a daily basis. According to Evers the majority of staff subscribed to the idea that they were members of an interdisciplinary team with the consultant geriatrician as the authoritative team leader. Few staff spontaneously mentioned that the patient or relatives contributed to the team but when asked specifically by Evers "the usual reply was that yes of course the patient was a member of the team" (p 209).

Evers' research, whilst potentially valuable in that she was endeavouring to define quality care, was badly flawed and indeed raises several real concerns. No data in the form of numbers or grades of staff, or the professions to which they belonged were included. A measure of patient/nurse dependency was mentioned but no explanation of which measure chosen was given or the rationale for the choice. The informal conversations with the staff and patients (unless tape recorded for later analysis) could not offer reliable information because of the researcher's lack of accurate recall and the inevitable bias in questioning which will occur without the use of a structured interview.

No mention was made of obtaining the patients informed consent or of any approach to an ethical committee in order to obtain permission to analyse the content of confidential written records. One can only hope that this was in fact done and that Evers merely omitted to include it in her paper, otherwise the staff who participated in the study could be accused of professional misconduct by not acting as the patients advocate. In her conclusions Evers seemed to have become very cynical and negative about the purpose of teamwork in care of the elderly. She believed that teamwork was a strategy for coping with uncertainty, a means of social control over patients and the sub-ordinate professions by doctors, a way of easing the pain of dealing with the lives of a low status social group.... the elderly sick and it helped pass the buck as the dirty work could be left to the other professions.

Feiger and Schmitt (1979) undertook a systematic longitudinal study of team interaction and attempted to show quantitively that particular aspects of team functioning enhanced the quality and efficiency of patient care in comparison with the more traditional fragmented care. Christensen and Lingle (1972) had attempted to prove a similar question by comparing the outcomes for stroke and fracture patients in a team versus a non team setting but no significant difference was found. Feiger and Schmitt (1979) focussed on three main areas in which they collected and analysed data on four multidisciplinary teams in order to test the teams cohesiveness and to see whether this correlated with differences in patient outcomes in each team. The patient sample in the study consisted of thirty elderly persons who were deemed to be chronically ill and all had a diagnosis of diabetes mellitus. No other information was given regarding the existence of additional medical problems. These thirty patients were allocated into the care of four interdisciplinary teams each containing a physician, two nurses and a dietitian. Each team was responsible for developing individualised plans of care for each of their patients. This plan had to demonstrate evidence of assessment of social, physical and emotional function. The team then had to plan and co-ordinate care in a way that was complementary to each other's role and would optimise positive patient outcomes. Once the care plan was devised the team was to meet on a monthly basis to discuss progress. Whilst it is recognised that these elderly patients were classified as chronically sick, a once monthly meeting seems to be woefully inadequate. These meetings were videotaped although some of the recordings were not of a sufficiently high quality to allow a proper analysis of the content. This resulted in an analysis of one group on seven occasions while another group was analysed on only four. The analysis consisted of identifying two types of interactions described as initiated or received. If a team member started a conversation they were awarded one unit of 'initiation', if that team member then included another member, that was an additional initiation credit. Each time the speaker introduced a new subject another initiation credit was awarded. Twelve categories were used to code the meetings:

1. Asks for information.	2. Gives information.	3. Asks for opinion.
4. Gives opinion.	5. Makes suggestion.	6. Gives direction (order).
7. Gives decision.	8. Gives education.	9. Supports or agrees.
10. Disapproves/disagrees.	11 Orientation.	12. Introduces humour.

Feiger and Schmitt (1979) believed that in a collegial group if there was no hierarchical differentiation the initiation rates would be approximately the same for all participants regardless of age, gender or occupation. This hypothesis had already been tested by Wessen (1966) who had measured the communication interactions that occurred both vertically and horizontally in a general hospital ward. He found that communication between the disciplines was nearly always initiated from the higher status occupation to the lower status. He obtained the same results within each discrete profession where the more senior member usually initiated the interaction. Bates (1969) again reported similar findings. Feiger and Schmitt (1979) in their analysis found that the mean percentage of interactions initiated by physicians equalled thirty one per cent, sixty one per cent by the two nurses collectively and nine per cent by the dietitian. In each of the health teams studied the physicians and nurses were reported to have an equally broad scope of expertise whereas the dietitian had a much narrower knowledge. It should be emphasised that the depth of knowledge was not measured, but Feiger and Schmitt suggested that the reason that the traditional hierarchical interactions did not materialise was due to the fact that the nurses had constant interaction with the patients themselves. Nurses, therefore had the most opportunity to glean information that would yield the most information.

The received interactions revealed a different ratio. Forty five percent were received by the physicians, forty two percent by the nurses and six percent by the dietitians. The remaining seven per cent was not attributed to any particular group. Interestingly these results which indicated a collegiate approach, became less persuasive over a period of time. By the end of the study the physicians had increased their number of initiating interactions and the nurses and dietitians had decreased their number. Feiger and Schmitt suggested that this may have been the result of the initial enthusiasm for a collegiate approach diminishing with a concommitant decrease in motivation. Their final results indicated that the traditional physician-nurse interaction pattern was re-emerging. In the analysis of the data from the specific teams, team three was found to be the most consistent throughout the period of the study where as team one was the least. Positive patient outcomes were then measured using the assessment schedule previously described.

The most collegiate team (number three) had cared for the patients who were judged to have the greatest number of positive outcomes whilst the least collegiate team (number one) had patients who were thought to have the greatest number of negative outcomes. Feiger and Schmitt concluded that because of the small numbers no definite statement could be made on the correlation between collegiate teams and positive outcomes of patient care. They believed nevertheless that there were indications that this may well be the case. Feiger and Schmitt recommended an extension of their study to include a much larger number. No evidence has been found that this was undertaken.

Janetekos and Schissel (1979), a social worker and nurse respectively, described the team approach they used in caring for patients in a medical rehabilitation clinic in Rochester USA. The two practitioners started sharing the information they had individually collected on specific client needs and joint assessment was undertaken. Janetekos extended his role as a social worker and started teaching interviewing skills to medical, nursing and social work students on an interdisciplinary basis. The purpose of this was to encourage the different disciplines to adopt a similar approach towards eliciting general information from a client whilst retaining the need to obtain specific information within the professional remit. An unexpected benefit was revealed through using this approach. Janetekos and Schissel found that 'patient manipulation' was reduced once the patient was aware that the professions were working collaboratively. Conjointly the team negotiated long and short term goals with the clients themselves, the philosophy being that individuals should be as active as possible about deciding their own health care. By focusing on client needs Janetekos and Schissel found that their knowledge, experience and practice overlapped. By agreeing that either of them could enter into the overlap in order to gain information which would then be shared, the workload diminished significantly. Clients expressed their appreciation of the fact that they were being treated as individuals and that there was a holistic approach to their problems. Janetekos and Schissel were obviously pleased with the success of their venture.

Snyder (1981) was particularly concerned with the quality of preparation for teamwork that American nurses received in their undergraduate training. She believed that it was especially relevant for nurses as they constituted the largest profession. In her study she used parameters that had been previously identified as essential preparation for teamwork. These consisted of group process skills (Aradine and Hansen 1970, Orem 1971), communication skills (Beloff and Willet 1968) and clarification of other professional roles (Mason and Parascandola 1972 and Rosenaur and Fuller 1973). Snyder (1981) completed a content analysis of three different nursing curriculum, examined their philosophies and developed a questionnaire which ascertained the students attitudes and experiences of health care teams. She then spent some time in the clinical areas as a non participatory observer in order to compare the results of the questionnaires with what actually occured in practice. Her content analysis revealed that "all three schools advocated interdisciplinary collaboration" (p 118) and that focus was made on the parameters described above. Overall the questionnaires returned supported the concept of health care teams (79% where N=169). Fewer nurses believed that they had been given any preparation in teamwork (59% where N=169). Snyder's observation confirmed the students opinions. Minimal interaction was evident in the clinical areas. Snyder proposed that a further study be undertaken; "to determine if personal variables such as self confidence, assertiveness and self esteem were correlated with the degree to which a student interacted with members of other health disciplines." (Snyder 1981 : 121)

No evidence has been found that such a study has been completed. It could be argued that the personality attributes described above enable a self confident, assertive individual with a high self esteem to interact with any group at will. Paradoxically an insecure, self conscious individual who lacks esteem is unlikely to interact with others spontaneously. A study such as the one Snyder suggests would be extremely difficult to undertake as a health care team is inevitably constituted by individuals with differing personality types. If a study was controlled to the extent that individuals were placed in teams depending on their personality this would yield biased results with the distinct possiblity of a strong team and a weak team emerging. Furthermore within each discrete team leaders and followers would still emerge. The team consisting of thos e individuals who lacked security and self esteem would still produce stronger and weaker members within the team itself. Engstrom (1986) as a Registered Nurse in Sweden, was concerned about the quality of information exchanged at the daily multi disciplinary team conferences (MTC) on a neurological unit. Engstrom explained that in Sweden "it is the registered nurses' responsibility to see to it that the patient's need for information is satisfied." (Ibid : 299)

For this reason registered nurses act as chairperson to the MTC. The patient's nurse was invited to report the patient's information problems. Engstrom described information problems as "the patients questions, ponderings, reflections and incorrect conclusions" (p 303). Berglund (1975) cited by Engstrom found that psychosocial problems were not given a priority in health care and that physicians overloaded the MTC with medical aspects of patient care. Patients were therefore given plenty of information regarding their medical problems but insufficient attention was being paid to their other needs. As the nurse had a collaborative function argued Engstrom, this was a further persuading factor in the decision to make the nurse chairperson. In earlier studies Engstrom (1984, 1986) had found that the information given to patients should be shared continuously and in good time so that the patient had time to reflect, ask further questions and receive further answers. She also reported that patients following discharge complained that they had received insufficient information regarding the psychosocial consequences of their disease and the prognosis.

The MTC consisted of physicians, registered nurses, enrolled nurses, counsellors, occupational therapists and physiotherapists. The team remit was to use the daily meeting as a forum for making decisions on or about each patient based on the biopsychosocial model. The conventional medical ward round was stopped but it was agreed that at the end of the meeting the opportunity would be given for the physicians to outline the medical directives. Engstrom tape recorded ten MTC in May 1982. She then analysed the contents using the following classifications ; investigations, treatment, prognosis, aspects of psychosocial and physical care. In all ten meetings the physicians made seventy two (mean score) utterances, the registered nurses made thirty three (mean score) utterances, with the other groups making respectively three, six, and one (mean score) utterances. The total number of patients discussed was one hundred and forty two. Engstrom then embarked on a training programme for the nurse chairpersons. She used problem solving activities, assertion training and enhancing leadership skills as the basis of her programme. The aim was to encourage the chairperson to facilitate the professions other than medicine to make their own utterances thereby theoretically increasing the number of communications concerning the psychosocial needs of patients without diminishing the number of utterances concerning medical needs. Having completed the training programme she then tape recorded a further ten MTC meetings. She used the same classifications for her content analysis. Statistical tests (Chi Square) were used in order to measure the differences between the two groups.

On this occasion one hundred and two patients were discussed in total. The results showed a clear difference. The number of utterances made by the physicians had reduced from seventy two to sixty three (mean score), registered nurses had increased from thirty three to seventy nine (mean score) and the other groups number of utterances had also increased. While the physicians made less utterances no statistical significance was found ($\chi 2 = 1.24$, $P< 0.05$) nevertheless Engstrom suggested that what had occured was an increase in the form of intervention from the other professions. The registered nurse interventions on pyschosocial matters for example, had increased from seventeen (mean score) to sixty seven (mean score). Interestingly Engstrom noted that neither before nor after training was an utterance made by any individual relating to cultural aspects of care. Engstrom concluded that problem solving and decision making should be the main strategies used at the MTC in order to achieve a holistic approach to care. She did not mention patient or relative contribution or participation at all, which was interesting in view of the emphasis on communication and meeting the psychological needs of the patient. This would not have pleased Evers (1977, 1981) who pleaded for patient and relative participation in health teams. Engstrom's study (1986), was persuasive on initial analysis. Further examination however indicated several fundamental flaws in the methodology. She did not mention any variables which may have affected the results. While it was made clear that fewer patients were discussed in the post training meetings (N=142 pre training, N=102 post training) the reader was given no indication of the severity of each patient's illness or whether any of the patients were re-admissions. Factors such as these would have a considerable influence on the results. There was no information about the individual members of the MTC. The initial recordings were taken in 1982 with the second batch of recordings in 1984. The constituent members of the MTC would undoubtedly have altered in two years and it could justifiably be argued that the group dynamics could have dramatically changed. These important omissions negate the efficacy of this study.

Dunlop and Hockley (1990) concentrated on the hospital/hospice interface and how a support team could improve the quality of care given to terminally patients and their families. They focused particularly on the hospital setting as they knew that more than fifty per cent of all cancer patients die in hospital. Some researchers have found that the figure is more than sixty per cent (Lunt and Hillier 1981). Dunlop and Hockley (1990) stated that without clear objectives no team could work cohesively. They suggested that topics such as the relief of distressing symptoms, counselling and support for both staff and relatives and death education should all be learned on an interdisciplinary basis. They were sure that a knowledge of psychology and sociology was a basic pre-requisite of terminal care. Each profession that had any involvement with caring for the terminally ill should be actively encouraged to share learning. They suggested that team review independent of team meetings was essential for effective interdisciplinary care. The review should be used as a forum for stress management and conflict resolution. An objective facilitator was also considered imperative. The effects of contact with the dying was emphasised. Evidence that nurses in particular come into contact with the dying very early in their training is available (Whitfield 1979, Broome 1990) although Ahmedzai (1982) reported that more than thirty per cent of medical students graduate without actively participating in caring for dying patients. McCue (1982) reviewed the emotions expressed by doctors when dealing with dying patients as being those of anger, avoidance, fear and despair. Degner and Beaton (1987) cited in Dunlop and Hockley (1990) found that the emphasis on teaching the biological sciences in medical schools left doctors ill prepared for the realities of the dying patient in clinical practice. Dickinson and Pearson 1980, Hoy et al (1984), Hoy 1985 and Nash (1984) suggested the adoption of interdisciplinary role play as a method of exposing medical students to the job of breaking bad news. Their position adds weight to the argument for introducing role play for situations such as caring for the dying at the beginning of each profession's curriculum.

In summary, evidence has been found of a number of initiatives in teamwork in the hospital setting. Most have been of a descriptive anecdotal nature which have on the whole described the perceived successes of teamwork. Little evidence has been found of an empirical nature which substantiates the claim that teamwork is the best strategy for achieving holistic quality care in a hospital setting. Nevertheless the rationale for its introduction and advancement would appear to be based on a sound philosophy and it begs the urgent attention of future research projects.

2.7.3 Teamwork in primary health care

The importance that is placed on effective teamwork in primary health care can be witnessed by the number of Government publications which demand evidence of its existence (Royal Commission on the NHS 1979, DHSS 1981, DHSS 1986a, DHSS 1986b, DHSS 1987, DHSS 1989). Over the last twenty five years it has become increasingly apparent that the concept of teamwork in primary health care has been adopted in a variety of ways. Indeed it has been suggested that the phrase 'teamwork' is vague and obscure in that it is interpreted quite differently by individual teams depending on the circumstances in which that team is functioning. The Central Council for the Education and Training of Social Workers (CCETSW) summarised this problem most succinctly; " Teamwork has become one of those nebulous phrases. Everyone would lend it support in the same way as everyone would vote for a sunny summer. Yet the precise meaning and content has become obscured." (CCETSW 1989: 8)

Many authors have addressed this issue and while most have centred their attention on the examination of teamwork in small geographical areas, the World Health Organisation in 1979 published a document which reflected its increasing concern about primary health care in the whole of the Third World. A detailed examination of health care structures in rural areas was undertaken and a general agreement reached that every health care worker should function with other personnel in a carefully composed team which reflected varying types of skill and knowledge. The WHO was entirely convinced that "The team as a whole has a greater impact than the sum of the contribution of its members. The concept of teamwork implies a co-ordinated delivery of health care" (WHO 1979b: 15).

Siegel (1974) had previously described the interdependent behaviour of a team as synergistic in that it "produces an effect that is greater than the effect produced by an individual's efforts".(Ibid: 342). The WHO advocated extending the membership of the primary health care team by including environmental health workers, agricultural workers and school teachers and implored that all educational programmes should reflect the interdisciplinary nature of health care by offering shared learning opportunities. They continued :

> The purpose of such training is to enable health team members to learn how to work efficiently together ..... Changes in the expectations and needs of the community should lead to parallel changes in the health delivery system itself and in the training of health team members.
>
> (WHO 1979b: 19)

Parker (1972) in a frequently referenced monograph examined the team approach to primary health care. She described many existing teams as 'professional confederations' many of which worked with minimal co-ordination. For this reason she regretted the fact that the word 'team' had been adopted into common usage as "it has come to mean everything and therefore nothing" (p 2). She explored the issues that surrounded the use of teams and stated emphatically that she was a strong advocate of the need for teamwork as the health needs of an individual could not be met by a single profession. Parker maintained that not only were different skill levels desirable but essential. The rationale for this she attributed to the "spiralling health care costs and inefficiency in the use of available resources" (p 5). Each individual practitioner should operate to the highest level at which they were effective as in this way resources could be fully utilised (a point also emphasised by McPherson et al in 1982). An interesting concept introduced by Parker (1972) was the idea that because of cultural and social differences in patient groups, health care professionals of similar cultures or social groups should be encouraged to work with minority groups. The need for nurse practitioners with particular responsibility for minority groups was recognised in the United Kingdom over a decade ago and there are now many health visitors and clinical specialists specifically appointed for this purpose.

Parker believed that in order to remain responsive to the constantly changing demands of the patients an effective team should be both flexible and dynamic. Nevertheless it should operate within a framework in which parameters were set. She prescribed a fixed structure in which core primary health care workers were identified to whom patients normally related. Where necessary additional personnel were then consulted. Without realising it, Parker (a Californian) was advocating the model adopted in the United Kingdom whereas in the USA each family directly consults a specialist. Furnham et al (1981) believed that the concept of teamwork in primary health care was only "an informal, voluntary and transitory liaison" (p 291) anyway and that it was the medical practitioner who was not only the undoubted team leader but also the person who called together a tailor made temporary team in order to meet a patients specific needs. Depending therefore on the doctor's willingness to delegate to allied professions, the team may or may not react positively. They concluded that the doctor was the "prime mover" (p 291) although they did point out the paradox that social workers and health visitors can be approached directly by a patient without reference to the doctor. Bowling (1981) examined delegation in general practice for her doctoral thesis. Her findings were later published in a book which has subsequently been widely quoted by other authors. Before concentrating on delegation itself, Bowling reviewed the development of health centres and health care teams. She defined a team as "a group of people who make different contributions towards the achievement of a common goal." (Bowling 1981: 29)

Bowling found no evidence of the ideally organised team and indeed suggested that such an ideal was as yet unknown. She warned that the presence of different professions under one roof did not constitute a team and continued that unless each discipline understood the purpose of teamwork and until effective communication channels were operative, the professions would not work together effectively. Gilmore, Bruce and Hunt (1974) found that lack of time and opportunity to meet led to mis-understandings between team members and that breakdown in communication was the major cause of problems encountered in primary health care. The blame was attributed to educational establishments' failure to promote integrated learning between the professions. Bowling (1981) seemed to re-inforce earlier findings by Dingwall (1976) in that the delicate issue of leadership caused resentment and resistance within the team itself. She identified traditional subservience by nurses to the medical practitioners and yet the issue of legal responsibility and accountability seemed insurmountable. For the last few years Practice Nurses have further complicated the issue as they are employed by the general practitioner and are therefore answerable to a member of another profession. Practice nurses (as with all registered nurses) are only licensed to practice through the UKCC and are therefore bound by the UKCC Code of Conduct (1992) (previously described). In the event of malpractice to whom is the practice nurse accountable? No definitive answer has yet been given but it could be argued that both the employing medical practitioner and the UKCC could decide that the individual nurse was unfit to practice. Waters, Sandeman and Lunn (1980) delegated many tasks to a practice nurse and stated that her contribution to their practice was invaluable. They argued that many of these tasks would not be delegated to the nurse if she was employed by a health authority because of the innumerable restrictive practices operated by health authorities. Whilst adding weight to the theory that a registered nurse is far more capable than health authorities are usually prepared to acknowledge, Waters, Sandeman and Lunn did not signify whom would take ultimate responsibility in the case of an accident. This highlights Batchelor and McFarlane's (1980) concern which was who would take responsiblility if anything went wrong? As they pointed out it is usual for a patient to sue an individual health authority if anyone other than a doctor made an error. In practice however the law states that each "professional is responsible for actions or omissions within his own sphere of competence and there is no difference in the legal status of responsibility" (Ibid: 13).

In primary health care this situation is manifestly complicated by the fact that so many other professions may be involved on an autonomous basis. Examples of these would include a dental surgeon, a pharmacist, an optician or a podiatrist. An individual client may consult any of these as well as consulting members of the core primary health care team in a health centre. Contradictory advice and treatment may be the end result and trying to attribute legal responsibility would be extremely difficult.

Parker (1972) advocated that the team must be allowed to function autonomously with control of its own resources, work area and support staff. In 1986 the Cumberledge Report recommended exactly the same approach in the UK. Parker felt that unrealistic expectations of a team led to frustration and a breakdown in morale. This she believed was due in part to the demands of individual consumers (the patients). She made a valid point when she wrote "it is the system which is continuing ..... the patient can step in and out as he or his advisors feel is necessary." (Parker 1972: 46)

Blackett et al (1957) had previously illustrated this point when they studied the social problems affecting the health of a small rural community. After a social worker was appointed to a practice he visited every family registered in that practice. The number of identified social problems directly contributing to ill health increased by 50%. Once solutions had been sought and the problems solved the number of visits to the medical practitioner decreased dramatically. Kane and Kane (1969) found that the majority of physicians believed that they could more than adequately care for patients without the contribution of other health care professions. It would appear that patients disagree if Silver (1968) is to be believed. He reported that 90% of his patients saw a combined approach to health care as a desirable trend. Both these reports must however be treated with some caution as no raw scores were published and consequently the validity of the results is at the very least questionable. Dingwall, cited in Clare and Corney (1982), focused on an analysis of the teamwork concept in primary health care. He suggested that successful organisation within a team hinged on the perceptions of individual team members in regard to relevant or irrelevant events. In other words was the problem worth solving or could it be disregarded? Dingwall described this as an internalised inclusion or exclusion. Dingwall found that the decrease in medical dominance had led to problems of instability in the team as there was no longer an acknowledged leader or expert. He wryly observed that whilst the nursing and social work professions had broken away from medical dominance, doctors still perceived themselves as being the most prestigious breed of health care worker. The expectations were that the medical contingency would continue to issue the orders and the other professions execute them. Navarro (1977) described this influence as unhealthy and drew attention to the problem by stating that 'class structure' militated against holistic care. Dingwall atttributed gender and male dominance as the predominant factor as traditionally most doctors were male and other health professions were female. Dingwall raised an interesting point when he observed that women rather than men were more likely to gain access to a client's home and that home visiting for health reasons rather than social reasons was more likely to be acceptable to the clients. He was rather pessimistic in his conclusions as to whether the true ethos of teamwork would ever be truly achieved.

Many authors have published papers pertaining to teamwork in primary health care. Most of these have been subjective descriptive accounts of small scale developments in health centres in either the UK or the USA (Brocklehurst 1966, Wallace 1966, Aradine and Hansen 1970, Beloff and Korper 1972, Tanner and Soulary 1972, Brooks 1973, Eskin 1974, Eskin 1975, Dingwall 1975, Lambert and Riphagen 1975, McCally et al 1977, Hendy 1978, Corney (cited in Clare and Corney 1982), Williams and Clare 1982, Hamel and Cope 1983, Craft and Brown 1985, Bumphrey 1989, Fraser Holland 1989, Josce 1989). In summary these authors report improved patient satisfaction when two or more health professions make the effort to increase collaboration. Examples were reviewed of effective teamwork in caring for the elderly in the community (Brocklehurst 1966, Eskin 1974, 1975, Strang et al 1983), families with predominantly social problems (Aradine and Hansen 1970, Beloff and Korper 1972, Tanner and Soulary 1972), mental health and mental handicap (Eskin 1974, 1975, Craft and Brown 1985). Other authors had concentrated on the existing conflict between one or more of the professions. As has been previously described, the relationship between social workers and health care workers seems to have held a particular fascination for many of the authors (Aradine and Hansen 1970, Beloff and Korper 1972, Tanner and Soulary 1972, Brooks 1973, Eskin 1974, 1975, Dingwall 1975, Lamberts and Riphagen 1975, Hendy 1978, Corney 1982, Williams and Clare 1982). A few had attempted to report findings of a more rigorous nature (McCally 1977, Beloff and Korper 1972, Williams and Clare 1982). On initial examination the paper by McCally et al (1977) seemed promising as the abstract indicated that they had conducted a survey of interprofessional learning activities in order to test their hypothesis that; " health professions students who share appropriate portions of their educational programme will perform more effectively as team members in the delivery of primary health care." (McCally et al 1977: 178)

Fifty four medical students and sixty nursing students participated in the study. McCally et al interviewed the students by telephone using a structured questionnaire. No measure of the reliability or validity of the questionnaire was made and no statistical analysis undertaken of the results obtained. Results were presented in percentages only although the reader was told previously that only 45 of the medical students aproached agreed to participate and 53 of the nurses. The content of the 8 item questionnaire was not revealed and repeated reading of the paper extracted only two identifiable statements which were presumably used as questions, whether interprofessional education was a recognised occurence in the students' programmes (80% of the medical students and 74% of the nurses confirmed that it was) and whether there was a specific individual, a specific programme or a specific committee which organised interprofessional education (50% of the medical students and 38% of the nurses replied positively). The paper must be heavily criticised for several reasons. It is impossible to assess the efficacy of their work as so much of the raw data has beeen omitted. They draw conclusions which cannot be verified as neither the questions nor the reponses have been included. The questionnaire apparently contained only yes/no responses. An element of bias cannot therefore be excluded particularly as no pilot study was conducted which would have tested the reliability and the validity of the instrument. Whilst Kindig (1975) had called for greater efforts to be made in gathering empirical evidence on interdisciplinary learning, it is suspected that he would not have been supportive of work of such poor quality.

Very few studies have been identified that merit detailed analysis in this review of the literature (Gilmore, Bruce and Hunt 1974, Milne 1980a, 1980b, 1980c, Bond et al 1987, Harding and Taylor 1990, Gregson, Cartlidge and Bond 1991, Hutchinson and Gordon 1992 being notable exceptions). An authorititative study which examined the work of health care teams was undertaken by Gilmore, Bruce and Hunt (1974). They collected extensive data over a one year period from three carefully selected health care teams. To substantiate their findings they also collected similar information from 36 similar teams. The main impetus for the research was to assess current health visitor training and to provide guidelines for future curriculum development. Prior to the commencement of the main project a pilot study was undertaken in Brighton in 1967/8, in which the work undertaken by health visitors and district nurses was assessed in situations which were considered by Gilmore et al to be conducive working conditions. 'Conducive' was defined as enabling "the development of innovative and integrative working methods" (p 13). The study co-incided with the inception of a team and a consequent induction course for the health visitors and district nurses prior to their commencing in the practice. The induction course addressed the issues of role clarification, research methods and topical medical subjects. Much of the study is not relevant to this current research, nevertheless some aspects have a particular significance and have been selectively included. Strict criteria were applied for the selection of the three main teams included in the study. These included that each team had to be "in the process of forming" (p 14), each team was to be based permanently on the same premises, the team co-ordinator had to be a nurse and the client population had to be at least twelve thousand in number. Ten inclusion criteria were originally identified but the researchers found only one team in the whole of England and Scotland that fulfilled all ten. The attempt to exclude all independent variables was patently unsuccessful. This adds credence to the claim by some authors that each team is a unique entity (Parker 1972, Dingwall 1976, Batchelor and McFarlane 1980). A further pilot study was undertaken in Scotland in order to assess effective teamwork and sufficient data was gathered through a questionnaire and an interview to persuade the researchers that this was the appropriate method for the main study. Their six randomly selected teams were invited to contribute information. Gilmore et al described these teams as similar in certain repects to the three main teams. Reviewing the criteria for these teams however revealed a major discrepancy; " members of the team should be working together for at least six months before the commencement of the survey, so that they would have had time to establish team relationships and working patterns." (Gilmore et al 1974: 16)

This would appear to be the complete antithesis of the original inclusion criteria, that of a team in the process of forming. Role conflict, interpersonal relationships and professional autonomy may well have already emerged by the time these teams were surveyed. Not surprisingly eighty two teams in England and Scotland fulfilled the criteria and from these thirty six were randomly selected. The number of personnel participating in the study was 174 general practitioners, 70 health visitors and 57 district nurses (N = 39 Teams including the 3 original teams). One researcher visited all 39 health centres and undertook 'personal discussions' with the participants. A forced choice questionnaire of 56 items was self administered by the respondents in all the teams. These 56 items were of a broad basis which was relevant to every team member, examples were cited as "assessment of clinical, social and emotional needs, communicating and co-operating" (p 18). Specific clinical skills which applied to one profession only were excluded.

The response rate for the returned questionnaires was described as 150 (79%) general practitioners, 70 (88%) health visitors and 58 (85%) district nurses. Analysis of the raw data did not seem to correspond with the original numbers given. Further examination of the report however yielded the fact that the three main teams in the study had not been included in the original numbers described. This caused confusion and misinterpretation for the reader and as such must be considered a weakness in the study. One of the most significant findings was that communication in all thirty nine teams consisted mainly on a one to one basis if and when the need arose, other strategies included the writing of memos, passing information via the receptionist and occasionally in a scheduled meeting. The type of information the receptionist was asked to convey from one person to another was not described but if any of this information was of a confidential nature the health professional disclosing this could be guilty of breaching confidentiality and thus be in a very vulnerable position legally.

Gilmore et al (1974) reported that considerable emphasis was placed on personal compatibility within teams by the team members themselves in ensuring effective teamwork. The general practitioners in particular and most of the health visitors and district nurses believed that the doctors should be involved in the selection of new members of nursing staff to the team. Interestingly participation by the nursing staff in the selection of new general practitioners was not seen to be essential. This rather negates the ideal of teamwork being dependent on good group dynamics as the opinions of a large part of the team are excluded. It also puts the general practitioner firmly into the role of the hierarchical leader of the team. The authors commented on the fact that many individuals were reluctant to admit the existence of any conflict in the team. This they suggested may be due to the possibility that individuals perceived an inadequacy in their own interpersonal skills (p 102). Further findings of relevance to this current review were the recommendations that receptionists and clerical staff should be included as an integral part of the primary health team and that each team must be permitted to generate and develop its own destiny from within. Any conflict within a team may be resolved more quickly and more effectively if an objective outsider is consulted.

As early as 1964 Swift and MacDougall were extolling the virtues of nurses attached to general practices. In an article describing the successful collaboration between general practitioners, health visitors and district nurses the authors (who were the general practitioners) categorically stated that the nurses were accepted as full and equal colleagues and "not in any way directed in what they do, but rather their help is enlisted when required." (p 1697). It appears from their detailed account that daily meetings took place between the medical and nursing staff. Positive regard was expressed for the contribution of the nursing staff. Many personnel working in health centres in 1993 would doubtless wish for such a positive attitude. Nearly thirty years ago this Hampshire practice seemed to be demonstrating a real commitment to teamwork. The study undertaken by Gilmore, Bruce and Hunt in 1974 certainly did not find much evidence of this on a nationwide basis. It should be emphasised however that an element of self flattery may have been present in Swift and MacDougalls paper. While recognising that an element of cynicism may be evident, it would have been very useful to have read an article written by the nurses employed in this practice which confirmed and endorsed the doctors comments!

In 1980 Milne completed a study in Aberdeen in which she explored the problems of duplication between some of the members of the primary health care team. She also examined the extent of role appreciation between student general practitioners, student health visitors, student district nurses and student social workers. Milne, a health visitor herself, undertook this work as the result of her increasing concern that "all was not as it should be within the primary health care team" (Milne 1980a: 61). Ignorance of roles, fear of erosion of responsibility and status were postulated by Milne to be the main cause of inefficiency and communication breakdown in primary health care teams. She debated at length the connotation of the word 'overlap' and suggested that it is both an expressive and emotive word when related to teamwork and professional roles. Some team members may perceive it as a desirable trait as it better utilises resources, whereas others perceive it as intrusive and threatening to their own expertise. Milne sub-divided 'overlap' into two categories, desirable and undesirable. Desirable overlap, Milne beleived, could be "complementary and therefore healthy for intelligent co-operation" (p 62). Undesirable overlap could be insidious leading to confusion and frustration within the team itself and most importantly to the patient who is the recipient of the overlap. Milne suggested that some of the current doubt that teamwork was not effective was due in part to the problem of overlap. This has also been expressed by Gilmore, Bruce and Hunt 1974, Ratoff 1974, Hicks 1978, Irvine 1979, Bond et al 1987, Harding and Taylor 1990, Gregson et al 1991. Overlap may in fact be the "root cause of defective communication" (Milne 1980a: 63). Other authors have made similar observations (Hunt 1972, Dingwall 1976, Hasler and Klinger 1976, Alaszewski 1977 and Bowling 1981). The debate seems to hinge yet again on professional identity, role conflict and the attempts by professional groups to extend their own areas of responsibility.

Milnes study aimed to demonstrate common functioning in the professions and therefore identify areas of overlap. She emphasised (1980c) the fact that the whole philosophy of team work should be to ensure that patients' needs were comprehensively met. Her research method involved a patient management questionnaire in which four fictitious case histories were described and open ended modified essay questions then formulated. Sixteen students from each of the four occupations previously described participated in the study (N = 64). The case histories were presented in such a way that the information was appropriate and realistic for all four professions. In order to compare the results with a 'normal' method of working, ie. a case conference, Milne divided her volunteers into two groups. Eight students from each profession formed the experimental group (N = 32). This group were invited to discuss the cases randomly with other members of the same group having previously completed the questionnaire. The control group were asked to refrain from discussion with members of their own group (N = 32). All 64 respondents were required to nominate the team members they considered most suited to make an assessment and to give the rationale for their choices (1980b).

In total 641 'assessors' were chosen by the 64 respondents. Milne reported that, apart from the district nurses who proposed health visitors on 53 occasions against themselves on 51 occasions, all groups significantly nominated themselves more often than they nominated the others (1980b). The general practitioner students, for example, nominated themselves 56 times but only nominated the other three groups collectively on 103 occasions. This, Milne concluded, was at least evidence of the other professions being perceived as relevant. She also suggested that these findings further supported the view that professional conservatism was present at the student stage. This supposition however can be refuted and represents a major flaw in Milne's study. Students undertaking training as general practitioners, health visitors and district nurses are all qualified practitioners in their own right. They have previously completed an extensive training, most of which has been experienced in the acute hospital sector. Numerous authors (annotated in section 2.6 Interprofessional Conflicts) have demonstrated that role set, interprofessional conflict, and the traditional hierarchical system are already in existence by the time students undertake post graduate continuing education. Paradoxically the social work students have not undertaken previous training and may not therefore have the same attitudes. The social work students are the only respondents in this study that can be really classified as 'students'.

Milne found that there was a high specifity of choice for some of the assessors identified. This was not entirely surprising as the general practitioner was chosen as the most appropriate person to deal with a person who had taken a drug overdose (a medical emergency) while the social worker was chosen as the most appropriate person to deal with a mother who had no money to buy clothes for her children (a social emergency). However Milne found instances where the students lacked conviction of their own potential (1980c: 584). When a family was in need of support and encouragement the nominations were much less clear. As the families specific problems were not described it is difficult to comment apart from the fact that this would seem to substantiate other authors who have suggested that the team leader (or link person) should depend on the current problem a family is experiencing (Ferguson and Corney 1970, Beloff and Korper 1972, Wise 1974, RCN 1975, Beynon 1978, Hutt 1980, Hutt 1986, Croen et al 1984). Many students in Milne's study considered themselves to be making the major contribution. Milne commented that this may be the result of teaching them that they can assess numerous problems in different situations. Health visitors' roles were seen as being complementary to the general practitioners' although when dealing with psycho-social care the social work students felt they had the monopoly whereas the other three groups saw this as a shared responsibility. Milne quite rightly suggested that very often it would be the professional who was first on the scene who would take prime responsibility by offering urgent intervention before seeking more informed help. Milne was obviously committed to improving the quality of patient care through team collaboration. She believed that whilst each profession guarded their role and what they perceived as 'their' responsibility, progress would not be made. She concluded that constant training and re-training was the key to success and that this was dependent on "the expectations and visions of the students and the young professionals" (Milne 1980b: 68).

A major study was completed in the middle of the last decade which has been reported in various books and journals (Bond et al 1985, Cartlidge and Bond

1986, Cartlidge 1987, Bond et al 1987, Cartlidge et al 1987a, Cartlidge et al 1987b and Gregson et al 1991). Although there are a plethora of reports they all describe the same study in which an attempt was made to determine "the extent of collaboration throughout England among district nurses, general practitioners and health visitors ..... and to develop indices of collaboration". Bond et al 1987: 158) The target population were pairs of professionals sharing the care of some patients. Each pair was described as a 'potential collaborative unit'. General practitioners were matched with either health visitors or district nurses. A random sample of twenty District Health Authorities (DHA) was produced after all the DHA's (N=199) had been stratified into the following categories, predominantly urban or rural, the number of general practitioners and the number of health centres within which they worked, the number of health visitors and district nurses attached to the health centres. Using the Chi Square test, Bond et al found no significant difference between the characteristics of the sampled and non sampled districts. Bond et al recognised that there could still be an inherent bias in the different health centres within each samples DHA. In order to minimise this they obtained lists of district nurses and health visitors which identified the number of hours each individual worked and whether each was attached to a small or large health centre. Three district nurses and three health visitors were then randomly selected from this group. Similarly 6 general practitioners were sampled after a comparable analysis. There were therefore 12 participants from each district in the initial stage of the project (N = 240). The clearest description of the five different research instruments used in the implementation stage of the project was given by Gregson et al (1991).

A short interview questionnaire was used to collect information regarding demographic data, organisation of individual activities, working environment and professional relationships, a prospective diary, a practice questionnaire which was completed by the general practitioner which elicited organisational data about management of the practice, a semantic differential attitudinal scale in which the respondents were asked to rate the professions of district nursing, health visiting and general practice with particular reference to their own profession and finally the researchers used a semi structured interview which involved the Director of Nursing Services with specific responsibility for community nursing. Sufficient data was collected from these instruments to expand the study. A second member for each collaborative unit was then identified and matched with one of the existing participants (N=480). Random sampling was again used and the final cohort was eighteen matched pairs from each of the twenty DHA's (N=360). In the final analysis 148 general practitioner/district nurse pairs and 161 general practitioner/health visitor pairs eventually completed the study (86% of the total where N=360). The structured interview questionnaire was used and the respondents were asked to rate the closeness of their working relationship with their matched pair on a five point taxonomy of collaboration.

This taxonomy was developed and first described by Armitage (1983), it is simple and well defined and is therefore worth directly reproducing. Having completed the data collection Bond et al (1987) met together to discuss the ratings given to each correspondent and then a judgement was made on the rating of each potential collaborative unit. Each respondent was asked to keep a diary in order to record what they actually did in the week following their interview; of particular importance was the number of patients seen, those referred and the age of these patients. The data obtained from these records revealed that while health visitors saw mainly young children, district nurses saw mainly elderly people and the doctors saw people from all age groups. Other data obtained was that health visitors attended more clinics and had more professional interactions with groups than the other respondents. The average number of general practitioners with whom both the district nurses and the health visitors worked was five but the range was from one to fifty. The district nurses and health visitors who worked with a large number of doctors tended to be working on a geographical basis rather than assigned to a health centre. The average length of time that the matched pairs had worked together was three years. More than a third of the respondents were based in the same building as their pair, although in heavily populated areas the nurses tended to be based some distance away. District nurses and general practitioners reported regular consultation between each other but the health visitors reported less regular communication. The results from the five point taxonomy confirmed the findings. The most frequent rating was level three 'communication'. Bond et al, identified the factors associated with higher levels of collaboration, these included mutual use of first names, clinics where both partners were present, mutual consultation of records, the length of time the pair had worked together, the number of chance meetings, shared decision making, being based in the same building and a high frequency of consultation and referrals.

Bond et al summarised this most interesting study by concluding that only 27% of general practitioner/district nurse pairs and 11% of general practitioner/health visitor pairs were rated as working in partial or full collaboration (levels four and five of the taxonomy). The majority of pairs were rated as working at level 3 - communication. They recommended that efforts should be made to increase the number of health centres in which the different professions could be based which would increase the levels of collaboration. Their final paragraph however warned that further research was needed which examined the "effectiveness of interprofessional collaboration on patient care" (p 161). This study is a good example of a well executed piece of research. Inherent bias had been minimised by stringent analysis followed by random sampling. Nevertheless several criticisms can be levelled. No indication was given of whether the same interviewer interviewed both of the matched pair. If this was the case it may have influenced the eventual rating on the taxonomy. There would have been less possibility of bias if a different researcher had interviewed each individual in

Table 2.3
A taxonomy of collaboration (Armitage 1983)

Stages of Collaboration	Definition
1. Isolation	Agents who never meet, talk or write to one another
2. Encounter	Agents who encounter or correspond but do not interact meaningfully
3. Communication	Agents whose encounters or correspondence includes the transference of information
4. Collaboration between two agents	Agents who act on that information sympathetically : participate in patterns of joint working : subscribe to the same objectives as others on a one to one basis in the same organisation
5. Collaboration throughout an organisation	Organisations in which the work of all members is fully integrated

a matched pair as there would be no previous knowledge or perceptions of the level of collaboration between the pair. The paper does not make it clear whether the structured interview questionnaire contained open ended questions. If this was the case how were the responses analysed? If the questions were mainly closed then the data collected may not be reliable and distribution of the questionnaires would have sufficed therefore dispensing with the need for time consuming interviews. If open ended questions were used then the case for having one interviewer to undertake each individual interview becomes stronger, as the interviewer can then use this information to generate related responses from the other paired partner. In spite of these identified flaws this study is one of the most credible found which examines collaboration and teamwork in primary health care.

On a much smaller scale Harding and Taylor (1990) aimed to "describe the nature of the relationship between pharmacists and general pracitioners in health centres" (p 464). Semi structured interviews was the method chosen. Thirteen general practitioners and ten pharmacists working in health centres were interviewed along with nine general practitioners and ten pharmacists who were not integrated. They had previously undertaken a study which had revealed a high level of consultation and collaboration between general practitioners and pharmacists who were based in the same building (Harding and Taylor 1988). The results of the 1990 study were most interesting. All respondents who worked within a health centre (N=23) perceived their mutual professional relationship as 'very good' or 'excellent' whereas the nine general practitioners and six of the ten pharmacists working independently answered the same question as 'satisfactory'. Within the health centres six of the doctors (N=13) and eight of the pharmacists (N=10) stated that face to face contact was routine whereas none of the independent practitioners stated that this was the case. Eleven of the integrated doctors (N=13) described the pharmacists within the health centres as having a marked effect on their choice of medication for prescription (an unexpected finding was that cost effective prescribing was also much greater in this group). Only three of the independent doctors (N=9) said that the community pharmacists had any influence whatsoever. Some dissonance was expressed by both groups of doctors on the pharmacists' role in providing information to patients regarding adverse reactions to their medication. The major advantage of an on-site pharmacy, perceived by all respondents, was that of easy access for the patient. The doctors also praised the on the spot advice available to them. Whilst acknowledging that the numbers in this study were very small and therefore inconclusive, Harding and Taylor were confident that the advantages of an integrated pharmacy in health centres was demonstrated and recommended that all health centres should adopt this strategy. The taxonomy described by Armitage (1983) would seem to be an appropriate tool to repeat Harding and Taylors' study on a larger scale. Only one other publication was identified that examined the role of the pharmacist in the health care team. Thompson et al (1988) discussed the attitudes that nurses and pharmacists had about each other and concluded that much improvement was needed.

The latest substantial study identified was one completed by Hutchinson and Gordon (1992) who noted in their introduction "Even today many members of teams would question whether they have a common purpose and whether they are understood by their colleagues from different disciplines" (Ibid : 32).

Northumberland Health Authority were aware that many of the problems described in the literature existed in their primary health care teams and in conjunction with the then Family Practitioner Committee (now the Family Health Services Authority, FHSA) debated the issue which ultimately lead to the formation of the Northumberland Primary Care Forum. Membership is held by general practitioners, community nurses, health visitors, midwives, practice nurses, public health officials, nurse managers and health service managers. It was decided in this forum to undertake a small survey of existing teamwork in Northumberland. Twenty practices were chosen of the fifty in the region as financial constraints did not allow a larger study. The county has a mixture of both rural and urban practices and so stratified sampling was undertaken.

The first stage was the identification of ten practices with no more than three doctors in post and ten with four or more doctors in post. According to the authors this tended to mean that the rural practices were included in the sample with three or less doctors. Either the practice manager or the receptionist was actively selected from the twenty practices. General practitioners, practice nurses, health visitors, midwives and district nurses were randomly selected one of each profession from each practice. The target population was 104. Fifty two responses were received from the large practice respondents (N=55) and forty one from the small practice respondents (N=49). The overall response range was therefore 90% (N=93) indicating an exceedingly high level of interest (Oppenheim 1992). The results were most revealing and many were pertinent to this current study. Approximately one third of the respondents confirmed that service provision objectives existed but only one sixth identified any training objectives. A fifth had not received any in service training during the past three years although almost a quarter had undertaken joint learning sessions at some stage. On a rating scale of 1 - 5 staff were asked to indicate their understanding of other team members roles and also to indicate their opinions of how well other team members understood their role. Most of the professions felt that they understood other professions roles well, but they all reported that the other professions did not understand other professions roles very well. Seventy nine respondents felt part of the team (N=93). The others all worked with more than one practice and were geographically isolated. Interestingly these respondents when asked to rank the features of teamwork they most highly valued placed 'understanding the roles of others, sharing expertise, joint training and integrated records' more highly than the rest of the respondents. Hutchinson and Gordon summarised their findings with the comment that membership of a team will never be standardised. They concluded with the challenge that "inflexibility; professional arrogance and jealousy; a need to be in charge; an ability to delegate; and failure to provide mutual support" (p 37) should all be confronted in order to enhance the ethos of teamwork. As they demonstrated the respondents in Northumberland saw role identity, relationships, effective communication and mutual understanding as the central tenets of successful teamwork. For those individuals that are already qualified, in service joint training would seem to be essential in order to enhance this. Future health professionals must however be given the opportunity to learn together from the beginning of their undergraduate training.

In conclusion teamwork in health care would seem to be not only desirable but essential in order to enhance the quality of care offered to patients. Since the Dawson Report was published in 1920 there has been a continual movement towards effective teamwork. It would appear that lack of communication, interprofessional conflict, territoriality, lack of mutual understanding and respect for other professions contributions in both the acute hospital sector and in primary health care have caused the continuing resistance to the concept of teamwork. Until this fundamental change occurs health professionals will only pay lip service to holistic care.

2.8 The behavioural sciences in health care

It is perhaps predictable that the majority of literature which considers the contribution of behavioural scientists in health care should have been written by sociologists and psychologists. Few health care professionals seem to have published papers on a similar theme. Nevertheless if the concept of holistic care is accepted then an understanding of an individual's psychosocial needs is essential. The most appropriate people to introduce these concepts are the behavioural scientists themselves. Bloom (1959, 1964), Samora et al (1961), Pattishall (1970), Gill (1975), Pattison (1975), Dervin and Harlock (1976), Baldwin (1976), Hartings and Counte (1977), Harlem (1977), Costello (1977), Knox et al (1979), Kahn et al (1979), Flaherty and Scharf (1979), Day (1979) Jeffrey (1980), Cassata (1980), Sharf et al (1982), Ley (1982), Field (1984), Irwin and Bamber (1984), Knox and Bouchier (1985), Northouse and Northouse (1985), Honeycutt and Lowe Worobey (1987), Mosley (1988), Ley (1988), Carroll and Munroe (1989) and Hughes (1991) are but a few of the authors who have appealed for the introduction of communication specialist teachers into health professionals' education. Mosley (1988) was convinced that there was "no more important tool of health care available to health professionals than human communication" (Ibid : 323).

He regretted the fact that the academic curriculum so often failed to include any formal teaching on communication skills. Harlem (1977) blamed the domination of the biological sciences and the disease process, whilst Day (1979) believed that medical schools in particular should evolve into socio-cultural institutions which influenced the potential of communication and consequently health care.

Dervin and Harlock (1976) identified ten themes in a content analysis of health communication literature published between 1965 and 1975. The themes can be summarised as follows:- the sociology of health and illness, the patients' definition of health and illness, the health professionals' definition of health and illness, patient behaviour in illness, the doctor/patient relationship, patient satisfaction, patient compliance, communication within the health professions, health promotion and health education. Costello (1977) was even more succinct in his summary, he described four functions of communication between patients and health professionals :- diagnoses, co-operation, counselling and education. Mosley (1988) agreed with Costello but added a few ideas of his own :- patient compliance and specific communication skills in dealing with patients of different ages, gender, culture and ethnic backgrounds.

Ley (1982) had selectively reviewed the literature on communication, compliance and patient satisfaction and concluded that a major source of patient complaint was dissatisfaction with the quality of communication received. Day (1979) suggested that psychology, sociology, linguistics and educational technology should be included in all health professions' curricula whilst Kreps and Thornton (1984) identified awareness, compassion, descriptiveness, receptiveness, adaptiveness and ethics as being the parameters upon which communication should be taught.

Northouse and Northouse (1985) were convinced that all this could be achieved only through an interdisciplinary approach to health care and cited the concept of teamwork as the exemplary model on which to base this. Mosley (1988) criticised the fact that most research to date on communication in health care had been limited to doctors and nurses. He called for a greater effort into researching the need for increased communication skills in the other professions. Examination of the literature has revealed a few descriptive studies concerning other disciplines but Mosley is correct in his statement that most attention has been paid to medicine and nursing.

The micro training approach for communication skills teaching has been used in many of the health care professions. Examples have been found in the teaching of counsellors (Uhlemann et al 1982, Naidoo 1983), medical students (Moreland 1971, 1974), nurses (Authier and Gustafson 1975, Carpenter and Kroth 1976, Spruce and Synder 1982, Wallace et al 1981), social workers (Hargie and Bamford 1984), physiotherapists (Dickson and Maxwell 1985), speech therapists (Saunders and Cave 1986), and health visitors Crute, Hargie and Ellis (1989). Micro training involves four phases, skill analysis, skill discrimination, skill practice and focused feedback. Desirable behaviours should be identified in advance and should be measured by an experienced communications lecturer prior to the commencement of the training and also on completion. All authors reported an increase in desirable skills behaviour by the end of the course.

Crute, Hargie and Ellis (1989) described a course undertaken by health visiting students (N=31). There was no indication whether these students were an assigned group or whether they were volunteers from a larger group. Crute, Hargie and Ellis identified 20 desirable behaviours prior to commencement of the course. The students were each asked to role play a home visit to an 'anxious pregnant woman'. The ten minute role play was videotaped and then the 'behaviours' were assigned into desirable/undesirable categories. An analysis was then made by the student and the lecturer, a discussion followed by a repeat role play was performed. Expert judges were asked to analyse both tapes without knowing which was the pre learning or the post learning tape. Crute et al admitted that the results may have been biased as the students were highly motivated (the micro skills course was included in the overall assessment strategy for the health visitor course), only one group of students participated in the experiment and no control group was used. In addition some students felt extremely threatened by the use of the videotape which may well have altered their behaviour. As the most senior member of staff role played the pregnant woman this might also be seen as an inhibiting factor for nervous students. In spite of these considerations Crute et al reported a 'significant improvement' in the desirable behaviours measured on the post learning video tape.

The Wilcoxon Matched Pairs Test was used to measure any significance. Highly significant changes were recorded in the following areas:- A decrease in undesirable behaviour such as fidgeting, interruptions, multiple questions and manipulation with an increase in desirable behaviours such as paraphrasing, explaining, probing and reflecting questioning. French (1983) warned however that the overuse of reflecting as a questioning technique may lead to the conversation degenerating into parrot like responses from the interviewer, which could then become undesirable behaviour. Overall Crute et al (1989) concluded that micro training was useful although they warned of the need to identify appropriate levels of skill as a pre-requisite. They observed that desirable behaviours such as leaning towards the patient could rapidly become an undesirable behaviour if it continued for too long or if it invaded the patient's personal space which meant that the strategy became threatening. Basic social skills were therefore seen as essential behaviours. The authors also recommended further research into measuring the interpersonal skills necessary for exemplary interaction between a professional and a client.

Van Dalen et al (1989) described a communication skills teaching course for medical students at Maastricht Medical School. Whilst the course is entirely unidisciplinary several important points emerge from this paper. A problem based approach to learning was adopted and by using a skills laboratory in the initial stages of learning real patients were not used as guinea pigs, a most important consideration in training health professionals. Students were also able to prepare for a whole range of hypothetical situations which may not always be readily available in clinical practice at any one time.

A series of simulated patient vignettes were presented to the students who then practiced their skills in dealing with the given situation. This method has previously been described by Dickens et al (1985). Both Dickens et al (1985) and Van Dalen et al (1989) emphasise the importance of immediate feedback and constructive criticism from both the tutorial staff and peer students. Van Dalen et al, stressed that the timing of the course was most important. They found that first and second year students were very enthusiastic and receptive whereas the third and forth year students were more varied in their responses. Van Dalen et al suggested that "greater medical knowledge seems to shift attention from communication skills" (Ibid :60).

Van Der Merwe's students in South Africa were not so well prepared. She advised all qualified doctors to communicate correctly during ward rounds. This she stated, would ensure that "students would learn to acquire the correct attitudes" (1989 : 47). It would also show them how to solve problems and how to question patients. If Irving and Bamber's (1984) findings are valid it would seem that the very last strategy that a medical student should adopt is to role model the doctor who has had no behavioural science training or skills training in communication (Knox and Bouchier 1985).

Several publications have been identified that specifically examine the doctor/patient relationship. Fitton and Acheson (HMSO 1979d) undertook a quantative analysis of the expectations of the relationship from the patient's perception. Some 80 patients who had booked appointments with their general practitioner were randomly allocated from two practices (N=160) and were described as Group A. They were interviewed in their own health centre prior to their consultation with the doctor. A further 80 patients randomly allocated from the same two practices (N=160) who had not made appointments were interviewed at home after being approached by the researchers in order to obtain consent and were described as Group B. There were therefore 320 patients who participated in total. The results confirmed some anticipated findings such as 123 patients complained that they had to wait too long for an appointment. There were also some unexpected findings. A surprising number (N=263) indicated that they would be satisfied with a nurse treating them for minor ailments rather than the doctor. Some 45 said that they would prefer to consult with a doctor first and then would not mind subsequently attending the nurse. Only one patient said that he/she would not contemplate this arrangement at all. If this bi-partite approach was adopted then here is further evidence of the need for exemplary communication skills between doctors and nurses.

An analysis was made of the 160 patients' symptoms and eventual diagnosis in Group A. There were 210 diagnoses of which 35 were categorised as 'mental' or 'psychological'. These were the most common categories, thus highlighting the importance of a conceptual understanding of psychology and sociology by every doctor, who must then demonstrate the ability to interact with the patient in order to ascertain the problem (p 66-67). Patients from both Group A and B were then questioned about how they perceived communication between themselves and their general practitioner. 184 felt that talking to the doctor was easy but 82 found that it was very difficult. When these 82 were asked the reasons why this was so, more than half (N=43) indicated that the major problem was the doctor's manner. Fitton and Acheson pointed out that almost all of these 43 patients came from Group B and therefore were interviewed at home. It would have been unethical to state whether an individual doctor could be identified as having a particularly difficult manner but such a disclosure may have raised an awareness in that individual that his/her interaction with the patients was not good. Fitton and Acheson concluded that all interaction between doctors and patients "is an exercise in communication" (p 84) and that it was therefore essential that every doctor understands the importance of a sound knowledge of psychology and sociology.

Stroller and Geerstma (1958) and Reynolds and Bice (1971) found that general practitioners neither wanted or indeed had the knowledge to treat the psychosocial problems of their patients. Stimson and Webb (1975) suggested that many doctors erected barriers between themselves and the patients when it came to psychosocial problems. In the general practitioners defence however, if Horder

(1977) and Gray (1980) are to be believed, the average consulting time between a patient and a doctor is only five to six minutes. It is therefore hardly surprising that patients do not reveal their real feelings to the doctor. Ley (1982) also concentrated on the quality of communication in the doctor/patient relationship and found that the main causes of patient dissatisfaction were poor transmission of information, poor understanding and low levels of recall of information by patients. As Ley pointed out "There does not appear to be any evidence that provision of additional information leads to adverse reactions by patients". (Ibid : 241)

Ley et al (1979b) concluded that sociodemographic changes, personality characteristics and the duration and severity of the illness did not effect patient compliance, providing the quality of communication between the doctor and the patient was good. Korsch et al (1968) had previously reached the same conclusion. Honeycutt and Lowe Worobey (1987) warned that effective communication skills were no longer a superfluous issue in health care but central to patient satisfaction. Without effective communication strategies there would be serious implications for the future of health care (p 217).

A Report entitled "Doctors in an Integrated Health Service" (HMSO 1971) summarised the need for a greater emphasis on the behavioural sciences in general practice most succinctly :

> The present and future of general practice lies in the social and psychological support of the patient in the community rather than developing more or sophisticated medical practice. In fact, any clinician whether specialist general practitioner needs to understand the patient as a whole man....... they become good clinicians only when they are sensitive also to personal and social need.
>
> (HMSO 1971 : 14)

This Report also concluded that it was essential at every level in the NHS to consult, exchange ideas and negotiate between every profession in order to "share the stimulus and scientific environment" (p 53) which contributed to the welfare of patients.

Jameton and Todes (1982) thought rather differently. As two humanities lecturers they questioned the contribution of the scientific environment and discussed the dichotomy between those who believed that a health professional was essentially a scientist and those who believed that they were "humanists in scientific clothing" (p 105). They recognised that students' basic interests lay in a curriculum rooted in clinical practice and argued that the inclusion of the humanities must therefore be seen as relevant to clinical practice. The study of law, ethics, economics, health policies, human development and aging, interviewing skills, the use of human values in decision making and the philosophy of health care were suggested as being appropriate topics for inclusion. Jameton and Todes had developed interdisciplinary workshops in bioethics. Anthropologists, lawyers and philosophers were appointed as the group leaders. They adopted a problem solving approach to hypothetical case histories in which students were asked to identify any ethical, legal and economic dilemmas present. These problems were then related to theoretical frameworks. The concept of patient rights was one such example given, with the right to treatment, the right to refuse treatment, the right to choose and the right to equality being debated.

The responsibilities of medical practice was another workshop title. Mock trials were arranged in which 'the defendant' had to contest the accusation of lack of informed consent or unethical behaviour. Confessional testimonies were used for discussion purposes using such examples as a substance abusing doctor, deliberate withdrawal of treatment of the terminally ill, the diversion of funds to bolster radical practice or research. Health and human rights were offered as elective seminars ; the right to health care, financing high technology care instead of primary health care, voluntary euthanasia, research on human subjects and cross cultural value differences were all debated at length. Jameton and Todes paper was most interesting but purely descriptive. No attempt was made to identify the number of students who participated, the disciplines who participated or any evaluation that took place. No conclusion can therefore be drawn about the effectiveness of such workshops. The course contents and the learning strategies employed would however seem to be sound.

Bloom (1959) considered the role of sociologists in medical education. He noted that in the USA medical education appeared to be facing a new kind of challenge - that of preparing "future physicians for a deeper understanding and skill with the interpersonal part of the doctor/patient relationship".(Bloom 1959 : 667). Bloom suggested that medical practice had evolved and a shift in emphasis had occurred from knowledge about the disease to questions about the patient, the patient's feelings and the environment in which he/she lived. Bloom felt that there would be an increasing need for social scientists knowledge and skills in medical schools. He described the freshmen's curriculum as consisting of three aspects of psychiatry ; the psychology of human behaviour, human development from childhood to old age and sociological aspects of human behaviour. Bloom discussed whether the sociologist should be viewed by the medical school as a colleague or a consultant. He concluded that 'consultant' was the better option as the specialist skills and knowledge could be 'consulted' thus allowing physicians to incorporate the sociologists teaching into their own teaching sessions by helping students apply theory to practice. In 1964 he further reported that an unprecedented interest in the psychological and social factors of health and illness was evident in medical schools. He discussed the increasing numbers of behavioural scientists employed by medical schools and referred to "permanent teaching and research installations" (Bloom 1964 : 820). Bloom described the two distinctly differing opinions of what the behavioural sciences meant to medical men, one being an isolationist disciplinary approach "restricted primarily to sociology, anthropology and social psychology" and the other being the view of an integrated biopsychosociological approach to man. Bloom, while praising the excellence of the scientific standards achieved in medical training, noted that a definite weakness in the system was the doctor/patient relationship. He believed that recognition of this fact had caused the sudden interest in the behavioural sciences just as the weakness in knowledge of the biological sciences had caused a much greater interest in physiology a century earlier. Bloom cited Reader and Goss (1959) who had reviewed the literature directly related to medicine and the behavioural sciences. Reader and Goss had identified topics such as attitudes and values towards health and illness, the social organisation of health personnel, the social roles played by health personnel when interacting with patients, professionalism, standards and competence and psychosocial factors influencing health. Bloom believed that these sort of concepts constituted the framework upon which the future relationship between doctors' and patients' would stand. The framework should be flexible and dynamic.

Pattishall (1970) traced the development of behavioural science teaching in medical schools. He reported that in 1914 the total time devoted to the behavioural sciences was one hour, in 1940 twenty hours, in 1951 fifty six hours and in 1966 an average of 96 hours. Pattishall described the struggle that behavioural scientists had experienced in even being accepted as a serious academic discipline. He analysed the types of behavioural science courses in existence in the USA medical schools and categorised them into four main groups :- 1. psychiatry based, 2. the introduction of the separate disciplines of psychology, sociology and anthropology, 3. a broad introduction to integrated behavioural sciences and 4. a behavioural science course. Pattishall found that category 4 was almost non existent. He differentiated this category from the others as being the one in which a scientific body of knowledge is presented to the student using the concept of a biopsychosocial approach to health care. Pattishall's thesis was persuasive in that the concept of a single causal factor in the disease process is no longer accepted and therefore the integrated approach should be encouraged.

Hartings and Counte (1977), a psychologist and sociologist respectively, reviewed the models that were currently available for teaching the behavioural sciences to medical students. Their aim was to identify the most effective model which they would then adopt at the Rush Medical School, Chicago. Their review yielded three basic models. The first and most commonly adopted was the inclusion of the behavioural sciences in the field of psychiatry. Hartings and Counte criticised this model as they believed that normality then became subsumed in abnormality. Pattison (1975) shared the same concerns. He was worried that "Behavioural science concepts tend to be identified in the medical students minds as psychiatric problems" (Pattison 1975 : 117).

Hartings and Counte (1977) rejected this model as they perceived that allegiances within a department of psychiatry could easily become disparate and "militate against needed collaboration in the teaching effort" (p 825). The second model they considered was a discrete department of behavioural sciences that operated entirely independently of the medical school. The advantage seemed to be that other disciplines apart from medicine could be unified into a teaching and research unit. These departments tended to be purely academic with no clinical responsibility. The major disadvantage with this model was that the medical students did not view the behavioural sciences as relevant to medical practice. In the final model a committee of behavioural scientists representing different departments was formed. The committee organised and delivered a behavioural science curriculum. Problems were encountered however through a lack of resources and through fluctuating interest and commitment by individual members of the committee. This Hartings and Counte suggested was hardly surprising as the teaching hours were dependent on volunteers undertaking extra teaching duties. The result was an ad hoc curriculum.

Not surprisingly the authors were not prepared to adopt any of the models per se. They developed their own model based on what they perceived to be the good points of all three. An independent autonomous behavioural science department was formed with the remit of teaching and research activities in conjunction with a clinical case load. The behavioural scientists had direct access to patient populations and participated in their therapy. Hartings and Counte perceived three advantages in this model. The teaching of the behavioural sciences and clinical activity stand as a discipline in its own right, theory is applied to practice and finally it unified the staff themselves. The behavioural sciences collectively constituted 148 hours of the curriculum and was organised into five discrete modules entitled :

1. Fundamentals of Behaviour (23 hours).
2. Observation and Communication (28 hours).
3. Behaviour in the Life Cycle (30 hours).
4. Behavioural Deviations (27 hours)
5. Mini Course Matrix (40 hours).

The mini course matrix was explained as four 10 hour electives in which the students chose from a variety of options available. The philosophy behind this was to enable students to pursue topics of particular interest and significance to them as individuals. In some of the modules the students had direct access to patients. This enabled them to develop their interviewing skills while gathering pertinent information relating to the patients' psychosocial history. Hartings and Counte were unable to draw conclusions about the success of their adopted model as only one group of students had completed this course. Initial findings had been encouraging. The students had evaluated the behavioural science course very positively and rated the learning as meaningful and appropriate. The effectiveness of the learning was borne out by the fact that the group of students achieved higher scores in the behavioural science component of the National Board of Medical Examiners examinations. A search for quantifiable information regarding this course was not successful. Hartings and Counte do not seem to have published further and so it is impossible to check the validity of these claims. On a subjective appraisal only it would appear that the model described had great potential.

Gill (1975) suggested that there were four questions which must be answered by behavioural scientists involved in medical education. These are what should be taught, which framework should be used, how the teaching should be distributed and which health disciplines should be taught together. He noted the increasing importance placed upon behavioural science as an emerging discipline in health care and attributed this to the increasing emphasis on health education and health promotion. The whole point of including the discipline in health professionals' education was to improve the quality of care. He identified five main constructs which he believed should constitute the framework of the behavioural science component in any health professions' curriculum. These were 1. the social context of health and illness, 2. data generation of health care problems on which treatment, prognosis and care can be based along with the identification and implementation of preventative measures, 3. the application of scientific knowledge from a holistic point of view, 4. an interdisciplinary approach to planning and managing care and 5. a regular and thorough review of comparative health care systems.

In order to meet the demands of these constructs, Gill recommended the adoption of the following propositions ; an adequate research base on which to base all teaching, an interdisciplinary approach, increased research projects relating to the behavioural sciences in health care and an identified behavioural science department or section within each faculty of health. By integrating the behavioural sciences throughout the curriculum, the application of theory could be applied to practice. Interdisciplinary groups led by adaptable, sensitive, dynamic facilitators, Gill believed, would mean that the best interests of both patient and professional would be maximised.

Kahn et al (1979) certainly did not confirm the Bloom (1964) or Pattishall (1970) findings or share their optimism. Indeed the work by Kahn et al seemed to demonstrate that little or no behavioural sciences were being taught in medical schools. The focus of their study was clearly identified. They investigated the number of medical schools in the USA which taught interpersonal skills, when and by whom they were taught, which teaching strategies were used and how these were evaluated. Some 111 medical schools were contacted by letter and asked whether interpersonal skills were included in the programme and 79 responded of which 76 (96%) replied in the affirmative. Kahn et al contacted the non respondents and found that most of them did not teach interpersonal skills. Of the 76 who had replied in the affirmative, 74 agreed to be interviewed by the researchers and 69 of these were identified as appropriate to be included in the study. (The inclusion and exclusion criteria were not described). Finally, 62 medical schools constituted the study group. Collation of the results revealed that >500 faculty members taught interpersonal skills (where N=62 faculties) and while 60 of the faculties stated that there was a special course in interpersonal skills the most common teaching method used was through the medium of commercial videos (N=450). The topics most frequently addressed were information gathering, psychological interventions, death and dying, counselling and crisis intervention. Psychiatrists, psychologists, social workers, sociologists, nurses and anthropologists were amongst the professions contributing to these teaching programmes. Psychiatrists contributed to all 62 faculty programmes. 54 of these programmes were informally assessed with the remainder not assessing the programmes at all. No faculty assessed the interpersonal skills programme formally and as such this part of the curriculum did not constitute part of the summative assessment. An interesting finding was that most (82%) had only introduced interpersonal skills into their programmes within the previous five years. This therefore completely undermines Bloom (1964) who had asserted that major progress had been made.

Kahn et al (1979) while appearing to be encouraged by the changes in attitude towards behavioural science teaching in medical education made an astute observation. As the majority of faculties had only introduced these programmes in the last five years most of the doctors in clinical practice would not have had the same exposure to the behavioural sciences. This had major implications for junior doctors and the medical students who would be viewing them as role models. As most of the teaching of interpersonal skills took place in the pre clinical years there was the risk that "if these skills are not systematically reinforced and applied in the clinical years, even if well learned earlier, they may be lost". (Kahn et al 1979 : 34). One result that Kahn et al did not draw attention to was the use of psychiatrists. It is interesting to reflect that as psychiatrists deal with the disorders of mental health then the traditional disease orientation may prevail even in the area of interpersonal skills teaching. An increased use of behavioural scientists may well reduce this risk. Flaherty and Scharf (1981) and Irwin and Bamber (1984) certainly advocated the introduction of such a strategy.

Irwin and Bamber (1984) evaluated medical students' communication skills. Reinforcing Kahn et al (1979), they recognised the importance of exemplary interpersonal skills in health professionals in order to increase patient satisfaction and also to improve their compliance to treatment. The importance of this has also been reported by Cartwright (1964), Raphael (1969), Knox et al (1979) and Engler et al (1981). Irwin and Bamber (1984) numerically evaluated medical students communication abilities by using a modified Verby scale (Verby et al 1979). Irwin and Bamber's scale consisted of 19 parameters of target behaviours and were scored on a scale of 1 to 4, a rating of 1 being described as poor or negative behaviours and a rating of 4 as very good or positive behaviours. The medical students had virtually no training in communication skills, partly Irwin and Bamber believed because of curriculum overload and also because it had been felt that the students would be better motivated to learn in the clinical areas. Some 73 medical students comprised the study group along with 11 trainers. Each student was asked to interview approximately 6 patients with a trainer observing. In total, 475 interviews were conducted by the 73 students. The results revealed two distinct groupings of communication skills; normal social communication and specific skills relating to patient/doctor interaction. While the students displayed normal behaviour in social communication, Irwin and Bamber noted that they lacked many of the specific skills that would be expected of them as doctors. They did not use confrontation appropriately and demonstrated avoidance behaviours. This reinforces the work by Hannay (1980) who believed that medical students did not confront patients as they were themselves confronted by people with multiple biopsychosocial problems. Knox et al (1979) reported that medical students tended to avoid addressing psychosocial problems and concentrate on the disease process. Similarly Irwin and Bamber (1984) described other desirable behaviours that were not evident. These included the picking up of non verbal clues, ability to clarify issues and the use of silence. They recommended the inclusion of these concepts in all teaching programmes. Knox and Bouchier (1985) described an introductory course in communication skills for preclinical students. 'Real' patients participated but Knox and Bouchier noted that the students' "lack of clinical knowledge did not interfere with their learning" (p 285). Knox and Bouchier had adopted a deliberate strategy of introducing this programme at the beginning of the students training and decided what to teach, when and by whom it should be taught, prior to writing the curriculum. They advocated the use of behavioural scientists. A point of interest in reviewing these publications was that neither Irwin and Bamber nor Knox and Bouchier reference each other. This is surprising as both medical schools are British and both were striving to achieve similar changes. Perhaps this is another example of a breakdown in communication.

Communication with the dying is a frequently reported problem for health professionals (Oken 1961, Glaser and Strauss 1968, Ward 1974, McIntosh 1977, Knight and Field 1981, Field 1984, Nash 1984, Nicklin 1987). Nash (1984) in a letter to the British Medical Journal drew attention to the need to expose medical students and young doctors to training in counselling and talking to dying patients. He maintained that role play in an interdisciplinary symposium had been an extremely valuable learning strategy in his own health authority. He concluded his letter with the significant statement "Understanding our own emotional reactions and that they exist, is the first step in helping these patients" (BMJ 1984 : 1996).

Nicklin (1987) in a short report of the research he undertook as part of his Masters degree in Education, reported a similar need. Using a 35 item scale to measure personal and professional attitudes to death and dying among doctors and nurses, he found that the basic training of both groups was woefully inadequate. One of Nicklin's recommendations was that "Interdisciplinary training, particularly in the area of interpersonal and communication skills could substantially improve attitudes" (Ibid : 58).

Field (1984), a sociologist, was also concerned with the amount of instruction UK medical students received on death and dying. The Royal Commission on Medical Education (HMSO -The Todd Report 1968) had contained no reference to death education for medical students at all. Field (1984) distributed 84 questionnaires to staff within the UK medical schools. Some 62 questionnaires were returned. The questionnaire was short and essentially exploratory so no concept definitions were included. The respondents included the clinical deans, lecturers in psychology and sociology. Total participation was 36 medical schools of which 27 reported some formal teaching on death and dying with a mean of six hours being spent on the subject overall. Several of the schools, Edinburgh, Southampton, Aberdeen and the London Hospital reported optional projects. At the Middlesex more than 60% of medical students experienced multi-disciplinary learning with nurses. In the pre-clinical years psychologists and sociologists were the usual lecturers and in the clinical years general practitioners and psychiatrists were the most frequently indicated. The most commonly used teaching method was the formal lecture although small group discussions were used during the clinical stage on occasions when appropriate. Field indicated that this tended to be when a student was already interacting with a dying patient. Respondents were asked to indicate which books were recommended to students. Most schools had no recommended reading lists.

The final question asked by Field involved the teachers' perceptions of the effectiveness of their teaching. While obviously subjective and informal it was generally reported that "medical students welcome teaching about death and dying, are enthusiastic about and interested in the topic" (Field 1984: 432). One school reported that students were dissatisfied because there was not enough time devoted to the subject. Five of the medical schools had undertaken formal evaluations. Edinburgh and Aberdeen gave their students questionnaires before and after the formal teaching sessions. The questionnaires were based on attitude scales and the post learning responses revealed a small change in attitude towards "greater disclosure of truth about terminal illness and diminution in fear of death" (Field 1984 : 432).

The London Hospital medical school reported changes that had been made in 1979 in order to improve the teaching as a result of student evaluations. The respondent in this particular instance was Dr Murray Parkes whose work on caring for the dying is internationally recognised. It is perhaps not surprising therefore that death education had a high priority at this particular medical school.

The predominance of lectures as the favoured teaching method is disturbing as it implies a one way didactic approach with little or no opportunity for discussion. Durlak (1978) and Maguire (1981) have both found that didactic teaching was less effective than other methods in death education. Maguire additionally found that the use of videotapes enhanced interviewing skills in a role play situation. Dickinson and Pearson (1980) examined physicians' attitudes towards dying patients and the effect that death education had upon those attitudes. Those physicians who had received formal instruction were more comfortable in dealing with the dying than those who had not.

Field and Howells (1986) reported their findings of a study which had examined medical students self reported worries about aspects of death and dying. 98 third year medical students completed a questionnaire in which open ended questions were used to try and ascertain "which aspects of the process of dying produce high fear" (p 148). Amongst the responses received were fear of own death, personal loss of significant others (>85% on both categories) but also more than 80% reported great fear of communicating with dying patients and of their own emotional problems when interacting with a dying person. Of the 76 students who expressed these latter worries, own helplessness was expressed by 97%. Field and Howells quoted one student who had written "Not knowing how to behave to the patient and possibly not being able to control myself emotionally watching someone else going through agony" (Field and Howells 1986 : 150).

The irony of the situation is that this is one of the most common concerns expressed by any health professional. Being given the opportunity to participate in sensitive small interdisciplinary groupwork may have reassured this student that this was a normal and perfectly understandable reaction and he/she may have been able to devise appropriate coping strategies. Field and Howells used Cochrans Q Test for statistical analysis. This is an appropriate test for comparing frequency data when observations are not independent. The concerns about the dying scored 78.22 (with a significance $p< 0.001$). Field and Howells concluded that this was a highly significant finding.

The evidence obtained by Field in 1984 of the situation in UK medical schools was alarming. It could be argued that the only statistically certain outcome for all human beings is that having been born they will all die. Inevitably many health professionals frequently encounter dying patients . Field and Howells (1986) identified a cause of great fear for most medical students in their study, that of communicating with the dying patient. It is not unreasonable to presume that these students are representive of all medical students and therefore it is a problem of magnitude. Evidence such as this must be used to increase the awareness of educators of the needs of students. A change in the amount, the quality and the teaching methods adopted is urgently needed.

It is generally felt that psychologists could contribute a great deal to enhancing the communication skills of the health care professions (HMSO 1979, The Trethowan Report). Trethowan and his colleagues believed that a holistic approach to care was paramount and that the only way that this could be realistically achieved was through integrated teamwork. Rather than considering psychology as an adjunct to the main stream health care professions the Report recommended that psychologists should adopt a central role.

The WHO agreed with this (WHO 1985). In 1984 a group of eminent psychologists met together in Geneva and considered the contribution that psychologists might make towards achieving the target for health for all by the year 2000. The group aimed to identify the potential advantages and benefits as well as the pit falls in becoming more closely integrated with the health professions. All participating members belonged to the European Federation of Professional Psychologists Associations (EFPPA) or the WHO. The consultation had been arranged as a result of a conversation held between the President of the EFPPA and the WHO Regional Officer for Mental Health in which they mutually discovered that neither organisation was aware of the policies, expertise and experience of the other. It was hoped therefore that this meeting would stimulate a cross fertilisation of ideas and a comprehensive exchange of information.

Dr Henderson (the WHO Regional Officer) outlined four of the WHO strategies. These were described as to ensure equity in health, to add years to life, to add life to years and to add health to life. The psychologists considered these strategies and tried to identify ways in which they could make a positive contribution towards achieving targets. It was felt that in order that progress could be made a change in attitudes, beliefs and behaviours had to take place in the population as a whole. The psychologists felt that they could make a particular contribution in the following areas ; social competence, positive self esteem, problem solving skills, emotion, self control and perceived control. These attributes they felt could be achieved by inducing behavioural changes through motivation and positive and negative reinforcement. Social influence was described as central to inducing attitudinal change and could be through conformity, compliance and obedience. Persuasion and instruction in the form of health education was also perceived as essential. In the general discussion which followed these findings an interesting statement was made; " People are often dissatisfied with their lives because of their failure to realise their full potential, psychologists are skilled in helping people to identify alternative goals more appropriate to their abilities and needs." (WHO 1985 : 8)

It seems a reasonable assumption therefore that psychologists would be invaluable in contributing to health care in two main areas. Not only are they the experts who could most appropriately introduce the theory behind client behaviour but could also contribute considerably to team building in health care by helping to reduce the interprofessional jealousies and conflicts which prevent a team from working collaboratively.

As the authors of this paper persuasively argue, psychology being both a discipline and a profession, is well placed to encourage the interaction of theory to practice. Psychology is orientated towards normal rather than abnormal behaviour thus the emphasis of psychology in health care and health promotion is entirely appropriate. It was ruefully observed that the majority of psychologists employed in health care were based in clinical areas as clinical psychologists with a client group already identified as needing intervention. It was recommended that more psychologists were employed in primary health care with educational psychologists concerning themselves with helping children acquire healthy life styles, occupational psychologists developing new roles in promoting work environments which reduce stress and the introduction of health promotion programmes in the work place. The meeting concluded with a firm agreement between the WHO and the EFPPA that closer collaboration was both desirable and essential.

The English National Board (1987) has recognised the need for behavioural scientists involvement in nurse education but warned that the theory practice gap could widen without the concommitant involvement of teachers of nursing. The Board suggested that the most appropriate way forward was for behavioural scientists to introduce the theory and then for the nurse teachers to help the students to apply that theory to clinical practice. This recommendation could be adopted in an interdisciplinary learning setting with a multidisciplinary group being introduced to the theory perhaps in a lecture, a single profession tutorial group applying the theory learned to clinical practice followed by an interdisciplinary tutorial group applying both the theory and the practice to a holistic approach to client care.

2.9 Integrated interdiscplinary learning frameworks

The final section of this literature review examines the small number of publications identified that have described in some detail suggested frameworks on which integrated interdisciplinary learning could be modelled. Never the less not all the models discussed are exemplary and indeed some potentially valuable suggestions are marred by inadequate and careless evaluations (Howard and Byl 1971, Mason and Parascandola 1972, Infante et al 1976, Darling and Ogg 1984 being illustrative examples of these). Papers which have concentrated on shared learning models involving collaboration between just two or three disciplines have been excluded as have those that describe specific post graduate initiatives such as short courses on pain management or care of the dying. Their contribution to quality health care is fully recognised but the review of the literature seems to suggest that most attention should be paid to examining the feasibility of introducing shared learning at the beginning of individuals' professional careers before they qualify. This is particularly relevant for the future of health care as the students of 1996 will be the professionals in the next millenium.

Milio (1979) suggested that the introduction of an integrative interdisciplinary core curriculum would contribute to the achievement of effective strategies for contemporary health care. She raised the issue of the continuing emphasis on 'disease' within professional training and argued that existing resources, both financial and manpower should be urgently diverted into health promotion, health education and primary care. Szasz (1970) accused health care professionals of using their talents inappropriately causing a fragmentation of the approach to human problems and a total waste of scarce resources :

> it is felt by observers of the health care scene that definite barriers exist between providers of health services which adversely influence the quality distribution and utilisation of the services and contribute to the rising cost of health care
>
> (Szasz 1970 : 386)

Szasz was convinced that the traditional educational methods encouraged and reinforced individual achievements at the expense of the principles of collaboration and co-operation. Combined with a reluctance to adopt the new philosophy of holistic care and teams which were "thrown together by administrative decisions" indiscriminately and inappropriately (p 386) no progress was likely to be made. Szasz was not entirely clear what constituted interdisciplinary learning. He certainly seemed to be quite clear what it was not! He did not perceive the physical presence of different health professions in the same place at the same time as shared learning. He insisted that it was vital that "the students are exposed to experiences which help them to learn to act together" (Szasz 1970 : 388). He also commented on the fact that all health care students share certain basic skills and knowledge and that this was the basis on which to build an interdisciplinary framework. Steinberg (1989) believed that consultation was educational in itself in that the core skills and knowledge allow a joint method of enquiry "into the fundamental nature of problems" (p 14). Szasz' enlightened comments and criticisms are just as relevant to the health care professions in 1996 as they were in 1970.

Hawkins (1972) believed that discussions about core curriculum for health care professionals was often hindered by a lack of an agreed definition. The Oxford Dictionary (1985) defines 'core' as a "central part of different character from what surrounds it" (p 210) and a 'curriculum' as a "course of study" (p 233). A core curriculum could then be described as a central integral part of a course of study. Hawkins (1972) was convinced that a core curriculum would help "provide the horizontal mobility that is desperately needed in the health field" (Hawkins 1972 : 167). He cited Wallenstein (1968) who had studied twelve allied health occupations using items of knowledge that could constitute a core curriculum. Wallenstein had identified commonalities in both the behavioural and biological sciences that were "essential or helpful in at least eight of the twelve occupations" (Hawkins 1972 : 168). Hawkins did not attempt to enumerate further on Wallenstein's work. The twelve professions studied and the commonalities within the curriculum were not disclosed. Efforts to obtain the original publication by Wallenstein have proved unsuccessful. Hawkins also cited Fullerton (1966) who studied twenty allied health professions. He identified 2,163 titles within the curriculum which would be suitable for shared learning. Fullerton was able with the consent of the educators from each profession to condense the titles to 126 in total. Of these 78 were found to be common to two or more professions. Fullerton appeared to concentrate particularly on the biological sciences according to Hawkins. Again efforts to trace the original source have been unsuccessful. Because the original sources have not been traced Hawkins report should be treated with some caution. Never the less it was surprising to find reports of similar analyses being completed more than twenty years ago. It must also be said that it was very disappointing that both Wallenstein and Fullerton's work has obviously been largely ignored and certainly neither author has been referenced in any substantive documents. The World Health Organisation for example should have been given the access to this information many years ago. If this had been the case then the whole of the educational strategies for the health professions over the past two decades may have been substantially altered. Pelligrino (1972) in the same year as Hawkins published observed :

> we are, of course very far from an idealised amalgamation of the health professions. Indeed the predominating tendencies appear to be all in the opposite direction.........towards separatist definitions of functions, ethics accreditation and education
>
> (Ibid : 213)

He continued that without a rapid reversal of the current trends optimal use of manpower would remain forever elusive.

Light (1969) stated the case even more strongly when refering to the "occupational tribes" he added that this entrenchment was adding to "communication pipe lines already clogged and showing signs of atherosclerosis" (p 114). He believed that the current state of the curriculum as it was then (and in certain instances remains) prevented manpower efficiency and the essential development and flexibility needed in health care. He supported the concept of a core curriculum for several reasons, there was a considerable saving in teacher time and cost, students would learn to learn together and to share information, the health team would be clarified at an earlier stage and there would be greater flexibility in career choice as the student could transfer to another discipline without too much difficulty. McCreary (1968), Kenneth (1969), Howard and Byl (1971), Leninger (1971), Mason and Parascandola (1972), McGaghie et al (1978), Owen (1982) and Ivey (1988) all reached similar conclusions.

Ivey et al (1988) made an extremely valuable contribution to the understanding of the nature of interdisciplinarity. They developed a continuum of interdisciplinary practice. They described parallel practice as occurring whenever a health care setting had more than one profession working within it. In this situation "Professional autonomy is at its height : shared expertise is at its nadir" (Ivey et al 1988 : 191)

Collaboration is the sharing of information between diverse professions "professional autonomy is quite high but the potential for shared expertise across professional boundaries has risen" (Ibid : 191).

Consultation is the seeking and reciprocating of advice between the professions on a one to one basis or in an interdisciplinary context, co-ordination incorporates a management function on a face to face basis through formal or informal channels. Ivey et al believed that multidisciplinary practice was a different phenomenon from interdisciplinary practice in that a multidisciplinary team can work in a co-ordinated and collaborative fashion but not meet face to face. They suggested that specific treatment units often operate at this level. Once case conferences and integrated learning begins then the interdisciplinary team starts to evolve "This type of collaborative practice maximises shared expertise and minimizes professional autonomy" (Ibid : 192).

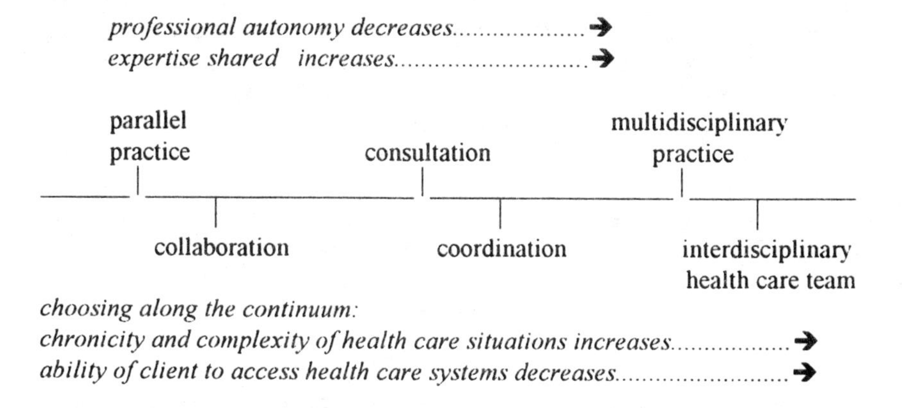

Figure 2.2 A continuum of interdisciplinary practice (Ivey et al 1988)

Ivey et al employed a teaching model upon which active interdisciplinary learning was the central tenet. Problem solving activities, role playing and field visits were the most commonly adopted learning strategies. This paper was purely descriptive and did not attempt to quantify the course itself. This seemed to be acceptable as the main thrust of the paper was obviously to further the debate on the concept of interdisciplinary education. The continuum for interdisciplinary practice is impressive and persuasive and should be considered for adoption in any interdisciplinary framework.

McGaghie et al (WHO 1978) warned that as well as ensuring academic quality in curriculum development attention should not be diverted "from the competence required to meet the real health needs of people" (p 11). The deficiencies of a subject centred curriculum has undesirable consequences for both the students and their future patients (p 15). They argued that a core curriculum is the only basis upon which integrated learning can be built. Concepts and operational definitions should be identified, learned and then built upon in a series of stages. The advantages, McGaghie et al believed, were that a core curriculum would make learning more meaningful and that the content could be constantly revised in order to reject obsolete information. These ideas would meet with the approval of cognitive psychologists who have advised the adoption of similar strategies in learning (Bruner et al 1956, Taylor 1964, Ausubel 1968).

McGaghie et al (1978) advocated the introduction of a competency based curriculum in which the core subjects are organised around measurable functions. It is based on the idea that the techniques used to produce learning can be subjected to testing with the intended outcome being an individual who can practice at a defined level of proficiency in accordance with local requirements and to meet local needs. If it is accepted that competence means the ability to perform to an expected standard then competency must be adopted as a construct which implies an holistic approach. A competent health professional therefore should be able to perform a particular function or satisfy a particular role in a diversity of settings over an extended period of time.

McGaghie et al (1978) concluded that it was meeting the needs of the community that should provide the "principle directional signals" in curriculum design. They maintained that it was wrong to highly train an individual for situations they would rarely, if ever, encounter whilst neglecting education relating to situations which would be met frequently. The educationalists responsible for developing the curriculum should consider the conditions and experience the graduates would face in the future and develop courses accordingly.

Towle (1991) produced a report summarising the findings of a study into the future of undergraduate medical education. The Inquiry was initiated by the Kings Fund in collaboration with St Bartholomews Medical School in London. Without reference to the work of McGaghie et al (1978) this report was the only one found that examined the current curriculum for UK medical students. The aim of the enquiry was; " To establish creative yet critical guidelines for the design of future undergraduate curricula in which clinical teaching is adapted to the changing needs and circumstances of health care." (Towle 1991 : 1-2)

Towle wrote of the 'widespread' recognition that the current curriculum was out of date and overcrowded with information which was irrelevant and inhibited medical students' creativity, problem solving abilities and critical thinking skills. A modified Delphi technique of three rounds was used to generate the data. 343 doctors were invited to take part with 213 (62%) responding in the first round, 192 (56%) responding in the second round and 28 (12%) providing additional comments in the final round. A clear consensus was reached on the urgent need for change. Within the section which explored clinical teaching the need for an increased emphasis in the following areas was identified (Towle 1991 : 10 -12) :

1. The understanding and application of concepts.
2. The importance of doctor/patient relationships, ensuring that students establish good relationships with patients, their families and other professionals involved in health care. Appropriate attitudes and good communication skills were described as essential qualities.
3. The holistic approach to individual patients. Psychosocial considerations were considered to be just as important as the biological ones when decision making.
4. The goal of health rather than the absence of disease. The maintenance of health and prevention of illness should be a central construct.
5. The need to think on a global, national and local level.
6. A wider perspective of medical practice should be addressed such as ethical, legal, social and economic issues.
7. Increased co-operation and collaboration between the professions involved in health care should be developed.

Agreement in summary was reached on the principles of future curriculum development. There should be :

1. A reduction in factual information.
2. Active learning thus encouraging an enquiring doctor.
3. Principles of medicine (core knowledge, skills and attitudes).
4. Development of general competences (critical thinking, problem solving, communication and management).
5. Integration at a vertical and horizontal level.
6. Early clinical contact.
7. A balance between hospital/community; curative/preventative care.
8. Wider aspects of health care.
9. Interprofessional collaboration.
10. Methods of learning/ teaching to support the aims of the curriculum.
11. Methods of assessment to support the above aims.

The widespread welcome given to this report is most encouraging. The medical profession is, and always has been, very powerful and vociferous in health care. If it has now adopted these findings and plans to implement them in full, then the future for closer interprofessional collaboration both in clinical practice and in education looks very promising.

Howard and Byl (1971) published an evaluation of the pitfalls they had experienced over a three year period since the introduction of an interdisciplinary core curriculum in the behavioural sciences. The curriculum was developed at the request of students from several disciplines and was entitled "Social Aspects of Health and Disease." The learning strategies adopted were ten, one hour lectures followed by 'small' interdisciplinary tutorial groups of two hours duration. In 1968 a large number of students had enrolled on the course (N=438). They represented the following disciplines : medicine (N=128), nursing (N=88), pharmacy (N=89), dentistry (N=75), physiotherapy (N=34) and dental hygienists (N=24). The 438 students were randomly assigned into an interdisciplinary mix of approximately 16 students in each group. Physicians (N=17), nurses (N=6) and dentists (N=4) were appointed group leaders.

Howard and Byl reported that in the second year of the experiment (with a different student population) several modifications to the programme were made. Lectures were extended to one and a half hours in duration and tutorial time was proportionately reduced by half an hour. In the third and final year of the experiment, again with a different and drastically reduced student group (N=75), the three hours were devoted to lectures and panel discussions.

Each year's course was evaluated by means of individual student questionnaires. In 1968 the response rate was 65%, in 1969 it was 42% and in 1970 it was 89%. Howard and Byl explained the high response rate in 1970 as being due to students being requested to submit a written assignment for assessment in conjunction with their completed evaluation forms. In 1968 of the 285 who returned the questionnaire 69% complained of a bias towards medical students with 53% commenting that medical students had dominated the group discussions. Only 53% felt that they had contributed as much to the discussion as they would have liked. Of the medical students 57% were 'very satisfied' with their own contribution while only 39% of nurses were 'very satisfied' with theirs. Overall 70% of the medical students rated the sessions as 'excellent' whereas only 16% of the dental and 25% of the pharmacy students rated the course in the same way.

As a result of these evaluations, the 1969 course was modified to increase the emphasis on the other disciplines. Although the response rate was lower (42%) only 45% thought that the course was medically biased in comparison with 69% the previous year. Some 31% thought that medical students had dominated the discussions compared with 53% in 1968, and 72% in total felt that they had contributed to the discussions compared with 57% in 1968. The third and final year, in 1970, yielded different results again when 36% said that the course was orientated towards all health professions (69% in 1968, 45% in 1969). Only 6% felt that the discussions were dominated by one profession and 78% reported that they had contributed as much as they desired.

In their conclusions Howard and Byl observed that medical students had become increasingly dissatisfied with the course while the other professions had reported increased satisfaction. In spite of this 76% of the medical students had voted for a continuation of the course. The two hour lectures were thought to be too long and the absence of tutorial groups were perceived by the students as a negative factor. The group leaders who were nurses (N=6) were rated lower than the group leaders who were doctors by the medical, dental and pharmacy students, but higher by the nurses, physiotherapy and dental hygiene students. Ironically all students, regardless of their professional bias, reported that the groups led by nurses had been the most effective in enabling students to fully participate in discussions as much as they wished.

Howard and Byl's own impressions of the three year experiment was that it had been 'mainly unsuccessful' and they concluded that they were "by no means wedded to the concept of multidisciplinary teaching in social medicine" (Howard and Byl 1971 : 781). This report, nonetheless, was full of flaws and as such is a useful publication as it highlights strategies which should be avoided. The first year of the experiment (1968) was heavily biased towards medical students (N=128). In a health team, if any bias exists, it is towards nurses with the medical staff frequently being the smallest in number. The stated aim of enhancing teamwork in this experiment is therefore null and void. Howard and Byl reported that the evaluations reflected a medical student dominance. This finding must surely be ignored because even if medical students do tend to dominate, the sheer number of them in this experiment would tend to ensure a dominating participation.

There were numerous dependent and independent variables in this research which were neither acknowledged nor addressed by the authors. In 1968 "a randomly selected interdisciplinary mix of about sixteen students" were chosen for each group (Howard and Byl 1971 : 773). If it was an interdisciplinary mix that was randomly allocated to twenty seven groups (Group leaders N=27), then in some groups no dental hygienists could have been present (N=24) with only one or two physiotherapy students participating (N=34). Whatever the final distribution four or five medical students would have been allocated to each tutorial group. This therefore means that the medical students would constitute 25% of the discussion in each group anyway if each group member contributed the same amount. Instead of building on the limited success of the tutorial group discussions reported by the 1968 group, the project team increased the amount of formal lecture time by 50% and decreased the tutorial time. There was no explanation for this change. Each year differed in content weighting as far as timing was concerned and had different numbers of students participating with a decreasing total annually. The presentation of results was therefore misleading and invalid. With the raw score differing (but not defined) in each year the percentages became meaningless. The 36% of the 75 students in 1970 who stated that the course was orientated towards all disciplines is not as meaningful as the 69% of the 438 who stated that it was in 1968. The two courses by the authors own admission were considerably different in content anyway.

The size of the discussion groups (N=16) was too large for meaningful learning to take place. Bruner (1966), Rogers (1969), Bolles (1979), Knowles (1984, 1986) and Boud and Griffin (1987) all suggest that the ideal number in a tutorial group is about ten persons. With sixteen students in a group the more extroverted, assertive students are likely to contribute more, whereas the more withdrawn, timid ones are likely to remain silent. The discussion is therefore more likely to be controlled by the dominant members of the group.

This paper in spite of the many flaws in the methodology has generated several unanswered questions which could be usefully explored in this current study. Questions could be asked of both staff and students which may clarify the ideal professional mix within an interdisciplinary tutorial group and also the preferred weighting of the teaching methods adopted.

Owen (1982) described the interdisciplinary learning initiatives taking place in Adelaide, Australia. The short course was specifically designed for final year students and used a structured, goal orientated framework. The stated aim was to maximise interaction between the students. He developed an evaluation questionnaire which categorised the students' impressions of the value of the course. In the same paper Owen heavily criticised the lack of empirical data on the real value of interdisciplinary learning and noted that most publications merely commented on the students' perceptions. He then compounded this by doing exactly the same. What was evident from his results however, was that of the 320 students who completed the questionnaire only 67 had found it 'generally unfavourable' and of these 23 were described as 'health administrators'. This can perhaps be explained by the fact that the other participating disciplines were all directly involved in 'hands on' care. It may be therefore that the health administrators did not see the relevance of much of the course although Owen did not comment on this.

Owen (1982) had several constructive comments to make for educators considering organising interdisciplinary courses. The choice of appropriate teaching methods was considered to be vital, with a combination of small group tutorials, traditional lectures, visits to relevant clinical areas, role play followed by interaction with 'real' patients and the opportunity for rapid feedback with the lecturers after any integrated learning being recommended. The content of any interdisciplinary course should be based on an analysis of what each discipline usually learned. This point was also made forcibly by Mase (1967). The differing levels of competence, interest and experience of the tutorial staff should not be ignored. The objectives of the course should be clearly identified and most importantly, presented to the students proir to the commencement of the course. Adequate time must be allowed to address the issues identifed and students should be presented with a challenge within the objectives in order that they experience a sense of achievement. Owen described this as 'avoiding the soft option'. Students' entry criteria, in the form of previous knowledge and experience must be taken into consideration and 'outside' lecturers must be briefed thoroughly.

Owen recommended that the planning team should minimise administrative difficulties and empirically evaluate their own performance as well as collating student evaluations. Owen suggested "Ask yourself how one would prove that any component........improves students' work performance or patient care (Owen 1982 : 54). He finally emphasised the importance of taking into account the local circumstances and available resources in any interdisciplinary developments.

McCreary (1968) and his colleagues encountered problems when implementing a major curriculum change in spite of "generous grants from......the Rockefeller Foundation and The John and Mary Markle Foundation" (Ibid : 1554). The grants had enabled them to design and commission a purpose built building which encompassed all the health professions' educational programmes and in addition to appoint a full time planning team.

The planning team was given three terms of reference - the identification of a core curriculum, the development of increased interdisciplinary learning in the clinical areas and to explore the possibility of clinical teaching on an interdisciplinary basis at an early stage in the curriculum.

Over a two year period the planning team made progress. An initial three month experience for all students from all disciplines was introduced, in which they jointly explored problems in community care. Clinical electives were undertaken on an interdisciplinary basis. Finally a core curriculum was developed which varied in length for each profession. This third and final development was not clearly explained. McCreary (1968) and his colleagues decided that different professions required three different levels of knowledge, the highest level for medical and dental students, the second for nurses and physiotherapists and the third for "dietitians and others" (p 1556). No mention was made of how and why they made these distinctions but it could be argued that while differing levels of knowledge in the biological sciences should exist an equal understanding of the behavioural sciences should be evident in all the health care professions. The planning team could not find an interdisciplinary learning model in existence and so had to rely on their own instincts when developing their programme. Thus the initiative evolved on a trail and error basis.

In 1992 although a few models have been identified, it would seem that each institution, considering the implementation of an interdisciplinary learning programme, should adapt and modify existing programmes in order to meet local unique circumstances.

Mason and Parascandola (1972) assumed that most health professionals accepted the need for interdisciplinary co-operation. They recognised that many qualified practitioners in most professions were actively working towards this goal, but suggested that the best way forward was that all students should start learning together at the beginning of their careers.

A multidisciplinary group of students commenced an introductory core curriculum. This new development was based on the following assumptions - if students learn how to function as team members they will operate as such, sharing learning experiences will be economically more efficient and interprofessional learning will increase interprofessional collaboration. Approximately 70 students enrolled on the first course. The aims of the course were stated as presenting a common body of knowledge enabling students to make informed choices about which career to follow, to stimulate interaction at an early stage for both students and staff and to provide a theoretical basis for future interdisciplinary learning.

The course content contained topics such as the philosophy of health care, teamwork, the organisation and delivery of health services in different settings, cultural and social factors affecting health, the role of the different health professions and the economics of health care. The format adopted was one of a series of whole group lectures followed by small group tutorials. Students were asked to evaluate each session. In addition, the students completed an unspecified attitudinal scale at the beginning and at the end of the course. Most of the students rated the course as 'good' to 'excellent'. Analysis of the attitudinal scales revealed an increased interaction between the students, an increased awareness of social and cultural influences in health care and a basic understanding of the concept of a health team. The problems encountered were minimal even though the students represented a wide variety of educational attainment to date. Mason and Parascandola also measured the success of the course by the fact that 260 students registered on the subsequent course.

The progress of the original approximately 70 students was monitored until they started working in a clinical setting with the aim of developing further interdisciplinary learning. A pilot study was undertaken in order to ascertain whether course proposals could be formulated which would identify the knowledge and skills needed by the students prior to commencing clinical practice. Students and staff collaboratively identified the desired learning outcomes and Mason and Parascandola were gratified to find that both groups seemed to have the same outcomes in mind. These included the identification of sociocultural and environmental factors which affect an individuals health status, planning a model of care on an interdisciplinary basis and the identification of external agencies which help contribute to a clients recovery.

In the initial stages of the pilot study itself 'clients' with long term health problems were used. The rationale for this was to enable students to plan intervention over a long period thereby having the opportunity to evaluate the effectiveness of the plan and change it if deemed necessary. Each student was given the responsibility of reporting the specific findings of his/her discipline at the staff - student conference. On alternate weeks the tutorial groups discussed group dynamics, role conflict and status differences, the reason for this being one of confronting potential or actual problems soon after they were identified. Mason and Parascandola (1972) reported that although the students were ill at ease with each other initially they subsequently developed a cohesion, rapport and an increase in self confidence. They also showed an increased interest in each others roles. As confidence increased they began to openly question and confront one another on particular issues and to discuss alternative approaches to client care.

The same attitudinal scale was completed by the students and compared with their written evaluations. Analysis of the scale supported the student evaluations and were positive in that the course had helped them clarify their ideas about groups, health teams and health care issues. All students and staff supported the continuance and extension of this course. Mason and Parascandola presented a convincing case but there were several flaws in their paper. No raw data was given whatsoever apart from the approximate number of students who participated in the study (N = "about 70" p : 729). Neither the disciplines involved nor the number of staff were given. The attitude scale used is not named nor described and it is therefore impossible to comment on its validity or reliability. The content analysis based on the written evaluations was not presented neither was the format the evaluations themselves took. Without access to this information the results must be treated with the greatest caution which is a pity as the philosophy of the course was impressive and the course contents seemed to be exciting and innovative. The assumption made regarding the economic efficiency of this course at the beginning of the paper was not referred to again. This may be simply due to an omission on the authors' part but it could be also due to a finding that indicated that it was less economically efficient.

In spite of these weaknesses Mason and Parascandola (1972) introduced the possibility of using a core curriculum at the introductory stage enabling students, planning to enter one of the health care professions, to make an informed choice regarding their career. A similar programme has subsequently been described in Finland by TEHY 1991a, 1991b.

The most illuminating author regarding an alternative curriculum for health care professionals was Leninger (1971). She published an excellent article in which she stated quite clearly her vision for the future of interdisciplinary education for the health professions. She addressed the challenges of curriculum development by suggesting different models which could be implemented.

Leninger (1971) believed that "interdisciplinary health education has received limited attention, yet it would seem to be a critical means for providing better health care to people" (Ibid : 787). She questioned whether there really was a shortage of manpower and suggested that it was the inappropriate use of talented personnel and resources that led to this impression being given. She noted that instead of increasing cohesiveness there was a worrying trend towards increasing diversity and specialism. While in no way trying to suggest that there was not a need for unique professional skills, Leninger postulated the reduction of interprofessional competitiveness so that the professions complemented rather than confronted one another. This, she suggested, could be best achieved through shared learning and the adoption of the shared goal of providing quality health care. Leninger felt that it was vital that undergraduate students learned to work together rather than at a later stage when they were qualified.

Leinger highlighted the attributes needed to make an interdisciplinary health curriculum work. These included commitment, time, effort, good interfaculty relationships with a dynamic and creative leadership, group effort and ownership, a willingness to take risks and a positive belief that each discipline has an unique contribution to make. Leninger predicted that increasing economic constraints would also lead to a greater demand for interdisciplinary learning. Planning and sharing educational resources (including tutorial staff) would become increasingly important. She acknowledged that many initiatives were already in existence but it was whether they "functioned as separate professional entities in a physical structure that houses different disciplines" (Leninger 1971: 788) that really concerned her. This criticism could be justifiably levelled in South East Wales in 1996.

Leninger, presuming that the reader accepted her observations, introduced the model that both the professionals and non professionals had described when questioned on their individual perceptions and expectations of health professionals. The typical response, according to Leninger, described a stratified pyramid model with the physician being at the apex and the others being viewed in varying subordinate roles in "rank, status, prestige, power and control" (1971 : p 788) (see Figure 2.3).

Leninger did not disclose how many people she questioned or indeed to which profession they belonged. A comparative study in which she measured the perceptions of a given number of personnel from each profession would have been of value. It must also be noted that Leninger was refering to health care in the USA. The results in The United Kingdom may have been different although this seems unlikely. The professions at the bottom of the pyramid would undoubtedly challenge their position which would increase the confrontation and conflict already in evidence. Leninger described most student training as linear and isolated in that each faculty prepared their own students within their own educational systems. Specific objectives and outcomes within each discrete profession Leninger described as the norm. This, she suggested, was costly, particularly as the same course content was often being taught to different disciplines at different times. She concluded "we need to reduce the educational costs and focus on the best use of faculty time and expertise" (Leninger 1971 : 790).

Leninger proposed the adoption of an interdisciplinary oval model (see Figure 2.4) The emphasis in this model is on the patient as the central focus with the broken lines suggesting the "open flow of ideas and opportunities between disciplines" (p 789). This, according to Leninger, would facilitate interdisciplinary learning and increase the self esteem of each professional group by enabling them to recognise the value of their unique contribution to patient care. This model would need an 'elected leader' who should be appointed on the

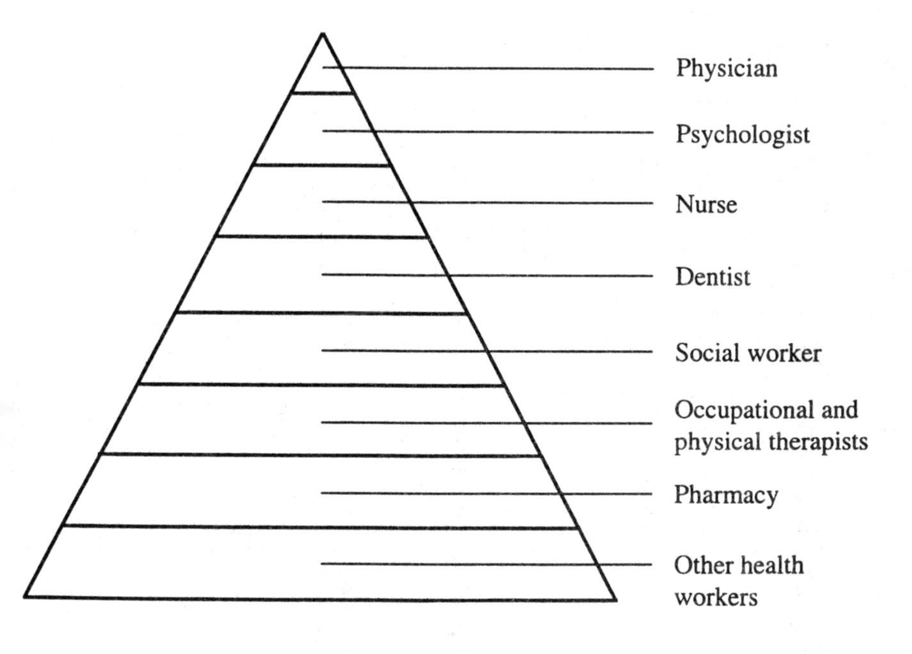

Figure 2.3 Stratified pyramid model (Leninger 1971)

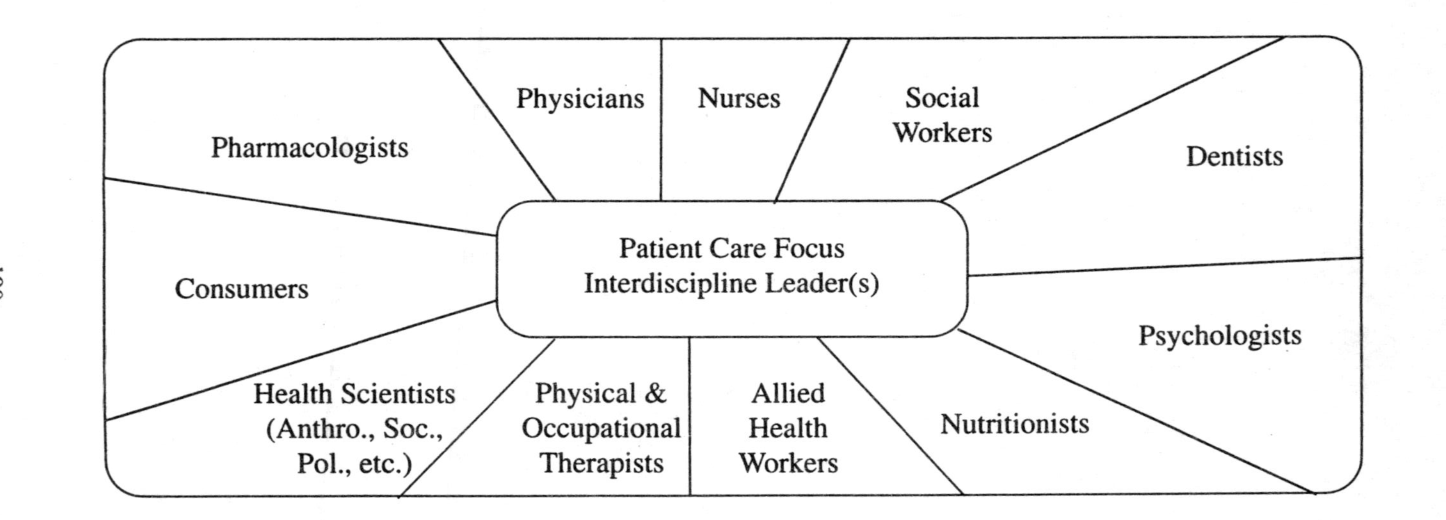

Figure 2.4 Interdisciplinary oval model (Leninger 1971)

criteria of openess, impartiality, objectivity, respect for others, organisational skills and commitment. If a person demonstrating these attributes could be identified then the profession to which he/she belonged would be of little relevance. Of particular interest in this model was the inclusion of the consumers. Leninger justified the inclusion of this group when she emphasised their unique contribution in the form of "concerns and ideas about health delivery services" (p 789).

An interdisciplinary cone model was another possibility explored by Leninger (see Figure 2.5). The vertical broken lines represent different disciplines with the arrows indicating the shared learning between disciplines. She suggested that there would be several advantages in adopting this model. Students would have the opportunity to learn and share knowledge on an interdisciplinary basis. There could be a core subject in which interdisciplinary seminars would have the effect of exploring each other's contributory roles in holistic health care. Leninger warned of the importance of the seminar leader maintaining an equal focus on each discipline and not demonstrating a bias towards their own profession. She asserted that the time for professional uniqueness was within the specialist tutorials. The first year being basic core courses would allow the students to move into another health discipline if they so wished "thus lateral and vertical career development and mobility would be possible in the model" (Leninger 1971 : 790).

This concept may be ideal however it would cause an administrative and educational nightmare. Staff/student ratios are based on the projected numbers of students on each course. It may well be the case that with no parameters set on the students in the introductory year, some disciplines would have too many applicants while others would not attract sufficient students. Manpower planning in the NHS has become increasingly important and consequently the number of students training for specific professions is closely monitored and the money released for these training programmes depends on the manpower predictions (Welsh Office 1990, HMSO 1990 Cmnd 555). Christman (1970) was very pessimistic in his outlook. He was convinced that the demands of the population was going to outstrip the production of trained manpower. He envisaged the time when a generic health professional would be caring for the patient. In the last few years in the United Kingdom, the introduction of National Vocational Qualifications (NVQ) for health care workers may be considered by some to have confirmed Christman's fears.

The interdisciplinary cone model (Figure 2.5) would encourage greater equity between the professions and Leninger (1971) suggests that it would ensure that no single profession would develop a feeling of superiority over the others. The Stratified Pyramid Model (illustrated in Figure 2.3) should be less evident amongst the professions trained using the interdisciplinary cone model than the others. The clustering of interdisciplinary courses described in the cone model would be reasonably predictable as some topics would be more relevant to nurses

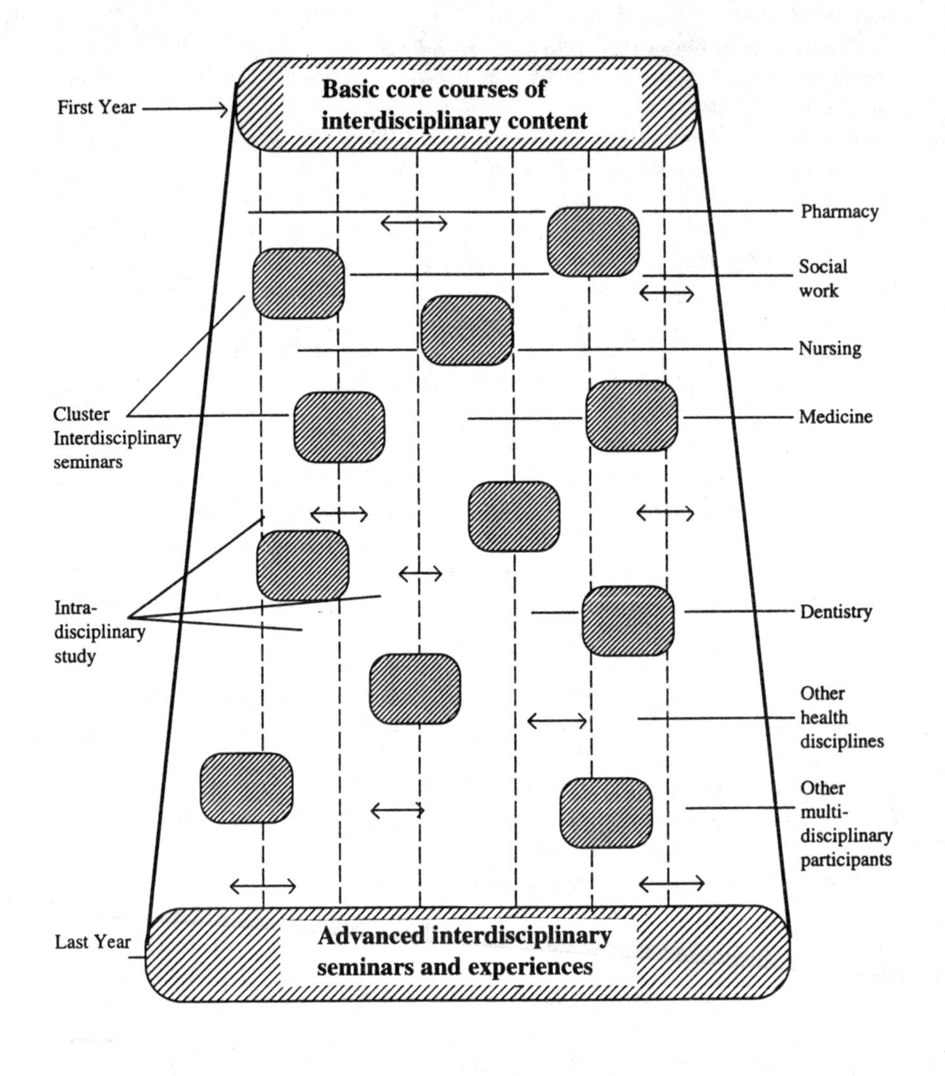

Figure 2.5 Interdisciplinary cone model (Leninger 1971)

and social workers than pharmacists for example.

Leninger also discussed the possibility of opting in and out of the model. Other disciplines such as humanities and social science students may well be interested in health problems and as such should be encouraged to participate. In the final year Leninger advocated an increased use of interdisciplinary seminars in which the students would "critically examine complex social and professional health problems that have led to problems in providing effective health care" (Leninger 1971 : 790).

Adopting such a strategy should mean that a common body of interdisciplinary knowledge emerged whilst ensuring that an element of refined specialist knowledge remains. In a wonderful analogy Leninger described health care disciplines as members of a symphony orchestra. Each has a specific tune to play but together what music they produce ! She made her convictions absolutely clear "it would not be prudent to completely and suddenly abolish our existing health disciplines. This would lead to chaos" (Leninger 1971 : 791).

Leninger, writing in 1971, can only be described as an educator with vision and courage. She demonstrated a very realistic grasp of interdisciplinary learning. In 1992 her ideas remain just as innovative and no evidence has been found of any institution adopting her ideas.

The final publication reviewed that identifies a core curriculum model was one written by Milio (1979). She was concerned with the quest for finding "more effective ways to deal with modern health problems" (p 152). She was convinced that the rationale for the introduction of a core curriculum could be based on contemporary illness patterns. This would then ensure that the training a health professional received would remain flexible and dynamic. Distinguishing between mental and physical health was no longer feasible. She introduced a most interesting discussion based on contemporary illness, in 1979, consisting of "relatively few types of conditions" (p 153). In the USA 75% of annual illness was "the result of fewer than 20 acute, chronic or death producing conditions" (p 153). She clustered these conditions and explained that they did not occur randomly as, for example, an individual with diabetes was more likely to have cardiovascular disease than a healthy member of the general population. In addition to this factors such as the inhalation of cigarette smoke increased the chances of ill health. Milio therefore suggested that a core curriculum could be based on primary, secondary and tertiary care which addressed the 20 conditions she identified. Health promotion and health education strategies she envisaged as assuming an ever more important role in health care. Too much time, she asserted, was spent by students from all disciplines "on learning the care of illness" (p 156). An attempt to share the many discipline specific research publications would be a major development in encouraging interdisciplinarity. Journals and textbooks should be adopted from every profession for the core curriculum.

Milio's model for a common core curriculum was very simple. She stated that it must be both integrative and interdisciplinary and should :

> encompass what all health professionals should know to effectively deal with modern health problems, including basic knowledge (a minimum level of awareness and understanding) and a perspective of a comprehensive and analytic nature from which and through which selected aspects could be developed in depth later.
>
> (Milio 1979 : 159)

From this philosophy Milio developed her objectives. These included that the students would become analytical in their approach, develop a critical consciousness and be stimulated to continually learn. The common core components thus became a series of questions rather than a set of answers. Milio suggested that the questions could be framed on the following :

1. What is modern illness ?
2. What are the major approaches to deal with modern illness ?
3. Why do certain strategies currently dominate ?
4. How might alternative strategies be developed and implemented ?

She believed that the answers could only be determined by complex mutual-casual decisions achieved through an integrated interdisciplinary approach. The adoption of this model would encourage staff and students from all disciplines to examine their own curriculum to assess how closely the content adhered to these four simple questions.

In 1992 these four questions remain just as crucial if not more so. The possibility of substituting the word 'illness' for 'education' in questions one and two would be of infinite help to the educators striving to produce quality courses for the health professions in order to meet the needs of the population they serve. This is absolutely vital because as Christman (1970) explained "The public will neither be content with superficial or one sided explanations about the gaps in care nor be willing to accept mediocrity in the quality of care" (Christman 1970 : 284).

2.10 Summary of the review of the literature

As stated at the beginning of this chapter, the impetus for this study was generated as a direct result of a growing awareness of the urgent need to address the problems of health professionals' education. The literature search yielded more than a thousand references to interdisciplinary initiatives in health care. Most have identifed the urgent need to increase interprofessional collaboration and co-operation and many have çhallenged the health care professions to solve the conflict, jealousy, cloistering and exclusivity in order that the needs of the patient become the central focus for everyone concerned with producing care of the highest quality. Although statutory requirements for each individual profession tend to constrain interdisciplinarity because of concerns with such issues as competence, accountability, confidentiality and responsibility, no evidence has been found which suggests that these problems are insurmountable.

Reports of developments in teamwork have had a high priority over the last twenty years and publications have been found which report such developments from all over the world. Opinions would appear to be divided as to when is the optimum time to introduce the professions to each other. On balance the general consensus would appear to be that interdisciplinary learning should commence at the very beginning of training and then be adopted as an integral part of a professional's continuing education. The importance of post graduate initiatives should not be minimised as most qualified professionals working in health care in 1996, all over the world, will have had little or no opportunity to experience the advantages of shared learning. Therefore for the forseable future, plans should be made for integrated interdisciplinary programmes to be introduced at all stages in a professional's career. Perhaps in the years to come, if interdisciplinary learning is assimilated into common educational practice, then advertised courses on health care issues will automatically be interdisciplinary unless specifically stated otherwise.

Manpower concerns, financial constraints, consumer demand and the recognition by many individuals within each profession has led to a greatly increased interest from all quarters. The implications of introducing interdisciplinary education are being considered by international, national and local organisations and paradoxically the implications of ignoring the concept is beginning to take a greater precedence. Some authors are committed to interdisciplinary education for purely altruistic reasons while others, mainly those who control the budget for health care, are more interested in the potential cost savings in both teaching personnel, student numbers and resources. It could be argued that the reasons for the upsurge in interest are purely academic. There is more than enough evidence to accommodate both diverse groups and certainly all the publications reviewed have indicated that the concept of holisitic patient care is more likely to be achieved through the adoption of an interdisciplinary learning strategy. There would appear to be no reason why an attempt to test the feasibility of introducing interdisciplinary learning at an undergraduate stage should not commence in South East Wales although this should not replace individual professional training programmes. Interdisciplinary learning should enhance and complement these programmes.

In spite of the number of publications identified which have described the success or otherwise of differing educational initiatives, many have been anecdotal reports. On initial reading some of the more rigorous papers have seemed promising. A critical analysis never the less has proved very disappointing. Many of the projects reported have been badly flawed in the methodology adopted. The use of volunteer students has in many cases invalidated the evaluation of a course, financial rewards have been used to increase student participation, the numbers of personnel participating in these studies have often been absent as have the raw scores in the evaluations of many of the so called successful programmes. Little attempt has been made to describe in detail the pitfalls of introducing such programmes and the content of the courses in many instances has been jealously guarded.

The importance of acknowledging each institution as unique, depending on the local population it serves, cannot be over emphasised. This does not mean however that guidelines could not be developed for other institutions to follow. Insularity is not a healthy strategy to adopt in seeking the highest quality for both education and health care. An interdisciplinary common core for health professionals may or may not be the ultimate aim in future developments but without doubt it is worthy of experimentation in some form. With the uniqueness of each local area in mind it may still be possible to utilise the work of previous researchers whose proposed frameworks for a core curriculum seem to have something to offer. The number of models identified have been minimal.

Only two authors (Leninger 1971 and Milio 1979) have been found who have described, in detail, frameworks upon which a realistic integrated interdisciplinary core curriculum could be based. The interdisciplinary cone model described by Leninger seems particularly powerful in its possibilities. This does not mean that the four core components identified by Milio are unworthy of serious consideration. Indeed it may be possible to adopt Leninger's model basing the course content on Milio's core components. The WHO (1988) document "Learning to Work Together For Health" clarifies the steps that should be taken when designing any integrated interdisciplinary learning programme. While the document is of vital importance to this study it does not identify a model core curriculum which should be adopted. For this reason the models suggested by Leninger (1971) and Milio (1979) formed the framework upon which the feasibility study continued in conjunction with the steps recommended by WHO (1988).

3 Design of the research

3.1 Introduction

The impetus for undertaking this study stemmed from an increasing personal awareness of the importance of interdisciplinarity in order to truly fulfil the concept of holistic patient/client care. The review of the pertinent literature revealed that urgent measures need to be taken if increased cooperation and collaboration both between and within the health and social care professions is to be achieved. The World Health Organisation has indicated that it wishes to encourage educational programmes for the professions "that will enable them to respond to the needs of the population they serve as part of efforts to achieve the goal of health for all...." (WHO 1988b : 5)

They proposed the introduction of interdisciplinary learning where students "learn together during certain periods of their education, with interaction as an important goal...." (Ibid : 6). In order to achieve this they suggested that interested individuals should examine the rationale and think through the implications of implementing such an innovation.

Two other documents published by the WHO also contributed significantly to the eventual research method chosen for this project (WHO 1987c and WHO 1987e). Two of these three documents included similar checklists as appendices which the WHO suggested could act as frameworks for the introduction of interdisciplinary learning (WHO 1987e and WHO 1988b). These have been included as Appendix 2.2 in this book. The third document (WHO 1987c) was less explicit but nevertheless was invaluable in helping identify the most appropriate research method. Within the document there was a chapter entitled "Getting Started". The authors suggested that before any innovation is attempted the external motives for change should be identified and that these motives should encompass broader aims than those within any discrete insitution. Having ascertained this the internal motives for change should then be addressed. An innovator should seek the support, in principle, of those people likely to be directly involved in the study and should identify others who strongly advocate the intended change, those who are risk takers, flexible and who would successfully promote the innovation. The curriculum of each profession which may be involved should be obtained and a content analysis of each should be completed. Financial support should be sought in the form of research grants, existing institutional budgets, or from any external agencies. The document advised not to plan for too long "while thoughtful planning and broad based input can relieve some anxiety, waiting too long can actually magnify doubts and paralyse dicision making." (WHO 1987c : 33) Traditional educators, they continued, wield great power and when the innovation is new it is most vulnerable to hostility and criticism.

Collectively these three documents suggested the adoption of many differing strategies in order to increase the chances of successfully implementing an innovative interdisciplinary programme. These can be summarised as follows ; involving different departments, institutions and outside agencies will diminish the researchers isolation and allow others to contribute productively to the project. Compromise is an important strategy to adopt. Defending and protecting the basic principles and values is vitally important but flexibility can be achieved on specific issues. Criticisms should be taken seriously and modifications made as a result of these. Student support is vital and the researcher should maintain a high profile with them. The evaluation methods adopted should be acceptable to both students and staff and the authors observed that most institutions demanded quantifiable results. The importance of emphasising the innovation as an experiment is highlighted with the concommitant need to be able to evaluate short term results. This would enable a long term strategy to be planned while the feasibility and effectiveness of such an innovation is still continuing. The aim of the innovation must be maintained as the central focus and extensive records should be kept of how and when changes occur, which strategies succeed and which fail and a written analysis of all developments should be made.

Establishing links with other institutions undertaking similar experiments is to be encouraged as a greater insight will be gained as a result of sharing experiences and making comparisons. Where possible the exchange of faculty staff and students, particularly on an international basis is seen as being an additional possibility. Affiliation with international or national networks would encourage external recognition and support for the innovation.

Maintaining the integrated interdisciplinary programme was described as a potentially excellent source of attracting external funding as it would be an ideal area for further experimentation and research. The programme therefore ultimately must prove it's worth to the institution in which it is operating as this may then encourage an extension of its philosophy.

The focus of this current study was to examine the feasibility of integrated, interdisciplinary learning of the behavioural sciences in the health and social care professions. Having reviewed the literature and having identified the three documents (WHO 1987c, 1987e and 1988b) referenced above as being central to any innovative changes intended, it was decided that the appropriate methodology for such a feasiblity study seemed to be action research.

3.2 Action research

Many references have been identified which examine the suitability of action research as a methodology in educational research (Lewin 1952 cited in Carr and Kemmis 1986, Halsey 1972 cited in Cohen and Manion 1992, Susman et al 1978, Barnes 1979, Cohen and Mannion 1980, Moore 1983, Kemmis cited in Boud et al 1985, Carr and Kemis 1986, Treece and Treece 1986, Stanford 1987, Burgess 1989, Kelly 1989, Tesch 1990, Parahoo 1991, Cohen and Manion 1992). Cohen and Manion perhaps summarised the most succinctly when to adopt action research as the methodology "Action research is appropriate whenever specific knowledge is required for a specific problem in a specific situation; or when a new approach is to be grafted on to an existing system." (Cohen and Manion 1992 : 226) They described action research as situational in that it diagnosed and attempted to solve specific problems. Moore (1983) also commented on the specificity of a situation; "Action research is conducted with the primary intention of solving a specific, immediate, concrete problem in a local setting. The development of theory or generalizable applications is not of concern." (Moore 1983 : 24).

Halsey (1972) cited in Cohen and Manion (1990) described the method as "a small scale intervention in the functioning of the real world and a close examination of the effects of such intervention" (Ibid : 217) Tesch (1990 : 66) described the method as a "transformative activity" which could therefore be described as a self examination, while Carr and Kemmis (1986 :183) decided that "action researchers are deliberately activist." They described this phenomena as emancipatory as "participants in a situation reach authentic understandings of their situation". (Ibid : 158)

Kemmis (1985) cited in Boud et al (1985) had previously developed this idea of emancipation when he discussed his understanding of action research. The aim he suggested was to emancipate "people from the dictates of taken for granted assumptions, habits, tradition, custom, domination and coercion and self deception." (Ibid : 145) As, according to Tesch (1990), the reason for undertaking emancipatory action research is to improve an unsatisfactory situation, action research is "successful to the degree in which the knowledge produced results in the improvement of practices." (Tesch 1990 : 66)

Stanford (1987) believed that it encouraged empowerment in people facing challenges or problems while Treece and Treece (1986) referred to the consumer orientation properties of action research. Susman et al (1987) suggested that it enabled a scientific contribution to problem solving. In health care it would seem that it aims to bridge the gap between theory and practice by continuously modifying the ongoing situation by evaluation (Stanford 1987, Cohen and Manion 1992). Both Stanford (1987) and Cohen and Manion (1992) identify collaboration between the researcher(s) and the participants in the study, as one of the key concepts of action research. Kelly (1989) adopted the term "simultaneous integrated action research" and concluded that it was imperative that the action and the research proceeded together. Implicit in this statement is that the researcher can not remain a neutral outsider but must be actively engaged in the situation he/she is studying. Heron (1985) expanded this theme by suggesting that this degree of cooperation means that it is a way of "doing research with people rather than on people." (p 128).

A potential problem therefore exists in the value laden involvement of the researcher. Barnes (1979) insisted that values needed to be made explicit and Kelly (1989) was convinced that without explicit commitment by the researcher for any proposed change then the impetus to undertake the project would not exist and the status quo would remain. Kelly was quick to point out; "To say that all research is value laden does not entail a disregard for traditional criteria of reliability and validity. On the contrary it takes them one stage further." (Kelly 1989 : 102).

Kelly recommended that a researcher should clearly state his/her own position as inevitably, she believed, the purpose of any research is to influence or alter the world in accordance with the values held (p 102). Parahoo (1991) made a similar statement. Kelly (1989) was convinced that although action researchers could be accused of interfering, the right to intervene should rest on the ability to persuade "teachers and other interested parties" (p 103), that the proposals were worth trying and of potential value. Of the greatest importance in action research is the need to retain a conviction that the assumption being made could be wrong and that any proposal may not be feasible after all. The whole exercise may even turn out to be counterproductive.

Kemmis (1985) cited in Boud et al (1985) was even more convinced that a researcher could not be value free or even "value neutral" (p 149) as critical thinking depended on the individual's ability to reflect, and values were the principles upon which this process depended. Kemmis argued that action research hinges on reflection and justified this in the statement "Reflection is not a purely internal psychological process : it is action oriented (sic) and historically embedded." (Ibid :140)

Kemmis believed that critical or meta thinking (p 141) was action orientated with the ultimate outcome being "informed committed action" or praxis. He made the interesting point that any outcome of reflection should have "meaning and significance in the social world" (p143). Carr and Kemmis (1986) expanded this idea when they debated authenticity. They decided that it occurs as a result of personal knowledge based on rational reflection of previous personal actions. Praxis can only apply to individual practices and Carr and

Kemis concluded that "Action research therefore cannot be other than research into ones own practice" (Carr and Kemmis 1986 : 191)

The aim of simultaneous action research should be to increase the awareness of respondents to issues they may not have previously considered. Carr and Kemmis (1986) described this process as extending and transforming the understanding of practitioners, while Kelly (1989) insisted that it is an ethical responsibility of a researcher to introduce practitioners to other points of view. Carr and Kemmis (1986 : 186) concluded that the use of "controlled intervention and practical judgement " is the correct strategy to adopt in action research.

The evolving nature of action research poses potential problems in that a formal contract explaining the exact nature and length of any involvement is impossible as the project should remain flexible and dynamic. A further problem in adopting action research as a methodology is deciding when the project is complete. The phrase "feasibility study" which was adopted for this current study addressed this dilemma. The findings of the study should enable a decision to be made of whether or not the introduction of integrated interdisciplinary learning is feasible.

Emancipatory action research is a collaborative process in which participants plan action based on self reflection, implement plans based on informed committed action or praxis, monitor progress and evaluate the success of the plan by collecting evidence (returning to reflection) and finally the formulation of further plans. Kemmis (1985) cited in Boud et al (1985) described this as a spiral of self reflection in which the participants are encouraged to develop insight into practical action. Kemmis suggested that emancipatory action researchers are ideologists in that they "articulate their own theories in their own language" (p 157) although subsequently Carr and Kemmis (1986) warned that although action researchers could be described as critical forces they also represent "a challenge to established authority" (p 206). Carr and Kemmis (1986) returned to the concept of a spiral of self reflection and quoted Lewin (1952) who first coined the phrase "action research". Lewin had described the process as one consisting entirely of planning, fact finding and execution. He based the methodology on the principles of independence, equality and cooperation. Heron (1985) aligned this spiral of reflection to an experiential learning cycle. Carr and Kemis (1986) agreed with this and added that action research should be also viewed as the "embodiment of democratic principles....." (p 164) thus ensuring ownership and empowerment of those involved. The spiral of reflection in conjunction with the embodiment of democratic principles thus is seen as the central tenet to action research.

To summarise, according to the literature, the two central aims of action research appear to be Improvement and Involvement.. However, within the context of this present study, true action research could not be used as no *actual* changes to the current situations could possibly be made because of lack of direct involvement and the multi-disciplinary, multi-institutional nature of the study.

The proposed research did have as a basic aim, the study of a situation in order to bring about a potential educational change which would improve the quality of patient care. In consequence, whilst a semi-modified form of action research could be used to gain initial data suitable for preparing research instruments, obtaining cooperation and gaining access to participants, the study would have to stop short of actual implementation of the findings. The data generated however, would enable direct implementation (improvement and involvement) by the participating professions and institutions if interdisciplinary learning was introduced.

3.3 Defining the population

The population in a research study refers to "the entire aggregation of cases that meets a designated set of criteria" (Polit and Hungler 1989 : 168). Authors agree that the inclusion criteria should be clearly defined and individuals who meet the criteria then become the target population (Gay 1976, Youngman 1979, Moore 1983, Treece and Treece 1986, Kerlinger 1986, Cormack 1987, Marshall and Rossman 1989, Robson and Foster 1989, Polit and Hungler 1989, Tesch 1990, Hicks 1990, Sommer and Sommer 1991, Streiner and Norman 1991, Judd et al 1991, Cohen and Manion 1992). Moore (1983) suggested that having identifed the target population the major demographic characteristics of that population should be compiled and then a sample large enough to represent those characteristics should be selected.

Data can be obtained from the target population on one occasion only or over a period of time. If the former method is adopted it is described as a cross sectional design with the latter being described as a longitudinal design. Polit and Hungler (1989 : 138) remarked that in a cross sectional design "the phenomena under investigation are captured" while Cohen and Manion (1992 :72) believed "it produces a snap shot of a population." In some instances the adoption of either method would be appropriate. An example of this being a comparison between first and third year students attitudes. A longitudinal approach could be used where the same cohort was tested in their first year and then two years later in their third year, alternatively data could be collected from different respondents in a first year group and a third year group. This then becomes a cross sectional survey. Treece and Treece (1986 : 182) described a survey as a "critical inspection of a particular situation, problem or question". The advantages of a cross sectional survey can be described as follows : It is practical, economical, relatively easy to manage, completed in a relatively short period of time, the variables are not altered by time, there are immediate results and potentially there is a larger sample. However there are inevitably weaknesses in adopting this method. These include the fact that society changes very quickly therefore responses regarding attitude, behaviours or characteristics may depend on trends and current thinking. The respondents may be asked to recall retrospectively a single incidence in time, which may introduce an element of bias and the researcher may not know if a confounding variable is present (Moore 1983, Treece and Treece 1986, Polit and Hungler 1989, Streiner and Norman 1991, Oppenheim 1992, Cohen and Manion 1992).

The adoption of the longitudinal approach also has several strengths and weaknesses. The strengths include the opportunity for the researcher to follow up each individual respondent, early trends can be noted and expanded upon, collecting data from the same cohort should increase the reliability of the results by reducing the number of independent variables. Unfortunately the greatest disadvantage of this type of survey is the length of time it takes to complete and "it may take many years before the results are known" (Treece and Treece 1986 : 220). It is therefore potentially more costly and there is the risk of losing some or many of the cohort. This has been described by Cohen and Manion (1992 : 73) as "sample mortality".

In a feasibility study the choice of a cross sectional survey approach is justified as it is in reality a pilot study to test the possibilities for future developments. If the results show that an innovation such as integrated interdisciplinary learning is feasible then a longitudinal survey would be an appropriate strategy to adopt to measure the long term progress of the new programme.

3.4 The sample

"A sample is a representative part of the whole" (Treece and Treece 1986 : 234). Polit and Hungler (1989) referred to a subset of the population. Accurate reflection of the target population would seem to be the key words in selecting the sample size which should be as large as possible as the larger the sample the more representative the results (Moore 1983, Kerlinger 1986, Judd et al 1991). If the number of subjects is too small bias will occur and the results would be invalidated. Nevertheless a large sample will not correct a faulty sampling design or guarantee representativeness. Various authors address the problems of a safe minimum and examples have been found that vary from a recommended fifteen subjects (Moore 1983) to twenty five (Hicks 1990) to thirty subjects (Cohen and Manion 1992). Treece and Treece (1986) insisted that adequate sampling depended on the level of insight the researcher had into the problem being investigated. This would ensure that most variables in the population would be recognised with regard to the key characteristics in the study.

Probability sampling occurs when each individual in the population has an equal chance of being selected whereas the hallmark of non probability sampling is that some people have a greater chance of selection than others. Data collected through non probability sampling has a greater chance of inaccuracy and non representativeness than that collected through probability sampling. In either case sampling errors and sampling bias can occur. Several authors distinguish between error and bias (Moore 1983, Robson and Foster 1989, Judd et al 1991). They suggest that sampling error is out of the control of the researcher and is due to the particular random sample obtained. This may be caused by freak chance. An example of this would be as the result of random sampling responses being obtained from nine men to every one woman when the population census indicated that there was nearly a fifty/fifty ratio. On the other hand sampling bias is usually the researchers fault and is caused by personal error, mathematical mistakes or inadequately designed research instruments such as a badly worded questionnaire. Sampling bias can therefore be reduced by the use of a pilot study which should identify such a problem.

Cohen and Manion (1992) and Treece and Treece (1986) did not differentiate between bias and error. Indeed Cohen and Manion (1992 : 105) commented that "sampling error is not necessarily the result of mistakes made in sampling" but may also be due to chance. Random sampling does however ensure to some degree that the results are reasonably representative and unbiased.

Stratified random sampling reduces the chance of obtaining a non typical sample. For this reason it is more accurate than random sampling in that the respondents are more uniform than the whole population. It is a "mutually exclusive segment of a population based on one or more characteristics" (Polit and Hungler 1989 : 170) or a combination of two or more inclusion criteria (Judd et al 1991 : 204). It allows for a more efficient use of time and resources and is therefore more cost efficient (Kerlinger 1986, Treece and Treece 1986, Hicks 1990). A potential problem in using random stratified sampling in a small target population is that too little data would be generated from some of the strata. This problem can be overcome by weighting the data in order to make the closest estimate to the overall population values (Moore 1983, Kerlinger 1986, Judd et al 1991).

The target population in this feasibility study comprised teachers and students from thirteen of the health and social care professions trained in South East Wales. It was of paramount importance that the views of each of these professions were sought if support for the study was to be universal. Therefore stratified random sampling was used to identify potential respondents for the focused interviews. In this way representatives from both the teaching staff and the student population of each profession were given the opportunity to participate in the study. Questionnaires were distributed to the entire target population of all staff and all students in every profession (Appendices 4.4 and 4.5).

3. 5 Dependent and independent variables

According to Moore (1983 : 21) "a variable is the opposite of a constant". A variable can have a range of different values or as few as two (de Vaus 1986 : 27). They must however have at least two properties, they must be measureable and they must be valid (Cohen and Manion 1992 : 204). Variables are unpredictable in that they are liable to change (Treece and Treece 1986 : 146) or take on different values (Kerlinger 1986 : 27, Polit and Hungler 1989 : 35). They can also be dependent or independent in different studies (Judd et al 1991 : 42). The independent variable is attributed as the cause and occurs before the dependent variable (Treece and Treece 1986 : 143). The dependent variable therefore cannot exist by itself. Oppenheim (1992 : 10) described dependent variables as those which "yield the predicted outcome". A dependent variable therefore varies according to an individuals performance or behaviour within a particular level or group of the independent variable. The independent variable stands alone and is not dependent on any other, it is a situation, characteristic or phenomenon within which an individual functions (Moore 1983 : 137).

In addition to these two main categories of variables other types of variables have to be taken into consideration. An intervening variable is the means by which an independent variable affects the dependent one. It cannot be measured and it cannot be controlled however it is a researchers responsibility to try to minimise potential intervening variables such as stress and anxiety (Kerlinger 1986, Judd et al 1991). Extraneous variables may lie outside the interest and control of the researcher, the educational levels and scholastic ability of respondents being possible examples of these (Moore 1983). Nevertheless in this current study the educational entry criteria of students were not extraneous. It was essential to know how many students had completed courses such as Advanced Levels in the behavioural sciences as this may have had an important influence on their opinions. Confounding variables interfere with the study design and data collection process by influencing the respondents (Treece and Treece 1986 : 157). This "can lead to a serious misinterpretation of the findings" (Oppenheim 1992 : 10). Organismic variables are not subject to manipulation, they are attributes such as gender, age, ethnic minority (Hicks 1990, Judd et al 1991). Organismic variables can therefore be identified through the comprehensive collection of demographic data at the beginning of a questionnaire.

3.6 Operational definition

An operational definition specifies precisely how to measure a variable in concrete steps so that anyone else could repeat the experiment and use the same measurements. It thus becomes "a specification of the operations that the researcher must perform in order to collect the required information" (Polit and Hungler 1989 : 37). Treece and Treece (1986 : 508) described an operational definition as converting the problem into an "empirically testable statement".

3.7 Concepts and constructs

A concept is an abstraction formed by generalisation of particulars, a class of objects or a general notion (Kerlinger 1986, Judd et al 1989, Oxford English Dictionary 1985) whereas a construct is deliberately and consciously invented or adopted for a specific scientific purpose (Kerlinger 1986). It is a mini theory to explain the relationships in aspects of behaviour that vary from individual to individual. (Moore 1983, Streiner and Norman 1991)

3.8 Validity

Vaughan and Morrow (1989) described validity as "The degree to which a measurement actually measures or detects what it is supposed to measure." (Ibid : 187) Streiner and Norman (1991) insisted that empirical evidence should be produced that demonstrated that what was intended was being measured. Validity will depend on how the concept it is designed to measure is defined. There are three main ways in which to assess validity.

1. Construct validity is "concerned not only with validating the measure but also the theory underlying the measure" (Holsti 1969 : 148). It is the interplay between the measurement of the constructs that constitute a theory and the degree to which the measurement tool conforms to the theory expectations. In the consideration of attributes such as values, reasoning and personal perceptions construct validity assumes a great importance (Moore 1983, de Vaus 1986, Treece and Treece 1986, Streiner and Norman 1991). De Vaus (1986 : 48) advised that care should be taken to avoid "developing a test so that it supports the theory" but Youngman (1979) pointed out that it was "the mere fact that it is needed in a piece of research implies that certain relationships involving the attribute concerned are already known or suspected" (Ibid : 182) Streiner and Norman (1991) suggested two reasons for developing a new instrument in order to measure a hypothetical construct, the construct is so novel that no instrument currently exists that will measure it, or if there are existing tools which only partly meet the need. They observed that construct validity is a continuing process of learning, in which new predictions are made and tested.

2. Content validity, sometimes described as face validity, is the accuracy or representativeness to which an instrument measures the situation being studied (Kerlinger 1986, Leedy 1989). Youngman (1979 : 181) believed that equating content validity with face validity gave "an unjustified credibility to a procedure". To support his statement Youngman cited Nunally (1967) who insisted that construct validity should be the over riding concern in test validation. Judd et al (1991) did not reference content validity at all but persisted in describing it as face validity whereas Moore (1983) used face validity and content validity interchangeably and described it as a professional appraisal. Content validity according to de Vaus (1986 : 48) "emphasises the extent to which the indicators measure the different aspects of the concept" while Streiner and Norman (1991 : 5), using the term interchangeably, postulated that it "simply indicates whether on the face of it the instrument appears to be assessing the desired qualities". This suggests that the outcome depends upon the application of the test rather than the test itself. It is most relevant for tests designed to measure knowledge in a specific content area and is based on judgement of whether the test represents a particular area of knowledge (Polit and Hungler (1989 : 247). Moore (1983) agreed with this. He suggested that content validity was most useful for testing skill and proficiency but least useful for testing personality domains. Treece and Treece (1986) reported that content validity was an important characteristic of check lists, inventories, evaluation instruments and interview schedules. They advised that in any study "every item should be related to the hypothesis and to the focus of the study" (Treece and Treece 1986 : 262). Streiner and Norman (1991) believed that expert judgement was essential if this was to be achieved.

3. *Criterion validity* is where the relationship between the test and one or more external variables is compared (Kerlinger 1986, Polit and Hungler 1989, Leedy 1989, Streiner and Norman 1991). De Vaus (1986) warned of a potential problem in comparing how respondents answered a new test in comparison with an existing test. As criterion validity indicates a high correlation between the two tests, if a low correlation is found this often meant that the conclusion was drawn that the new test was invalid. This de Vaus concluded, may not in fact be the case as in examining new concepts existing tests may not be the precise measures to use.

3.9 Reliability

Streiner and Norman (1991 : 8) Stated that reliability "simply assesses that a test is measuring something in a reproducible fashion; it says nothing about *what* is being measured" In action research altering strategies within a flexible and dynamic study cannot and should not be replicated in other studies and this should be made clear in the written report. Nevertheless records should be kept of each planning decision and the rationale behind it for subsequent critical examination. All data should be kept in an easily retrievable form. Marshall and Rossman (1989) advised an action researcher not to try and control the conditions in which the research was taking place but to concentrate instead on "recording the complexity of situational contexts and interrelations as they occur" (Ibid : 148) Marshall (1985) cited in Marshall and Rossman (1989) advised that the following rules should be applied in these situations ; data collection methods should be explicit; data should be used to document analytical constructs ; negative findings should be discussed and accounted for ; personal biases and assumptions should be admitted ; methods of data collection and analysis should be publicised : a change of strategy or focus should be clearly documented : competing problems and their proposed solutions should be recorded ; all data should be preserved : the respondents reliability should be measured and any generalisations should be made explicit.

3.10 Content analysis

Classical content analysis involves "making replicable and valid inferences from data to their context" (Krippendorf 1980 : 21). It requires objectivity, reliability, systematic application and consistency by the analyst (Holsti 1969, Kerlinger 1986, Polit and Hungler 1989, Judd et al 1991). Treece and Treece (1986 : 349) observed that it is a "precise, authoritative procedure" which examines and quantifies a specific topic. Kerlinger (1986 : 479) described this as defining "U" or the universe of a phenomena. In other words the phenomena to be coded must be chosen. The analyst must not inhibit or enhance the possibility of obtaining particular findings and so the coding categories must be made from either a simple binary system or from multi-category systems. A choice must be made among the categories to be coded whether every reference should be noted or just a representative sample. Categories should not be established prior to the analysis itself but should emerge from the data. The results may lead to a reconceptualisation which then require additional analysis. Tesch (1990) warned however, that although the method is largely numeric, any conclusions are not only statistical but substantive, while Holsti (1969 : 11) recommended that the "content analyst should use qualitative and quantitative methods to supplement each other". Marshall and Rossman (1989) suggested that content analysis should aim at producing descriptive information, cross validating research findings or testing a hypothesis. They described it as a flexible method that allows the analyst to arrange components best suited to meet the requirements of the study. They were convinced that it is an art as well as a science which can be used effectively to supplement other research methods.

Cohen and Manion (1992 : 61) suggested the method could be used in the analysis of educational documents. They believed that the categories could only be determined after an initial inspection of the documents and should only cover the main areas of content. If an enumeration of recorded occurences is made these then become classified as units of analysis. A unit of analysis may consist of a sentence, a paragraph, a theme or as little as a single word (Polit and Hungler 1989, Tesch 1990, Cohen and Manion 1992). Treece and Treece (1986) were less specific when they wrote that it consisted of "The reviewing of the content of some form of communication for consistent use of word or idea". (Ibid : 503)

The process of content analysis is time consuming, classification of the units of analysis may be ambiguous, the analysts interpretation may be subjective and the documents being analysed may only consist of what "was thought important enough to write down" (Wiseman and Aron 1972 : 149). To minimise these weaknesses the researcher should create a rationale showing that the analysis is relevant and necessary to the problem being studied (Holsti 1969). Evidence of expert opinion should be cited or a theory or model which has evolved from previous research should be identified (Moore 1983, Marshall and Rossman 1989, Tesch 1990). If no appropriate instrument already exists then one should be devised.

A content analysis of each curriculum in order to ascertain the behavioural science component seemed to be the most appropriate method to choose in spite of the inherent problems identified. As each curriculum was unique to the development team in each discipline it was necessary to analyse each document for the key concepts.

3.11 Interviews

According to Kahn and Cannell (1957), quoted by Marshall and Rossman (1989 : 82), an interview "is a conversation with a purpose". Kerlinger (1986) described it as a face to face encounter while Wiseman and Aron (1972 : 43) likened it to a "fishing expedition". Authors generally agree however that it is a method of collecting data as a result of an interaction between two or more people in order to obtain information (Wiseman and Aron 1972, Youngman 1978, Moore 1983, Treece and Treece 1986, Kerlinger 1986, Polit and Hungler 1989, Robson and Foster 1989, Judd et al 1991, Cohen and Manion 1992, Oppenheim 1992).

Two opposing views have been voiced on the popularity of individual interviews as a means of collecting data. Burns cited in Robson and Foster (1989 : 47) noted that because of the cost implications the individual interview had been "a relatively neglected technique in recent years". Burns argued that only when personal, intimate or threatening topics were involved should individual interviews take precedence over group interviews. She did concede however that if the purpose of the interview was to generate data for a subsequent inclusion in a questionnaire it may be preferable to conduct a one to one interview. Paradoxically Treece and Treece (1986) described interviews as the second most popular way of data collection with questionnaires being the most popular.

An interview has three main purposes. It can be an exploratory device to help identify variables, to suggest hypotheses and to guide future developments in a research project. It can be the main instrument of data collection in research or finally it can supplement other methods by following up unexpected results and validate the other methods used. Whatever the purpose, the interview must be subjected to the same stringent criteria as all other data collection methods. Reliability, validity and researcher objectivity are paramount as is the necessity to obtain informed consent from the respondent with the assurance of concommitant confidentiality. Data collected at interview may be difficult to validate so in a focused interview the careful formulation of the questions is vital.

Oppenheim (1992) identified three interacting variables in the interviewing process, the interviewer, the respondent and the interview schedule or questionnaire. Robson and Foster (1989) did not dispute these but added that the territory on which the interview was conducted was also extremely important. They recommended that the interview should be conducted on neutral territory which would minimise the bias towards either the interviewer or the respondent.

There are many limitations in the use of interviewing as a data collection method. These should be identified, accepted and where possible resolved. Interviews must involve personal interaction, the respondent therefore is not anonymous although confidentiality can be guaranteed (Kerlinger 1986, Cohen and Manion 1992). Mutual cooperation and rapport are essential otherwise the respondent may refrain from giving information (Robson and Foster 1989, Marshall and Robson 1989, Judd et al 1991). Judgement, common sense, training, experience, good listening skills, an awareness of non verbal communication strategies are all essential interviewing skills (Hoinville et al 1987, Robson and Foster 1989, Polit and Hungler 1989, Judd et al 1991, Streiner and Norman 1991, Oppenheim 1992). The social/ethnic characteristics of the interviewer may afford bias in the respondents answers because of stereotyping, prejudice or role set (Wisemann and Aron 1972, Weiss 1975, Kerlinger 1986, Hoinville et al 1987, Marshall and Rossman 1989, Robson and Foster 1989, Judd et al 1991, Streiner and Norman 1991, Cohen and Manion 1992, Oppenheim 1992). Inappropriate questions may be asked because of lack of interviewer expertise (Kerlinger 1986, Marshall and Rossman 1989) or the answers given by the respondents may be misinterpreted by the interviewer for the same reason (Oppenheim 1992, Robson and Foster 1989). Interviewing is more expensive, time consuming and resource demanding than many other data collection methods (Wiseman and Aron 1972, Kerlinger 1986, Robson and Foster 1989, Judd et al 1991, Streiner and Norman 1991, Cohen and Manion 1992, Oppenheim 1992).

In defence of the interview as a research method there are also many advantages in its adoption. According to Oppenheim (1992 : 32) "an undisputed advantage" is the "richness and spontaneity of the information collected ....". while the greatest advantage is the flexiblity of this method (Wiseman and Aron 1972, Polit and Hungler 1989, Judd et al 1991, Streiner and Norman 1991, Oppenheim 1992). Oppenheim (1992 : 31) added a caveat to this statement however, he asserted that this was only possible "in the hands of a skilled interviewer". Several authors commented that the response rate was likely to be higher and a large amount of data could be assimilated quickly (Marshall and Rossman 1989, Polit and Hungler 1989, Judd et al 1991, Streiner and Norman 1991). An additional bonus is that this technique allows immediate follow up questions, interviewers can determine whether the respondents have understood the questions and can also probe inadequate responses (Marshall and Rossman 1989,

Polit and Hungler 1989, Judd et al 1991, Streiner and Norman 1991). Additional information may also be obtained through observation of the respondents non verbal communication (Polit and Hungler 1989).

In summary, the use of individual face to face interviews as a data collection method, while fraught with many potential problems, is appropriate if the intention of the interviewer is to generate information which can subsequently be incorporated into a questionnaire which is to be distributed widely. The focused interview schedule must be developed with as much caution as the questionnaire itself and must be tested in a pilot study before commencement of the main interviews.

The review of the literature generated many questions which could be incorporated into a questionnaire. Nevertheless it was necessary to attempt to generate as much information as possible pertaining to the unique situation in which the feasibility study was taking place. It was decided that individual focused interviews with both staff and students from each discipline would be the best way to achieve this. The analysed information would then form the basis of the questionnaire.

3.12 Questionnaires

"An ideal questionnaire possesses the same properties as a good law" observed Cohen and Manion (1992 : 106). They quoted Davidson (1970) who wrote "it is clear,unambiguous and uniformly workable". Oppenheim (1992 : 2) described it as "essentially a scientific instrument for measurement and collection of particular kinds of data". A questionnaire should have a specific design for the specific study in mind and should always have the mode of analysis built in (Youngman 1978). Hicks (1990 : 74) described it as a "complex science in its own right" and insisted that it must be tested for bias, sequencing, clarity, reliability and validity in a pilot study before the main data collection commenced. A questionnaire should be highly structured so that the respondents can be asked the same set of questions. The answers obtained should be amenable to quantitative and where appropriate statistical analysis (De Vaus 1986). All questionnaires rely on the honesty and accuracy of the responses and it should be remembered that the values and internalised beliefs of the respondents may be difficult to obtain (Marshall and Rossman 1989).

Leedy (1989) suggested that the first principle in designing a questionnaire should be to inspect the assumptions underlying the questions. Questions should be realisitic and fit in with "the realities of life" (p 143) and essentially they should elicit facts that provide information for action. Oppenheim (1992) believed that a questionnaire should be developed specifically to explore the relationships between particular variables. Cohen and Manion (1992) suggested the use of a flow chart in order to clarify the sequencing of the questions. By adopting this method the range and quality of the potential responses may be able to be anticipated. They advised that leading, highbrow, complex, irritating and negative questions should be avoided (p 108). They also recommended avoiding open ended questions in self completing questionnaires (p 109). Oppenheim (1992) on the other hand suggested that free response questions could usefully be used at the pilot study stage and that these may then generate further information which could be redesigned into forced choice responses in the main study. There are several advantages in the use of forced choice questions; they are quicker to answer, easier to code, they are less discriminatory, they minimise interviewer bias, they demand an immediate response and allow for greater anonymity. However, the quality of the respondents potential answers are lost as they are unable to voice an opinion. For this reason alone it is wise to include some open ended questions or to invite the respondent to make additional comments in appropriate places.

In this current feasibility study the use of focused interviews to generate questions for the questionnaire meant that free responses were encouraged at the interview stage, with the specific intention of developing a final self completion questionnaire amenable to statistical analysis, which meant that the questions were predominantly forced choice. Nevertheless the opportunity for the respondents to make additional comments was also included.

Most authors emphasised the importance of the visual appearance of the questionnaire. It should be well organised, comprehensively worded, attractive to view, with clear instructions and with an example question and completed response. A covering letter is vital in which the purpose of the study is explained, the invitation to participate is clear, an assurance of confidentiality should be given along with the right to refuse and the opportunity to withdraw at any stage. It was also recommended that the letter should be terminated with thanks being given to the potential respondents along with the offer to send an abstract of the results on completion of the study. Finally the name, position and contact address of the researcher should be clearly identified (Oppenheim 1992, Youngman 1979, Moore 1983, Treece and Treece 1986, Kerlinger 1986, Cormack 1987, Marshall and Rossman 1989, Polit and Hungler 1989, Judd et al 1991, Cohen and Manion 1992). This advice was adhered to as closely as possible in both the questionnaire itself and in the explanatory letter which accompanied it (see Appendix 3.1).

3.13 The pilot study

The purpose of a pilot study is to test the feasibility of the main study and usually focuses on the efficacy of the research instruments used. Youngman (1978 : 26) believed that it "is an integral part of any research", Polit and Hungler (1989 : 399) described it as a "small scale version, or trial run...." while Marshall and Rossman claimed that it lent credence to the main study's credibility. The Open University (1989 Book 4 : 53) claimed that it prevented "the temptation to cut corners" which "could easily be a short cut to disaster" while Hoinville et al (1987) observed that it was a relatively inexpensive way to avoid errors. Youngman (1979 : 4) summarised the purpose of a pilot study as one of testing the instrument, modifying it if necessary and obtaining validation. It should therefore help the main project to run efficiently and smoothly and should also indicate the amount of time that should be allocated for example, to conduct an interview or complete a questionnaire. Although it is a form of trial run the research instruments should be thought to be in the final draft. Treece and Treece (1986) suggested that a thorough methodologist should tabulate the data in order to detect unforeseen problems. Ambiguity, areas of omission, lack of comprehension, failure to elicit appropriate information are all indications that the research instrument needs refining (Youngman 1979, Treece and Treece 1986, Kerlinger et al 1986, Hoinville et al 1987, Polit and Hungler 1989, Hicks 1990, Cohen and Manion 1992, Oppenheim 1992) When interviewing, responses that appear the most frequently should be retained for future consideration. Hoinville et al (1987) recommended recording interviews at the pilot stage so that the exact questions and the exact responses could be exactly recalled for subsequent examination. Judd et al (1991) observed that the pilot study could also reveal new and previously unthought of possibilities.

The number of respondents in a pilot study should be large enough to reveal any of the ambiguities, inappropriate questions and areas of omission previously described. The numbers will in reality depend on the amount of time available to complete the entire study and the resource implications. As in the main study, written and verbal explanation should be given to potential participants in a pilot study, the opportunity to refuse to participate or withdraw at any stage shoud be upheld and confidentiality should be guaranteed. Written informed consent should be obtained wherever possible.

3.14 Informed consent

The principles of informed consent are that participation is voluntary, that the respondent can withdraw consent at any time without detriment to him/herself, that personal autonomy will remain and that confidentiality will be respected and maintained both during and after completion of the study (Weiss 1975, Barnes 1979, Klein 1984, 1985, Treece and Treece 1986, Kerlinger 1986, Carr and Kemis 1986, Burns and Grove 1987, Stanford 1987, Quinn and Smith 1987, Hoinville et al 1987, Cormack 1987, Polit and Hungler 1989, Burgess 1989, Sommer and Sommer 1991, Parahoo 1991, Smith 1992).

The doctrine of these principles becomes even more important when adopting action research as the methodology in a project. As action research implicitly means that the researcher is actively engaged in the situation being studied this may lead to potential respondents feeling obliged or even coerced into participating. Hoinville et al suggested that "in all such cases the absolute right to refuse should be asserted". (Hoinville et al 1987 :187)

Burgess (1989) advised researchers to remain constantly aware of their potential to be intrusive while Smith (1980) cited by Burgess (1989) believed that people should only agree to participate once they are satisfied with the exact aims and purpose of the research and have, in their opinion, received sufficient information to enable them to give informed consent. Klein (1984) was quite sure of the rights of individuals. " An individual of sound mind has the right to make his/her own decisions and plot his/her own destiny. To imply otherwise is a value judgement of another." (Ibid : 58)

Klein (1984) maintained that individuals had the right to with-hold themselves and their possessions from public scrutiny. Quinn and Smith (1987) re-inforced this when they remarked that informed consent legally protected an individuals right to autonomy and as they emphasised "a decision is free when it is made without pressure or coercion from others" (p 78). Informed consent should be obtained wherever possible in writing (Treece and Treece 1986, Polit and Hungler 1989). Polit and Hungler (1989) decided that any consent form should contain the following elements :

1. The purpose of the study.
2. The procedures to be followed.
3. The nature and extent of the subjects' time commitment.
4. The type of information to be obtained.
5. A description of possible physical or emotional discomforts.
6. The methods used to protect the participants'privacy.
7. The names of people to contact for answers to questions about the study.
8. A clear statement that participation is voluntary and that non participation or termination will not result in any penalties.
9. A description of the possible gains and benefits of the research.

(Polit and Hungler 1989 : 24)

Polit and Hungler pointed out that even after informed consent has been given the researcher has an ethical obligation to look after a respondent's welfare (p 129) while Simons (1989) cited in Burgess (1989) warned that as soon as any of the original aims and purposes change in a study, consent should be regained after a further explanation has been given.

In this current study such advice was adhered to as closely as possible. Informed consent was gained in writing from each member of staff and each student from every discipline who participated in the interviews (see Appendix 3.2). An explanatory letter was sent with the questionnaire to the target population requesting their co-operation (see Appendix 3.1). Respondents who exercised their right not to participate were asked to return the blank questionnaire in the envelope provided.

3.15 Confidentiality and anonymity

Examination of relevant publications pertaining to the concepts of confidentiality and anonymity revealed that some authors use the words interchangeably (Barnes 1979, Kerlinger 1986, Hoinville et al 1987, Judd et al 1991). Even the Oxford English Dictionary (1982) defines anonymity as an "undeclared source" and confidentiality as "entrusted with secrets". Simon (1989) cited in Burgess (1989) seemed completely confused as he wrote of anonymity offering individuals some privacy and protection of their identification but also that anonymity allowed explicit discussion and reporting of contentious issues. In the minds of many ethicists and researchers there is a clear distinction between the two. Sometimes it is possible to maintain both but in educational research maintaining confidentiality is usually the chosen option and certainly the easiest to achieve.

Judd et al (1991) believed that the over-riding responsibility of a researcher was to maintain participants anonymity at all times "unless specific arrangements to the contrary are made with the participants themselves" (p 520). This advice seeems to be perfectly acceptable but if Eraut (1984), Streiner and Norman (1989) and Polit and Hungler (1989) are correct in their assertions, Judd et al (1991) are describing confidentiality and not anonymity. The above authors make a clear distinction between the two concepts. Anonymity they maintain, can only be assured when nobody (including the researcher) can identify the respondent. This is possible in such instances as distributing questionnaires randomly to a population. If the questionnaires contain no demographic data which would enable identification and are returned anonymously then a respondent could be assured that anonymity was possible. Confidentiality is more easily adhered to as the researcher can reassure the respondent in writing or in a face to face interaction that he/she will not be identified in any way. Nevertheless the researcher has personally contacted that individual and consequently the respondent in no longer anonymous to the researcher. The promise of maintaining absolute confidentiality by the researcher regarding the identity of respondents is therefore of paramount importance. As interviews and questionnaires were some of the methods used to generate data in this study anonymity could not be promised as some interaction took place between the researcher and the respondents. Confidentiality however was guaranteed.

Barnes (1979) remarked that confidentiality is at risk of compromise as soon as an individual is in possession of information that would not normally be disclosed. Streiner and Norman (1989) noted however that "Promises of confidentiality for non sensitive material does not appear to materially increase compliance ; although it is probably safest to ensure anonymity". (Ibid : 154)

Judd et al (1991) also commented on intimate and sensitive material. They suggested that the greater the sensitivity of the information gained the greater the transgression in revealing it. This point is arguable altruistically in that a promise to maintain confidentiality is a promise and therefore confidentiality must be maintained even if the information gained could be considered by some to be trivia. Value judgements must not be used by researchers in deciding what is sensitive and what is not. Judd et al described as questionable practice the procedure of precoding questionnaires in order to identify the locality of a respondent as this deviated from ethical principles. This presented a problem in this current study as it was necessary to involve both staff and students in the data collection on more than one occasion. Two options were available, the first being that the respondents were invited to choose their own identification number whch would enable a greater degree of anonymity. The most feasible option however was to use random stratified sampling of the students within each discipline through access to their college registration numbers. This served two purposes. Primarily it meant that a representative sample from each discipline could be approached anonymously in the first instance and secondly that the recruitment of 'interested volunteers' could be minimised therefore reducing the element of bias so heavily criticised in the review of the literature.

Limiting access to data was also considered vital. Raw data was kept by the researcher and only when necessary disclosed to the academic supervisor. No other individuals had access to the data. Treece and Treece (1986) advocated the creation of a link file in which the identification numbers of the respondents were kept. Names and addresses of respondents should be kept entirely separately with nothing to link the two together. It was therefore planned that all data collected would be kept in separate, locked files. In this study this was of the greatest importance as the data was collected in identifiable institutions. Judd et al (1991) advised researchers that in these circumstances arrangements should be made in advance to ensure that confidentiality could be maintained or else be prepared to justify the non disclosure of raw data. In an internal study changing the names of places and organisations was not possible if a credible feasibility study was to be completed. It was important therefore to be sensitive to the fact that the results may in some way be perceived as compromising by the organisations concerned. Eraut (1984) suggested that if this threatened to be the case then the organisations or any accountable individual therein should be forewarned. Eraut (1984) described this as 'controlled leakage' while in political terms it is frequently described as 'damage limitation'. It was therefore important to gain the co-operation and consent of the management within each institution before the data collection began.

3.16 Summary of the research design

Holsti (1969 : 24) stated that "A research design is a plan for collecting and analyzing data in order to answer the investigators problem". A flow chart was designed with the intention of acting as a guide throughout the study. It was acknowledged however, that as a result of reflection at each stage the research plan could change. The flow chart is presented as Figure 3.1 on the next page.

Figure 3.1 Flow chart for research method

1. Review of the pertinent literature
⇓
2. Content analysis of the relevant curriculum
⇓
3. Identify core concepts
⇓
4. Content analysis of reading lists
⇓
5. Contact Statutory & Professional Bodies to ascertain support
⇓
6. Visit existing interdisciplinary programmes in Finland, Sweden & France
⇓
7. Conduct unstructured interviews in above countries
⇓
8. Generate questions for interviews based on literature review & findings from overseas visits
⇓
9. Pilot interviews of teachers & students
⇓
10. Analyse data to produce main study interview schedules
⇓
11. Main study interviews using stratified random sampling of teachers & students in each discipline
⇓
12. Analyse data to construct questionnaires
⇓
13. Pilot questionnaires for teachers & students
⇓
14. Analyse data to produce main study questionnaires
⇓
15. Main study questionnaires for all teachers & students in each discipline
⇓
16. Analyse data
⇓
17. Decide if interdisciplinary learning is feasible
⇓
18. If positive outcome propose appropriate core curriculum
⇓
19. Write research report

4 Description of the research instruments and measurement techniques

4.1 Introduction

The adoption of modified form of action research as the appropriate methodology enabled a research plan to be formulated which encompassed several methodologies. It was nevertheless important to remember that each stage should be followed by a period of reflection in order that later decisions could be based on informed action.

4.2. Content analysis of the curriculum and indicative reading lists

The essential starting point was to undertake a content analysis of the curricula from fourteen existing undergraduate programmes in South East Wales. The rationale for this action was the need to identify whether there were sufficient commonalities within each curriculum to continue with the study. Identification of potential common themes addressed in at least two of the disciplines was undertaken. The content analysis was assisted by means of a computer spread sheet which was designed to encompass each discipline against the list of topics derived from the curriculum analysis. Wherever possible the exact terminology was transposed from each curriculum on to the spread sheet. In some instances, however, it was necessary to adopt the phrase which was used most frequently. An example of this was the use of the terms "ethnicity", "ethnic minorities" and "ethnic issues". The term "ethnicity" was adopted as this was used the most frequently Use of the spread sheet also enabled raw scores to be calculated and statistical analysis to be undertaken using a computer. Content validity was checked by requesting each course leader to examine the analysis pertaining to their individual curriculum. This prevented the introduction of any possible influence from the other disciplines results. A 100% response was obtained and minor alterations were made. This included the deletion of a few entries and the inclusion of others.

A content analysis of the recommended reading lists, where available, for each curriculum was also completed to try and obtain further evidence of common themes. An Excel spread sheet was again identified as the most appropriate manner in which to collate the data. The information was transferred from the reading lists using the Harvard method of referencing. The completed content analysis of the fourteen curricula and the recommended reading lists are presented in Chapter 5 (Sections 5.2 and 5.3) of this book. Initial interpretation of the raw data displayed in the content analysis indicated that the Statutory and Professional Bodies should be contacted at this stage.

4.3 The opinions of the statutory and professional bodies

It was decided that the opinions of the Statutory and Professional Bodies responsible for each health and social care discipline should be ascertained. The rationale for this decision was that as each Statutory Body validates the curriculum of each profession, it was of paramount importance to know whether any potential innovation within a validated curriculum would be approved. To this end a letter was sent to each Statutory Body comprising the General Medical Council (GMC), the General Dental Council (GDC), the United Kingdom Central Council for Nurses, Midwives and Health Visitors (UKCC), the Council for Professions Supplementary to Medicine (CPSM) and the Central Council for Education and Training in Social Work (CCETSW). In addition, opinions were sought from the British Medical Association (BMA), the British Dental Association (BDA), the Chartered Society of Physiotherapists (CSP), the College of Occupational Therapists (COT), the College of Radiographers and the Royal College of Nursing (RCN). A response was received from each Statutory and Professional Body contacted. Each respondent indicated provisional approval for such an initiative and were all most helpful in the additional information which they provided. Several respondents included guidelines for curriculum development for each profession. Nevertheless all respondents emphasised that while such an initiative would be supported, the most important consideration would always remain competence in each specific profession. This stated reservation was anticipated and welcomed as the need to maintain specific professional competencies has not been challenged. The introduction of any integrated interdisciplinary learning was intended to enhance rather than detract from specific professional competence. Each respondent emphasised the importance of involving the Statutory Bodies at an early stage in any potential major changes in the curriculum if this study proved that such a change was feasible and desirable.

Evidence of provisional support given can be demonstrated by directly quoting the following personal, important communications :

"The Council and Boards welcome any moves which strengthen the institutional base of a course.....provided it would not be at the cost of lowering standards or of weakening the provision and approach."

(CPSM 1992)

"This is a matter to which the Council has given considerable attention over the last year and our position is that we would wish to support interdisciplinary and multidisciplinary learning where appropriate, within the context of the profession - specific qualifications."

(UKCC 1992)

"The growth of interdisciplinary or 'shared' learning is already an established fact in physiotherapy education............You will realise from the above that the Society supports the concept of shared and interdisciplinary learning but obviously any individual venture which involved physiotherapy education would require both our approval and that of the statutory body, the Council for Professions Supplementary to Medicine, with whom we work in tandem."

(The Chartered Society of Physiotherapy 1992)

"The College of Occupational Therapists supports progress in those areas you have quoted which lend themselves to interdisciplinary development.....Provided that the curriculum observes the standards for professional education laid down by the World Federation of Occupational Therapy, the College supports individual insitutional course development in pre-registration education."

(College of Occupational Therapists 1992)

"....the principle of a collaborative approach to health care provisions is to be nurtured and advanced. Shared teaching and learning is a way forward in this venture. The potential gains for all those involved in the provision of health care are enormous and most importantly the care of patients and clients should be enhanced as a consequence."

(Royal College of Nursing 1992)

The response received from the Central Council for Education and Training in Social Work (CCETSW) indicated that one of the strategic objectives for this Statutory Body is to "Identify and promote relevant links between social work and the training provisions of other bodies" this, the letter continued, was to be achieved through :

" Multi-disciplinary staff development and training, supporting and promoting joint training and shared learning, contributing to training of related professions or occupations."

(CCETSW 1993)

The General Medical Council responded in a long informative letter and also enclosed several additional documents. One of these documents discussed integrated, interdisciplinary education from an entirely different perspective within the medical curriculum itself. The General Medical Council Education Committee wished to encourage "integrated and interdisciplinary teaching throughout the undergraduate curriculum". (GMC 1980 : 14) An example of integrated interdisciplinary learning however, was given as teaching by anatomists, physiologists and biochemists. The document continued;

"....... interdisciplinary teaching can illuminate overlapping areas of different disciplines and specialities and thus help to keep teachers abreast of advancing knowledge in fields other than their own."

(GMC 1980 : 14-15)

From this perspective the General Medical Committee in 1992 in a personal communication responded that it :

"......does not generally have in mind an approach of the kind you envisage,whereby students intending to make a career in a variety of health care and related professions, including medicine, receive part of their teaching in common, and join together in learning programmes designed for their mutual benefit."

(GMC 1992)

In spite of the seemingly negative response the letter continued with the observation that :

"......the Education Committee is not prescriptive in its approach and seeks to encourage innnovation on the of medical schools in the design and implementation of their curricula. Although the Recommendations provide broad general guidelines for the medical schools, the precise means whereby individual schools provide the training regarded as requisite for a medical student is a matter for the schools themselves."

(GMC 1992)

The General Medical Council Education Committee indicated that they would be happy to consider any firm proposals if approached by the Curriculum Committee of the Medical School participating in this study.

4.4 Visits to countries where interdisciplinary learning exists

The review of the literature indicated that several centres had existing interdisciplinary learning in the health and social care professions. Of these the national curriculum in Finland, the programme in The Faculty of Health Sciences, Linkoping, Sweden and the programme at the Universitie de Paris Nord, Bobigny, France seemed to be appropriate for an in depth investigation. The award of a Smith and Nephew Scholarship enabled a visit to all three countries in the autumn of 1992 and the spring of 1993. The purpose of these visits was to informally interview teachers and students involved in these programmes and to be a non participant observer in some of the interdisciplinary sessions. Difficulty with the Finnish and Swedish languages in particular was anticipated but nevertheless an interview check list for teachers and another for students was developed with the intention of asking similar questions in each country wherever possible (see Appendix 4.1). It was recognised that the checklist would need to be flexible as the words chosen to question the respondents would depend on their ability to speak English. The information generated from these interviews and the non participant observation of the interdisciplinary groups, it was hoped, would form the basis of the structured interview schedule in the main study. The questions included in the interview checklist were generated from the review of the literature. The demographic data was kept to a minimum as it was believed that questions such as age and qualifications may be deemed intrusive and irrelevant. This was particularly important as different cultures may have different values regarding the disclosure of personal data.

For this reason the demographic questions that were asked of the teaching staff consisted only of confirmation of their profession, the number of years they had been in clinical practice before starting to teach, the number of years they had been teaching and their teaching specialisation.

The remaining questions related to their experiences in participating in interdisciplinary teaching. In order to generate as much information as possible the majority of the questions were open ended. It was vital that these questions were asked in clear simple English with no ambiguity. The questions explored such issues as :

1. The advantages and disadvantages of interdisciplinary learning.
2. The learning strategies adopted in the programme.
3. The preparation the teachers had received prior to the introduction of inter-disciplinary learning and what preparation in hindsight would have been helpful.
4. Any problems of integration between any of the disciplines for either teachers or students.
5. Any topics which were thought to be unsuitable for interdisciplinary learning apart from profession specific competencies.
6. Any personal reservations the individual may have about shared learning with the other professions.

A similar approach was adopted for the student's interview schedule. The demographic data consisted of confirmation of the profession for which they were training and in which year of training they were currently in. Again the remainder of the open ended questions concentrated on interdisciplinary learning and sought the students' opinions on issues such as :

1. The topics which they were learning together.
2. Their preferred learning methods.

3. The advantages and disadvantages of interdisciplinary learning.
4. Whether there were any problems in learning with any other professions and if so which ones.
5. Any topics which were unsuitable for shared learning apart from profession specific competencies.
6. Any personal reservations the individual may have about shared learning with the other professions.

It was decided that these interview schedules would be used whenever feasible and appropriate. It was not possible to predict the number of respondents, the disciplines or the reliability of the schedule itself in advance of the visits to Finland, Sweden and France. It was also recognised that any potential respondents would not represent a random sample but would be self selecting in that the students had registered on the programmes knowing that a degree of interdisciplinary learning was undertaken and the staff who had been employed prior to introduction had been volunteers and those that had been employed since had specifically applied to advertisements which mentioned interdisciplinary learning. A further limitation was that it would only be possible to interview those teachers and students who had a reasonable command of the English language.

4.4.1 The situation in Finland

The National Board of Education based in Helsinki advises the Ministry of Health about the education of health professionals. In conjunction with the health union TEHY, a national core curriculum has been devised for students prior to entering the health professions. This one year course appeared to have similarities to the United Kingdom National Vocational Qualifications. In 1992 more than twenty percent of the working population was unemployed in Finland and it was believed by the National Board of Education that many of the students undertaking the core curriculum would not subsequently continue into any health profession training. The Government manpower predictions for the health professions were continually being revised downwards and as a result the number of students entering these professions was being severely curtailed. Each institution which offered the national curriculum was empowered to develop its own course content providing it met the criteria laid down by the National Board of Education.

A disappointing finding was that once the students commence professional training no interdisciplinary learning was undertaken at all. This means that the only time that shared learning takes place is before a student could possibly have any notion of their own role in holistic health care let alone the role of the other professions. Although a number of Faculties of Health Sciences were visited around the country in both Universities and Institutes of Higher Education no evidence was found of any of the professions sharing learning in spite of several different professions sharing the same facilities on the same campus. The opportunity to observe several different teaching sessions was readily available in each centre visited. Each situation observed revealed individual professions learning in isolation at the undergraduate stage. The teaching strategies adopted were mostly didactic lessons with little or no interaction between the lecturer and the students except for the opportunity to ask questions at the end of a session. Some group work was observed and on occasions the library was used by the students as a resource.

In view of these findings it was decided that it was totally inappropriate to interview either the lecturers or students using the interview schedule. Discussions with many individuals and different professional groups however revealed a desire to explore the issues surrounding interdisciplinary learning and a willingness to promote the concept within each faculty. This current feasibility study had generated a great deal of interest amongst the lecturers in all centres which resulted in the opportunity to visit other institutions by invitation to discuss the findings to date and further invitations to return with the results of the completed study in order to act in an advisory capacity. In summary, although a large amount of useful information regarding health care in Finland and the training of health and social care professions was obtained, regretably it did not contribute any additional insight into integrated interdisciplinary programmes. A full analysis of the visit to Finland was completed and submitted as part of a report to the Smith and Nephew Foundation (Tope 1993).

4.4.2 The situation in Linkoping, Sweden

As has been described in the review of the literature, the Faculty of Health Sciences, University of Linkoping, Sweden is seen as one of the pioneer establishments in the introduction of interdisciplinary problem - based learning. The first ten weeks of training for all the health and social care professions is completed on this premise and forms the introductory course entitled "Man and Society". Students representing medicine, nursing, occupational therapy, physiotherapy, medical laboratory technicians and social work are assigned into interdisciplinary groups. Using a problem solving approach the students, with the help of a lecturer who facilitates the group, work their way through the syllabus with each student having to contribute to the student led tutorials and seminars. The lecturer may belong to any of the professions described above. Assessment is undertaken through individual project presentation, group project presentation and also in an unseen written examination for all students at the end of the ten weeks. Once the ten week course is completed the students then separate into the specific professional training. Further opportunities for interdisciplinary learning are however an integral part of each curriculum throughout undergraduate training. All facilities are shared and there was no evidence of elitism or isolationalism between any of the professions.

The opportunity to observe the interdisciplinary groups in action at a variety of stages in training was readily available as was the opportunity to interview both lecturers and students involved in the programme. The total number of staff interviewed was 11 and the total number of students was 38. Representation of the disciplines were :

Teaching Staff - Medicine (N=2), Nursing (N=5), Occupational Therapy (N=2), Physiotherapy (N=1), Nutrition and Dietetics (N=1). All teaching staff with the exception of one doctor were female.

Students - Medicine (N=6, 3 female, 3 male), Nursing (N=9 all female), Occupational Therapy (N=6 all female), Physiotherapy (N=12, 5 female, 7 male), Social Work (N=3, all female), Medical Laboratory Technicians (N=2, both female).

Analysis of the Interviews 1. Teaching Staff The majority of staff were employed on a full time basis and all, with the exception of one of the medical staff, had spent at least five years in clinical practice before commencing their teaching careers. Most had experience of teaching students within their own specific profession before becoming involved in the interdisciplinary programme. Every member of staff (N=11) interviewed continued to be fully involved with teaching on their profession specific curriculum as well as teaching on an interdisciplinary basis with the exception of one individual (a nurse teacher) who was the co-ordinator of the ten week introductory course and therefore had a correspondingly reduced work load as far as the rest of the nursing curriculum was concerned. Predictably the teachers areas of teaching specialisation reflected their own specific professional training in varying degrees, although it was evident that before the interdisciplinary programme had commenced each individual had made every effort to increase the depth and most importantly the breadth of their knowledge. All staff were fully cognisant of the number of hours that the students learned on an interdisciplinary basis and it was agreed that in addition to the ten week introductory course, a further six formal hours per semester was devoted to interdisciplinary learning. Many staff commented, without prompting, that this was nothing like enough and were keen to highlight the fact that the new curriculum would incorporate much more shared learning. In addition, several staff commented that many students on a voluntary and informal basis met each other regularly in interdisciplinary groups in order to maintain momentum. The favoured teaching strategies were small group tutorials using case studies, role play and student led seminars although lectures to large groups of students were common and perceived as very valuable providing they were followed by tutorials.

The teachers were unanimous in their opinions regarding the advantages of interdisciplinary learning. The most frequently cited advantages were "the understanding of each others' role and contribution to care", "reduced conflict", "increased respect", "enhanced teamwork" and this "encouraged everyone to work together in order to enhance the quality of care given to the patient". All those interviewed mentioned the patient and quality care. Paradoxically the disadvantages of interdisciplinary learning related to organisation and planning of the curriculum, "an administrative nightmare", "time consuming", "staff with traditional views do not co-operate", "arguments over whose training budget should pay for guest speakers". Nevertheless all staff were convinced that many of these difficulties were resolving over a period of time and were keen to give advice on how to circumvent these problems. Several staff commented that the main disadvantage was that there was "not enough" shared learning in the current programme. No member of staff had noticed any problems of integration between any of the disciplines and none had any reservations about continuing and extending the interdisciplinary component within each curriculum.

Analysis of the interviews 2. The students The total number of students interviewed was 38. The majority of these were in the first year of training (N=21). Of the remainder 10 were in the second year and 7 were in the third year. Their responses to the questions on most occasions reflected many of the teachers opinions. They all preferred problem based learning, small group tutorials, seminars, hypothetical case studies and role playing. The advantages of interdisciplinary learning included "helps us understand each other", "the patient has a better deal", "helps us work as a team", "everything" and "patient centred". In many instances no disadvantages were identified. Most students commented that they wanted more shared learning although one second year student was concerned that professional identity may be lost. The seemingly limited response from the students regarding the disadvantages of interdisciplinary learning may be justified by comparing it with the teachers responses which highlighted the difficulties of administration and organisation. The students, as the consumers of the course, would not necessarily be aware of these difficulties. There were no topics identified as unsuitable for interdisciplinary learning although some students commented that it was necessary for some of the professions to examine some topics in greater depth than the others. No student reported any reservations about learning with other professions.

In summary the opinions of both the staff and the students were very positive about the value of interdisciplinary learning. The level of commitment to, and enthusiasm for, the programme was much in evidence. Nevertheless, the results should be treated with some caution because, as has been previously identified in Section 4.4, most of the staff and all of the students had opted to commence this curriculum and therefore constitute a biased sample. The opportunity to visit Linkoping to collect data was invaluable and certainly most of the responses complimented the findings of many of the publications analysed in the review of the literature.

4.4.3 The situation in Bobigny, France

The visit to the Universite Paris XIII, Bobigny took place in March 1993. The literature had described the existing interdisciplinary programmes in detail (D'Ivernois, Cornillot and Zomer cited in WHO 1986c). The aim of this visit, in keeping with the visits to Finland and Sweden, was to gather as much information as possible relating to these programmes and to talk with the teaching staff and the students participating. Within the first hour of arrival it became obvious that the interdisciplinary programmes described in the literature had been amended beyond all recognition. The current one is described as the "DEUG Soins" and is the only one in existence in France. The DEUG Soins is in fact only one of a number of modules which must be completed by the medical, dental and nursing students undertaking professional training in Bobigny. The module is compulsory and is included in the first year. Other modules are designed for each specific profession and comprise compulsory and optional ones. Paramedical training has now been transferred to other Universities in Paris and consequently the amount of interdisciplinary learning has been severely curtailed. Additional information obtained included the fact that there are 13 medical schools in Paris alone and also that the nurse education programme in Bobigny is the only one in France that is offered within a University. The academic entry criteria to the undergraduate programmes in Bobigny was therefore comparatively easy for medical students because of the number of medical schools from which to choose and paradoxically difficult for nursing students because of the unique status. No interviews with prospective students is undertaken and a total of 450 students commence each year in Bobigny.

The initial impression gained was that the "innovatory" programme offered in Bobigny did not fulfil the promise that the literature suggested. However, it was decided that the opportunity to interview the teachers and staff should not be missed. A number of appointments were therefore made. A major difficulty was encountered in that none of the students or staff spoke English and consequently all conversations were conducted by the researcher in French. This meant that the exchange of information may have been misunderstood on occasions and the selection of words and phrases was necessarily limited. An attempt was made to address this problem by meeting Professor Attali (an endocrinologist) who also has a teaching and administrative responsibility for the DEUG Soins. This meeting took place on the final day of the visit and the conversation took take place in English. Professor Attali was able to confirm that the information obtained had been understood correctly and added further observations of his own.

Nine students were interviewed in total, two of whom were in their final year of training, four in the second year of training and three currently undertaking the

DEUG Soins module in the first year. One of the most important pieces of information to emerge was that the content of the DEUG Soins alters every year as a result of the teaching staff evaluations. All nine students stated that there was no formal opportunity for the students to evaluate the module either in writing or verbally. This meant that students' opinions did not contribute to future developments within the programme. In addition, the annual implementation of a new DEUG Soins meant that at no stage could the validity of this module be measured at the end of a students three or five year training as the module content would have been altered accordingly each year. A further limitation of the Bobigny programme is the teaching strategies that have been adopted. The students and teaching staff agreed that the most common method used was that of the formal lecture which students from the three professions attended. Small group tutorials frequently followed the lectures but these were always profession specific and not interdisciplinary. If the word "interdisciplinary" is accepted as meaning "interaction" between the participating professions, then it seems that the Bobigny programme is not interdisciplinary. The students all agreed that minimal interaction takes place between the professions. Students do not lead seminars, undertake problem based learning, or spend much time in self directed learning. This last finding was explained by Professor Attali who described the library facilities as extremely limited. The number of journals published in French are minimal for the medical and dental staff and there appeared to be no nursing journals published in France at all. A suggestion that the French Canadian nursing journals may be of some use was gratefully received. Journals published in the English language were not generally purchased as so few of the staff or students could read English.

The students also revealed that the assessment strategy within the DEUG Soins module, differed for each profession. There was therefore no need for the students from the three professions to work together in order to successfully complete the module. The content of the module seemed to be most appropriate for shared learning and consisted of a total of 120 hours in which the students were taught (mainly through lectures) law, ethics, health care organisation and administration, psychology, anthropology, sociology and culture. The opportunities for a limited degree of interdisciplinary learning seemed to be present but the teaching staff did not seem to know how to implement such opportunities. An explanation for this was offered by Professor Attali who revealed that there are no formal continuing education programmes for the health care professions and that the teaching staff, in the nursing profession in particular, are recruited for their enthusiasm and interest in teaching, rather than for their clinical expertise and academic careers. In essence this means that individuals could start a teaching career with no more knowledge or clinical expertise than that of a newly qualified staff nurse in the United Kingdom. It was therefore not surprising that the delivery of these educational programmes seemed haphazard and piecemeal. The education of health professionals in

France and most particularly the nursing profession seems to be outdated, outmoded and unsuitable to meet the demands of holistic care. The delivery of the programmes seemed to reflect those in existence in the 1960's in the United Kingdom. The teaching staff expressed their anxieties about how to meet the criteria laid down by the E.C. which will ensure France can participate in a free exchange of health professionals with the other EC countries.

In summary, the visit to Bobigny was a major disappointment as far as interdisciplinary learning programmes are concerned. Rather than being innovative, the educational programmes for the health care professions seemed to be outdated. As Bobigny is obviously viewed as a centre of excellence in France, there is even more cause for concern for those programmes in other universities and cities. Educationally the visit was very enlightening with the added bonus of being able to share the developments in educational programmes within the United Kingdom. As in Finland, the French were very keen to obtain as much information as possible, which may help their considerable problems. The information obtained from this visit was inadequate and inappropriate to include in the main study questionnaires.

4.5 The pilot study

The information generated from the interviews conducted in Sweden in conjunction with the analysis of the pertinent literature was considered to be sufficient to allow the designing of suitable questions for the interview schedules for both teachers and students in the main study. The interview schedules contained mainly open ended questions but also some forced choice responses. Similar themes were explored to the ones adopted in Sweden but on this occasion most of the questions were formulated on the predicted advantages and disadvantages of interdisciplinary learning or any anticipated problems between the professions. In addition it was considered necessary to clarify whether teachers had experienced interdisciplinary learning as a student or had taught on such a programme and also whether they saw a knowledge of the behavioural sciences as being essential for the health and social care professions. Their opinions were also sought as to the most appropriate time to introduce shared learning. The questions on the two interview schedules were designed to complement each other, thus allowing more accurate comparison between the teachers' responses with those of the students. It was anticipated that each interview would take approximately thirty minutes to complete.

A summary of the research proposal and copies of the interview schedule with its accompanying letter was sent to the Ethics Committee of the Health Authority in which some of the participating educational institutions are based. Full approval was given to proceed with the study.

4.5.1 The teacher's interview schedule

The absolute necessity to undertake a pilot study was demonstrated during the first interview. The respondent answering the questions from the teachers questionnaire highlighted the ambiguity of question number 2. "How many years were you in clinical practice before you started teaching ?" She queried whether this included time spent as a student before qualifying and any post graduate courses undertaken. It was decided on reflection that this question should be rewritten to read "After you qualified how many years did you spend in clinical practice, including any post graduate courses before you commenced your teaching career ?". The second pilot study also exposed a potential anomaly. Initially question number 8 had been written as "Do you agree/disagree that the behavioural sciences are basic to the health and social care professions ?" One respondent suggested that the words "a knowledge of" should be included whilst another suggested that the adoption of the word "essential" rather than "basic" would be preferable. After further reflection question 8 was rewritten to read "Do you agree/disagree that a knowledge of the behavioural sciences is essential for the health and social care professions ?" Questions 9 and 10 were also rewritten to incorporate the word "essential". The third and final draft of the interview schedule was then tested (N = 10) and no further anomalies were revealed. It was therefore decided that the schedule was sufficiently reliable to adopt in the main study (See Appendix 4.2). The anticipated time taken for each interview was reasonably accurate with the shortest interview taking twenty minutes and the longest taking forty five.

4.5.2 The student's interview schedule

The weaknesses highlighted in the first two teacher interview schedules enabled immediate remedial action to be taken with the students interview schedule even before the initial testing took place. This meant that the first draft of the schedule for the students reflected the third draft of the teachers version. An initial pilot study was undertaken (N=5) (Appendix 4.3) Each respondent answered the questions with seemingly little difficulty and no alterations to the structure or content of the interview schedule were suggested. It was therefore decided that the instrument was sufficiently reliable to adopt for the main study (Appendix 4.3). The completion time was approximately thirty minutes.

4.5.3 The teacher's questionnaire

In order to obtain an accurate picture of the opinions of the teaching staff within each profession, it was decided to distribute a questionnaire to every member of staff in post on a given date. The target population was therefore more than 370. It was not possible to predict the finite number in post as staff establishment records are produced retrospectively. The questions were formulated from three main sources. The review of the literature had highlighted many issues which could usefully be explored. In addition, the information generated from the interviews with the teaching staff in Linkoping, Sweden and with the random stratified sample of teachers in South East Wales had identified still more. With a target population of this size the design of the questionnaire was crucial as it was recognised that the analysis would need to be completed on a data sheet. It was also believed that the return rate would improve if the questions were designed in such a way that respondents were able to tick the answers wherever possible. Nevertheless some questions invited additional responses. An explanatory letter (see Appendix 3.1) was enclosed with each questionnaire along with a self addressed envelope which could be mailed through the internal postal system.

The first draft of the questionnaire was distributed as a pilot study (N=40). It was decided that, if possible, the target population in the main study should be totally excluded from the pilot study. Two lecturers (one in Wales the other in England) were contacted and asked whether they would be prepared to distribute and collect the pilot questionnaires to members of staff within their own colleges. Both agreed and consequently twenty questionnaires were posted to each individual.

The return rate for the pilot study questionnaires was 34 (85%) within the specified period. Analysis of these revealed no major flaws with all respondents indicating that they had understood all the questions. It was necessary however to make some minor modifications to several questions. The word "chiropody" was added to "podiatry" in the lists of professions (see Questions 1, 7b, 10a and 13a). The rationale for this being that no respondent indicated that podiatrists could share learning with any of the other professions. It was suspected that this may be due to a lack of understanding of who podiatrists actually were. Subsequent enquiries to the colleges in which the pilot study took place proved this to be the case. The traditional term "chiropody" was still used. It was therefore decided to include both terms in an attempt to allow the respondents in the main study to make an informed decision.

Question 6 also yielded some interesting answers. Respondents were asked if they had any additional areas of knowledge that they could teach apart from their own professional expertise. Whilst most included topics such as psychology of counselling or computing skills, a few included diverse hobbies. It was decided that the word "relevant" should be inserted into the question in an attempt to obtain more specific information.

Two individuals noted that midwives had not been included as a separate category. On reflection it was decided that this should continue to be the case for the following reasons. In the institutions, in which the main study was to take place, there was no direct entry to midwifery training. All student midwives had previously qualified as Registered Nurses and therefore could be classified as post graduate students. As the focus of this study was on interdisciplinary learning at an undergraduate, level post graduate students were not included at all. A further reason for not classifying midwives separately was that with the diversity within both the medical and nursing professions it could be argued that sub classifications within both should also be included. In order to make the data manageable it was decided that this was not feasible within this study. In conclusion the questionnaire appeared to be both valid and reliable and with the modifications made was adopted for the main study (See Appendix 4.4).

4.5.4 The student's questionnaire

A similar strategy was adopted for the students questionnaire. The target population was every student in each year of every profession who was registered in the educational institutions on a given date. The lists of names were obtained from the administrator of each institution after permission had been granted by members of the senior academic staff. The target population in this instance was more than 1600. The number was again approximate as the lists are produced retrospectively. A staged distribution of the questionnaires and explanatory letter was delivered by hand to each student year in each profession. Arrangements were made to collect the questionnaires forty five minutes later.

The first draft of the questionnaire was distributed in the institutions where the main study took place (Appendix 4.9). The respondents in the pilot study were final year students in three of the professions who were awaiting their results. These students therefore, if successful, would not be indexed when the main study instrument was distributed. The adoption of this strategy enabled the target population for the main study to remain unaffected. A total of 65 questionnaires were distributed for the pilot study with 64 (98%) being completed. Only 4 students indicated that they had experienced a problem in understanding a question while another 2 commented that they had been unable to answer the question regarding their age as there was no column for the age of twenty ! This was rectified in the main study questionnaire. One of the students queried whether question number 7 (Have you experienced any shared learning with any of the other health and social professions) meant in the clinical areas or in a classroom. While no other student raised the issue, it seemed to be a very valid point. The question was ambiguous. On reflection it was decided to include the words "Excluding the clinical areas" in the main study. The rationale for this decision was based on the need to measure meaningful interaction between the professions rather than in circumstances such as a consultants ward round where medical students and sometimes students from the other professions observe the interaction between the patient and the doctor.

The other question that caused some confusion for 3 of the students was question 13a in which they were asked "are there any topics apart from specialist practitioner areas" which they would reject as unsuitable for shared learning. All 3 asked what was meant by the term "specialist practitioner". This was an interesting response as none of the teachers had questionned this term. It was decided to clarify the question by deleting "specialist practitioner" and inserting the term "apart from knowledge specific to your own profession". Following these amendments the main study student questionnaire was distributed (Appendix 4.5).

4.6 Proposal for an interdisciplinary workshop

The literature reviewed suggested that an appropriate strategy to adopt would be an interdisciplinary workshop for teaching staff who may be involved in any future shared learning initiatives. Discussion with the random stratified sample of teaching staff interviewed in the main study revealed that such a workshop would be welcomed. It was therefore necessary to try and obtain funding for such an event. It was important that a suitable venue was identifed which constituted a neutral territory for all potential participants. To this end a letter was written to The Director, NHS Wales, The Welsh Office, in which the rationale and the aims of the proposed workshop were explained and a request for financial support was made. The Director was also invited to be the key note speaker. A positive response from the Director was received at the beginning of January 1993 with the sum of £1500 being allocated and with his agreement to attend as the key note speaker. Consequently immediate planning of the workshop commenced. A hotel with excellent workshop facilities was booked and the potential delegates identified. All teaching staff who had participated in the interviews were invited thus ensuring a representative interdisciplinary mix. In addition the Principals of each participating Institution and representatives from the Welsh Office received an invitation. The estimated number of delegates was therefore approximately fifty people.

Arrangements had been made previously for members of the teaching staff from Linkoping, Sweden to visit Cardiff in March 1993 to explore possible teacher/student exchanges through 'Erasmus'. An invitation was therefore issued to them asking them if they would be prepared to share their experiences with the delegates. They indicated that they would be delighted to participate.

The content of the workshop was obviously of vital importance if this stage of the research was to be successful. Active participation by the delegates was essential if the workshop was to be of an interdisciplinary nature. It was decided that with the key note speaker's address and with the lecturers from Sweden also giving a presentation that this should consitute the formal input to the workshop. The opportunity to present the results of the content analysis of the curriculum was too good to miss. The most appropriate way to present this seemed to be by revealing the results of all the curriculum analyses (but not the profession to which each was attributed) to interdisciplinary working groups. Each group would then be asked to decide which analysis matched the professions participating in this research. The overall results would then be disclosed to all delegates and discussion invited.

The afternoon was designed to encourage the interdisciplinary working groups to interact with each other using problem solving exercises. The rationale for this strategy was based on the need to illustrate the potential for shared learning between the different professions. Each working group was given a hypothetical case study. They were asked to make an assessment of the patient/clients needs and by using a problem solving approach identify a plan of action on an interdisciplinary basis. In addition each group was asked to suggest areas where shared learning may have been useful using the broad themes identified from the results of the content analysis.

An evaluation of the day was undertaken by distributing a questionnaire to each delegate which was completed before departure. The evaluations completed anonymously, indicated that the majority of delegates had very much enjoyed the day. Nonetheless the general opinion was that there was too much information given in the time available and that insufficient time was allocated for the interdisciplinary group work. It had been anticipated that this would be the case but unfortunately there was no further time available. Many respondents (RS = 28) commented to the effect that they had gained a much better insight into the contribution to health care that the other professions make. The positive comments made by the respondents justified the expense of this workshop and several lessons were learned regarding the amount of time that would be needed if teachers were being prepared for teaching on an interdisciplinary basis. The implications for the preparation of teachers is discussed at length in Chapter 6, Section 6.14.

5 The results

5.1 Introduction

Owing to the diversity of the data collection methods adopted in this study, the results are presented in the same order as the data was collected. The order therefore complements the flow chart included at the end of Chapter 3 and also the sub-sections within Chapter 4.

5.2 Content analysis of the fourteen curricula

The original intention was to identify concepts that could be categorised within the academic disciplines of psychology and sociology. It quickly became evident that this could not be achieved as many other concepts were included in the defined behavioural science section of some curricula while others had adopted an integrated approach with no defined behavioural science section. Consequently it was decided that the other concepts could not be excluded from the analysis. Examples of these included "ethics, law and practice, management and research methods". The rationale for the inclusion of these by the respondents was not understood at this stage of the study but it was believed that one possible explanation could be that the term "behavioural sciences" was interpreted by some teachers as including these addditional concepts. To explore this idea a question was included in the teachers interview schedule (see Section 5.4, Question 7) in which the respondents were asked which broad topics would they include in the term "behavioural sciences". The diversity of responses indicated that teachers do include topics other than psychology and sociology in the term "behavioural sciences". The following results therefore include some topics which may not be considered as strictly reflecting the academic disciplines of psychology and sociology. A more detailed interpretation of the content analysis is undertaken in Chapter 6, Section 6.2 where the implications of the results are discussed.

Table 5.1 Content analysis of fourteen curricula

Professional curriculum YES = 1, NO = 0

SYLLABUS CONTENT	SPEECH THERAPY	PODIATRY	DENTAL TECHNOLOGY	RADIOGRAPHY	DENTAL HYGIENIST/D.S.A.	OPERATING DEPT. PRACT.	NURSING PROJECT 2000	NUTRITION & DIETETICS	SOCIAL WORK	PHYSIOTHERAPY	OCCUPATIONAL THERAPY	MEDICINE	DENTISTRY	NURSING PRE-REG. B.N.	TOTALS
AGEING PROCESS	1	1	0	1	0	0	1	1	1	1	1	1	1	1	**11**
AGGRESSION	0	0	0	0	0	0	1	1	1	0	1	1	0	1	**6**
ANDRAGOGY / ADULT LEARNING	1	0	0	0	0	0	1	0	1	1	1	1	0	1	**7**
ASSERTIVENESS	1	1	0	0	0	0	1	1	1	0	1	1	0	1	**8**
ATTRACTION	1	0	0	0	0	0	1	1	0	1	1	0	0	1	**6**
ATTITUDES	1	1	0	1	1	1	1	1	1	1	1	1	1	1	**13**
BEHAVIOURIST APPROACH	1	1	0	0	1	0	1	1	0	1	1	1	1	1	**10**
BEREAVEMENT	1	1	0	0	0	1	1	1	1	1	1	1	0	1	**10**
BIOLOGIGAL APPROACH	1	1	0	0	0	0	1	0	0	1	1	1	0	1	**7**
BODY IMAGE	1	1	1	1	0	1	1	1	1	1	1	1	1	1	**13**
BUDGETING	0	1	1	1	0	1	0	1	1	0	0	0	1	0	**7**
CHILD HEALTH	1	1	0	0	1	0	1	0	1	1	1	1	1	1	**10**
CLIENT ASSESSMENT	0	1	0	0	1	1	1	0	1	1	1	1	1	1	**10**
COGNITIVE APPROACH	1	1	0	0	0	0	1	1	0	1	1	1	0	1	**8**
COGNITIVE DEVELOPMENT	0	0	0	0	0	0	1	1	1	1	1	1	0	1	**7**
COMP.HEALTH THERAPY	1	0	0	0	0	0	1	1	0	1	1	0	0	1	**6**
COMPETENCIES	0	1	0	1	1	1	1	1	1	1	1	1	0	1	**11**
COMPUTING SKILLS	1	1	1	1	0	0	1	1	1	0	1	1	1	1	**11**
CONCEPT FORMATION	1	1	1	1	0	0	1	1	1	1	1	1	0	1	**11**
CONCEPTS,HEALTH/ILLNESS	1	1	0	1	1	1	1	1	0	1	1	1	1	1	**12**
CONFIDENTIALITY	1	1	0	1	1	1	1	1	1	1	1	1	1	1	**13**
CONFLICT RESOLUTION	1	1	0	0	0	0	1	1	1	0	1	1	0	1	**8**
COPING MECHANISMS	1	0	0	0	1	0	1	1	1	1	1	1	1	1	**10**
COUNSELLING	1	1	0	1	1	1	1	1	1	1	0	0	1	1	**11**
CULTURAL VALUES	1	1	0	0	1	1	1	1	1	1	1	1	1	1	**12**
DECISION MAKING	1	1	1	1	1	1	1	1	1	1	1	1	0	1	**13**
DIFFERING GROUPS	1	1	1	1	1	1	1	1	1	1	1	1	1	1	**14**
DISABILITY	1	1	0	0	1	1	1	1	1	1	1	1	1	1	**12**
ECON OF HEALTH CARE	0	1	0	1	0	0	1	1	0	1	1	0	1	1	**8**
EMPLOYMENT	0	1	0	1	0	1	1	1	1	0	1	0	0	1	**8**
ETHICS	0	1	0	1	1	1	1	1	1	1	1	1	1	1	**12**
ETHNICITY	1	1	0	0	1	1	1	1	1	1	1	1	0	1	**11**
EVALUATION OF CHANGE	1	1	1	1	1	1	1	1	1	1	1	1	0	1	**13**
FAMILY GROUPS	1	0	0	0	1	0	1	1	1	0	1	1	1	1	**9**
FAMILY NEEDS	1	0	0	1	1	0	1	1	1	0	1	1	1	1	**10**
FAMILY THERAPY	1	0	0	0	0	0	0	0	1	0	0	0	0	1	**3**
FIRST AID	0	1	0	1	1	1	1	0	0	1	0	0	1	1	**8**
GENDER	1	0	0	0	0	1	1	1	1	0	1	1	0	1	**8**
GRIEF	1	1	0	0	0	0	1	1	1	1	1	1	0	1	**9**
GRIEVANCES	1	0	0	1	0	1	1	1	0	1	0	0	0	0	**6**
GROUP DYNAMICS	1	1	1	1	1	1	1	1	1	1	1	1	1	1	**14**
GROUP THERAPY	1	0	0	0	0	0	0	1	1	0	1	0	0	1	**5**
HEALTH BEHAVIOURS	1	1	0	1	1	1	1	1	0	1	1	1	1	1	**12**
PAGE TOTALS	**34**	**31**	**8**	**21**	**21**	**22**	**40**	**37**	**33**	**32**	**38**	**33**	**22**	**41**	

SYLLABUS CONTENT	SPEECH THERAPY	PODIATRY	DENTAL TECHNOLOGY	RADIOGRAPHY	DENTAL HYGIENIST/D.S.A.	OPERATING DEPT. PRACT.	NURSING PROJECT 2000	NUTRITION & DIETETICS	SOCIAL WORK	PHYSIOTHERAPY	OCCUPATIONAL THERAPY	MEDICINE	DENTISTRY	NURSING PRE-REG. B.N.	TOTALS
HEALTH BELIEFS	1	1	0	1	1	0	1	1	0	1	1	1	1	1	**11**
HEALTH PROMOTION	0	1	0	1	1	0	1	1	0	1	1	1	1	1	**10**
HEALTH/SAFETY AT WORK	1	1	1	1	1	1	1	1	0	1	1	0	1	1	**12**
HOLISTIC CARE	1	1	0	1	1	1	1	0	0	1	1	1	1	1	**11**
HUMANIST APPROACH	1	0	0	0	0	0	1	1	0	0	1	0	0	1	**5**
I.Q.TEST	1	0	0	0	0	0	1	0	0	0	0	0	0	0	**2**
ILLNESS PERCEPTION	1	1	0	1	0	1	1	1	0	1	1	1	1	1	**11**
IMAGERY	1	0	0	0	0	0	0	0	0	1	1	1	0	0	**4**
IMPLEMENTING CHANGE	1	1	0	1	1	1	1	0	1	1	1	1	1	1	**12**
INDIVIDUALITY	1	0	0	0	1	1	1	0	1	1	1	1	1	1	**10**
INFORMATION TECHNOLOGY	1	1	1	1	0	1	1	1	1	0	1	0	1	1	**11**
INFORMED CONSENT	0	1	0	1	1	1	1	0	1	1	1	1	1	1	**11**
INTELLIGENCE	1	0	0	0	0	0	1	0	1	0	1	1	1	0	**6**
INTERDISCIPLINARY	1	1	1	1	1	1	1	1	1	1	1	1	0	1	**13**
INTERPERSON PERCEPTIONS	1	1	1	1	0	1	1	1	1	1	1	1	1	1	**13**
INTERVIEWING	1	1	1	1	1	1	1	1	1	1	1	1	1	1	**14**
KELLY'S CONSTRUCT THEORY	1	0	0	0	0	0	0	0	0	0	0	0	0	1	**2**
LAW & PRACTICE	0	1	0	1	0	1	1	1	1	1	1	1	1	1	**11**
LEADERSHIP	1	0	0	1	0	1	1	1	1	0	1	0	0	1	**8**
LEARNING DIFFICULTIES	1	1	0	0	1	0	1	1	1	1	1	1	1	1	**11**
LEARNING STYLES	1	0	1	1	1	1	1	1	1	1	1	0	1	1	**12**
LISTENING	1	1	0	1	1	1	1	1	1	1	1	1	1	1	**13**
LISTENING SKILLS	1	1	1	1	1	1	1	1	1	1	1	1	1	1	**14**
LITERATURE REVIEWS	1	1	1	1	0	1	1	1	1	1	1	0	1	1	**12**
MANAGING CHANGE	1	1	0	1	1	1	1	1	1	1	1	1	1	1	**13**
MEMORY	1	0	0	0	0	0	1	1	0	0	1	1	1	1	**7**
MINORITY GROUPS	1	1	0	0	1	1	1	1	1	1	1	1	1	1	**12**
MORAL DEVELOPMENT	1	0	0	0	0	0	1	1	1	0	1	0	0	1	**6**
MOTIVATION	1	1	0	1	1	1	1	1	0	1	1	1	1	1	**12**
NATURE/NURTURE	1	0	0	0	0	0	1	0	0	1	1	1	1	1	**7**
NON-VERBAL COMMUNICATION	1	1	1	1	1	1	1	1	1	1	1	1	1	1	**14**
ORGANISATION THEORY	1	0	1	1	0	1	1	1	1	1	1	0	0	1	**10**
PARTNERSHIP	0	0	0	0	0	0	1	0	1	1	1	1	1	1	**7**
PATIENT CHOICE	0	1	0	0	1	1	1	1	1	1	1	1	1	1	**11**
PATIENT DIGNITY	0	0	0	1	0	1	1	0	0	1	1	1	1	1	**8**
PATIENT & ENVIRONMENT	0	1	0	1	1	1	1	1	1	1	1	1	1	1	**12**
PATIENT RIGHTS	0	1	0	0	1	1	1	1	1	1	1	1	1	1	**11**
PEDAGOGY	1	1	0	0	0	0	1	0	1	0	1	0	0	1	**6**
PERCEPTION	1	1	1	1	1	1	1	1	1	1	1	1	1	1	**14**
PERSONAL ORGANISATION	1	1	1	1	0	1	1	1	1	1	1	0	1	1	**12**
POWER	1	0	0	1	0	0	1	1	1	0	0	1	0	1	**7**
PRESENTATION SKILLS	1	1	1	1	1	1	1	1	1	1	1	0	0	1	**12**
PROBLEM SOLVING	1	1	1	1	0	1	1	1	1	1	1	1	0	1	**12**
PROFESSIONAL BODIES	1	1	1	1	1	1	1	1	1	1	1	1	1	1	**14**
PROFESSIONALISM	1	1	0	1	0	1	1	1	1	1	1	1	1	1	**12**
PSYCHOLOGY & AGEING	1	1	0	1	0	0	1	1	1	1	1	1	1	1	**11**
PAGE TOTALS	**38**	**27**	**15**	**27**	**17**	**24**	**41**	**33**	**33**	**34**	**39**	**30**	**24**	**42**	

SYLLABUS CONTENT	SPEECHTHERAPY	PODIATRY	DENTAL TECHNOLOGY	RADIOGRAPHY	DENTAL HYGIENIST/D.S.A.	OPERATING DEPT. PRACT	NURSING PROJECT 2000	NUTRITION & DIETETICS	SOCIAL WORK	PHYSIOTHERAPY	OCCUPATIONAL THERAPY	MEDICINE	DENTISTRY	NURSING PRE-REG, B.N.	TOTALS
PSYCHOANALYTIC APPROACH	1	0	0	0	0	0	1	1	0	0	1	1	0	1	**6**
PSYCHOLOGY OF PAIN	1	1	0	0	0	1	1	1	0	1	1	1	1	1	**10**
QUALITY ASSURANCE	0	1	0	1	0	1	1	1	1	1	1	0	1	1	**10**
QUESTIONNAIRE DESIGN	1	1	0	1	0	0	1	0	1	1	1	0	0	1	**8**
QUESTIONS CLOSED	1	1	0	1	0	1	1	1	1	1	1	1	1	1	**12**
QUESTIONS OPEN	1	1	0	1	1	1	1	1	1	1	1	1	1	1	**13**
REFLECTIVE QUESTIONING	1	1	0	1	1	1	1	1	1	1	1	1	1	1	**13**
RESEARCH METHODS	1	1	0	1	0	1	1	1	1	1	1	1	1	1	**12**
RESEARCH SAMPLING	1	1	0	1	0	0	1	1	1	1	1	0	1	1	**10**
RISK TAKING	1	0	0	0	0	0	1	0	1	0	0	1	0	0	**4**
ROLE	1	1	1	1	1	1	1	1	1	1	1	1	1	1	**14**
SEXUALITY	1	0	0	0	0	1	1	0	1	0	1	1	0	1	**7**
SOCIAL DEVELOPMENT	1	0	0	0	1	0	1	1	1	0	1	1	1	1	**9**
SOCIAL SKILLS	1	1	1	1	1	1	1	0	1	0	1	1	1	1	**12**
STAFF.DEVEL.TRAINING	1	1	1	0	0	1	1	0	1	1	0	0	1	0	**8**
STATISTICS	1	1	1	1	0	0	1	1	1	1	1	1	1	1	**12**
STEREOTYPING	1	0	0	0	0	0	1	1	1	1	1	1	1	1	**9**
STRESS	1	1	0	1	1	1	1	1	1	1	1	1	1	1	**13**
STUDY SKILLS	1	1	1	1	1	1	1	0	1	1	1	1	1	1	**13**
SUBSTANCE ABUSE	1	0	0	0	0	1	1	1	1	1	1	1	0	0	**8**
TASK & FUNCTION	1	0	1	1	0	1	1	0	1	1	1	0	0	1	**9**
TEAM WORK	1	1	1	1	1	1	1	1	1	1	1	0	1	1	**13**
THEORY & PRACTICE	0	0	0	0	0	1	1	0	1	1	1	1	0	1	7
VERBAL COMMUNICATION	1	1	1	1	1	1	1	1	1	1	1	1	1	1	**14**
WORK RELATED STRESS	1	0	0	1	1	1	1	1	1	1	1	1	1	1	**12**
WRITING REPORTS	1	0	1	1	0	1	1	1	1	1	1	0	1	1	**11**
PAGE TOTALS	**24**	**16**	**9**	**17**	**10**	**19**	**26**	**18**	**24**	**21**	**24**	**19**	**9**	**22**	
GRAND TOTALS	**95**	**74**	**32**	**65**	**48**	**65**	**107**	**88**	**90**	**87**	**101**	**82**	**55**	**105**	

5. 3 Content analysis of the available recommended reading lists

The content analysis of the reading lists was completed with difficulty as many of the course documents did not contain real indicators of what core reading material is recommended. It is acknowledged that the analysis does not reflect an accurate picture but nonetheless it does raise issues about libraries and the duplication of resources. The results are discussed in detail in Chapter 6 and the content analysis is presented overleaf as Table 5.2.

Table 5.2 Content analysis of the available recommended reading lists

AUTHOR(S)	DATE	TITLE	DENTAL TECHNOLOGY	RADIOGRAPHY	DENTAL HYGIENIST / D.S.A.	OPERATING DEPT. PRACT	NURSING PROJECT 2000	NUTRITION & DIETETICS	SOCIAL WORK	PHYSIOTHERAPY	OCCUPATIONAL THERAPY	MEDICINE	DENTISTRY	NURSING PRE-REG B.N.	TOTALS
ABERCROMBIE.A, WARD.B.	1988	CONTEMPORARY BRITISH SOCIETY									1				1
ALLSOP.J.	1984	HEALTH POLICY & THE N.H.S.					1								1
ARGYLE.M.	1983	PSYCHOLOGY OF INTERPERSONAL BEHAVIOUR					1							1	2
ARGYLE.M.	1988	BODILY COMMUNICATION													1
ARGYLE.M. (ED)	1981	SOCIAL SKILLS & HEALTH					1								1
ARGYLE.M, HENDERSON.M.	1985	ANATOMY OF RELATIONSHIPS									1				1
ARMSTRONG.D.A.	1983	AN OUTLINE OF SOCIOLOGY					1				1				2
ARMSTRONG.M.	1988	HOW TO BE AN EVEN BETTER MANAGER									1				1
ARONSON.E.	1984	THE SOCIAL ANIMAL					1					1		1	3
ATKINSON, ATKINSON & HILDGARD	1983	INTRODUCTION TO PSYCHOLOGY												1	1
BADDLEY.A.	1987	WORKING MEMORY													1
BALINT.M.	1964	THE DOCTOR HIS PATIENT & THE ILLNESS					1								1
BALY M.	1984	PROFESSIONAL RESPONSIBILITY					1								1
BANNISTER. D, FRANSELLA. F.	1986	INQUIRING MAN												1	1
BARBER.J, KRATZ.C.	1980	TOWARDS TEAMCARE												1	1
BARLEY.N.	1983	INNOCENT ANTHROPOLOGIST					1								1
BARON.R, BYRNE.D.	1987	SOCIAL PSYCHOLOGY					1							1	2
BAUGH.B.	1982	INTRODUCTION TO SOCIAL SERVICES					1								1
BEARD.R, HARTLEY.J.	1984	TEACHING AND LEARNING IN H.E.												1	1
BEAUCHAMP.T.L., CHILDRESS.J.F.	1983	PRINCIPLES OF BIOMEDICAL ETHICS					1								1
BECKER.M.H.	1974	THE HEALTH BUILDING MODE					1								1
BEE.H.	1989	THE DEVELOPING CHILD					1								1
BEE.H.L., MITCHELL.S.K.	1984	THE DEVELOPING PERSON					1								1
BELL.C., NEWBY.H.	1972	COMMUNITY STUDIES					1							1	2
BELL.J.	1988	DOING YOUR RESEARCH PROJECT		1							1			1	3
BENJAMIN.A.	1981	THE HELPING INTERVIEW		1											1
BERNE E.	1968	GAMES PEOPLE PLAY												1	1
BETTLEHEIM.B.	1971	CHILDREN OF THE DREAM					1								1
BILTON., et al.	1987	INTRODUCTORY SOCIOLOGY												1	1
BLACK J.	1986	PAEDIATRICS AMONG ETHNIC MINORITIES					1								1
BLACK.N., et al.	1984	HEALTH &DISEASE:A READER					1							1	2
BLACKLOCK.H.M.	1970	AN INTRODUCTION TO SOCIAL RESEARCH									1				1
BLACKMAN.M.E.	1989	PSYCH. OF PHYSICALLY ILL PATIENT													1
BLAND.N.	1988	AN INTRODUCTION TO MEDICAL STATISTICS									1				1
BLAXTER M.	1980	THE MEANING OF DISABILITY					1								1
BLINDIS.M., JACKSON.E.	1982	NON-VERBAL COMMUNICATION WITH PATIENTS		1											1
BLOOMFIELD.R., FOLLIS.P.	1974	THE HEALTH TEAM IN ACTION					1								1
BOGDAM.R., TAYLOR.S.	1975	INTRO.TO QUAL. RESEARCH METHODS					1								1
BOLGER.A.W.	1982	COUNSELLING IN BRITAIN					1								1
BOND.J., BOND.S.	1986	SOCIOLOGY AND HEALTH CARE					1								1
BOND.J., BOND.S.	1986	SOCIOLOGY & HEALTH CARE						1			1				2
BORGER. & SEABOURNE.	1982	PSYCHOLOGY OF LEARNING					1								1
BOUD.D.J.	1981	DEVELOPING STUDENT AUTONOMY												1	1
BOUD. et al	1985	REFLECTION. TURNING EXPERIENCE												1	1
BOWER.T.	1982	DEVELOPMENT IN INFANCY													1
BOWKER J.	1983	WORLDS OF FAITH					1								1
BOWLBY.J.	1965	CHILD CARE & THE GROWTH OF LOVE					1								1
BRADFORD-HILL.A.	1987	A SHORT TEXTBOOK OF MEDICAL STATS.		1											1
BRANDES.D, PHILLIPS.H.	1977	GAMESTERS HANDBOOK													1
BREARLY.G., BUCKLEY.P.	1986	INTRODUCING COUNSELLING SKILLS									1				1

Author	Date	Title	Den.Tech	Rad	Den.Hyg	ODP	Nur (P2k)	Diet	Soc.W	Physio	Occ.T	Med	Den	Nur. (BN)	Totals
BRECHIN. et al	1981	HANDICAP IN THE SOCIAL WORLD					1								1
BRIMBLECOMBE.G.	1987	CHILDREN IN HEALTH AND DISEASE												1	1
BRITTON.T.	1989	INTRODUCTORY SOCIOLOGY					1								1
BROCKINGTON.C.F.	1985	HEALTH OF THE DEVELOPING WORLD					1								1
BROOKFIELD.S.	1987	DEVELOPING CRITICAL THINKERS												1	1
BROWN .A.	1986	GROUP WORK							1						1
BROWN.M.	1983	THE UNFOLDING SELF					1								1
BROWN.M.	1985	INTRO.TO SOCIAL ADMIN. IN BRITAIN					1								1
BROWN.R,	1986	SOCIAL PSYCHOLOGY					1								1
BROWN.R.	1988	GROUP PROCESSES						1							1
BRUHN.J., CORDOVA.D.A.	1977	DEVELOPMENTAL APPROACH												1	1
BRUMFITT.S.	1986	COUNSELLING													1
BRUNER et al	1966	STUDIES IN COGNITIVE GROWTH					1								1
BRYMAN.A.	1988	QUANTITY & QUALITY IN SOCIAL RESEARCH												1	1
BULMER.M.	1982	THE USES OF SOCIAL RESEARCH							1						1
BULMER.M.	1987	SOCIAL BASIS OF COMMUNITY CARE									1				1
BURGESS.P.	1984	IN THE FIELD.					1								1
BURNARD.P.	1989	COUNSELLING SKILLS FOR HEALTH PROFS.					1	1						1	3
BURNARD.P., MORRISON.P.	1990	NURSING RESEARCH IN ACTION		1											1
BURNS.R.B.	1986	CHILD DEVELOPMENT					1								1
BURTON.G. DIMBLEBY.R.	1988	BETWEEN OURSELVES.						1							1
BUTLER.A. (ED)	1985	AGEING					1								1
BUTTERWORTH.E., WEIR.D.	1976	SOCIOLOGY OF MODERN BRITAIN					1								1
BUZAN.A.	1982	USE YOUR HEAD									1				1
CAHOON.M.	1987	R3ECENT ADVANCES IN NURSING		1			1							1	3
CAHOON.M.	1987	RESEARCH METHODOLOGY					1							1	2
CALAN.M.	1987	HEALTH &ILLNESS.					1								1
CALNAN.J.	1983	TALKING WITH PATIENTS									1				1
CAMPBELL.M.J., MACHIN.D.	1990	MEDICAL STATISTICS		1				1							2
CANTER.D.	1985	FACET THEORY												1	1
CAPLOW.T. et al	1983	THE SOCIOLOGY OF WORK									1				1
CAPRON.H.L.	1987	COMPUTERS						1							1
CAPSTICK.I.	1985	PATIENT COMPLAINTS & LITIGATION													1
CARKUFF R.	1980	THE ART OF HELPING				1									1
CARTER.R., MARTIN.J.N.T.	1984	SYSTEMS MANAGEMENT & CHANGE									1				1
CARVER.V., LIDDIARD.P.	1978	AN AGEING POPULATION												1	1
CASEY.F.	1985	HOW TO STUDY: A PRACTICAL GUIDE							1						1
CHALLEN.C. et al	1988	RESEARCH FOR STUDENTS & SUPERVISORS		1											1
CHALMERS.A.F.	1982	WHAT IS THIS THING .					1								1
CHAPMAN.M.	1986	PLAIN FIGURES						1							1
CHELL.E.	1987	PSYCH. OF BEHAVIOUR IN ORGANISATIONS							1						1
CLARKE.J., et al	1987	IDEOLOGIES OF WELFARE					1								1
CLAUS.K., BAILEY.J.	1977	POWER &INFLUENCE IN HEALTH CARE.					1								1
CLAXTON.G.	1984	LIVE & LEARN												1	1
COATES.H., KING.A.	1982	PATIENT ASSESSMENT								1					1
COHEN.G.	1987	SOCIAL CHANGE & THE LIFE FORCE					1								1
COHEN.G.. et al	1986	MEMORY : A COGNITIVE APPROACH													1
COHEN.L., MANION.L.	1989	RESEARCH METHODS IN EDUCATION		1											1
COLE.T.	1986	WHOSE WELFARE					1								1
COPP.L.A.	1986	PERSPECTIVES ON PAIN												1	1
COPPERMAN.H.	1983	DYING AT HOME					1								1
CORMACK.D.	1984	THE RESEARCH PROCESS					1				1				2
CORNWELL.J.	1984	HARD EARNED LIVES					1								1
COSWELL. D.F.S.	1982	SUCCESS IN STATISTICS		1											1
COUTTS.L.C., HARDY.L.K.	1985	TEACHING FOR HEALTH					1								1
COX.T.	1986	STRESS									1				1
CUFF.E.C., PAYNE.G.C.F.	1984	PERSPECTIVES IN SOCIOLOGY												1	1
DALE.P.	1986	DANGEROUS FAMILIES												1	1
DALLOS.R., PROCTOR.H.	1984	FAMILY PROCESSES AN INTERACTIONAL VIEW												1	1

Author	Date		Den.Tech	Radio	Den.Hyg	ODP	Nur. (P2k)	Diet	Soc.W	Physio	Occ.T	Med	Den	Nur. (BA)	Totals
DANIEL.W.W.	1987	BIOSTATISTICS													1
DANZIGER.K.	1971	SOCIALIZATION					1								1
DASEN.P	1988	HEALTH &CROSS CULTURAL PSYCHOLOGY					1								1
DAWSON.S.	1986	ANALYSING ORGANISATIONS					1				1				2
DE BONO.E.	1981	MANAGEMENT:PROBLEM SOLVING					1								1
DeGILIO et al	1989	THE MANAGEMENT MANUAL									1				1
DELAMONT.S.	1980	THE SOCIOLOGY OF WOMEN												1	1
DERLAGA.V.J., JANDA.L.H.	1982	PERSONAL ADJUSTMENT					1								1
DeVITO.J.	1986	THE INTERPERSONAL COMMUNICATION BOOK		1											1
DIMOND.B.	1989	LEGAL ASPECTS.					1				1				2
DIXON.B.R.et al	1987	HANDBOOK OF SOCIAL SCIENCE RESEARCH						1							1
DONALDSON.R.J., DONALDSON.L.J.	1988	ESSENTIAL COMMUNITY MEDICINE					1								1
DOWNIE.R.S.	1987	HEALTHY RESPECT													1
DOWNIE.R.S., TELFER.E.	1980	CARING & CURING					1								1
DRYDEN.W.	1987	COUNSELLING INDIVIDUALS							1						1
DRYDEN.W.	1988	GROUP THERAPY									1				1
DRYDEN.W. (ED)	1984	INDIVIDUAL THERAPY IN BRITAIN						1							1
DUCK.S.	1988	RELATING TO OTHERS					1								1
DUSEK.J.B.	1987	ADOLESCENT DEVELOPMENT & BEHAVIOUR													1
EGAN.G.	1976	INTERPERSONAL LIVING					1								1
EGAN.G.	1986	THE SKILLED HELPER					1	1	1					1	4
ELLIS.A.W, YOUNG.A.W.	1988	COGNITIVE NEUROPSYCHOLOGY													1
ELLIS .R.	1988	PROFESSIONAL COMPETENCE & QUAL. ASS					1				1				2
ELLIS.R., WHITTINGTON.D.	1983	NEW DIRECTIONS IN SOCIAL SKILLS.		1							1				2
ELWES.L.	1985	PROMOTING HEALTH						1							1
ENELOW.A.J., SWISHER.S.N.	1986	INTERVIEWING & PATIENT CARE		1											1
ERIKSON.E.	1968	CHILDHOOD & SOCIETY					1		1						2
ERKSON.E.	1959	IDENTITY & THE LIFE CYCLE					1								1
EVANS K.M.	1984	PLANNING SMALL SCALE RESEARCH					1								1
EVANS.D.W.	1986	PEOPLE COMMUNICATIONS & ORGANISATIONS													1
EVANS.G.(ED)	1984	ENVIRONMENTAL STRESS					1								1
EYELS.J., WOODS.J.K.	1983	SOCIAL GEOGRAPHY OF MEDICINE & HEALTH					1							1	2
EYSENCK.H,	1984	A HANDBOOK OF COGNITIVE PSYCHOLOGY					1								1
EYESENCK.H.	1975	SENSE & NONSENSE.					1								1
FAIRBURN S.	1987	PSYCHOLOGY ETHICS CHANGE					1								1
FAULDER C.	1985	INFORMED CONSENT					1								1
FAULDER.C.	1985	WHOSE BODY IS IT					1								1
FELNER.R., et al	1983	PREVENTIVE PSYCHOLOGY					1								1
FIELD.F.	1981	INEQUALITY IN BRITAIN					1								1
FIELDING.P., BERMAN.P.C.	1990	SURVIVING IN GENERAL MANAGEMENT									1				1
FINCH.J, GROVES.D.	1983	A LABOUR OF LOVE												1	1
FINCH.J.D.	1984	ASPECTS OF LAW								1	1				2
FITZGERALD M.	1977	WELFARE IN ACTION							1						1
FITZPATRICK.R., HINTON.J.	1984	THE EXPERIENCE OF ILLNESS								1				1	2
FLETCHER.R.	1973	FAMILY & MARRIAGE IN BRITAIN												1	1
FLYNN.N.	1990	PUBLIC SECTOR MANAGEMENT							1						1
FODOR.J.	1983	MODULARITY OF MIND								1					1
FONAGY.P., HIGGIT.A.	1984	PERSONALITY THEORY &CLINICAL PRACTICE						1							1
FORGAS.J.B.	1985	INTERPERSONAL BEHAVIOUR.												1	1
FORGAS.J.P.	1981	SOCIAL COGNITION.		1											1
FREEDMAN.M.	1988	CURRENT LEGAL PROBLEMS					1								1
FREEMAN.M.D.A.	1988	MEDICINE ETHICS & LAW													1
FREIDMAN.G.D.	1987	PRIMER OF EPIDEMIOLOGY					1								1
FREUD.A.	1966	NORMALITY & PATHOLOGY.					1								1
FREUD.S.	1923	THE EGO & THE ID					1								1
FULDER S.	1989	HANDBOOK OF COMPLEMENTARY MEDICINE					1								1
FURNHAM.A., BOCHNER.S.	1986	CULTURE SHOCK					1								1
GAHAGN.J.	1984	SOCIAL INTERACTION & ITS MANAGEMENT					1								1
GARRETT.G	1983	HEALTH NEEDS OF THE ELDERLY									1				1

Authors	Date	Title	Den.Tech	Radio	Den.Hyg	ODP	Nur.(P2k)	Diet	Soc.W	Physio	Occ.T	Med	Den	Nur. (BN)	Totals
GATCHEL.R.J.	1989	AN INTRODUCTION TO HEALTH PSYCHOLOGY												1	1
GERGEN.K.J., GERGEN.M.M.,	1985	SOCIAL PSYCHOLOGY					1								1
GERHARDT.U	1989	IDEAS ABOUT ILLNESS									1				1
GESSELL.A.	1971	FIRST FIVE YEARS OF LIFE					1								1
GIBBS.G.	1986	TEACHING STUDENTS TO LEARN		1											1
GIDDENS.A.	1989	SOCIOLOGY					1	1			1				3
GILLIS.L.	1972	HUMAN BEHAVIOUR INILLNESS					1								1
GLASER.B., STRAUSS.A.	1965	AWARENESS OF DYING												1	1
GLASER.B., STRAUSS.A.	1968	TIME FOR DYING												1	1
GLOVER.D., STRAWBRIDGES.	1985	SOCIOLOGY OF KNOWLEDGE					1								1
GOFFMAN.E.	1971	THE PRESENTATION OF SELF												1	1
GOFFMAN.E.	1968	STIGMA					1							1	1
GOLDSTONE.L.A.	1985	UNDERSTANDING MEDICAL STATISTICS		1											1
GORE.S.M., ATTMAN.D.G.	1982	STATISTICS IN PRACTICE		1											1
GRAHAM H.	1985	HEALTH AND WELFARE					1								1
GRAHAM.H.	1984	WOMEN & ILLNESS					1							1	2
GRAHAM.H.	1984	WOMEN HEALTH & THE FAMILY					1							1	2
GRAY.J.A.	1988	PSYCHOLOGY OF FEAR & STRESS												1	1
GREEN.S.A.	1984	MIND & BODY : PSYCH. OF PHYSICAL ILLNESS													1
GREENE.J., DOLIVEIRA.M.	1982	LEARNING TO USE STATS. TESTS									1				1
GRIFFITHS.D,	1981	PSYCHOLOGY & MEDICINE										1			1
GREENHOUGH.W. (ED)	1973	THE NATURE & NURTURE OF BEHAVIOUR					1								1
GUBA.E.G., LINCOLN.Y.S.	1985	EFFECTIVE EVALUATION												1	1
GUNNING.R.	1986	TECHNIQUE OF CLEAR WRITING						1							1
HAKIN.K.	1987	RESEARCH DESIGN							1						1
HALL.C., LINDZAY.G.	1978	THEORIES OF PERSONALITY												1	1
HAM.C.	1985	HEALTH POLICY IN BRITAIN					1			1					3
HANDY C.	1985	UNDERSTANDING ORGANISATIONS					1								1
HARALAMBOS.M.	1985	SOCIOLOGY :THEMES & PERSPECTIVES							1					1	2
HARALAMBOS.M.	1985	SOCIOLOGY NEW DIRECTIONS												1	1
HARE.R.M.	1981	MORAL THINKING					1								1
HARGIE.O.	1986	HANDBOOK OF COMMUNICATION SKILLS		1			1								2
HARGIE.O., et al	1987	SOCIAL SKILLS IN INTERPERSONAL COMMUN.		1											1
HARLOW.E.	1967	PRACTICAL COMMUNICATION					1				1				2
HARRIS T.	1973	I'M O.K. YOU'RE O.K.					1								1
HARRIS.J.	1985	THE VALUE OF LIFE					1								1
HARRISON.P.	1983	INSIDE THE INNER CITY												1	1
HART.N.	1988	SOCIOLOGY OF HEALTH & MEDICINE												1	1
HAWKINS.P., SHOHET.R.	1989	SUPERVISION IN THE HELPING PROFESSIONS												1	1
HAWTON.K., et al	1989	COGNITIVE BEHAVIOUR THERAPY.													1
HAYNES.M.	1987	MAKE EVERY MINUTE COUNT		1											1
HAYNES.R., SACKETT.D.	1976	COMPLIANCE WITH THERAPEUTIC REGIMES					1								1
HAYSLETT.H.T.	1974	STATS.MADE SIMPLE									1				1
HEIM.A.	1985	INTELLIGENCE & PERSONALITY					1								1
HELMAN C.	1984	CULTURE HEALTH AND ILLNESS					1							1	2
HENLEY A.	1983	ASIANS IN BRITAIN							1						1
HERON.J.	1989	SIX CATEGORY INTERVENTION ANALYSIS												1	1
HEWSTONE.M. et al	1988	INTRODUCTION TO SOCIAL PSYCHOLOGY							1						1
HICKS.H.G., GILLET.C.R.	1981	MANAGEMENT						1							1
HILGARD.E.R., et al	1990	INTRODUCTION TO PSYCHOLOGY					1				1				2
HOLDSWORTH A.	1988	OUT OF THE DOLLS HOUSE							1						1
HOOYMAN .N. ET AL	1989	SOCIAL GERONTOLOGY: MULTIDISCIPLINARY P.					1								1
HOWARD.K., SHARP.J.A.	1983	MANAGEMENT OF A STUDENTS RESEARCH PROJ.		1							1				2
HUDSON.B.L., MACDONALD.G.M.	1986	BEHAVIOURAL SOCIAL WORK: AN INTRODUCTION							1						1
HULMES E.	1989	EDUCATION AND CULTURAL DIVERSITY							1						1
HUNTER.I.	1964	MEMORY					1								1
IRVINE.J. et al	1984	DEMYSTIFYING SOCIAL STATISTICS					1								1
IVEY.A.	1980	COUNSELLING & PSYCHOTHERAPY					1								1
IVEY.A.E.	1983	INTENTIONAL INTERVEIWING &COUNSELLING					1								1

Author	Date	Title	Den.Tech	Radio	Den.Hyg	ODP	Nur (P2k)	Diet	Soc.W	Physio	Occ.T	Med	Den	Nur (BN)	Totals
JAMIESON.A., et al	1984	DEALING WITH DRUG MISUSE							1						1
JANISSE.M.P.	1988	INDIVIDUAL DIFFERENCES												1	1
JARVIS.P	1983	PROFESSIONAL EDUCATION					1								1
JESPERSSEN.E., PEGG.P.	1988	USING PSYCHOSOCIAL COUNSELLING.					1								1
JOHNSON.J.A.	1986	WELLNESS AS CONTEXT FOR LIVING									1				1
JOHNSON.N.	1987	WELFARE STATE INTRANSITION					1								1
JOLLEY.J.	1987	MISSED BEGINNINGS					1								1
JORDAN B.	1987	RETHINKING WELFARE							1						1
KAPLAN.L	1978	ONENESS & SEPERATENESS.					1								1
KARPF A.	1988	DOCTORING THE MEDIA							1						1
KAYFELZ.J., SHIE.R.C.	1987	ACADEMICALLY SPEAKING		1											1
KENNEDY.I.	1981	THE UNMASKING OF MEDICINE					1								1
KENNEDY.I.	1988	TREAT ME RIGHT					1								1
KENT.G., DALGLEISH.M.	1986	PSYCHOLOGY & MEDICAL CARE					1								1
KHAN V.S.	1979	MINORITY FAMILIES IN BRITAIN							1						1
KIELHOFNER.G. (ED)	1985	A MODEL OF HUMAN OCCUPATION					1				1				1
KIMERSLEY.P.	1973	HAZARDS AT WORK					1								1
KIMMEL.D.C.	1980	ADULTHOOD &AGEING					1								1
KING.M., et al	1983	IRRESISTIBLE COMMUNICATION					1								1
KLINE.P.	1979	PSYCHOMETRICS & PSYCHOLOGY					1								1
KNAPP.M	1984	THE ECONOMICS OF HEALTH CARE							1						1
KNOWLES M.	1984	THE ADULT LEARNER							1						1
KOCH.H.C.H.	1988	GENERAL MANAGEMENT IN THE HEALTH SERVICE									1				1
KOHLER RIESSMAN C.	1989	WOMEN AND MEDICALISATION							1						1
KOLB.D.A., et al (Eds)	1984	ORGANISATIONAL PSYCHOLOGY												1	1
KRISTAL.L.	1979	UNDERSTANDING PSYCHOLOGY					1								1
KUBLER ROSS.E.	1986	ON DEATH AND DYING												1	1
LAKE.T., ACHESON.F.	1988	ROOM TO LISTEN ROOM TO TALK												1	1
LAMB.M.	1976	ROLE OF THE FATHER.					1								1
LAZURUS.R., FOLKMAN.S.	1984	STRESS APPRAISAL & COPING					1								1
LEGGE.D.	1975	INTRO. TO PSYCHOLOGICAL MEDICINE					1								1
LEIGH.A.	1984	20 BETTER WAYS TO MANAGE									1				1
LEIGH.H., REISER.M.F.	1980	THE PATIENT:								1					1
LEY.P.	1987	COMMUNICATIONING WITH PATIENTS					1								1
LISHMAN.J	1983	COLLABORATION & CONFLICT							1						1
LOFLAND.J., LOFLAND.L.H.	1984	ANALYSING SOCIAL SETTINGS												1	1
LOLAS.F., MAYER.H. (Eds)	1987	PERSPECTIVES ON STRESS					1	1							2
LONEY M.	1987	THE STATE OR THE MARKET:							1						1
LONG.A.F.	1985	RESEARCH INTO HEALTH &ILLNESS.						1							1
LONG.A., HARRISON.S.	1985	HEALTH SERVICE PERFORMANCE									1				1
LONSDALE.S.	1985	WORK & INEQUALITY					1				1				2
MACE.C.A.	1968	THE PSYCHOLOGY OF STUDY												1	1
MACK.J. LANSLEY.	1985	POOR BRITAIN							1						1
MACKIE.J.L.	1977	ETHICS INVENTING RIGHT &WRONG					1								1
MADDERS.J.	1989	STRESS & RELAXATION									1				1
MADDOX. H.	1988	HOW TO STUDY		1											1
MADDOX.R.B.	1987	EFFECTIVE PERFORMANCE APPRAISALS									1				1
MAITLIN.M.W.	1989	COGNITION												1	1
MANGEN S.	1982	SOCIOLOGY AND MENTAL HEALTH												1	1
MANN.P.	1976	METHODS OF SOCIOLOGICAL ENQUIRY							1						1
MARES.P., et al	1985	HEALTH CARE IN MULTI RACIAL BRITAIN												1	1
MARRIS.P.	1974	LOSS & CHANGE					1								1
MARTIN.P., BATESON.P.	1986	MEASURING BEHAVIOUR							1						1
MASLOW.A.	1968	TOWARD A PSYCHOLOGY.					1								1
MASSIE.J.L.	1987	ESSENTIALS OF MANAGEMENT												1	1
MATTHEWS.A.	1988	ESSENTIAL PSYCH. FOR MEDICAL PRACTICE										1			1
MAYO.B.	1986	PHILOSOPHY OF RIGHT &WRONG					1								1
MAYON - WHITE.B. (ED)	1986	PLANNING & MANAGING CHANGE												1	1
McGHEE. J.W.	1985	INTRODUCTORY STATISTICS		1											1

Author	Date	Title	Den.Tech	Radio	Den.Hyg	ODP	Nur (P2k)	Diet	Soc.W	Physio	Occ.T	Med	Den	Nur (BN)	Totals
McLAUGHAN.N.	1978	GROUP WORK LEARNING & PRACTICE							1						1
McNEIL.P.	1990	RESEARCH METHODS							1						1
MEADOWS.S.	1986	UNDERSTANDING CHILD DEVELOPMENT							1						1
MEARNS.D., DRYDEN.W.	1990	EXPERIENCE OF COUNSELLING IN ACTION					1								1
MELTZER.H., NORD.W.R.	1982	MAKING ORGANISATIONS					1								1
MILES.A.	1987	THE MENTALLY ILL									1				1
MILLER.D., FARMER.R.	1982	EPIDEMIOLOGY OF DISEASES					1								1
MITCHELL.L.	1977	SIMPLE RELAXATION													1
MORGAN.M. ET AL	1985	SOCIOLOGICAL APPROACHES.					1								1
MORRICE.J.K.W.	1976	CRISIS INTERVENTION					1								1
MOSS.R.TSU.V	1977	COPING WITH PHYSICAL ILLNESS												1	1
MURGATROYD.S., WOLFE.R.	1982	COPING WITH CRISIS					1								1
MURGATROYD.S.	1986	COUNSELLING & HELPING												1	1
NAGEL.T.	1989	WHAT DOES IT ALL MEAN					1								1
NEAVE.H.R.	1981	ELEMENTARY STATISTICS TABLE		1											1
NELKIN.D., BROWN.M.S.	1984	WORKERS AT RISK					1								1
NELSON - JONES.R.	1982	THEORY & PRACTICE OF COUNSELLING PSYCH.							1						1
NELSON-JONES.R.	1988	PRACTICAL COUNSELLING &HELPING SKILLS							1						1
NELSON.M.J.	1989	MANAGING HEALTH PROFESSIONALS									1				1
NEUBERGER J.	1987	CARING FOR DYING PEOPLE OF DIFF. FAITHS												1	1
NEW.C., DAVID.M.	1985	FOR THE CHILDRENS SAKE					1								1
NIVEN.N.	1989	HEALTH PSYCHOLOGY.					1	1						1	3
O'NEILL.P.	1983	HEALTH CRISIS 2000					1								1
OPEN UNIVERSITY	1985	STUDYING HEALTH &DISEASE					1								1
OPEN UNIVERSITY	1985	THE HEALTH OF NATIONS					1								1
ORME.J.E.	1984	ABNORMAL & CLINICAL PSYCHOLOGY						1							1
OTT.L., MENDENHALL.W.	1985	UNDERSTANDING STATISTICS		1											1
PARKER.S.R.	1976	SOCIOLOGY OF LEISURE									1				1
PARKES.C.M.	1975	BEREAVEMENT					1								1
PARKIN.A.	1986	HUMAN MEMORY & ITS PATHOLOGY												1	1
PARTRIDGE.C., BARNETT.R.	1986	RESEARCH GUIDELINES								1					1
PASCALL.G.	1986	SOCIAL POLICY, A FEMINISTS ANALYSIS					1								1
PATRICK D., SCAMBLER G.	1986	SOCIOLOGY AS APPLIED TO MEDICINE												1	1
PATRICK.D., SCAMBLER.G.	1988	SOCIOLOGY AS APPLIED TO MEDICINE					1			1					2
PAYNE.R.	1987	STRESS IN HEALTH PROFESSIONALS													1
PENNEBAKER.J.	1982	PSYCHOLOGY OF PHYSICAL SYMPTOMS					1								1
PENNININGTON.D.C.	1986	ESSENTIAL SOCIAL PSYCHOLOGY							1						1
PERLS F.	1969	GESTALDT THERAPY VERBATIM												1	1
PERVIN.L.A.	1989	PERSONALITY: THEORY & RESEARCH						1							1
PETRILLO.M.	1980	EMOTIONAL CARE OF THE HOSPITALISED CHILD												1	1
PHILLIPS.M., DAWSON.J.	1985	DOCTORS DILEMMAS.					1								1
PHILLIPSON.C., WALKER.A.	1986	AGEING &SOCIAL POLICY					1								1
PHILP.T.	1983	MAKING PERFORMANCE APPRAISAL WORK					1								1
PIAGET.J.	1973	THE CHILDS CONCEPTION.					1								1
PIPKIN.R.E.	1984	MEDICAL STATISTICS MADE EASY										1			1
POSTILLO.R.	1984	HEALTH PROF/PATIENT INTERACTION									1				1
PRITCHARD M.J.	1986	MEDICINE AND THE BEHAVIOURAL SCIENCES										1			1
PUNER.M.	1979	TO THE GOOD LONG LIFE					1								1
PURTILLO.R.B., CASSELL.C	1981	ETHICAL DIMENSIONS IN HEALTH PROFS.								1					1
RACK P.	1982	CULTURE AND MENTAL DISORDER							1						1
RAPOPORT.R.N.	1982	FAMILIES IN BRITAIN												1	1
RAPHAEL.D.D.	1987	MORAL PHILOSOPHY					1								1
RATHWELL S.	1985	TOWARDS A NEW UNDERSTANDING							1						1
REASON.P.	1981	HUMAN ENQUIRY					1								1
REID.N.G., BOORE.J.R.F.	1987	RESEARCH METHOD & STATS. IN HEALTH CARE					1	1			1				3
RICHARDS., LIGHT.P.	1986	CHILDREN OF SOCIAL WORLDS					1								1
RICHMAN.J.	1987	MEDICINE & HEALTH					1								1
ROBERTSON-ELIOT.F.	1986	THE FAMILY CHANGE OR CONTINUITY												1	1
RISEBOROUGH.W., WALTER.M.	1988	MANAGEMENT IN HEALTH CARE								1					1

Author	Date	Title	Den.Tech	Radio	Den.Hyg	ODP	Nur.(P2k)	Diet	Soc.W	Physio	Occ.T	Med	Dentist	Nur.(BN)	Totals
ROBINSON.D.	1973	PATIENTS PRACTICIONERS &MEDICAL CARE					1								1
ROBINSON.R	1988	PEOPLE IN ORGANISATIONS													1
ROBSON.C.	1983	EXPERIMENTAL DESIGN &STATS.					1				1				2
ROGERS C.	1965	CLIENT CENTERED THERAPY												1	1
ROGERS. C.R.	1976	ON BECOMING A PERSON					1							1	2
ROTH.I.	1990	INTRODUCTION TO PSYCHOLOGY							1						1
ROWLAND.J, COOPER.P.	1983	ENVIRONMENT & HEALTH					1								1
ROWNTREE .D.	1989	LEARN HOW TO STUDY		1											1
ROWNTREE.D.	1981	STATISTICS WITHOUT TEARS		1											1
RUST.J., GOLOMBOK.S.	1989	MODERN PSCHOMETRICS										1			1
SAMPSON.C.	1985	THE NEGLECTED ETHIC					1								1
SANTS.J., BUTCHER.H.	1974	DEVELOPMENTAL PSYCHOLOGY					1								1
SATIR.V.	1972	PEOPLEMAKING					1								1
SCAMMELL.B.	1990	COMMUNICATION SKILLS		1											1
SEAMAN.C., VERHONICK.P.J	1982	RESEARCH METHODS FOR UNDERGRADUATES		1											1
SEEDHOUSE .D.	1986	HEALTH.FOUNDATIONS FOR ACHEIVEMENT					1							1	2
SEEDHOUSE.D.	1988	ETHICS:HEART OF HEALTH CARE					1							1	2
SEEDHOUSE.D.	1989	CHANGING IDEAS IN HEALTH CARE												1	1
SEEDHOUSE.D.	1989	ETHICS IN HEALTH EDUCATION													1
SHACKELTON.FLETCHER	1984	INDIVIDUAL DIFFERENCES					1								1
SHACKMAN J.	1984	THE RIGHT TO BE UNDERSTOOD							1						1
SHAEFF.W.R.	1990	MARKETING IN THE N.H.S.									1				1
SHAR.C.D.	1986	INTRODUCING QUALITY ASSURANCE									1				1
SHEARER.A.	1981	DISABILITY. WHOSE HANDICAP?												1	1
SHERIDAN.M.D.	1981	FROM BIRTH TO FIVE YEARS									1				2
SHOTTER.J.	1975	IMAGES OF MAN												1	1
SIMPSON.A.	1988	INVITATION TO LAW					1								1
SINCLAIR.D.	1988	HUMAN GROWTH AFTER BIRTH									1				1
SMART.J.J.C., WILLIAMS.B.	1973	UTILITARIANISM					1								1
SMITH V.M., BASS T.	1982	COMMUNICATION FOR THE HEALTH CARE TEAM												1	1
SMITH.A.	1985	RECENT ADVANCES INCOMMUNITY MEDICINE					1								1
SMITH.M.M., et al	1987	COGNITION IN ACTION					1								1
SMITH.R.M	1983	LEARNING HOW TO LEARN									1				1
SMITH.V.M., BASS.T.	1982	COMMUNICATIONS FOR HEALTHCARE TEAMS		1										1	2
SPENCE.S.	1987	SOCIAL SKILL TRAINING							1						1
SPINELLI.E.	1989	THE INTERPRETED WORLD												1	1
STACEY.M.	1988	SOCIOLOGY OF HEALTH &HEALING					1								1
STACEY.M., CURRER.C (Eds)	1986	CONCEPTS OF HEALTH,ILLNESS & DISEASE					1								1
STEDEFORD.A.	1984	FACING DEATH					1								1
STERN.D.	1985	INTERPERSONAL WORLD OF THE INFANT					1								1
STEVENSON .O.	1989	AGE & VULNERABILITY					1								1
STEWART.D.M.	1987	HANDBOOK OF MANAGEMENT SKILLS						1							1
STEWART.W.	1985	COUNSELLING IN REHABILITATION									1				1
STOODLEY.K.O.C.	1984	APPLIED STATISTICAL TECHNIQUES		1											1
STOPFORD.B.	1987	UNDERSTANDING DISABILITY												1	1
STORANDT.M.	1988	CLINICAL PSYCHOLOGY OF AGEING										1			1
SUGARMAN.L.	1986	LIFESPAN DEVELOPMENT					1		1						2
SUTTON.C.	1987	HANDBOOK OF RESEARCH.							1						1
SYLVA.K, LUNT.I.	1982	CHILD DEVELOPMENT							1					1	2
TANNER.J.M.	1981	CONTROL OF GROWTH									1				1
TAYLOR.P.W.	1975	PRINCIPLES OF ETHICS					1								1
TAYLOR.S., BOGDAN.R.	1984	INTRODUCTION TO QUALITATIVE RESEARCH												1	1
TELFER.E.	1980	CARING & CURING					1								1
THANE.P.	1982	FOUNDATIONS OF THE WELFARE STATE					1								1
THIROUX.J.P.	1986	ETHICS THEORY & PRACTICE					1								1
THOMPSON.R.	1959	PSYCHOLOGY OF THINKING					1								1
THOMPSON.T.L.	1986	COMMUNICATION FOR HEALTH PROFESSIONALS		1											1
THOMPSON.K., TUNSTALL.J.	1971	SOCIOLOGICAL PERSPECTIVES												1	1

Author(s)	Date	Title	Den.Tech.	Radiog.	Den.hyg.	ODP	Nur(P2k)	Diet.	Soc.Wor.	Physio	Occ.Ther.	Med	Denm	Nur(BN)	TOTALS
TINKER.A.	1986	THE ELDERLY IN MODERN SOCIETY					1								1
TOWNSEND P.	1979	POVERTY IN THE U.K.							1						1
TOWNSEND P. et al	1988	BLACK REPORT AND THE HEALTH DIVIDE												1	1
TOWNSEND P. et al	1988	INEQUALITIES IN HEALTH							1						1
TROWER.P. et al	1988	COGNITIVE BEHAVIOURAL COUNSELLING									1				1
TUCKETT .D. (ED)	1976	INTRO. TO MEDICAL SOCIOLOGY										1			1
TURK.C., KIRKMAN.J.	1989	EFFECTIVE WRITING						1							1
TURLA.P., HAWKINS.K.L.	1987	TIME MANAGEMENT MADE EASY		1											1
TURNER.B.S.	1987	MEDICAL POWER &SOCIAL KNOWLEDGE					1								1
TWINING.C.	1988	HELPING OLDER PEOPLE													1
VALLE.R.S., HALLING.H.S	1989	EXISTENTIAL PHENOMENOLOGICAL PERSPECT.												1	1
VANDER-ZANDEN	1985	HUMAN DEVELOPMENT					1								1
VERNON.M.	1971	PSYCHOLOGY OF PERCEPTION					1								1
VICTOR.C.	1987	OLD AGE IN MODERN SOCIETY									1				2
WALTON.W.	1984	MANAGEMENT & MANAGING					1								1
WATSON J.L.	1977	BETWEEN TWO CULTURES							1						1
WEINMANN.J.	1987	AN OUTLINE OF PSYCHOLOGY						1		1					2
WEYANT.J.M.	1986	APPLIED SOCIAL PSYCHOLOGY												1	1
WHITAKER.D.	1985	USING GROUPS TO HELP PEOPLE							1					1	2
WHO	1978	PRIMARY HEALTH CARE										1			1
WICKENS.C.D.	1984	ENGINEERING PSYCHOLOGY												1	1
WILLCOX.S.G., SUTTON.M.	1985	UNDERSTANDING DEATH & DYING					1								1
WILLIAMS.B.	1972	MORALITY					1								1
WILLIS.L., LINWOOD.M.	1984	MEASURIHNG THE QUALITY OF CARE												1	1
WILSON.B.J.	1979	STRESS IN HOSPITALS					1								1
WILSON.M.	1975	HEALTH IS FOR PEOPLE					1								1
WOOD.D.	1988	HOW CHILDREN THINK & LEARN													1
WORSLEY.P.	1988	THE NEW INTRODUCTORY SOCIOLOGY												1	1

5. 4 The structured interviews

5.4.1 The Teaching Staff

Thirty one teaching staff were invited by letter to participate in an interview (see Appendix 3.2). Twenty nine (93.55%) were willing to be interviewed with one respondent (a medical practitioner) declining to participate and the other (a nurse) failing to return the form. Appointments were made to suit the respondents convenience and choice of venue and the interviews were completed over a seven week period. Most of the respondents were identified by random stratified sampling of the staff lists supplied by the participating institutions. The only exception occurred when the teaching team consisted of just two people. Both agreed to be interviewed.

Table 5.3
Question 1 Distribution of teacher respondents by profession

Profession	N =29
Dentistry	2
Dental Hygienists/DSA	2
Dental Technology	2
Medicine	2
Nursing (B.N)	2
Nursing (Project 2000)	3
Nutrition & Dietetics	2
Occupational Therapy	2
Operating Department Practitioner	2
Physiotherapy	2
Podiatry	2
Radiography	2
Social Work	2
Speech Therapy	2

The majority of the respondents (N=16) were in practice for five or six years before commencing their teaching careers. The reasons for this finding are not clear although it may be due in part to prescribed career pathways by some Statutory Bodies. The number of years in practice reported by each respondent are listed in Appendix 5.1

Table 5.4
Question 2. Years in practice before commencing teaching career

Years in practice	N =29
Less than one year	1
One to five years	10
Six to ten years	11
Eleven to fifteen years	4
More than fifteen years	3

Table 5.5
Question 3 Number of years in teaching

Years in Teaching	N =29
Less than one year	1
One to five years	6
Six to ten years	8
Eleven to fifteen years	4
More than fifteen years	10

The number of years in teaching reported by each respondent are listed in Appendix 5.1.

Question 4 Areas of teaching specialisation
The respondents were asked to identify any subjects/topics that they were able to teach in addition to profession specific subjects. Only eight people described themselves as unable to teach other topics. The majority (N =21) identified a variety of topics some of which, it could be argued, are not only of direct relevance to profession specific knowledge but also indicate an expertise in certain fields within the profession itself. Examples of this include a speech therapist who listed "cerebral palsy", and a physiotherapist who listed "the elderly, paediatrics and neurology". However a number of respondents (N = 13) identified topics which were neither profession specific nor exclusively within the realms of health and social care. These included philosophy, ethics, law, psychology, sociology, counselling, research methods, computing skills and management. A complete list of responses to this question is included in Appendix 5.2

Question 5 Previous experience of teaching other professions

The respondents (N=29) were asked whether they had any experience of teaching professions other than their own. This question elicited 24 positive responses and five negative responses. The responses are reported verbatim which accounts for the variety of terms describing the various professions (Table 5.6)

Experience of interdisciplinary teaching was very limited and mainly confined to a "one off " situation and was described as speaking at conferences or study days. The topics taught by all respondents tended to be related to their own specific professional expertise. Several respondents commented that they tended to be invited to speak to a single profession on a particular subject which they then repeated to another single profession on a different occasion. The respondents who had no experience of teaching other professions besides their own would like the opportunity if it arose. This statement can be substantiated by cross referencing the responses with the results obtained in Question 14 in which the respondents were asked whether given the opportunity they would be willing to participate in interdisciplinary teaching.

Question 6 Experience of learning with other professions

The teachers (N=29) were asked whether they had any experience of learning with other professions. All 29 confirmed that they had but only two (Respondents 10 and 14) had done so at an undergraduate level and one of those was with students on a very closely related training. The amount and type of interdisciplinary learning that had been experienced varied widely. Some of the respondents (N=9) had registered on Masters degrees which were interdisciplinary. Interdisciplinary teaching courses such as the FETC, the PGCE and the B.Ed were also identified (N=7). Interdisciplinary management courses were described by a few (N=5). Thirteen respondents reported their experience of learning with other disciplines as consisting of attendance at multidisciplinary conferences with Respondent 16 making the revealing comment; "I have sat in the same lecture room as physios, radiographers, orthoptists on study days if that's what you mean!"

It seemed that all respondents had elected to attend either courses or conferences with one or other of the professions. This "elective" element of attendance may suggest that others may choose not to attend and consequently may not be exposed to any interaction in a learning capacity with the other health and social care professionals at all. In spite of the finding that only two teachers had experienced shared learning with other professions at an undergraduate level all 29 (100.00%) believed that interdisciplinary learning should begin at an undergraduate level with 23 (79.31%) stating that it should commence right at the beginning of training and continue for life (See Question 19). The individual responses are listed as Appendix 5.3

Table 5.6
Experience of teaching other professions

(N=29)	Profession.	Other professions taught.
1	Dentist	DH/DSA, nurses, environmental health officers, residential care workers, hairdressers.
2	Dentist	DH/DSA, medical students.
3	DH/DSA	Nurses, health visitors, district nurses.
4	DH/DSA	Nursery nurses, nurses, play group leaders, teachers.
5	Dent. Tech.	No experience.
6	Dent. Tech.	No experience.
7	Medicine	Nurses and all paramedical professions.
8	Medicine	Nurses and all paramedical professions.
9	Nursing	Nursing auxilliaries.
10	Nursing	Health visitors, midwives, counsellors, psychologists.
11	Nursing	Managers, physiotherapy, occ. therapy, medical students
12	Nursing	Nursery nurses, liberal studies students.
13	Nursing	Medicine, physiotherapy, occ. therapy, radiography, health visitors, ODP's, administrators.
14	Nut. & Diet	Nursery nurses, hotel and catering students.
15	Nut. & Diet	No experience.
16	Occ. Ther.	Management, field work students (interdisciplinary basis)
17	Occ. Ther.	Nut. & Diet., radiography, physiotherapy, medical physicists, nurses & social workers.
18	ODP	Nurses.
19	ODP	Nurses, medical students, physiotherapy, administrators.
20	Physio.	Nurses, teachers, voluntary workers.
21	Physio.	Radiographers, nurses, MLSO's
22	Podiatry	Physiotherapy, occ. therapy, nurses, dentists, speech therapy,
23	Podiatry	Interdisciplinary retirement courses, nurses, physiotherapy, occ.therapy.
24	Radio.	No experience.
25	Radio.	Nurses, physiotherapy, orthoptics, podiatrists, medicine, technicians.
26	Social Work	Community psychiatric nurses, counsellors, care staff, voluntary sector.
27	Social Work	Housing students, nursery nurses, health visitors.
28	Speech Th.	Nursery nurses, teachers, physiotherapy,occ.therapy,nurses.
29	Speech. Th.	SocialWorkers,teachers,parents,dentists,medics,physios'

Question 7 Subject areas which would be included in behavioural sciences
The teachers were asked their opinions regarding the broad topics which constituted the behavioural sciences. All 29 identified psychology and sociology as being core subjects but most added additional topics (see Appendix 5.4). This supports the supposition made and the difficulties encountered during the initial content analysis of the fourteen curriculum where it was suspected that the term "behavioural sciences" tended to be interpreted loosely. Two comments made by Respondents 2 & 7 respectively illustrated this point most effectively when they commented "it seems everything is lumped in these days" and "anything and everything that can't be described as a life science". Respondent 27 spontaneously noted that she was "unhappy with the word 'behavioural', a negative connotation and a limiting concept". Ethics, philosophy, law and management were all mentioned frequently with Respondent 8 observing that "these cannot be isolated from psychology and sociology". A full analysis of the responses to this question are presented in Appendix 5.4.

Question 8 A knowledge of the behavioural sciences is essential in health and social care
Teachers were asked whether they agreed or disagreed with the above statement. All 29 (100.00%) agreed that a level of knowledge was essential. Some made additional observations such as "absolutely essential" (Respondents 7 & 12) "strongly" (Respondents 8 & 29) "absolutely definitely" (Respondent 18), "I've no problem in agreeing with that" (Respondent 25), "it's a key issue to care" (Respondent 26). Respondent 16 added the observation that "different levels of knowledge might be required". This, it could be argued could also be true of different specialisations within each profession.

Question 9 Disagreed that a knowledge of the behavioural sciences was essential
This question was included in the interview schedule for respondents who disagreed that a knowledge of the behavioural sciences were essential to all health and social professions (Question 8). In the event the 29 respondents all agreed with the statement and so the exploration of why they felt it was not essential was redundant.

Question 10 Should the health and social care professions study these subjects together?
This question was perhaps *the* key question. A negative response would have been an early indication of a rejection of the whole ethos of shared learning and was therefore central to the whole study. All 29 respondents (100.00%) replied "Yes" and additional spontaneous comments such as "without a shadow of a doubt" (Respondent 5) were made by several individuals. The teachers were also asked to identify the potential advantages and disadvantages of such an initiative. Content analysis was completed and these results are presented as Tables 5.7/8 .

Table 5.7
Advantages of learning the behavioural sciences together

Advantages Identified	(N=29)
Breakdown professional isolation.	14
Reduce conflict "professions might even speak to each other".	8
Reduce arrogance in some of the professions.	7
Breakdown existing jealousies.	3
Increase respect for each other.	9
Contribute to a holistic approach to care.	13
Increase teamwork	22
Increase quality of care "patients would have a better deal"	15
Learn what other professions do.	11
Learn from other professions.	12
A cross fertilisation of ideas and knowledge.	7
Broaden everyones outlook	3
The best use of resources.	7
Increase the opportunities for the teaching staff	3
Facilitate the development of problem solving skills	2
"A new way of looking at an old problem"	1
"Reflect the All Wales Strategy on partnership, added value and quality of service"	1

Most respondents listed several advantages and all suggested at least one.

Table 5.8
Disadvantages of learning the behavioural sciences together

Disadvantages identified	(N=29)
Possible difficulties with mixed ability learning.	7
Attitudes of students higher up in the hierarchy.	2
Organisational nightmare for the teaching staff.	8
Financial difficulties ie "who pays for what"	5.
"Professional uniqueness may be lost" & " a blurring of roles"	4
"May highlight inadequacies in the system"	1
"Possibly times when things not directly applicable"	1
"May be accountability problems"	1
"May end up teaching very large groups"	2
"Statutory & Professional Bodies might object"	1
"Staff resistance"	2
"Student expectations"	2
"May increase tension for staff because of numbers involved"	1

Several of the respondents (N=4) said that they would prefer to use the word "difficulty" rather than "disadvantage" as difficulties were more easily overcome. In total, five respondents could not think of any disadvantages, with Respondent 6 admonishing the interviewer with the words "dont think negatively, think positively"

.

Question 11 Reservations about teaching other professions

This question explored any potential reservations the teachers may have had about teaching professions other than their own. The rationale for the inclusion of this question was that if the majority of teachers expressed reservations it was likely that the idea of teaching on an interdisciplinary basis would reveal even more. Although 24 respondents had previously confirmed that they had taught other professions (see Question 5) this did not necessarily mean that they had no hesitation in doing so. Of the 29 respondents 26 reported that they had no reservations at all. Spontaneous additional comments included "I love to when I'm asked" (Respondent 2) and "No, I've enjoyed it and made every effort to do it well" (Respondent 19). One response was particularly revealing. Respondent 24 had no experience in teaching other disciplines (see Question 5) but never the less if given the opportunity she would have no reservations and would be "dead chuffed". Of the three respondents who expressed reservations two had no previous experience (Respondents 5 and 9) and the other (Respondent 1) qualified her statement by commenting "only with the medical profession because of the hierarchy". Interestingly this respondent previously had taught many of the other professions (see Table 5.6). The reservation expressed by Respondent 5 was that he was "not a qualified lecturer" however he subsequently said (see Question 14) that regarding interdisciplinary teaching he would "probably find it a challenge and very interesting". Respondent 9 had reservations "because of my own knowledge base". He too however commented (see Question 14) that "given the right situation and topics it would be an interesting experience". Very few reservations were therefore expressed and these would not prevent the respondents from teaching professions other than their own.

Questions 12 & 13 The words most frequently used by teachers to describe shared learning between the professions and their rationale for choosing these words

Most respondents had not thought about the nomenclature before the interview and the consensus seemed to be that it really did not matter providing shared learning took place. The results are presented in Table 5.9.

Table 5.9
The nomenclature most frequently used

Nomenclature	(N=29)	Additional comments
Multidisciplinary	8	"it's as good as any"
Shared Learning	3	
Interdisciplinary	2	"it means interaction"
Holistic	1	
Interprofessional	1	
Do not know (don't mind)	14	"they are all fashion words" "anything will do" "never thought about it" (N=8)

Most respondents had difficulty in differentiating between the terms. Only Respondent 13 described multidisciplinary as "the coming together of many professions" while she saw interdisciplinary as "interaction and integration between the professions". The remainder gave a variety of similar responses such as "they all mean much the same" and "I think they are all synonymous". Respondent 27 did not like any of the words that included the term "disciplinary" as she believed that they had negative and restrictive connotations. This respondent had given a similar response to the term "Behavioural" (see Question 7). On explanation of the rationale for adopting the word "interdisciplinary implying *interaction* between each profession" 28 respondents felt that it was justifiable to try and encourage the adoption of the word "interdisciplinary".

Question 14 How interested would the teachers be in participating in interdisciplinary teaching?

Of the 29 teachers questionned 26 would be "very interested" in being given the opportunity to teach on an interdisciplinary basis. The remaining three respondents would be "quite interested". As most of the respondents were identified through random stratified sampling this was an encouraging finding although the sample was much too small to draw any firm conclusions. If the responses were representative of all the teaching staff in the health and social care professions in South East Wales it would suggest that there is a high level of interest. The questionnaire that was to be distributed to the total population of teachers within the three participating Institutions may subsequently prove or disprove this hypothesis. Additional individual responses are presented as Appendix 5. 5.

Question 15 Would teachers need special preparation to prepare them for interdisciplinary teaching?

The response to this question was an unanimous "Yes" (N=29). A variety of suggestions were made regarding the teachers needs with some respondents commenting that team building exercises would be the essential starting point inorder to address the existing conflict and isolation. The number of responses to each item are presented as Table 5.10.

Table 5.10
The preparation needed before commencing interdisciplinary teaching

Suggestions for preparation of teachers	(N=29)
An indication of what would be important for the other professions ie what they would expect.	13
The opportunity to discuss each others roles and contributions to patient/client care	14
The opportunity to practice learning methods with the other teachers, ie using a case study approach.	7
Mutually agreed objectives for each session	12
A clear brief for each session ie interdisciplinary mix, number of students, stage of training.	8
Team building exercises between the teachers themselves ie the chance to examine conflict, stereotyping , mutual respect.	6
The opportunity to observe others at work in practice	2

Question 16 Excluding profession specific competencies where there any topics which were thought to be unsuitable for interdisciplinary learning ?

Of the 29 respondents only three people identified topics which they deemed unsuitable. Respondent 11 replied "life sciences would be difficult because of the different levels of knowledge needed". Respondent 16 identified "the basic life sciences" and Respondent 25 replied "yes, the biological sciences". All three did not believe there would be any particular problems with interdisciplinary learning of the behavioural sciences. Many of the respondents who replied "no" to this question added the caveat that *provided profession specific competencies and knowledge stayed* they could not think of any topics which would be unsuitable. The individual responses are presented in Appendix 5.6.

Question 17 Teachers opinions on their own professions sharing learning with the other professions

The teachers were invited to identify the other professions with whom they believed their own profession could appropriately share learning. From a checklist of the 13 professions participating in this study, a "Yes/No/Uncertain" response was requested from each respondent (see Teachers Interview Schedule - Appendix 4.5). As each respondents own profession was excluded from the checklist the maximum number of responses possible was 12. The combined opinions of all the professions about the appropriateness of sharing learning with any one single profession was also calculated. As in most instances two members of each profession were interviewed the maximum number of responses that could be made was 27. The exception to this being the nursing profession where five teachers were interviewed. The maximum number of responses in this case could only be 24. Table 5.11 displays the results of Question 17 with the total score of each respondent recorded at the end of each row and the total score of all respondents pertaining to each profession at the bottom of each column. Where respondents were undecided the result is displayed as "?". In many instances (N=11) the respondents commented that the reason that they were undecided was due to their uncertainty of what the profession in question actually did. These individual comments are presented in Appendix 5.7. Of the 29 respondents 18 (62.07%) identified a minimum of ten other professions which could usefully share learning with their own profession. Of these, six respondents (20.69% where N=29) had selected *all* twelve other professions. The remaining eleven respondents selected between six and nine of the other professions. In effect all respondents (N=29) selected at least 50% of the other professions as being suitable for a shared learning initiative with their own profession. As the number of "uncertain" responses may possibly be due to lack of knowledge about the roles of the other professions (a problem identified by the respondents themselves) then it could be suggested that with a deeper understanding of each others profession the number of positive responses would further increase.

Question 18 Did respondents think that there may be any specific problems in any of these professions learning together and if so which ones ?

The majority of respondents did not think that there would be any specific problems (N=17) however two of these did add "there shouldn't be any but you would only find out by trial and error" (Respondent 7), "not if you start at the beginning of training but there would be if you started later on" (Respondent 13). Of the 12 teachers who thought there may be problems their comments ranged from specific anxieties with one particular profession, with Respondent 6- (dental technology) believing that "there may be hierarchical difficulties with dentists" and Respondent 11 (nursing) observing that "medical students may have a built in arrogance" to general observations about group dynamics.

Table 5.11
The teacher's opinions on their own professions sharing learning with others

Other Professions ⇒ Respondents ⇓	A	B	C	D	E	F	G	H	I	J	K	L	M	TOTAL SCORE
1. Dentist	1	*	1	1	1	1	*	1	1	1	1	1	1	11
2. Dentist	1	*	1	1	1	1	1	1	?	1	1	1	1	11
3. DH/DSA	1	1	1	?	1	1	?	1	1	1	1	*	1	10
4. DH/DSA	1	1	1	1	1	1	1	1	1	1	1	*	1	12
5. Den.Tec.	1	1	1	1	1	1	0	1	0	1	*	1	?	9
6. Den.Tec.	1	1	1	?	1	1	0	1	1	1	*	1	?	9
7. Medicine	*	1	1	1	1	1	1	1	1	1	1	1	1	12
8. Medicine	*	1	1	1	1	1	1	1	1	1	1	1	1	12
9. Nurse (BN)	1	1	*	1	1	1	0	1	1	1	0	1	1	10
10. Nurse (BN)	1	?	*	1	1	1	?	1	1	?	0	1	1	8
11. Nurse (P2k)	1	1	*	1	1	1	1	1	1	1	0	1	1	11
12. Nurse (P2k)	1	1	*	1	1	1	1	1	1	1	1	1	1	12
13. Nurse (P2k)	1	1	*	1	1	1	1	1	1	1	1	1	1	12
14. N & D	1	1	1	?	?	1	0	1	0	*	1	1	1	8
15. N & D	1	1	1	1	1	1	0	1	1	*	1	1	1	11
16. Occ. Therapy	1	0	1	1	1	*	0	1	1	1	0	1	?	8
17. Occ. Therapy	1	0	1	1	1	*	0	1	0	1	0	1	1	7
18. ODP	1	1	1	1	1	0	*	0	0	?	1	0	1	7
19. ODP	1	1	1	1	1	?	*	0	0	?	?	?	1	6
20. Physio.	1	1	1	1	*	1	1	1	1	1	1	1	1	12
21. Physio.	1	1	1	1	*	1	?	1	1	1	?	?	1	9
22. Podiatry	1	1	1	1	1	1	1	1	*	1	0	0	1	10
23. Podiatry	1	1	1	1	1	1	?	1	*	1	0	1	1	10
24. Radiog.	1	1	1	*	1	1	1	1	0	1	1	1	1	11
25. Radiog.	1	?	1	*	1	1	1	1	1	1	1	1	1	11
26. Social Work	1	1	1	1	1	1	1	1	1	1	0	1	*	11
27. Social Work	1	?	1	1	1	1	1	1	1	1	0	1	*	10
28. Speech Ther.	1	1	1	?	1	1	0	*	1	1	0	1	1	9
29. Speech Ther.	1	1	1	1	1	1	?	*	0	1	1	*	1	9
TOTAL SCORE	27	22	24	23	26	25	13	25	19	24	15	21	24	

Key to above table, see next page.

KEY :-
A = Medicine B = Dentistry C = Nursing D = Radiography
E = Physiotherapy F = Occ. Therapy G = Op. Dept. Practitioner
H = Speech Therapy I = Podiatry J = Nutrition & Dietetics
K = Dental Technologists L = DSA/Dental Hygienists M = Social Work
YES = 1 ; NO = 0 ; UNDECIDED = ? ; NOT APPLICABLE = *
Nurse (BN) = Bachelor of Nursing Nurse (P2k) = Project 2000

and "a general reluctance to share and transfer knowledge and skills" (Respondent 17 - occupational therapy) with Respondent 27 (social work) expressing concern that "there may be too much emphasis on the medical model and not enough on holistic care".

Question 19 At which stage of training did the teachers think interdisciplinary learning commence ?

The teachers were asked to choose from four alternatives, at the beginning, in themiddle, or at the end of training or should interdisciplinary learning commenceafter qualification. After making their choice they were invited to give theirrationale for their decision.

Table 5.12
When should interdisciplinary learning commence ?

Stage of Training	(N=29)
From the beginning	23
In the middle	3
At the end	3
Post qualification	0

Each teacher's (N=23) rationale for introducing interdisciplinary learning at the beginning was similar in that they believed that teamwork, communication, better understanding of each others roles, reducing interprofessional conflict and increasing co-operation would only be achieved by enabling students to be part of an interdisciplinary team from the start of their careers. Many teachers commented that it should be "throughout" the whole of training and should continue after qualification. (This option was therefore subsequently included in the teachers questionnnaire). Respondent 13 commented that interdisciplinary learning should commence "right at the beginning. If they learn separately and then come together it ties in with professional isolation. They should be socialised to grow up together.....joint knowledge is power."

The three teachers who opted for the "middle of training" all rationalised their decision on the students need to "settle down" and "concentrate on finding their own role". For the three who chose the "end of training" option the rationale was similar to those who had chosen the "middle of training", this being the need for "students to find their professional identity". The individual responses to this question are reported in Appendix 5.8 .

Question 20 *Which teaching/learning methods did teachers think would be the best to adopt in interdisciplinary learning?*

This question elicited a predictably wide number of responses with the majority of teachers qualifying their answers with the observation that it would depend on the topic, the number of students, the time available, the number of staff available and the number of professions represented within the student population. "Student centred, student led" featured frequently in the responses with the term "interactive" being mentioned by several. Table 5.13. shows the number of responses to this question with Appendix 5.9 displaying each individuals comments.

Table 5.13
Preferred teaching methods for interdisciplinary learning

Teaching/learning Methods	(N=29)
Mixed tutorials	20
Case studies	17
Student led seminars	13
Workshops	12
Problem based learning	10
Role play	10
Lectures*	9
Visits to client areas	2

* The nine teachers who identified lectures as being appropriate teaching strategies all qualified this by emphasising that lectures must always be followed immediately by tutorials.

5.4.2 The students

Thirty nine students were invited by letter to participate in an interview (see Appendix 3.2). This represented a random stratified sample of one student from each year of each course. Twenty two students were willing to be interviewed (56.00 %). Two students were unwilling to be interviewed. The remaining fifteen did not respond. One explanation for this may be due to the fact that many of the students were on clinical placements throughout the United Kingdom at the time the letters were sent and it was subsequently realised that these letters had been placed within the colleges in the student post rooms and had remained there for as long as eight weeks. Appointments were made to suit the respondent's convenience and choice of venue. The interviews were completed over a period of one month.

Question 1 For which profession were the students training ?
With the exception of dental technology at least one student was interviewed from each profession.

Table 5.14
The distribution of student respondents : by profession

Profession	N = 22
Dentistry	1
Dental Hygienists/DSA	1
Dental Technology	0
Medicine	1
Nursing (BN)	3
Nursing (Project 2000)	1
Nutrition & Dietetics	2
Occupational Therapy	3
Operating Department Practitioner	2
Physiotherapy	2
Podiatry	1
Radiography	2
Social Work	1
Speech Therapy	2

Question 2 In which year of training were the students ?
The respondents were asked to identify which year of training they were currently undertaking. The results in Table 5.15 are presented by individual respondent. It should be noted that Respondent 1 (the dental student) and Respondent 3 (the medical student) described themselves as being in the third and fourth years respectively. In essence this means that the dental student was in his first clinical year and the medical student was in his second clinical year. Pre-clinical training had been completed in a University College not included in this study. There were no dental technology students interviewed.

Table 5.15
The year of training : by respondent

Resp. No.	Profession	Year
1	Dentistry	3
2	Dental Hygienist/DSA	2
3	Medicine	4
4	Nursing (BN)	1
5	Nursing (BN)	2
6	Nursing (BN)	3
7	Nursing (Project 2000)	1
8	Nutrition & Dietetics	1
9	Nutrition & Dietetics	3
10	Occupational Therapy	1
11	Occuaptional Therapy	2
12	Occupational Therapy	3
13	Operating Dept. Pract.	1
14	Operating Dept. Pract.	2
15	Physiotherapy	2
16	Physiotherapy	3
17	Podiatry	1
18	Radiography	2
19	Radiography	3
20	Social Work	2
21	Speech Therapy	2
22	Speech Therapy	3

Question 3 Had the students experienced shared learning during their training ?
All respondents were asked whether they had ever experienced shared learning with any of the other professions. Of the 22 respondents 17 had no experience and five had some. Respondents 1 & 4 (the dental and medical student) both identified pre-clinical physiology as a shared learning experience. Dental and medical students attend the same classes. Respondent 21 (the second year speech therapy student) had shared learning with psychology students. Respondent 22 (the third year speech therapy student) had not, the reason for this being due to the introduction in 1991, of a new degree in which psychology and speech therapy students share learning during the first year. Respondent 22 had completed the first year prior to this date. Respondent 17 (a first year podiatry student) had work experience with physiotherapists and occupational therapists prior to the commencement of her training. She commented that the experience had been invaluable. Never the less she had not shared learning while a podiatry student. Respondent 19 (a third year radiography student) had shared learning

with physiotherapy and occupational therapy students. This was during a first aid course which was taught by a nurse teacher.

Question 4 What does the term behavioural sciences mean ?
Question 4 aimed to determine what the term "behavioural sciences" meant to the respondents. A number of suggestions were made. Fourteen respondents explicitly stated psychology and sociology, while a further five respondents implicitly mentioned these. An example of this being Respondent 21 (a speech therapy student) who stated; "it is how people behave and why they behave in the way they do, ... the environment and community in which an individual lives and the effect that has on their behaviour."

Further suggestions included ethics, anthropology, philosophy, physiology, psychiatry, teamwork, health care and law. One student responded "I have no idea, I've never heard the term". An explanation was offered to this individual in order that the respondent could continue with the interview in an informed way. Individual responses are presented in Appendix 5.10.

Question 5 Is a knowledge of the behavioural sciences essential ?
The students were asked whether they agreed or disagreed with the statement that "a knowledge of the behavioural sciences was essential for the health and social care". professions. All 22 agreed that such a knowledge was essential with some adding additional comments to re-inforce the point. Respondent 20 (a social work student) believed that it was " the central focus of care" while Respondent 16 (a physiotherapy student) stated "you can't practice without it".

Because of the 100% agreement in Question 5, *Questions 6 and 7 were not required.* The students were asked whether they thought there would be any advantages in learning the behavioural sciences with professions other than their own. All 22 stated "yes" . In addition they were asked to identify the advantages and disadvantages of such a development. The advantages are presented as Table 5.16 and the disadvantages as Table 5.17. (Many students identified several advantages and several disadvantages).

Question 8 Reservations about learning with other professions
The students were asked whether they would have any reservations about sharing learning with other professions and if so what these reservations were. Twenty one students had no reservations. Some of these spontaneously added comments such as "Not at all. I think it is an excellent idea" (Respondent 1), "I would love to, it is odd you should ask me that, as we were talking about it the other day, the idea of teamwork is non existent in this college" (Respondent 11), "I would feel very positive about it" (Respondent 20). The student who expressed reservations (Respondent 9) when asked to identify what these were commented "from my own personal point of view I think dietetics is not taken seriously enough, we are looked down upon".

Table 5.16
Advantages of learning the behavioural sciences together

Advantages	(N = 22)
Increase teamwork	19
Better understanding of each others roles	14
Improve holistic patient care	8
Give a broader outlook	7
Less isolation from the other professions	7
Learn from the other professions	4
Cheaper, less expensive	2
Breakdown the barriers. Increase respect for others.	2
"Demonstrate that we are all basically the same"	1
"We would learn to work in harmony as we should"	1

Table 5.17
Disadvantages of learning the behavioural sciences together

Disadvantages	(N =22)
Some students will think they are better than others.	3
May lose some professional identity	3
Harder to tailor learning for individuals	1
May not be relevant to every profession	5
I don't really know there are any.	12
Some students may not want to mix	1
Organisation difficulties	1
Some students may lack confidence	2

Table 5.18
The nomenclature used

Nomenclature	(N = 22)	Additional Comments
Multidisciplinary	8	
Interdisciplinary	2	"Integrated, interactive".
Multiprofessional	2	
Shared learning	1	"Combined, all together"
Never thought about it	9	"It doesn't matter a bit"

Questions 9 & 10 The words the students use to describe shared learning & what they understand by the term shared learning.

Several students expressed surprise at these questions as they had never thought about the terminology before. Reflecting the opinions of the teaching staff, the students believed that the nomenclature was irrelevant providing shared learning took place.

Question 11 How interested would the students be in being given the opportunity to share learning with the other professions.

Generally the response to this question was very favourable. the majority stated that they would be "very interested". Several students justified their response with additional comments.

Table 5.19
The level of interest in shared learning

Level of Interest	(N = 22)	Additional Comments
Very interested	15	"It would be great", "It is a real pity I've missed the boat", " I would really love it","Fantastic"
Quite interested	6	"I would certainly give it a go",
Not at all interested	1	"It's not my scene"

Question 12 Did the students feel that teachers would require special preparation ?

Of the 22 students interviewed, 18 felt that the teachers would require special preparation although the type of preparation suggested as appropriate varied considerably. Several students spontaneously identified that it would "very much depend on the individual teacher" and the "knowledge and insight each teacher has into the other professions". Of the four students who did not feel there was a need for special preparation, one physiotherapy student commented "all teachers should be governed by the same aims, that of improving patient care" . The most frequent comment made by the students (N = 11) was that all teachers involved in any interdisciplinary initiative, must be able to facilitate interaction between the students from the different professions in the tutorial groups. If the teacher was a skilled group leader and ensured that every student was encouraged to contribute to the discussion then specific knowledge of each profession was not thought to be of great importance. Five students mentioned that if students take responsibility for their own application of theory to practice then it was probable that they would learn more from any interdisciplinary tutorials than profession specific ones. When asked to explain why this may be so the medical student replied " I would get a much better picture of who the patient is, what makes him tick, rather than just concentrating on what's wrong with him". All 18 students believed that any teacher involved in interdisciplinary tutorials should be given the opportunity to meet with teachers from the other professions in order that a general agreement of the structure and content of the sessions was reached before any such programme was started.

Question 13 See next page.

Table 5.20

Question 14. Student's opinions on their own professions sharing learning with the others

Other Profession ⇒ / Respondents ⇓	A	B	C	D	E	F	G	H	I	J	K	L	M	Total Score
1. Dentist	1	*	1	1	?	1	1	1	0	1	1	1	1	10
2. DSA/DH	0	1	1	1	1	1	0	1	0	1	1	*	0	8
3. Medicine	*	1	1	1	1	1	1	1	1	1	1	1	1	12
4. Nursing	1	1	*	1	1	1	1	1	1	1	1	1	1	12
5. Nursing	1	1	*	1	1	1	1	1	1	1	0	1	1	11
6. Nursing	1	0	*	1	1	1	1	1	0	1	0	0	1	8
7. Nursing	1	1	*	1	1	1	?	1	0	1	0	0	1	8
8. Nut & Diet.	1	1	1	0	1	1	0	1	0	*	1	0	1	8
9. Nut. & Diet.	1	1	1	1	1	1	?	1	1	*	0	0	1	9
10. Occup. Therapy	1	0	1	0	1	*	1	1	0	1	0	0	1	7
11. Occup. Therapy	1	0	1	0	1	*	0	1	1	1	0	0	1	7
12. Occup. Therapy	1	0	1	1	1	*	0	1	1	1	0	0	1	8
13. ODP	1	?	1	1	1	1	*	0	1	1	1	1	1	10
14. ODP	1	0	1	1	1	0	*	0	0	0	0	0	0	3
15. Physiotherapy	1	0	1	0	*	1	0	1	1	1	0	0	0	6
16. Physiotherapy	1	1	1	1	*	1	1	1	1	1	1	1	1	12
17. Podiatry	1	0	1	1	1	1	?	0	*	1	0	0	1	7
18. Radiography	1	1	1	*	1	1	?	1	1	1	1	1	1	11
19. Radiography	1	1	1	*	1	1	?	1	0	1	0	0	1	8
20. Social Work	1	?	1	0	1	1	0	1	1	1	0	0	*	7
21. Speech Therapy	1	1	1	1	1	1	0	*	1	1	1	1	1	11
22. Speech Therapy	1	1	1	0	1	1	?	*	1	0	1	1	1	9
TOTAL SCORE	19	13	18	15	19	18	7	17	13	18	10	9	18	

Key:-
A = Medicine B = Dentistry C = Nursing D = Radiography
E = Physiotherapy F = Occ. Therapy G = Op. Dept. Practitioner
H = Speech Therapy I = Podiatry J = Nutrition & Dietetics
K = Dental Technology L = DSA/Dental Hygienist M = Social Work
YES = 1 NO = 0 UNDECIDED = ? NOT APPLICABLE = *

Question 13 Were there any topics (apart from profession specific ones) that students believed would be unsuitable for interdisciplinary learning ?
The majority of students (N = 17) could not identify any topics, although nine emphasised the need to continue with profession specific learning as well as interdisciplinary learning. All five students who responded "yes", identified the biological sciences as a potential difficulty. The reason for this being, they suggested, the different depth and breadth of knowledge required by the different professions. The students had varied opinions regarding the professions with whom they believed it would be appropriate to learn. The results are presented in Table 5. 20 overleaf.

Question 14 See Table 5.20 on previous page.

Question 15 Did the students think there may be any specific problems in learning together and if so which ones ?
This question provoked a mixed response. Thirteen students did not think there would be any problems but nine believed there may be. Of these seven identified a potential problem in sharing learning with medical students. The rationale given for this was very similar for each respondent and consisted of anxieties that the medical students would feel superior to all other students. One respondent, a radiography student, commented "medical students think they are totally right on all occasions" while another respondent (a nurse) observed " the medical students wouldn't like it, they are so territorial, they have the power and don't want to share it with anyone else". Several of the students did however remark that given the opportunity to learn together these conflicts may be overcome.

Table 5.21
Question 16 When should interdisciplinary learning commence ?

Stage of training	(N = 22)
From the beginning	17
In the middle	5
At the end	0
Post qualification	0

The majority of students felt that it was essential that interdisciplinary learning was introduced right at the beginning of training and then continued throughout. The reasons for this decision were similar and included such responses as "we are absolutely ignorant about each others practice and the jobs we all do. For this reason patient care isn't as good as it could be. It would improve the camaraderie between us all and get rid of all the biases and prejudices" (third year nursing student). The third year radiography student commented "people wouldn't develop prejudices, they wont be biased, we will work together". Interestingly the medical student commented that "by adopting this idea we wouldn't feel so isolated from everybody else". When asked whether he felt that medical students deliberately isolated themselves he replied "for some that may be the case but for most of us that is a myth" . He then added the comment "anyway we don't mean to be like that at the beginning but some of the senior medical staff teach us to behave as superior". The five students who opted for "the middle of training" all believed that they needed to understand their own profession first. Of these five students, three however commented that some of the core subjects could be learned at the beginning of training with all the other professions providing that everyone was given the opportunity to have profession specific learning at the same time. The five students represented five of the professions included in this study (radiography, social work, dentistry, occupational therapy, speech therapy). There was therefore no single professional group which believed that interdisciplinary learning should be delayed until the middle of training.

Question 17 Which learning methods would the students prefer to adopt on an interdisciplinary basis ?

The responses elicited to this question were most interesting in that the students most readily identified what they did not want. Lectures it would seem are not generally well received. Seven students overtly stated that they did not like formal lectures as there was no interaction, they were unable to learn anything from each other and two used the expression "they are too didactic". Only one student (an ODP) stated that lectures were his preferred choice. The other students identified a variety of preferred methods and these are presented in Table 5.22.

Table 5.22
Preferred learning methods for interdisciplinary learning

Teaching/Learning Methods	(N = 22)
Mixed tutorials	19
Seminars	15
Workshops	11
Case studies	21
Role play	5
Visits to client areas	16
Lectures	2
Problem based learning	17

5.5 The questionnaires

As previously described in Chapter 4, the random stratified structured interviews with the 29 teaching staff and the 22 students generated responses that were subsequently transcribed into questions which formed the basis of the two main questionnaires (see Appendices 4.8 and 4.10). Following the pilot studies, the questionnaires were distributed to all teaching staff and students from the thirteen professions training in South East Wales who participated in this study. The data collection was completed over a 10 week period in the Spring of 1993. In total, 300 teaching staff and 1,383 students completed the questionnaires. The overall results are presented as Appendices 5.11 and 5.12.

In presenting the results of the quantatative data obtained from the questionnaires the following points should be noted :-

1. All tables contain numeric and percentage values where appropriate. Percentage scores have been included to ensure consistency and to enable direct comparisons to be made even when the sample sizes are small.

2. Where indicated, results have been subjected to tests of significance and the levels of probability are quoted in the results as follows :-

- Not significant $P > 10\%$
- Not very significant $P > 5\%$
- Significant $P < 5\%$
- Highly significant $P < 1\%$
- Very highly significant $P < 0.1\%$

It was suggested by a statistician that a 5% level was acceptable as statistically significant throughout the presentation of these results due to the nature of the data collection instrument used. The chi-square statistic was selected as being an accurate and reliable non-parametric test of significance especially suited for large samples.

The total number of respondents (N = 1683) and the concomitant data generated suggested that the most appropriate way to present the results would be in the following sections :

5.5.1 The teaching staff from all professions

5.5.2 The students from all professions

5.5.3 A profile of the teachers and students by individual professions

There were three key questions in both the teacher and the student questionnaires however, that serve as an appropriate introduction to the overall results of the main study :-

- How many respondents believed there should be some interdisciplinary learning between the health and social care professions.
- How interested were the respondents in being involved in such a development.
- At which stage should interdisciplinary learning take place, if at all.

Table 5.23
Number of teacher and student respondents : by profession

Profession	Teachers (N =300)	Students (N = 1383)
Dentists	40	93
DSA/D. Hygienists	4	37
Dental Technicians	6	30
Medicine	107	269
Nursing	97	396
Nutrition & Dietetics	4	45
Occupational Therapy	7	89
Operating Dept. Pract.	2	25
Physiotherapy	10	101
Podiatry	8	63
Radiography	6	52
Social Work	7	130
Speech Therapy	2	54
Total	300	1383

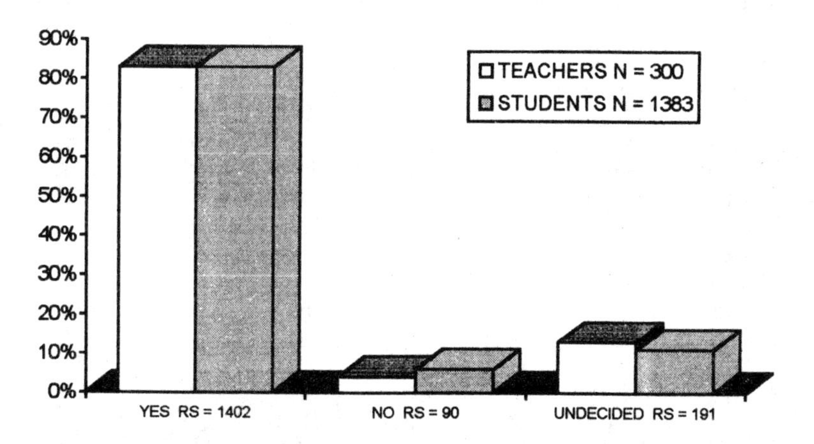

Figure 5.1 Should there be some interdisciplinary learning between the health and social care professions ? : By percentage

Table 5.24
Should there be some interdisciplinary learning between the health and social care professions ? : all professions

Response	Teachers	%	Students	%	Total	%
Yes	249	82.99	1153	83.37	1402	83.30
No	12	3.99	78	5.64	90	5.35
Undecided	39	12.99	152	10.98	191	11.35
Totals	300	100.00	1383	100.00	1683	100.00

Of the 1683 respondents 1402 (83.30%) believed there should be some interdisciplinary learning, 90 (5.35%) thought there should not and the remaining 191 (11.35%) were uncertain. There was no significant differences between the opinions of the teachers and students ($\chi^2 = 2.12$, df = 2, p > 5%). The results by individual profession are presented in Table 5.25

Table 5.25
Should there be some interdisciplinary learning ? : by profession

Profession		Teachers (N=300)			Students (N = 1383)	
Response	Yes	No	Undecided	Yes	No	Undecided
Dentists	36	1	3	71	11	11
DSA/DH	4	0	0	28	2	6
Den.Tec.	5	0	1	27	0	3
Medicine	83	5	19	177	42	47
Nursing	83	5	8	344	9	38
Nut&Diet	4	0	0	42	1	2
Occ. Ther	5	0	2	84	0	5
ODP	2	0	0	21	1	3
Physio.	6	0	4	71	5	24
Podiatry	7	1	0	60	1	2
Radio.	4	0	2	45	5	2
S. Work	7	0	0	124	1	5
Sp. Ther.	2	0	0	47	0	7
Totals	249 82.99%	12 3.99%	39 12.99%	1150 83.37%	78 5.64%	155 10.98%

The teachers and students in the sample demonstrated similar patterns of opinions, in that more than 80% in both groups thought that the opportunity to learn on an interdisciplinary basis should be available.

The second key question asked how interested the teachers would be in interdisciplinary teaching and how interested the students would be in interdisciplinary learning.

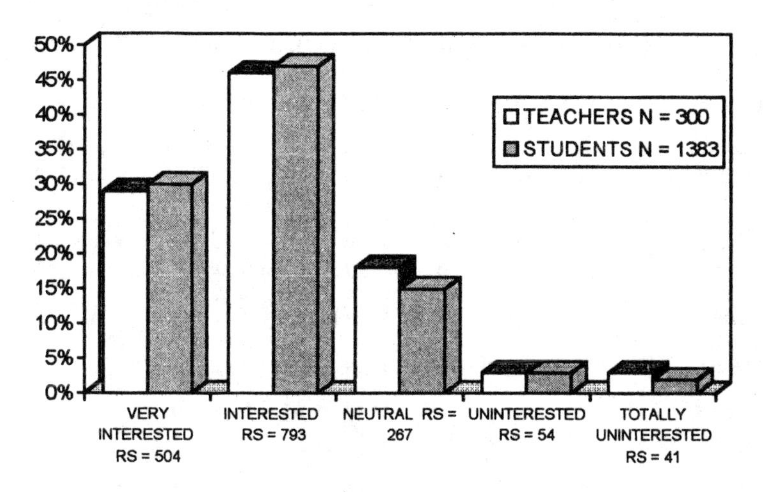

Figure 5.2 The level of interest in interdisciplinary learning : By percentage

Table 5.26
Level of interest in interdisciplinary teaching and learning

Level of interest	Teachers (N = 300)	%	Students (N = 1383)	%	Total (N = 1683)	%
Very Interested	87	28.99	417	30.15	504	29.95
Interested	139	46.33	654	47.29	793	47.12
Neutral	54	17.99	213	15.40	267	15.86
Uninterested	10	3.33	44	3.18	54	3.21
Totally Uninterested	9	2.99	32	2.31	41	2.44

Of the 1683 respondents, 504 (29.95%) were "very interested" with a further 793 (47.12%) being "interested" in the concept. With 267 (15.86%) expressing neutrality this meant that only 54 (3.21%) were "uninterested" with the remaining 41 (2.44%) being "totally uninterested". There was no significant difference between the results of the teachers and the students ($\chi^2 = 1.64$, df = 4, $p > 5\%$) with a significant Spearman Rank Coefficient of Rs = 1.00, n = 5, p <

5%) The teachers and students results by individual professions are presented as Tables 5.27 and 5. 28

Table 5.27
Level of interest in interdisciplinary teaching : all teachers

Profession	N =	V. I	%	I	%	N	%	U	%	T.U	%
Dentists	40	9	22.50	22	55.00	7	17.50	0	0.00	2	5.00
DSA/DH	4	0	0.00	3	75.00	1	25.00	0	0.00	0	0.00
Den.Tec.	6	0	0.00	6	100.0	0	0.00	0	0.00	0	0.00
Medicine	107	23	21.50	46	43.00	29	27.10	5	4.67	5	4.67
Nursing	97	41	42.27	41	42.27	8	8.25	3	3.09	2	2.06
N & D	4	0	0.00	4	100.0	0	0.00	0	0.00	0	0.00
Occ. Ther.	7	2	28.57	4	57.14	1	14.29	0	0.00	0	0.00
ODP	2	0	0.00	1	50.00	1	50.00	0	0.00	0	0.00
Physio	10	1	10.00	3	30.00	4	40.00	2	20.0	0	0.00
Podiatry	8	2	25.00	6	75.00	0	0.00	0	0.00	0	0.00
Radio.	6	3	50.00	1	16.67	2	33.33	0	0.00	0	0.00
Soc. Work	7	5	71.43	2	28.57	0	0.00	0	0.00	0	0.00
Sp. Ther.	2	1	50.00	0	0.00	1	50.00	0	0.00	0	0.00
Totals	300	87	29.00	139	46.33	54	18.00	10	3.33	9	3.00

Key to Tables 5.27 and 5.28
V.I = Very Interested   I. = Interested   N. = Neutral
U. = Uninterested   T.U. = Totally Uninterested

Table 5.28
The level of interest in interdisciplinary learning : all students

Profession	N =	V.I.	%	I.	%	N.	%	U.	%	T.U	%
Dentists	93	15	16.13	53	56.99	19	20.43	4	4.30	2	2.15
DSA/DH	37	9	24.32	17	45.95	7	18.92	1	2.70	2	5.41
Den. Tec.	30	8	26.67	16	53.33	3	10.00	1	3.33	1	3.33
Medicine	269	25	9.29	118	43.87	82	30.48	18	6.69	18	6.69
Nursing	396	117	29.55	201	50.76	56	14.14	5	1.26	5	1.26
N & D	45	25	55.56	18	40.00	1	2.22	1	2.22	0	0.00
Occ. Ther.	89	37	41.57	49	55.06	3	3.37	0	0.00	0	0.00
ODP	25	7	28.00	13	52.00	5	20.00	0	0.00	0	0.00
Physio.	101	20	19.80	54	53.47	17	16.83	7	6.93	2	1.98
Podiatry	63	33	52.38	23	36.51	6	9.52	1	1.59	0	0.00
Radio.	52	15	28.85	25	48.08	9	17.31	2	3.85	1	1.92
Soc. Work	130	78	60.00	47	36.15	2	1.54	1	0.77	1	0.77
Sp. Ther.	54	28	51.85	20	37.04	3	5.56	3	5.56	0	0.00
Totals	1383	417	30.15	654	47.28	213	15.40	44	3.18	32	2.31

The third key question centred on when interdisciplinary learning should take place. The same question was included in both the teacher and student questionnaires. The results are presented in Figure 5.3 and Table 5. 29.

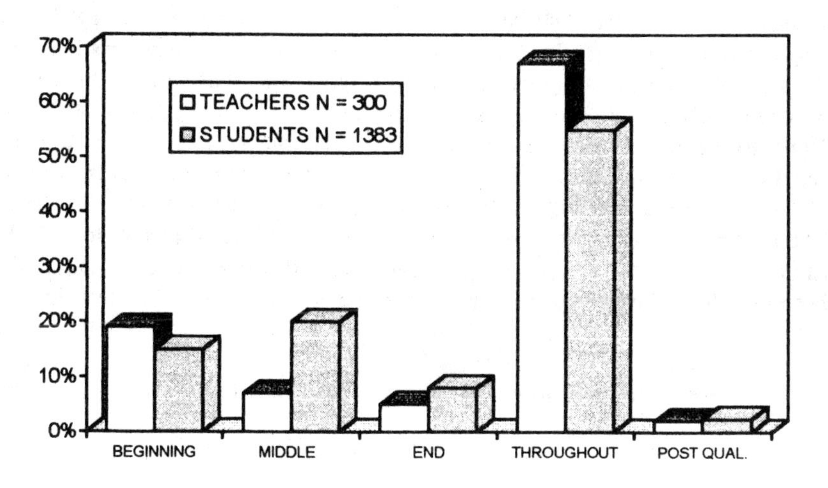

Figure 5. 3 When interdisciplinary learning should take place : By percentage

Table 5.29
When interdisciplinary learning should take place : Teacher and student responses

Response	Teachers (N = 300)	%	Students (N = 1383)	%	Total (N = 1683)	%
Beginning	56	18.67	201	14.53	257	15.27
Middle	21	6.99	276	19.96	297	17.64
End	15	5.00	108	7.81	124	7.37
Throughout	201	66.99	764	55.24	965	57.34
Post Qual.	7	2.33	33	2.39	38	2.26

There was a highly significant difference between the teacher and student responses for the "middle of training" and "throughout training".
($\chi^2 = 34.80$, df = 4, $p < 0.1\%$).

5.5.1 The teaching staff

It was planned to distribute 382 questionnaires through the internal post to all the teaching staff from the thirteen participating professions who were listed as teachers in September 1992 within the three Institutions involved. It was recognised that as the distribution did not take place until March 1993 some teachers would have left South East Wales, while others were new appointments. This made it likely that anyone who had joined the staff during the current academic year did not receive a questionnaire. A number of medical staff were Honorary Lecturers in clinical practice (N = 37) and in fact had no teaching input in South East Wales. After discussion with a senior member of the College of Medicine it was decided that these 37 questionnaires should not be distributed. The total number of questionnaires distributed was reduced therefore to 345. By the closing date 300 completed questionnaires and 6 blank questionnaires had been returned. This meant that a positive response rate of 86.96% was achieved.

Table 5.30
The teaching respondents : by profession

Profession	N = 300
Dentists	40
DSA/DH	4
Dental Technology	6
Medicine	107
Nursing	97
Nutrition & Dietetics	4
Occupational Therapy	7
Operating Dept. Practitioner	2
Physiotherapy	10
Podiatry	8
Radiography	6
Social Work	7
Speech Therapy	2

5.5.1.2 Biographic data of the teachers

Table 5.31
Gender of the teachers : by profession

Profession	N = 300	Male	%	Female	%
Dentists	40	29	72.50	11	11
DSA/DH	4	0	0.00	4	4
Den. Tech.	6	5	83.33	1	1
Medicine	107	80	74.77	27	27
Nursing	97	29	29.89	68	70.10
Nut. & Diet.	4	0	0.00	4	100.00
Occ. Therapy	7	2	28.57	5	71.43
ODP	2	2	100.00	0	0.00
Physiotherapy	9	3	33.33	6	66.67
Podiatry	8	4	50.00	4	50.00
Radiography	6	3	50.00	3	50.00
Social Work	7	3	42.86	4	57.14
Speech Therapy	2	0	0.00	2	100.00
Totals	298*	159 (52.99%)		139 (46.33%)	

* Two teachers did not respond to this question.

The results demonstrate that in this sample there are more male teachers than females. Some of the professions however have no male teachers at all.

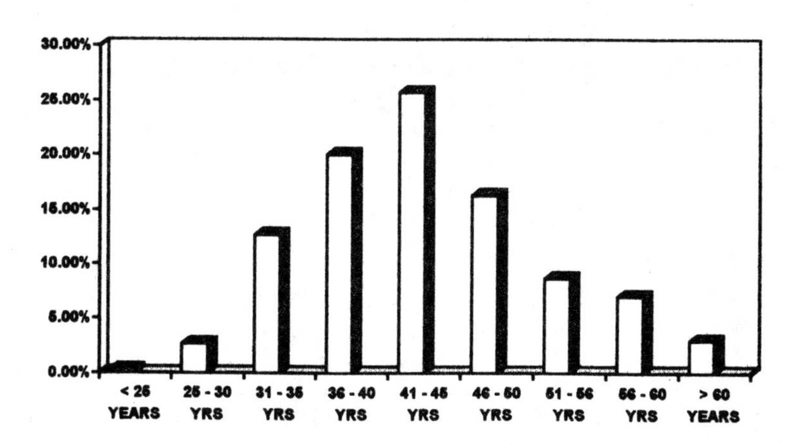

Figure 5.4 Age of the teachers (N = 300) : By percentage

Table 5.32
Age of the teachers : by profession

Profession	< 25 years	25 - 30 years	31 - 35 years	36 - 40 years	41 - 45 years	46 - 50 years	51 - 55 years	56 - 60 years	> 60 years
Dentists	0	2	4	9	12	8	0	1	3
DSA/DH	0	0	2	0	0	0	0	1	0
Den. Tech.	0	2	1	0	2	0	0	1	0
Medicine	0	0	11	21	18	20	19	12	4
Nursing	0	0	16	23	27	13	5	6	0
N. & Diet	0	0	0	1	1	2	0	0	0
Occ. Ther.	0	1	2	0	3	1	0	0	0
ODP	1	0	0	0	1	0	0	0	0
Physio.	0	1	0	3	4	1	0	0	1
Podiatry	0	0	0	0	5	2	0	0	1
Radio.	0	0	2	2	0	1	1	0	0
Soc. Work	0	2	0	1	3	1	0	0	0
Sp. Ther.	0	0	0	0	1	0	1	0	0
Total (N = 300)	1	8	38	60	77	49	26	21	9
%	0.33	2.66	12.66	19.99	25.66	16.33	8.66	6.99	2.99

Table 5.33
Years in clinical practice before commencing teaching career : all professions

Years in Practice	< 1 years	1 - 5 years	6-10 years	11-15 years	16 - 20 years	21 - 25 years	> 25 years
Dentists	4	20	8	4	3	0	0
DSA/DH	0	3	0	1	0	0	0
Den. Tech.	0	1	4	1	0	0	0
Medicine	25	55	23	2	0	0	1
Nursing	0	26	42	18	10	0	0
Nut & Diet.	1	2	1	0	0	0	0
Occ. Therapy	0	0	3	4	0	0	0
ODP	0	2	0	0	0	0	0
Physiotherapy	0	4	0	4	2	0	0
Podiatry	1	3	4	0	0	0	0
Radiography	0	1	4	1	0	0	0
Social Work	1	1	1	4	0	0	0
Sp. Therapy	0	1	0	1	0	0	0
Totals (N = 300)	32	119	90	40	15	0	1
%	10.67	39.67	30.00	13.33	5.00	0.00	0.33

An unexpectedly high percentage (23.36%) of the medical profession indicated that they had practised for less than one year before commencing their teaching careers. It may be assumed that these 25 respondents previously had completed their pre-registration year after obtaining their degree but before starting teaching. Only seven teachers from the other professions had practised for less than one year before commencing teaching. On reflection it would have been useful to have included a question asking whether teachers had obtained relevant qualifications prior to commencing their professional training. This may have indicated whether these respondents had additional related expertise which enabled an immediate commencement of their teaching careers.

The high number of nurse teachers (RS = 42) who had been in clinical practice for 6 - 10 years before commencing their teaching careers can be explained by the regulations which originally were laid down by the General Nursing Council for England and Wales and continued in 1983 by the UKCC. These demand a minimum of 3 years full time clinical practice which includes a senior post plus an additional advanced nursing qualification before statutory teacher training can commence (UKCC PS & D 88/03). In this respect nursing/midwifery is unique in as much that the teaching qualification is mandatory and is recorded on the professional Register.

There was a highly difference in the number of years between medical practitioners and nurses experience in clinical practice before commencing teaching ($\chi^2 = 48.91$, df = 2, $p < 0.1\%$)

Table 5.34
Number of years in teaching : by profession

Profession	>1 year	1 - 5 years	6 -10 years	11 -15 years	16 -20 years	21 - 25 years	>25 years
Dentists	0	9	12	10	3	1	5
DSA/DH	0	1	2	0	1	0	0
Den. Tech.	0	3	0	2	0	0	1
Medicine	1	20	23	18	18	17	9
Nursing	2	27	23	28	10	4	2
Nut & Diet.	0	0	0	1	1	1	1
Occ. Ther.	0	4	2	0	1	0	0
ODP	0	1	0	0	0	1	0
Physio.	2	2	3	1	0	2	0
Podiatry	0	0	1	1	3	2	1
Radiography	0	3	1	0	1	1	0
Soc. Work	3	2	2	0	0	0	0
Sp. Ther.	0	0	0	1	0	1	0
Totals (N=300)	8	72	69	62	38	30	19
%	2.67	24.00	23.00	20.67	12.67	10.00	6.33

All teaching staff were asked to identify any additional subjects which they were able to teach. In total 111 (36.99%) identified additional subjects. Of these 111 respondents only 29.73% were dentists or medical practitioners with the remaining 78 being nurse teachers or from the professions allied to medicine. The explanation for this finding may be the move towards all
graduate status for teachers of nursing and teachers for the professions allied to medicine. Many of these teachers have consequently completed degree courses which have a direct relevance to their professions and they are now teaching these subjects to their students. As both the medical and dental professions have had an all graduate training for many years, implicitly all teaching staff are already graduates when they start their teaching careers.

Table 5.35
Respondents who can teach additional related subjects : by profession

Profession	N = 300	Responses (RS = 112)	% of N= 300
Dentists	40	8	20.00
DSA/DH	4	0	0.00
Den. Tech.	6	1	16.66
Medicine	107	25	23.36
Nursing	96	52	53.61
Nut. & Diet.	4	3	75.00
Occ. Ther.	7	5	71.43
ODP	2	2	100.00
Physio.	10	5	50.00
Podiatry	8	4	50.00
Radio.	6	2	33.33
Social Work	7	4	57.14
Speech Therapy	2	1	50.00

The additional related subjects by profession are displayed in Chapter 5, Section 5.5.3.
The teachers were asked if they had previously had the opportunity to teach other health and social care professions. The inclusion of the word "opportunity" was believed to be important as a subsequent question asked how interested teachers would be in interdisciplinary teaching. The level of interest would not necessarily reflect the current opportunities available for the teachers to obtain this experience. This proved to be the case as can be seen in Table 5.36 and Table 5.46. Further analysis of the questionnaires revealed that only two of the 19 teachers who declared that they were either "uninterested" or "totally

uninterested" had been given the opportunity to teach other professions. This raises the interesting question of whether these individuals may have responded differently if they had been given the opportunity to teach professions other than their own.

Table 5.36
The number of teachers who had taught professions other than their own : by profession

Profession	N = 300	Response (RS = 231)	% of N = 300
Dentists	40	30	75.00
DSA/DH	4	3	75.00
Den. Tech.	6	4	66.66
Medicine	107	96	89.72
Nursing	97	60	61.86
Nut. & Diet.	4	4	100.00
Occ. Therapy	7	7	100.00
ODP	2	1	50.00
Physio.	10	9	90.00
Podiatry	8	3	37.50
Radio.	6	5	83.33
Social Work	7	7	100.00
Sp. Therapy	2	2	100.00

The respondents were also asked to identify which of the other professions they had taught. Many had taught professions which could be interpreted as "closely related" to their own. An example of this being the dental surgeons. Of the 30 who had taught at least one other profession, 27 had taught dental hygienists, 12 had taught dental technologists, 13 had taught nutritionists and dieticians and six had taught speech therapists (Several respondents indicated that they had taught all of these). Paradoxically it was much less likely that these other professions had taught dental students. Only one nutrition and dietetics lecturer and two dental technologists had taught dental students. This may be the result of the perceived hierarchical professional structure described in the review of the literature. The results of individual profession's experiences of teaching other professions are described in Section 5.5.3
All teachers were asked whether they had ever participated in learning with any other professions and if so whether it was before or after they qualified.

Table 5.37
Had teachers participated in any shared learning and if so when ? : by profession

Profession	N = 300	Yes	Pre Qual	Post Qual.
Dentists	40	24	11	13
DSA/DH	4	4	2	2
Den. Tech.	6	3	2	4
Medicine	107	54	17	37
Nursing	97	70	6	64
Nut. & Diet.	4	2	1	1
Occ. Therapy	7	7	0	7
ODP	2	2	0	2
Physiotherapy	10	7	2*	7
Podiatry	8	3	0	3
Radiography	6	5	1*	5
Social Work	7	3	0	3
Speech Therapy	2	2	0	2
Total		186	42	150
%		61.99%	13.99%	49.99%

* These respondents indicated they had experienced shared learning at both a pre and post qualification stage.

Of the 300 teacher respondents 186 (61.99%) had experienced some shared learning with other professions. However of these only 42 (13.99%) had done so prior to qualifying (11 were dentists and 17 were medical practitioners who indicated that they had done so during their pre-clinical years). There was no evidence that these professions had experienced shared learning other than with each other. The six nurse teachers who indicated that they had shared learning pre qualifying had all done so in subjects such as "liberal studies". The results of this question confirm that the majority of learning between the professions takes place after individuals qualify. A similar trend to the previous results could be identified in that for example, dentists tend to learn with dental hygienists, speech therapists, nutritionists and dietitians or dental technicians. This may be as the result of attending conferences of shared professional interest. The results by individual profession are presented in Section 5.5.3.

Due to the many different and seemingly interchangeable words used in the literature relating to shared learning in the health and social care professions the nomenclature used by the teaching staff participating in this study was of interest.

Table 5.38
The nomenclature most frequently used by teachers

Term Used	(N = 300)	%
No specific term	94	31.33
Multidisciplinary	128	42.67
Interdisciplinary	38	12.67
Multiprofessional	18	6.00
Interprofessional	12	4.00
Pluridisciplinary	1	0.33
Other terms	9	3.00

The respondents who indicated that they used "other terms" all stated that they tended to refer to "shared learning". While it would appear that the most frequently adopted word is "multidisciplinary" a large number of individuals use no specific term.

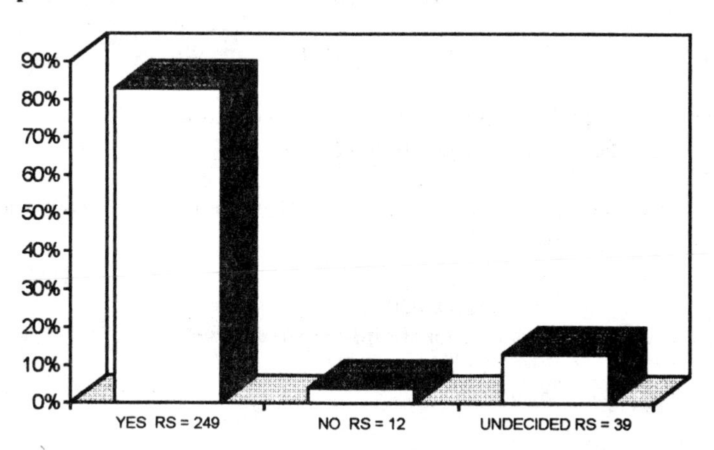

Figure 5.5 Did the teachers believe that there should be some interdisciplinary learning between the professions ? (N = 300)

In spite of the substantial percentage of teachers (82.99%) who believed that there should be some interdisciplinary learning, it was thought that they may well have reservations about its introduction. It was important to discover whether the teachers believed that any potential advantages out weighed any potential disadvantages. The questions were open ended and invited the respondents to identify what in their opinions were the advantages and disadvantages of interdisciplinary learning.

Table 5.39
Would there be advantages in interdisciplinary learning?

Profession	N=	Yes	%	No	%	Undecided	%
Dentists	40	36	90.00	1	2.50	3	7.50
DSA/DH	4	4	100.0	0	0.00	0	0.00
Den. Tec.	6	4	66.66	0	0.00	2	33.33
Medicine	106*	84	78.50	4	3.74	18	16.82
Nursing	95**	84	86.60	3	3.09	8	8.25
Nut. & Diet.	4	4	100.00	0	0.00	0	0.00
Occ. Therapy	7	5	71.43	0	0.00	2	28.57
ODP	2	2	100.0	0	0.00	0	0.00
Physiotherapy	10	4	40.00	0	0.00	6	60.00
Podiatry	8	7	87.50	0	0.00	1	0.00
Radiography	6	5	83.33	0	0.00	1	0.00
Social Work	7	7	100.0	0	0.00	0	0.00
Speech Therapy	2	2	100.0	0	0.00	0	0.00
Total	297	248	82.67	8	2.67	41	13.67

* One medical practitioner did not respond to this question
** Two nurses did not respond to this question.

The suggested advantages were analysed and classified into four main categories which are displayed as Table 5.40.

Table 5.40
Advantages of interdisciplinary learning

Advantages	RS =177*
Increase understanding of each others roles & contribution	157
Increase teamwork & collaboration	113
Broaden horizons, cross fertilise ideas	92
Make better use of time & scarce resources	42

* Of the 300 respondents, 248 indicated that they thought that there would be advantages. Only 177 however, listed what they believed these may be. Many respondents listed more than one advantage.

Although more disadvantages seemed to be evident the number of respondents who identified these were far fewer.

Table 5.41
Disadvantages of interdisciplinary learning

Disadvantages	RS = 61*
Time constraints	18
Organisational difficulties	22
Irrelevant material	58
Hierarchical domination & prejudice	26
Loss of professional identity	11
Different academic ability	21
Different knowledge base	1
Too many students in a class	0**

* The number of individuals who identified potential disadvantages was 61.

Many of these 61 respondents listed several potential disadvantages. The respondents who listed "time constraints" and the "organisational difficulties" were distributed fairly evenly over the level of interest responses. The individuals who listed "irrelevant material" (RS = 58), "hierarchical domination and prejudice" (RS = 26) and "loss of professional identity" (RS = 11) tended to declare that they were either "uninterested" or "totally uninterested" in shared learning.

** This category has been included to enable comparison with the results from the student population (see Section 5.5.2)

An unexpected response referred to "the threat of redundancy" and "the loss of teachers jobs" (RS = 23). Even more unexpected was the fact that each of these respondents was a teacher of nurses (100.00%). It is suggested that this may not have occurred 7 years ago when nurse teachers were as secure in their jobs as all other teachers of the health and social care professions. The introduction of the Project 2000 training for nurses has meant the amalgamation of former schools of nursing into large colleges of nursing and midwifery. In a second phase these new colleges are becoming affiliated, amalgamated or integrated into Universities, or Institutes of Higher Education. These changes, together with a large reduction in student numbers and the concomitant threat of teaching staff redundancies explains this response.

Table 5.42
At which stage should it take place ?

Profession	N =	Beginning	Middle	End	Throughout	Post Qual.*
Dentists	40	4	3	2	30	2
DSA/DH	4	2	0	0	2	0
Den. Tec.	6	0	0	0	6	0
Medicine	107	21	12	2	70	3
Nursing	97	22	2	4	69	0
Nut.& Diet	4	0	1	0	3	0
Occ. Ther.	7	0	1	2	3	0
ODP	2	0	1	0	1	0
Physio.	10	0	0	4	4	1
Podiatry	8	3	1	1	2	1
Radio.	6	2	0	0	4	0
Soc. Work	7	2	0	1	5	0
Sp. Ther.	2	0	0	0	2	0
Total (N =299) **	300	56 (18.73%)	21 (7.02%)	16 (5.35%)	201 (67.22%)	7 (2.34%)

*Of the 42 respondents who indicated that shared learning should take place after qualifying, the majority (RS = 35) also indicated that it should take place throughout. Several of these respondents further emphasised the point by adding additional comments such as "It should start from day one and continue for the rest of ones career" (Medic Resp. 53). Only 7 respondents therefore chose post qualifying as the only option.

**One medical practitioner (Resp 17) replied "it is not necessary for it to take place at all !"

Tests for significance between the responses of the nurse teachers and the medical teachers indicated that there was no difference in the opinions of the two groups ($\chi^2 = 8.11$, df = 4, p > 5%, Yates Correction applied).
The overall response to this question by all the professions is displayed as Figure 5. 6.

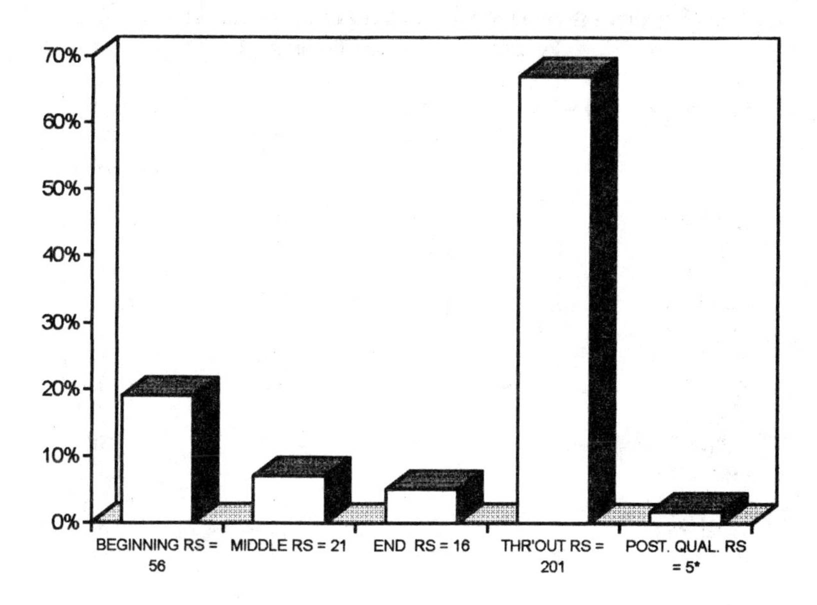

**Figure 5.6 When should interdisciplinary learning take place ?
All teachers (N = 300)**

*This response reflects the 7 teachers who selected "post qualification" only.

The teachers were asked to identify other professions with which their own profession could share learning. When collating the results it was necesssary to calculate the potential raw scores against the actual raw scores by each profession. The response rate from each profession was deducted from the overall 300 responses. For example the number of dentists who responded was 40. This was subtracted from 300 therefore giving a potential response rate of 260. The results of the other professions opinions of the potential for sharing learning with dentists was therefore calculated from a raw score of 260. Similarly in the case of the speech therapy lecturers (N = 2) the potential response rate was 300 minus 2 which equalled 298.

Table 5.43
With which other professions could interdisciplinary learning take place ? : All professions

Profession	N = 300	Potential Responses	Actual Responses	% of Potential Responses
Dentists	40	260	103	39.62
DSA/DH	4	296	91	30.74
Den. Tec.	6	294	71	24.15
Medicine	107	193	147	76.17
Nursing	97	203	158	77.83
Nut. & Diet.	4	296	170	57.43
Occ. Ther.	7	293	166	56.66
ODP	2	298	81	27.18
Physio.	10	290	178	61.38
Podiatry	8	292	95	32.53
Radiography	6	294	132	44.90
Social Work	7	293	195	66.55
Sp. Therapy	2	298	157	52.68

The responses by individual professions are presented in Section 5.5.3. Overall the teachers seemed to believe that there was the potential for some shared learning with many of the professions participating in this study. Nurses were chosen the most frequently (77.83%) by the other respondents, followed by the medical practitioners (76.17%). Social workers were ranked in third place (66.55%) overall. All teachers were also asked whether they envisaged any particular problems in shared learning between their own profession and any of the others and if so what these problems would be. In total 105 respondents believed there would be some problems. Most of these problems related to the different knowledge base required by each profession and the relevance of all the subject material. These problems had previously been identified in response to the question which asked what the disadvantages of interdisciplinary learning would be. An interesting result was that of the 21 respondents who referred to "interprofessional rivalry" "professional dominance" and "elitism" , five were from the medical profession.

Two comments were particularly revealing, "Everyone will gang up on the doctors" (Medical Resp. 23). "The airing of ingrained prejudice leading to a breakdown in communication may occur on occasions, i.e. what can a middle aged white male doctor expect to know about anything" (Medical Resp. 107).

Further analysis of this respondents questionnaire revealed him to be a male middle aged doctor who was "very interested" in participating in interdisciplinary teaching. A possible explanation is that he might have experienced ingrained prejudice against him from the other professions.

A subsequent question asked the teachers to identify which broad subject areas could be learned on an interdisciplinary basis. These subject areas were those suggested by the teachers and students in the structured interviews as possibly comprising the behavioural sciences (see Section 5.4).

Table 5.44
Suitable subjects for interdisciplinary learning

Subjects	Yes (N=299)	%	No (N=299)	%
Psychology	277	92.64	22	7.36
Sociology	265	88.63	28	9.36
Ethics	281	93.98	14	4.68
Law & Practice	266	88.96	29	9.70
Research Methods	244	81.60	55	18.39
Management	259	86.62	40	13.38
Economics of health & social care	262	87.62	37	12.37
Health Promotion	277	92.64	16	5.35
Study Skills	260	86.96	39	13.04
Quality Issues	264	88.29	35	11.71
Structural Organisation	270	90.30	29	9.70
Computing Skills	274	91.64	25	8.36

The responses indicate that all of the topics, identified by the student population as "behavioural sciences", are deemed to be potentially suitable for interdisciplinary learning by more than 85% of the teacher respondents in this study.

In addition, the teachers were asked whether (apart from those relating to profession specific training) they rejected any other topics. The results are presented in Table 5. 45

Further analysis of these 46 questionnaires revealed some very interesting findings. Some of the respondents (RS = 5) mistakenly listed profession specific topics as being unsuitable, (an example of this being Medical Resp. 44 who identified "the histology of tumours"). Many of the 46 respondents were concerned about the life sciences because of the different levels of knowledge needed (four of the six physiotherapy teachers came into this category). The most interesting finding was that where a respondent had rejected many topics, if their response to the subsequent question of how interested they were in interdisciplinary learning was compared it seemed that those who were "neutral", "uninterested" or "totally uninterested" were the people who rejected the greatest number of topics. Of the 46 people who rejected additional topics 41 (89.13%) had declared themselves to be either "uninterested" or "totally uninterested".

Table 5.45
Rejected topics : by profession

Profession	N =300	Rejected Topics (RS = 46)	% of N
Dentists	40	0	0.00
DSA/DH	4	1	25.00
Den. Tec.	6	0	0.00
Medicine	107	12	11.21
Nursing	97	20	20.62
Nut. & Diet	4	2	50.00
Occ. Therapy	7	2	28.57
ODP	2	0	0.00
Physiotherapy	10	6	60.00
Podiatry	8	2	25.00
Radiography	6	1	16.67
Social Work	7	0	0.00
Speech Therapy	2	0	0.00

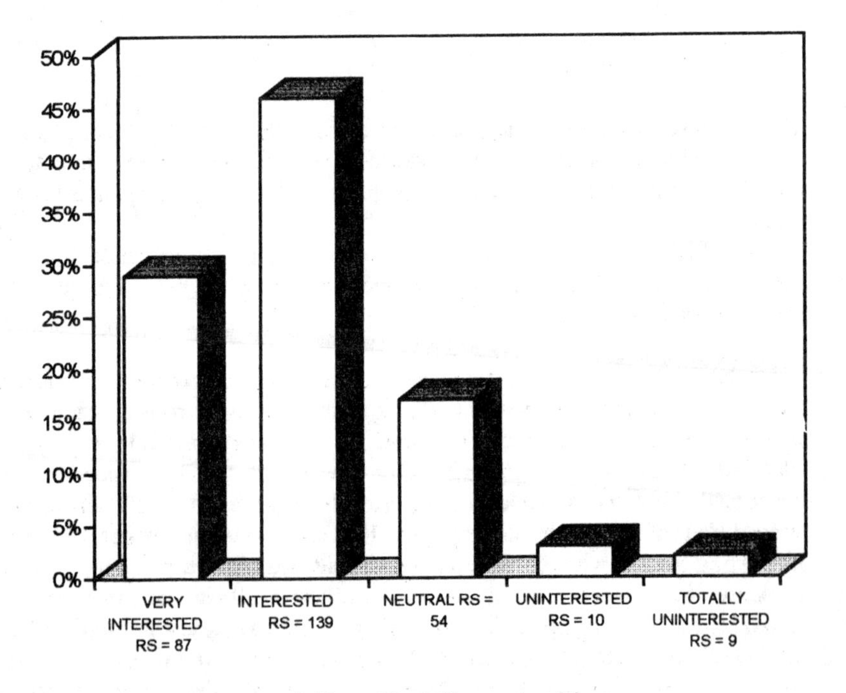

Figure 5.7 Level of interest in interdisciplinary teaching All teachers (N = 300)

Table 5.46
Level of interest in interdisciplinary teaching : by profession

Profession	N =	Very Interested	Interested	Neutral	Uninterested	Totally Uninterested
Dentists	40	9	22	7	0	2
DSA/DH	4	0	3	1	0	0
Den. Tech.	6	0	6	3	0	0
Medicine	107	23	46	29	5	5
Nursing	97	41	41	8	3	2
Nut & Diet	4	0	4	0	0	0
Occ. Ther.	7	2	4	1	0	0
ODP	2	0	1	1	0	0
Physio.	10	1	3	4	2	0
Podiatry	8	2	6	0	0	0
Radio.	6	3	1	2	0	0
Soc. Work	7	5	2	0	0	0
Sp. Ther.	2	1	0	1	0	0
Total	300	87	139	54	10	9
%		28.99	46.33	17.99	3.33	2.99

Of the 300 respondents 226 (75.33%) were "interested" or "very interested" in interdisciplinary teaching. Only 19 (6.33%) described themselves as "uninterested" or "totally uninterested". This finding was not only unexpected but also very encouraging in that if such an initiative was introduced it would appear that many teachers would possibly volunteer to be involved. Indeed a surprising number of individuals (including fifteen from the medical profession) signed their questionnaires and requested that they were directly approached if any definite plans were made.

The difference in the responses between the medical practitioners and the nurses was highly significant in that nurses were much more interested in interdisciplinary teaching than their medical colleagues, ($\chi^2 = 17.46$, df = 4, $p < 0.1\%$ Yates correction applied). More than 64% of the medical profession nevertheless, were "very interested" or "interested" in interdisciplinary teaching (RS = 69).

More than half of the teachers (53.00%) stated that they would benefit from special preparation if they were to be involved in interdisciplinary teaching. Many teachers listed several benefits. The results are presented in Table 5. 47.

Table 5.47
Perceived benefits of special preparation for interdisciplinary teaching : all professions

Rationale	RS = 159
Break down existing barriers	26
Gain insight into each others work	65
Opportunity to clearly identify areas of responsibility	8
Opportunity to experience interdisciplinary learning	23
Opportunity to practice interdisciplinary teaching	31
Clear identification of objectives, expected outcomes, assessment strategies etc.	92

One medical practitioner (Resp. 16) made the interesting and pertinent comment "You should know where to start otherwise the foundations will not hold up the house."

The implications of these perceived benefits will be discussed in Chapter 6, Section 6.11. The findings are however a clear indication that interdisciplinary learning could not be introduced without careful preparation of the teachers involved.

5.5.2 The students

As previously described in Chapter 4, permission was obtained from the deans of the faculties involved to collect data from the student population. Access to each year group of each profession was negotiated with the course directors and a mutually convenient time was identified within the time table when the questionnaires could be distributed and collected. The purpose of the research was given in a verbal explanation to each group of students along with an invitation to participate in the study. All students were advised that participation was voluntary and confidentiality and anonymity would be maintained. If students did not wish to participate they were requested to return the blank questionnaire into the box provided. The researcher then withdrew thereby leaving the students to complete the questionnaires if they so wished. The questionnaires were collected 45 minutes later. The number of student respondents by individual profession are displayed in Table 5.48.

The total number of respondents equals the number of students present on each data collection day and who completed the questionnaires plus one group of nutrition and dietetics students and one group of speech therapy students who were not directly accessible in college. These students were contacted therefore through a postal questionnaire with an accompanying letter and stamped addressed envelope.

Table 5.48
The student respondents : by profession

Profession	N = 1383	%
Dentists	93	6.72
DSA/DH	37	2.68
Den. Technology	30	2.17
Medicine	269	19.45
Nursing	396	28.63
Nutrition & Dietetics	45	3.25
Occupational Therapy	89	6.44
Operating Dept. Pract.	25	1.81
Physiotherapy	101	7.30
Podiatry	63	4.56
Radiography	52	3.76
Social Work	130	9.40
Speech Therapy	54	3.90

Of the total student population only 22 blank questionnaires were returned when the questionnaires were completed in college (98.4% response rate). The postal response rate was not so high. Of the 31 questionnaires sent by post, 24 were returned (77.41%). This means that the completion rate (N = 1383) was 96.26%. The 22 students who returned blank questionnaires appeared to be random as they represented most years from most professions with one or two blank questionnaires being returned in each sample.

5.5.2.2 Biographic data of the students

Of the 1383 students who completed the questionnaire, 364 (26.32%) were male and 1018 (73.61%) were female. One student did not complete this question.

An unexpected finding was that the percentage of female medical students (54.65%) was greater than the percentage of males (44.61%). The other finding of interest was the predominance of males amongst dental technology (60.00%) and operating department practitioner (64.00%) students. One explanation for this may be that males choose to enter training programmes which contain a high technological content. Nevertheless Table 5.49 shows that in this sample more females (73.61%) than males (26.32%) enter the health and social care professions. (See Table 5.49)

Table 5.49
Gender of the students : by profession

Profession	N =	Male	%	Female	%
Dentists	93	53	56.99	40	43.01
DSA/DH	37	0	0.00	37	100.00
Den. Tech.	30	18	60.00	12	40.00
Medicine	269	120	44.61	147	54.65
Nursing	396	63	15.91	333	84.09
Nut. & Diet.	45	1	2.22	44	97.78
Occ. Therapy	89	9	10.11	80	89.89
ODP	25	16	64.00	9	36.00
Physiotherapy	101	23	22.77	78	77.23
Podiatry	63	15	23.81	47	74.60
Radiography	52	10	19.23	42	80.77
Social Work	130	35	26.92	95	73.02
Sp. Therapy	54	1	1.85	53	98.15
Total	1363	364		1019	

Table 5.50
Age of the students : by profession

Profession	< 20 yrs	21- 25 yrs	25- 30 yrs	31- 35 yrs	36- 40 yrs	41- 45 yrs	46- 50 yrs	51- 55 yrs	> 55 yrs	N = 1383
Dentists	23*	62	6	1	0	0	0	0	0	93
DSA/DH	16	15	2	3	0	0	0	0	0	37
Den. Tech.	10	11	4	3	0	1	0	0	0	30
Medicine	5*	239	16	7	0	0	0	0	0	269
Nursing	159	128	40	31	24	6	2	0	0	396
Nut. & Diet.	11	27	3	1	1	1	0	0	0	45
Occ. Therapy	21	36	13	6	2	7	3	0	0	89
ODP	0	14	8	2	1	0	0	0	0	25
Physiotherapy	42	29	18	6	4	0	1	0	0	101
Podiatry	19	18	9	7	6	3	1	0	0	63
Radiography	29	16	5	1	1	0	0	0	0	52
Social Work	0	13	35	34	17	20	8	2	0	130
Sp. Therapy	17	22	1	4	2	4	3	0	0	54 **
Totals	352	630	160	106	56	42	18	2	0	1366
%	25.4	45.5	11.5	7.66	4.05	3.04	1.30	0.14	0.0	

* The majority of dental and medical students less than 20 years of age did not participate as they were in preclinical years in a different University College.
** Seventeen students did not disclose their age.

The majority of students training in South East Wales were less than 25 years of age (RS = 982, 71.00%). Of the 384 students who were more than 25 years of age, 116 (30.21%) were training to be social workers. There are several explanations for this finding which are discussed in detail in Chapter 6, Section 6.4. The second oldest group of students were the nurses with 63 (15.91%) being more than 31 years of age.

It was not considered appropriate to present the students year stage of training overall as the length of training varies considerably throughout the thirteen professions. Nonetheless the students year stage of training by individual profession is subsequently presented in Section 5.5.3.

The students were asked to indicate whether they had undertaken any previous courses that they considered relevant to their current training. They were asked to exclude their school qualifications as it was believed that most of these would have been entry criteria for training. The overall results can be seen in Table 5.51. The results by individual profession are presented in Section 5.5.3.

Table 5.51
Previous relevant courses : by profession (N = 1383)

Profession	N=	RS = 358	. % of N
Dentists	93	9	9.65
DSA/DH	37	1	2.70
Den. Tech.	30	10	33.33
Medicine	269	46	17.10
Nursing	396	121	30.56
Nut. & Diet.	45	5	11.11
Occ. Therapy	89	21	23.60
ODP	25	7	28.00
Physiotherapy	101	22	21.78
Podiatry	63	20	31.75
Radiography	52	9	17.3
Social Work	130	77*	59.23*
Speech Therapy	54	10	18.52

* Tables 5.51 & 5.52. This result has been previously explained following Table 5.50. The students were also asked to indicate whether they had any previous related work experience prior to commencing their training and what this work entailed. The question did not indicate what was considered "relevant work" as it was thought that the students should decide whether the experience was relevant.

Table 5.52
Relevant work experience : by profession (N = 1383)

Profession	N =	RS = 820	% of N
Dentists	93	25	26.88
DSA/DH	37	25	67.57
Den. Tech.	30	11	36.67
Medicine	269	122	45.35
Nursing	396	256	64.65
Nut. & Diet.	45	27	60.00
Occ. Therapy	89	62	69.67
ODP	25	20	80.00
Physiotherapy	101	60	59.41
Podiatry	63	38	60.32
Radiography	52	17	32.69
Social Work	130	123*	94.62
Speech Therapy	54	34	62.96

* Previously explained following Table 5.50

The results show that 59.29 % of all students have gained relevant work experience prior to commencing their training. The work experience described varied considerably although most could be attributed to either voluntary work or paid jobs pertaining to health or social care. The work experience described by the students is presented by individual profession in Section 5.5.3.

Experiences of shared learning during training

Very few students had experienced shared learning on their current courses apart from the medical and dental students who had shared some sessions with each other in their pre-clinical years and 15 of the 18 first year speech therapy students who had commenced a new degree course where speech therapy and psychology students share teaching sessions in the first year. In-depth analysis of the responses revealed that many of those who had experienced shared learning had either gained a previous qualification such as the seven podiatry students who already had Registered Nurse qualifications or they had gained work experience in health and social care fields. The shared learning seemed to have taken place in patient/client areas such as in ward rounds or case conferences. Although 68 (73.12% where N = 93) dental students and 62 (23.05% where N = 269) medical students confirmed that they had shared some learning, 25 (26.88%) dental students and 205 (76.21%) medical students said they had not. The reason for this is not known. Perhaps the medical students, in particular, did not view this preclinical training as shared learning at all. The overall results are presented as Table 5.53.

Table 5.53
Students shared learning experience : by profession (N = 1383)

Profession	N =	RS = 336	% of N
Dentists	93	68	73.12
DSA/DH	37	3	8.11
Den. Tech.	30	11	36.67
Medicine	269	62	23.05
Nursing	396	79	19.95
Nut. & Diet.	45	3	6.67
Occ. Therapy	89	8	9.00
ODP	25	6	24.00
Physiotherapy	101	7	6.93
Podiatry	63	12	19.05
Radiography	52	9	17.31
Social Work	130	61	46.92
Speech Therapy	54	15	27.78

The structured interviews which had been conducted with a sample of the students (N = 22) indicated that many were unsure which subjects constituted the behavioural sciences. The main study questionnaire distributed to the total student population therefore included
a question which listed broad subject areas which the students were asked to decide whether should be included or not.

Table 5.54
Subjects students would include in the behavioural sciences : all professions (N = 1383)*

Subject	Yes	%	No	%	Undecided	%
Psychology	1341	96.96	8	0.58	23	1.66
Sociology	1238	89.52	47	3.40	87	6.29
Ethics	758	54.81	237	17.14	377	27.26
Law & Prac.	480	34.71	572	41.36	321	23.21
Management	518	37.45	545	39.41	298	21.55
Health Prom	918	66.38	230	16.63	221	15.98
Study Skills	538	38.90	522	37.74	311	22.49
Quality Ass.	431	31.16	397	28.71	544	39.33

* Not every student totally completed this question. Nevertheless all 1383 respondents completed at least part of it. The raw score therefore equalled 1383 and the percentages were calculated accordingly.

The students understanding of the term "behavioural sciences" was very varied. While psychology (96.96%) and sociology (89.52%) seemed to be recognised as behavioural sciences by most students, 54.81% also included ethics and 66.38% included health promotion. More than one third of the sample also included law and practice, management and study skills.

Apart from psychology and sociology many students were undecided about the other subjects. One explanation for this may be due to the number of course documents that included the above topics in a section identified as "The Behavioural Sciences". This factor was identified during the content analysis stage of this study (see Chapters 4.2 and 5.2).

The students were also asked whether they thought that there would be advantages in introducing shared learning and if so what these would be. They were also asked to list any disadvantages which may result. These questions were worded exactly the same as those on the teachers' questionnaire, the rationale for this being that the advantages and disadvantages perceived by the students may have revealed an entirely different perspective from that of the teachers. Table 5. 55 displays the results.

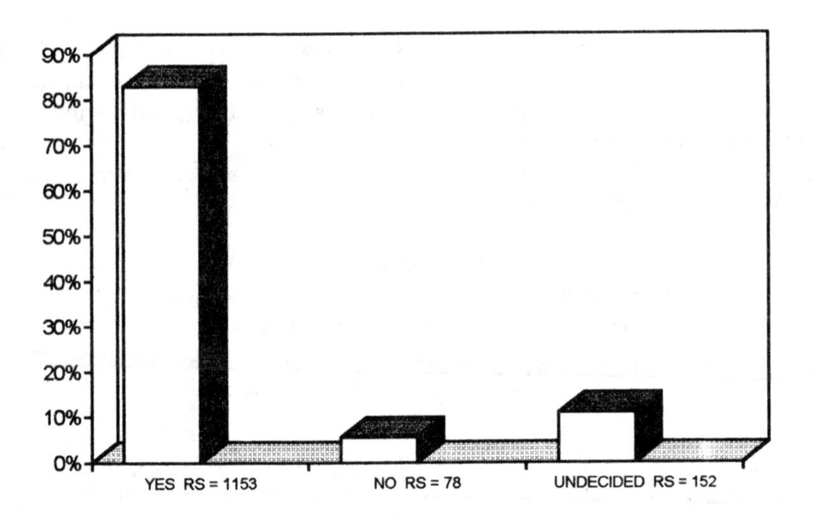

Figure 5.8 Did the students believe there should be some shared learning between the professions ? By percentages (N = 1383)

(The students opinions by individual profession are presented in Section 5.5 Table 5.28.)

Table 5.55
Would there be advantages in interdisciplinary learning ?
: by profession

Profession	N =	Yes	%	No	%	Un-decided	%
Dentists	93	65	69.89	8	8.60	20	21.51
DSA/DH	37	28	75.68	1	2.70	8	21.62
Den. Tech.	30	26	86.67	1	3.33	3	10.00
Medicine	269	177	65.80	42	15.61	47	17.47
Nursing	396	329	83.08	10	2.53	57	14.39
Nut. & Diet	45	41	91.11	0	0.00	4	8.89
Occ. Therapy	89	86	96.62	0	0.00	3	3.37
ODP	25	20	80.00	1	4.00	4	16.00
Physiotherapy	101	87	86.14	4	4.00	10	9.90
Podiatry	63	60	95.24	1	1.59	2	3.17
Radiography	52	42	80.77	5	9.62	5	9.62
Social Work	130	123	94.62	1	0.77	6	4.62
Sp. Therapy	54	51	94.44	0	0.00	3	5.56
Total	1383	1121	81.06	78	5.64	175	12.65

Of the 1383 student respondents 1121 (81.06%) believed there would be advantages with 175 (12.65%) being undecided. Only 78 (5.64%) thought there would be no advantages at all. Of these 42 (53.85% where RS = 78) were medical students. The percentage of dental students who believed there would be no advantages gained was also higher than the other student groups (8.60% where N = 93) The students' suggestions for the potential advantages of interdisciplinary learning were analysed and categorised in the same way as the responses from the teaching staff (see section 5.5.1. Table 5.40)

There were several highly significant differences observed in these results. The medical students were the least likely to identify any advantages when compared with the nursing students ($\chi^2 = 42.42$, df = 2, $p < 0.1\%$) and the physiotherapy students ($\chi^2 = 14.92$, df = 2, $p < 0.1\%$) but there was no significant difference between the medical students and the dental students opinions ($\chi^2 = 3.21$, df =2, $p > 5\%$). The opinions of the physiotherapy students and the occupational students were similar ($\chi^2 = 5.42$, df = 2, $p > 5\%$) but the opinions of the nurses and social workers differed in that more social workers thought there would be advantages ($\chi^2 = 10.23$, df = 2, $p < 1\%$).

Table 5.56
Advantages of interdisciplinary learning : all professions

Advantages	RS = 1089
Increase understanding of each others roles & contribution.	699
Increase teamwork & collaboration	704
Broaden horizons, cross fertilise ideas	387
Make better use of time & scarce resources	14

Many students mentioned that they did not know what the other professions actually did. One final year medical student observed; " When I qualify I wont (sic) have any real idea of what the others do. Surely this is essential from the patients point of view. I am really sorry I shall miss the opportunity to participate in your study." (Respondent 17) A total of 1089 students listed potential advantages with many listing several.

The number of students who listed potential disadvantages were fewer in number but there was a more diverse response. Although many of the disadvantages identified were the same as those identified by the teachers (see Table 5.41) there were others that did not feature in the teachers' responses at all. A few students were totally against any form of interdisciplinary learning and made some revealing comments:- "I am totally against any form of shared learning. I cannot see any overlap at all" (Nursing Resp 296), "Everybody would steal everybody elses ideas" (Nursing Resp. 78) and "Any time spent with medical students is a waste of time!" (Occ. Therapy Resp. 60).

Table 5.57
Disadvantages of interdisciplinary learning : all professions

Disadvantages	RS = 485
Time constraints	60
Organisational difficulties	3
Irrelevant material	143
Hierarchical domination & prejudice	65
Loss of professional identity	71
Different academic ability	23
Different knowledge base	29
Too many students in a class	74*
None	173**

* This response was totally unexpected. No mention was made in the briefing to the students about how any interdisciplinary learning programme would be implemented. It would seem that the 74 students who identified this as a disadvantage were under the impression that very large numbers of students may be clustered together. No teacher identified this as a potential disadvantage (see Table 5.41)

** If a student wrote comments in the space provided such as "none" or "none at all" or "I cannot think of any" this response was counted. In a total, 173 students wrote such comments.

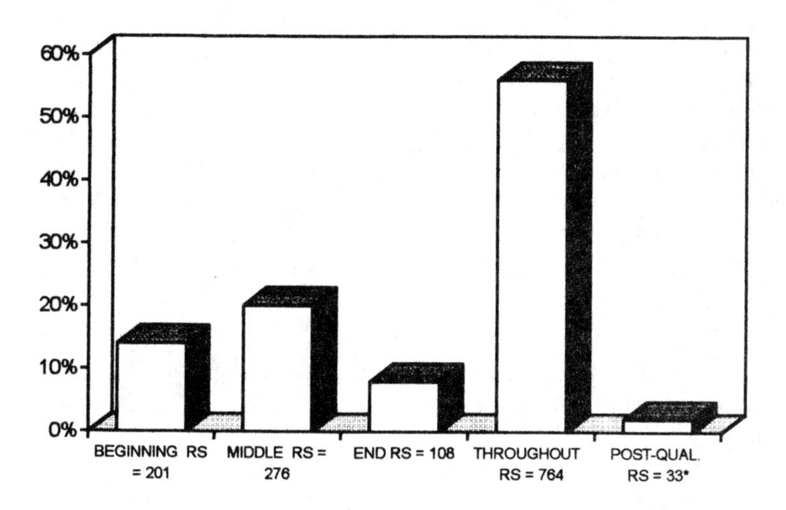

Figure 5.9 The stage of training when interdisciplinary learning should be introduced (N = 1383)

* This represents the 33 students who selected "post qualifying" as their only response.

The majority of students chose "throughout training" (55.10%). More students (20.68% where N = 1383) chose the "middle of training" as their preferred option than did the teachers (7.02% where N = 300). Statistical tests indicated that this was a highly significant finding ($\chi^2 = 17.63$, df = 4, $p < 0.1\%$).

Table 5.58
The stage at which interdisciplinary learning should take place : by profession

Profession	N =	Beginning	Middle	End	Throughout	Post. Qual
Dentists	93	5	16	7	61	4
DSA/DH	37	9	9	2	15	2
Den. Tech	30	2	9	4	15	1
Medicine	269	37	69	33	119	7
Nursing	396	51	81	23	239	7
Nut.& Diet.	45	7	6	8	22	2
Occ. Ther.	89	17	15	2	59	0
ODP	25	7	5	2	10	4
Physio.	101	19	20	5	49	8
Podiatry	63	8	18	5	35	0
Radiog.	52	19	7	5	20	1
Social Work	130	17	20	7	85	0
Sp. Therapy	54	3	11	5	33	2
Totals	1383	194	286	108	762	38*
%		14.02	20.68	7.81	55.10	2.75

* In total 1350 students chose one of the categories at a pre-qualification stage. A number also selected post qualification as well. Only 38 (2.75%) chose post qualification only.

The students were asked to identify the other professions with which their own profession could share learning. As in the analysis of the teacher questionnaires the potential response rate was calculated against the actual response rate. For example of the total number of student responses (N = 1383), 93 were dental students. The figure of 93 was therefore subtracted from the overall response rate in order to calculate the number of students who thought it would be useful to share some learning with dental students. (See Table 5. 59, next page)

Table 5.59
With which other professions could interdisciplinary learning take place ? : by profession

Profession	N = 1383	Potential Response	Actual Response	% of Potential Response
Dentists	93	1290	316	24.50
DSA/DH	37	1346	341	25.33
Den. Tech.	30	1353	164	12.12
Medicine	248	1135	866	76.30
Nursing	396	987	725	73.45
Nut. & Diet.	45	1338	826	61.73
Occ. Therapy	101	1294	878	67.85
ODP	25	1358	361	26.58
Physiotherapy	101	1282	852	66.46
Podiatry	63	1320	287	21.74
Radiography	52	1331	526	39.52
Social Work	130	1253	817	65.20
Speech Therapy	54	1329	712	53.57

The students responses by individual profession are presented in Section 5.5.3.

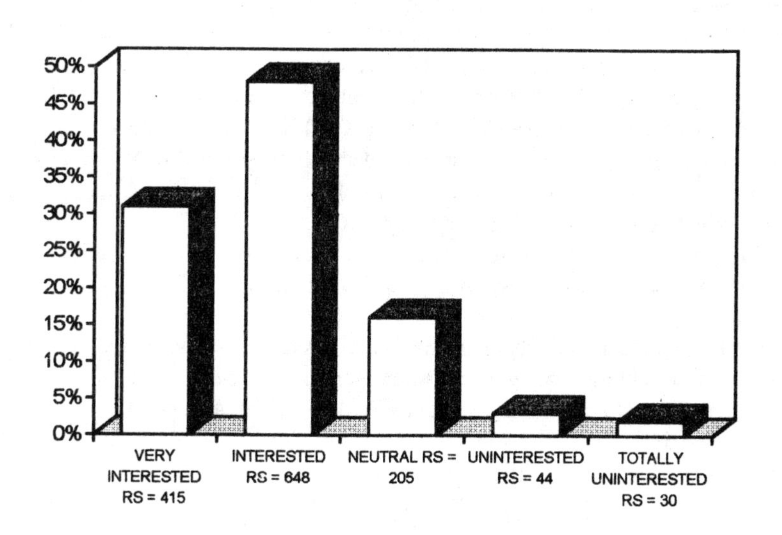

Figure 5.10 The students level of interest in interdisciplinary learning (N = 1383)

As the level of student interest in interdisciplinary learning was high, the learning strategies that students thought would be suitable for such an initiative was crucial. The students were asked to indicate the suitability of a variety of learning strategies which were described in the different curricula. The results are presented in Table 5.60

Table 5.60
Preferred interdisciplinary learning methods : all professions
(N = 1383)

Learning Method	Yes	%	No	%	Undecided	%
Mixed Tutorials	888	64.21	214	15.47	253	18.29
Workshops	911	65.87	195	14.10	236	17.06
Case Studies	891	64.42	222	16.05	262	18.94
Seminars	801	57.92	231	16.70	298	21.55
Problem based learning	795	57.48	192	13.88	390	28.20
Role Play	456*	32.97	560	40.49	337	24.37
Lectures	712	51.48	346	25.02	297	21.48
Visits to client areas	1045	75.56	134	9.69	176	12.73

* This result is distorted by one of the professions' student population. Social Work students were the only group who indicated that role play was an acceptable learning method. In this group 81 students (62.31% where N =130) gave a positive response. In all other professions more than two thirds of the students rejected role play as an acceptable learning method. This was a highly significant finding (χ^2 = 580.57, df = 2, p < 0.1%). Another significant finding was the number of students who were undecided about the use of problem based learning (χ^2 = 68.52, df =2, p< 0.1%). The interpretation of these findings which will be discussed in detail in Chapter 6.

The most popular learning strategy directly involved the client/patient. Interdisciplinary learning involving visits to client areas (75.56%) was strongly endorsed.

For the final question the students were asked to decide which topics were potentially suitable for study on an interdisciplinary basis. A list of 11 subjects were included. The results are presented as Table 5.61, next page.

Table 5.61
Suitable topics for interdisciplinary learning:
All professions (N = 1383)

Topics	Yes	%	No	%
Psychology	1173	84.82	170	12.29
Sociology	1098	79.39	241	17.43
Ethics	1087	78.60	257	18.58
Law & Practice	831	60.09	518	37.45
Research	778	58.03	571	41.29
Management	774	55.97	575	41.58
Economics of care	948	68.55	401	28.99
Health Promotion	1054	76.21	195	14.10
Study skills	783	56.62	566	40.93
Quality Issues	776	56.11	573	41.43
Structural Organisation	1047	75.70	301	21.76
Computing Skills	1089	78.74	295	21.33

More than 50% of all students believed that all these topics could be taught on an interdisciplinary basis. Psychology (84.82%), sociology (79.39%), ethics (78.60%) and health promotion (76.21%) were thought to be suitable by the majority of the sample. The overall results however show a less positive response to introducing all these topics on an interdisciplinary basis than the results of the teaching respondents. (see Table 5.44)

Table 5.62
Comparison between teacher's and student's opinions
on suitable subjects for interdisciplinary learning

Topics	Teachers (N = 300)	%	Students (N = 1383)	%
Psychology	277	92.64	1173	84.82
Sociology	265	88.63	1098	79.39
Ethics	281	93.98	1087	78.60
Law & Practice	266	88.96	831	60.09
Research	244	81.60	778	56.25
Management	259	86.62	774	55.97
Econ. of care	262	87.62	948	68.55
Health Promotion	277	92.64	1054	76.21
Study skills	260	86.96	783	56.62
Quality Issues	264	88.29	776	56.11
Structural Organisation	270	90.30	1087	75.70

There were several highly significant findings in this set of results which indicated that the teachers were more positive than the students about many of these subjects being introduced on an interdisciplinary basis. The significant findings were as follows :-

Law and Practice :	($\chi^2 = 16.90$,	df = 1,	$p < 0.1\%$)
Research :	($\chi^2 = 14.48$,	df = 1,	$p < 0.1\%$)
Management :	($\chi^2 = 20.57$,	df = 1,	$p < 0.1\%$)
Economics of Care :	($\chi^2 = 6.59$,	df = 1,	$p < 5\%$)
Health Promotion :	($\chi^2 = 4.28$,	df = 1,	$p < 5\%$)
Study Skills :	($\chi^2 = 19.90$,	df = 1,	$p < 0.1\%$)
Quality Issues :	($\chi^2 = 22.37$,	df = 1,	$p < 0.1\%$)

5.5.3 The results by individual profession

5.5.3.1 The Dentists

Forty teaching staff completed the questionnaire, all of whom were qualified dental surgeons. One respondent was also a medical practitioner. Twenty nine (72.50%) were male and eleven female (17.50%). Ninety three students completed the questionnaire. Fifty three (56.99 %) were male and forty female (43.01%). The biographic data of each set of respondents is presented separately.

Biographic data of the teaching staff

Table 5.63
Age of the teaching staff

Age Group	N = 40	%
Under 25 years	0	0.00
25 - 30 years	2	5.00
31 - 35 years	4	10.00
36 - 40 years	9	22.50
41 - 45 years	12	30.00
46 - 50 years	8	20.00
51 - 55 years	0	0.00
56 - 60 years	1	2.50
Over 60 years	3	7.50

Table 5.64
Years in practice before commencing teaching career

No. of years in practice	N = 40	%
Less than one year	4	10.00
1 - 5 years	20	50.00
6 - 10 years	8	20.00
11 - 15 years	5	12.50
16 - 20 years	3	7.50
21 - 25 years	0	0.00
Over 25 years	0	0.00

Table 5.65
Number of years in teaching

No. of years in teaching	N = 40	%
Less than one year	0	0.00
1 - 5 years	9	22.50
6 - 10 years	12	30.00
11 - 15 years	10	25.00
16 - 20 years	3	7.50
21 - 25 years	1	2.50
Over 25 years	5	12.50

Nine respondents indicated that they were able to teach subjects in addition to those related specifically to dental practice. These subjects were described as 'medico-legal studies', 'marketing', 'behavioural sciences' (RS = 2), 'disability', 'health education/promotion' (RS = 2), 'communication skills', 'law', 'statistics', 'computing sciences', 'resuscitation training' and with one respondent mentioning 'fly fishing' (!)

Thirty dentists (where N = 40) had experienced teaching professions other than their own. The respondents were invited to identify which professions.

Table 5.66
Experience of teaching other professions

Different profs. taught	RS = 30	%
DSA/Den. Hygienist	27	89.99
Dental Tech.	12	39.99
Medicine	8	26.67
Nursing	13	43.33
Nutrition & Dietetics	3	9.99
Occ. Therapy	1	3.33
O.D.P	2	6.66
Physiotherapy	0	0.00
Podiatry	1	3.33
Radiography	1	3.33
Social Work	1	3.33
Speech Therapy	6	19.99
"Other Professions"	11	36.67

The 11 dentists who had taught "other professions" variously described these as being with pre and post graduate pharmacy students (RS = 5), orthoptists, health promotion officers, medical photographers, "dental health to a wide variety of professions" a marketing course for general studies students and an English language and hygiene course in Africa.

The respondents were also asked whether they had participated in any shared learning with any other professions and if so whether this was before or after they qualified. Twenty four (60.00% where N = 40) confirmed that they previously had shared learning. Of these 24 only 11 (27.50 %) had done so at an undergraduate level. All 11 described learning with medical students at the pre-clinical stage of training. (This practice continues in 1993 as was evidenced by the dental and medical students responses in this study). There was no evidence of any other shared learning at an undergraduate level. The overall results are presented in Table 5. 67, next page.

Table 5.67
Teacher's shared learning experiences

Other Profession	RS = 24	% (N=40)
DSA/Dental Hygienist	6	15.00
Dental Tech.	5	12.50
Medicine	24 *	60.00 *
Nursing	5	12.50
Nutrition & Diet.	2	5.00
Occ. Therapy	1	2.50
ODP	1	2.50
Physiotherapy	1	2.50
Podiatry	0	0.00
Radiography	2	5.00
Social Work	1	2.50
Speech Therapy	2	5.00
"Other Profession"	1	2.50

*Of the 24 respondents who indicated they had at some stage learned with medical practitioners, eleven had done so at the undergraduate stage. The one teacher who had learned with "other profession" indicated that this was with Health Promotion Officers.

Biographic data of the dental students. (N=93)

Table 5.68
Age of the students

Age Group	N=93	%
20 years or less	23	24.73
21 - 25 years	62	66.67
26 - 30 years	6	6.45
31 - 35 years	1	1.07
36 - 40 years	0	0.00
41 - 45 years	0	0.00
46 - 50 years	0	0.00
51 -55 years	0	0.00
Over 55 years	0	0.00

The majority of dental students it would appear, are recruited directly after completing secondary school. There were very few mature students in the sample, with only one being more than 30 years of age.

Table 5.69
Students year stage of training

Year of Training	N = 93	%
1	0 *	0.00
2	0 *	0.00
3	18	19.35
4	33	35.48
5	42	45.16
6	0 **	0.00

* The 1st and 2nd year students complete their pre -clinical training in a University college which has not been included in this study. For this reason these students were excluded.

** A date and time was arranged to meet the twelve students in their sixth year. Unfortunately no student attended. A possible explanation could be that these students had previously been referred in their final examinations and the re-sit examinations were very close. It would be understandable that completing questionnaires would not take a high priority.

Previous courses relevant to the dental profession
The students were asked whether they had undertaken any courses which they perceived as relevant to their current training. Only nine (9.67%) of the 93 respondents had completed previous courses. Three students were already graduates, one with a degree in Biochemistry, one with a degree in Biology and another with a degree in Pharmaceutical Sciences. Another student had completed three years of medical training and then transferred to dental training. The remaining courses ranged from Dental Surgery Assistant training (RS = 1), a pre nursing course (RS = 1), a BTEC medical physics course (RS = 1) and first aid courses (RS = 2). The student with the degree in Pharmaceutical Sciences had also worked as a pharmacist. This individual was the one student who was over 30 years of age. The relatively small number of students who had completed courses was predictable in that the age distribution indicated that this would be the case.

Work experience relevant to the dental profession.

Of the 93 respondents, 25 indicated that they had gained relevant work experience. The majority (RS = 16) had worked on a voluntary basis usually with children with special needs. Other work experience included care assistants (RS = 3), an ophthalmic receptionist, a dental surgery assistant, an occupational therapy assistant, a medical technician, a pharmacy assistant and the mature student who had worked as a pharmacist. Of the 25 who had previous relevant work experience, 21 (84.00%) were female. Analysis for statistical probability produced a highly significant result (χ^2 = 13. 26, df = 1, p < 0.1%) indicating that the results could not have occured by chance. Female dental students are more likely to have gained work experience relevant to their training than their male colleagues.

Previous experience of learning with other professions.

The students were asked whether they had been given the opportunity of learning with other professions. Of the 93 respondents 68 confirmed that they had. The majority (RS = 58) indicated that they had shared some learning with medical students. As previously explained this occurs within the first two pre clinical years in another University College. This question therefore should have provoked a greater positive response as all dental students complete the pre clinical course. The professions with whom the dental students had shared learning are presented as Table 5. 70

Table 5.70
Student's shared learning experiences

Professions Involved	N=93	%
DSA/DH	0	0.00
Dental Tech.	6	6.45
Medicine	58	62.36
Nursing	1	1.08
Nutrition & Diet.	1	1.08
Occ. Therapy	0	0.00
ODP	0	0.00
Physiotherapy	0	0.00
Podiatry	0	0.00
Radiography	1	1.08
Social Work	0	0.00
Speech Therapy	0	0.00
Other professions	4	4.30

A limitation has been identified regarding the results obtained from this question. The question should have made clear that the information wanted related to any shared learning on the course that the student was undertaking currently. It is suspected that some of the responses presented above relate to courses previously undertaken by the students. The justification for this assumption is made because the students (apart from those who indicated shared learning with the medical students) had all previously completed courses. Of the four respondents who indicated "other professions" three identified these as "neurophysiologists" (all three had completed science degrees), the student who indicated that shared learning had occurred with the nursing profession had completed a pre nursing course and the student who indicated radiography had trained as a medical technician. While not conclusive it does seem to indicate that very little or no shared learning takes place between the dental students and others apart from medical students in the pre clinical years.

The samples opinions regarding the concept of interdisciplinary learning

It seemed appropriate when presenting the results of both the teachers and students questionnaires to display these in combination where ever possible. The rationale for this decision was based on the need for the opinions of both the teaching staff and the students to be seen as being of equal importance for any future developments.

Two of the fundamental questions central to the whole study were whether the teaching staff and students sampled from each of the participating professions believed that there should be some interdisciplinary learning between them and if so at which stage of training this should take place. Overall the opinions of those representing the dental profession were very positive.

Table 5.71
Should there be interdisciplinary learning ?

Response	Teachers (N=40)	%	Students (N=93)	%	Total (N = 133)	%
Yes	36	90.00	71	76.34	107	80.45
No	1	2.50	11	11.83	12	9.02
Undecided	3	7.50	11	11.83	14	10.53

There was no significant difference between the opinions of the teachers and the students. ($\chi^2 = 2.96$, df = 2, $p > 5\%$)

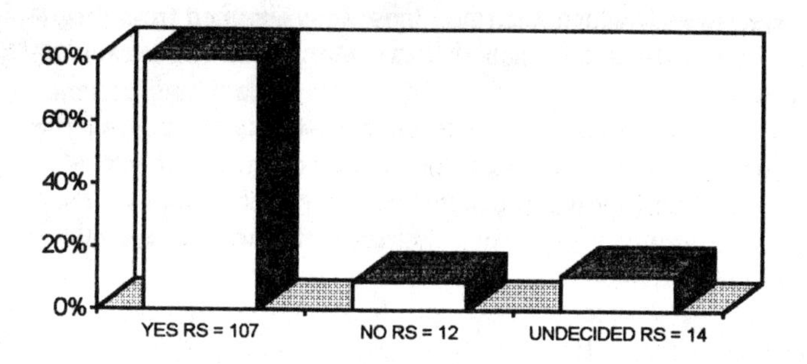

Figure 5.11 Should there be some shared learning ? : By percentage

Table 5.72
At which stage should it take place ?

Response	Teachers (N =40)	%	Students (N = 93)	%	Totals (N = 133)	%
At the beginning	4	10.00	5	5.38	9	6.77
In the middle	3	7.50	16	17.20	19	14.29
At the end	2	5.00	7	7.53	9	6.77
Throughout	30	75.00	61	65.59	91	68.42
Post Qual.	2	5.00	2	2.15	4	3.01

The teachers and the students opinions were similar in that the majority thought that interdisciplinary learning should take place throughout training. Proportionately more students than teachers selected the middle of training but no significant difference was found (χ^2 = 2.85, df = 4, p = > 5% with Yates correction applied)

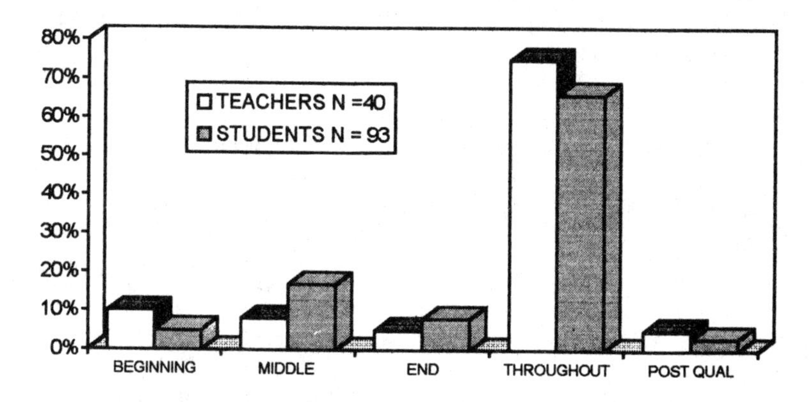

Figure 5.12 At which stage should it take place ? : By percentage

* Several respondents indicated at the "post qualification stage" as well as "throughout". Only two teachers and two students responded "post qualification" only.

The majority of teachers and students sampled indicated a belief that there should be some interdisciplinary learning between the health and social care professions. In addition most respondents also suggested that this should take place throughout training. They were also asked to give the rationale for their decisions. Examples of these were :

1. *At the beginning*
   "It would provide a common core of knowledge which would breakdown professional barriers before they become established." (Teacher resp. 13) "Everthing is common in the beginning and we are not set in our ways." (Student resp. 90)
2. *In the middle*
   "Early enough to prevent entrenched ideas developing." (Teacher Resp. 19) "So you have enough time to settle in but before we are corrupted by experience." (Student resp. 26)
3. *At the end*
   "Need to understand your own profession before you can share with others." (Teacher resp. 20) "Able to appreciate the relevance of what you are being taught." (Student resp. 51)
4. *Throughout*
   "Education is a process designed for life, it must be integral throughout." (Teacher resp. 37) "People skills are crucially important throughout a caring career." (Student resp. 9)
5. *Post Qualification*
   "Until one has a good working knowledge of ones subject it is difficult to interact with others. Merely attending the same lecture is not shared learning." (Teacher resp. 2) "Then it is entirely up to you, if you want to or not." (Student resp. 74)

Table 5.73
Would there be advantages in interdisciplinary learning?

Response	Teachers (N = 40)	%	Students (N = 93)	%	Totals (N = 133)	%
Yes	36	90.0	75	80.65	111	83.46
No	1	2.50	8	8.60	9	6.77
Undecided	3	7.50	10	10.75	13	9.77

Tests for significance revealed no differences between the teacher and student results ($\chi^2 = 1.43$, df = 2, p > 5%).

Table 5.74
Advantages of interdisciplinary learning

Response	Teachers (RS = 30) *	Students RS = 47) *	%
Increase understanding of each others' role	22	28	50
Increase teamwork & collaboration	16	31	47
Broaden horizons, cross fertilise ideas	9	21	30
Make better use of time & scarce resources	4	0	4

* Of the 40 teaching staff who completed the questionnnaire, 30 listed the reasons why they thought there would be advantages. Similarly with the 93 students who participated 47 listed reasons.

** Many respondents listed more than one reason. The raw scores are therefore calculated against the total population (N =133).

One student (Resp. 72) observed "I would *really* be able to understand the patient I am dealing with".

Both sets of respondents also were asked to list any disadvantages which they could identify. In total 16 teaching staff and 23 students listed disadvantages. A similar analysis was undertaken but it proved more difficult to classify precisely. For this reason there are eight different categories.

Table 5.75
Disadvantages of interdisciplinary learning

Responses	Teachers (RS = 16)	Students (RS = 23)	Totals (N = 133)
Time constraints	2	1	3
Organisation difficulties	6	5	11
Irrelevant material	5	10	15
Hierarchical domination & prejudice	2	2	4
Loss of prof. identity	0	2	2
Different academic ability	1	1	2
Different knowledge base	0	0	0
Too many students in a class	0	2	2

Interestingly each respondent only gave one disadvantage. Of the 16 teachers who responded to this question, two (where RS = 2) subsequently indicated that they were totally uninterested in any interdisciplinary learning. The same pattern emerged with the students. Of the 23 who listed disadvantages six (where RS = 6) subsequently indicated that they were either uninterested or totally uninterested in interdisciplinary learning.

The teachers and the students were asked to indicate their level of interest in interdisciplinary learning. The teachers were asked how interested they would be in participating as a teacher in any future developments and the students were asked how interested they would be in participating as a learner in any such initiative. It was believed that these questions constituted the central focus of the entire study as a neutral or negative response would indicate that there was likely to be resistance or even hostility to any interdisciplinary developments.

Table 5.76
Level of interest in interdisciplinary learning

Level of Interest	Teachers (N = 40)	%	Students (N = 93)	%	Total (N = 133)	%
Very Interested	9	22.50	15	16.13	24	18.05
Interested	22	55.00	53	56.99	75	56.39
Neutral	7	17.50	19	20.43	26	19.55
Uninterested	0	0.00	4	4.30	4	3.01
Totally Uninterested	2	5.00	2	2.15	4	3.01

The two sets of responses were very similar and no significant difference was found ($\chi^2 = 1.46$, df = 4, p > 5% Yates correction applied).

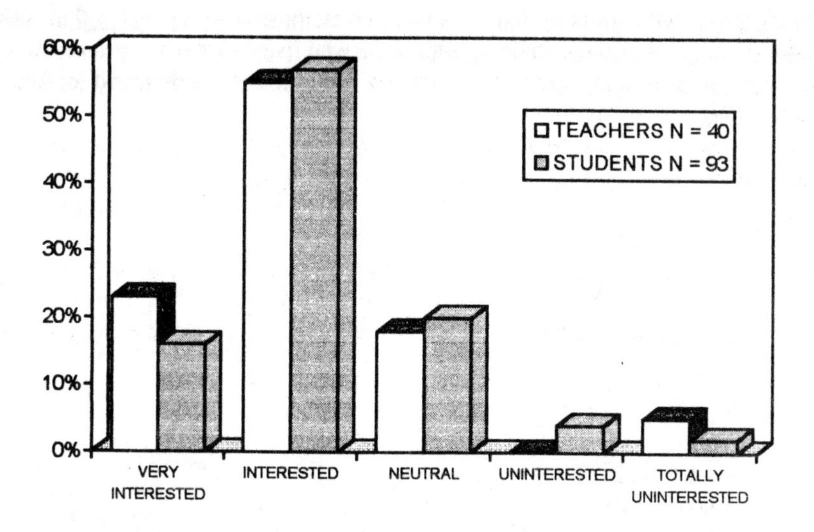

Figure 5.13 Level of interest in interdisciplinary learning : By percentage

Of the 133 respondents 99 (74.44%) indicated that they were "interested" or "very interested" in the concept.

From a list of core subjects (identified from the content analysis of the 14 curricula) the respondents were asked to indicate whether they believed that the subjects were suitable or unsuitable for interdisciplinary learning.

Table 5.77
Subjects suitable for interdisciplinary learning

Subject	Teachers (N = 40)	%	Students (N =93)	%	Totals (N = 133)	%
Psychology	40	100.0	83	89.25	123	92.48
Sociology	36	90.00	77	82.80	113	84.96
Ethics	37	92.50	67	72.04	104	78.20
Law & Practice	34	85.00	60	64.52	94	70.68
Research Methods	34	85.00	44	47.31	78	58.65
Management	33	82.50	62	66.67	95	71.43
Economics of Care	31	77.50	72	77.42	103	77.44
Health Promotion	37	92.50	84	90.32	121	90.98
Study Skills	32	80.00	47	50.54	79	59.40
Quality Issues	31	77.50	49	52.69	80	60.15
Structural Organisation	34	85.00	71	76.34	105	78.95
Computing Skills	36	90.00	82	88.17	118	88.72

The teachers and students were very similar in their opinions regarding which subjects would be suitable for interdisciplinary learning. The only anomaly was in the research category where significantly more teachers identified as appropriate ($\chi^2 = 3.94$, df =1, $p < 5\%$)

The students had previously indicated from a list of 8 subjects which ones they thought should be included in the term "behavioural sciences".

Table 5.78
Subjects students included in the behavioural sciences

Subjects	Yes	%	No	%	Undecided	%
Psychology	91	97.85	1	1.08	1	1.08
Sociology	83	89.25	2	2.15	8	8.60
Ethics	62	66.67	20	21.51	11	11.83
Law & Practice	35	37.63	41	44.08	17	18.28
Management	45	48.39	34	36.56	14	15.05
Health Promotion	73	78.49	14	15.05	6	6.45
Study Skills	34	36.56	43	46.24	16	17.20
Quality Issues	27	29.03	22	23.66	44	47.31

From these results it can be seen that there is a lot of indecision about what constitutes the behavioural sciences. This confirms the findings obtained in the structured interviews previously conducted with the students from all the professions (N = 22). Many students appear to be unsure what the term behavioural sciences means. Most know that psychology and sociology are included but a significant number included many other topics which would not be considered by the purists as a behavioural science. However when compared with Table 5.78 above, there is an indication that additional subjects other than the behavioural sciences could be included in any future interdisciplinary developments.

Table 5.79
Dental students preferred interdisciplinary learning methods

Learning Method	Yes	%	No	%	Uncertain	%
Tutorials	73	78.49	10	10.75	10	10.75
Workshops	49	52.69	18	19.35	26	27.95
Case Studies	76	81.72	8	8.60	9	9.78
Problem Based Learning	47	50.54	20	21.51	26	27.95
Role Play	38	40.86	38	40.86	17	18.28
Lectures	46	49.46	29	31.18	18	19.35
Visits to client areas	78	83.87	7	7.53	8	8.60

Many of the suggested interdisciplinary learning methods were accepted by the students. Role play however was rejected by the majority. This result was highly significant ($\chi^2 = 15.61$, df = 2, p = < 0.1%). This finding along with the significant results of the other professions will be discussed in Chapter 6.

The students were asked what would be appropriate learning methods in any future developments. This invoked a most interesting response from an educational point of view. It was realised subsequently that this question most probably elicited students preferred learning styles rather than the suitability for shared learning. It would seem that dental students would welcome visits to clinical areas (78.49%), case studies (81.72%), mixed tutorials (78.49%) and seminars (73.12%) but were not so keen on role play (40.86%), problem based learning (50.54%) or lectures (49.46%). The most negative response evoked was that relating to role playing. It is not known whether this was because the students in this population sample had experienced this learning style and rejected it as unsuitable, whether they had no experience in role playing, or whether they actively dislike role playing. Students' preferred learning styles therefore may directly conflict with teachers ideas of what consitutes appropriate teaching methods. It is suspected that the results for problem based learning and workshops may be misleading in that 27.95% were "undecided" in both categories. This may be due to a lack of experience in both of these learning styles. It would have been useful therefore to have ascertained the teaching/learning methods used by the dental school by inserting a suitable question in both the teacher and student questionnaires.

The teachers and the students were asked to select which other professions they believed could undertake some interdisciplinary learning in conjunction with their own.

Table 5.80
Other professions suitable for interdisciplinary learning with dentists

Other Prof.	Teachers (N = 40)	%	Students (N = 93)	%	Total (N = 133)	%
DSA/DH	30	75.00	82	88.17	112	84.21
Den. Tec.	27	67.50	61	65.59	88	66.17
Medicine	30	75.00	82	88.17	112	84.21
Nursing	29	72.50	37	39.78	66	49.62
N.& D	30	75.00	62	66.67	92	69.17
Occ. Th	7	17.50	21	22.58	28	21.05
ODP	6	15.00	13	13.98	19	14.29
Physio	7	17.50	17	18.28	24	18.05
Podiatry	6	15.00	4	4.30	10	7.52
Radio.	20	50.00	59	63.44	79	59.40
S. W.	17	42.50	40	43.01	57	42.86
Sp. Th.	22	55.00	45	48.39	67	50.38

The results show similar opinions between the teachers and the students in the sample for many of the professions. The desire to learn with the medical profession is evident (84.21%) and also predictable as this already exists in pre clinical training. Of particular interest is the fact that the same percentage of respondents (84.21%) expressed the view that some shared learning should occur with dental hygienists and dental surgery assistants. A significant percentage also identified nutritionists and dietitians (69.17%) and dental technicians (66.17%). Speech therapists however, were selected by only 50.38 % of the respondents which was only slightly more than the nursing profession (49.62%). The social workers were identified by 42.86 % of the respondents. This was a particularly interesting result as it seems to indicate that the dental profession is well aware of the social needs of their client population and many would find it useful to share some learning with social workers at an undergraduate stage. Only one student (Resp 70) was disparaging about the inclusion of social workers "Social workers are *not* of any relevance to any of the other groups as they have no medical or scientific knowledge." This student was "totally uninterested" in the concept of interdisciplinary learning and also rejected the relevance of the behavioural sciences in dentistry, " I am here to treat patients not worry about the way they think and act". It is surprising that this student chose to enter a profession where interpersonal skills are of such importance.

5.5.3.2 The dental hygienists and dental surgery assistants

The number of staff and students in this school is small. However the opinions of these respondents were as important as those in the larger schools. In total four teachers (100%) and 37 students completed the questionnaires. All respondents were female (N = 41).

Biographic data of the teaching staff

The age group of the teachers was evenly distributed between 31 years and 60 years. Three of the teachers had been in practice less than five years before they started their formal teaching careers while the other teacher had practiced between 11 and 15 years. The number of years of teaching experience varied from less than 5 years (RS = 1), 6-10 years (RS = 2) and 11-15 years (RS = 1). The four teachers did not consider themselves to have other related areas of knowledge, but three had experienced teaching students other than their own. One respondent had taught occupational therapists, physiotherapists and dental technicians while all four had taught nurses. All four teachers had experienced some shared learning with other professions with two of them indicating that this had originally taken place before qualification. Both had identifed Operating Department Practitioners with one also including occupational therapy, physiotherapy and radiography. The other two respondents had shared learning with nurses after qualification with one of them also learning with social workers.

Biographic data of the students

Nearly half the students were less than 20 years of age (RS =16) with a further 15 being between 21 and 25 years of age. Of the remaining five students, two were aged between 26 and 30 years and three between 31 and 35 years. The majority of student respondents were in their first year (RS = 29). Of these 14 were training as dental hygienists and 15 as dental surgery assistants. The eight second year students were training as dental hygienists.

Several of the students (RS = 6) had undertaken courses which they considered relevant to their current training. These courses were "first aid courses" (RS = 2), Dental Health Cert. (RS = 1), Dental Therapist (RS = 1), BTEC Science (RS = 1), Pre nursing course (RS = 1). A number had also obtained relevant work experience. Many of the dental hygienist students had previously completed a dental surgery assistant training (RS = 14), one had worked as a dental therapist, other occupations were described as "sales rep in dental field", voluntary work as carers (RS = 4), Red Cross, nursery nursing, pharmacy assistant, care assistants (RS = 3).

Of the 37 dental surgery asssistants and dental hygienists 15 had experienced shared learning. The most frequent profession idenitified was that of dentistry (RS = 8) with three identifying nursing, one describing pharmacists and two social workers and another speech therapists. Further analysis of the data revealed that all of these respondents were the ones that had previous work experience. The care assistants had learned with the nurses, the voluntary work carers had learned with the social workers and the speech therapists and the pharmacy assistant with the pharmacists. It would seem that during their training DSA and dental hygiene students learn as an isolated professional group apart from some unspecified contact with the dental students. It would seem likely that this occurs in the clinical areas.

Opinions regarding the concept of interdisciplinary learning

The four teachers all used different words for shared learning, however all four believed that some shared learning should take place between the health and social care professions.

Table 5.81
Should there be interdisciplinary learning ?

Response	Teachers (N = 4)	%	Students (N = 37)	%	Total (N = 41)	%
Yes	4	100.0	29	73.38	33	80.49
No	0	100.0	2	5.41	2	4.88
Undecided	0	100.0	6	16.22	6	14.63

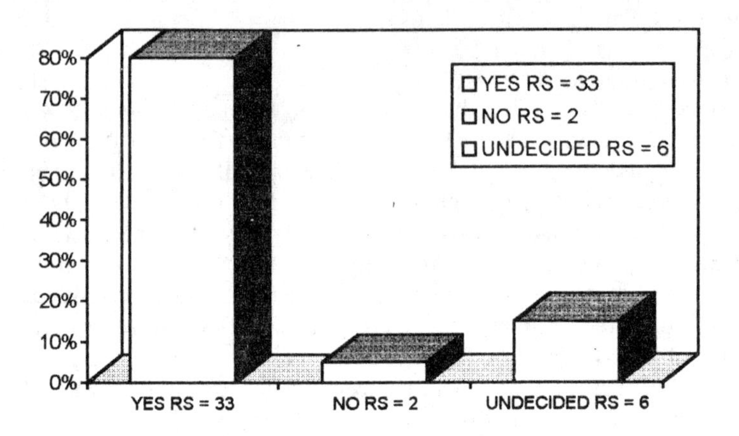

Figure 5.14 Should there be some shared learning ? : By percentage

Potential advantages in shared learning were identified by two of the teachers and 28 of the students. None of the teachers identified any disadvantages but 13 of the students listed some. The advantages all centred on increased collaboration, teamwork and insight into the other professions contributions. All 13 students who listed disadvantages raised anxieties about the relevance of all the topics which may be covered. One student in spite of this commented , "A more open and realistic approach between us all is bound to be better for the patient" (Student Resp. 10). There were diverse opinions regarding when interdisciplinary learning should be introduced.

Table 5. 82
At which stage should it take place ?

Response	Teachers (N = 4)	%	Students (N = 37)	%	Total (N = 41)	%
Beginning	2	50.00	9	24.33	11	26.83
Middle	0	0.00	9	24.33	9	21.95
End	0	0.00	2	5.41	2	4.88
Throughout	2	50.00	15	40.54	17	41.46
Post Qual	0	0.00	2	5.41	2	4.88

The students (RS = 15) who thought that "throughout" would be most appropriate all gave similar reasons such as "enhance teamwork", "becomes a normal thing". The two who chose post qualification both gave "time constraints" as the reason for their choice. The nine who selected "the beginning" commented on the need to "get into the habit", "get used to the other professions" and similar reasons. Those students (RS = 9) who chose "the middle" all wanted to get to grips with their own subject first, "so I would be able to cope with something new" (Resp 7). The level of interest expressed in interdisciplinary teaching and learning again produced a diversity of opinions although on the whole the teachers and the students were either "very interested" or "interested" (70.73% where N = 41).

Table 5.83
Level of interest in interdisciplinary learning

Response	Teachers (N = 4)	%	Students (N =37)	%	Total (N =41)	%
Very Interested	0	0.00	9	24.32	9	21.95
Interested	3	75.0	17	45.95	20	48.78
Neutral	1	25.0	7	18.92	8	19.51
Uninterested	0	0.00	1	2.71	1	2.44
Totally Uninterest.	0	0.00	2	5.41	2	4.88

The students were unsure in many instances as to which subjects constituted the behavioural sciences. The results are displayed in Table 5.84

Table 5.84
Subjects included in the behavioural sciences

Subject	Yes	%	No	%	Undecided	%
Psychology	36	97.30	0	0.00	1	2.71
Sociology	34	91.89	1	2.71	2	5.41
Ethics	18	48.65	4	10.81	15	40.54
Law & Prac.	16	43.24	10	27.03	11	29.73
Management	17	45.95	13	35.14	7	18.92
Health Prom	28	75.66	0	0.00	9	24.32
Study Skills	17	45.95	6	16.22	14	37.84
Qual. Issues	13	35.14	8	21.62	16	43.24

The staff and students were asked to select from the list of core subjects which ones would be suitable on an interdisciplinary basis. The results are displayed in Table 5.85.

Table 5.85
Subjects suitable for interdisciplinary learning

Core Subject	Teachers (N=4)	%	Students (N=37)	%	Totals (N=41)	%
Psychology	3	75.0	35	94.59	38	92.68
Sociology	4	100.0	29	78.38	33	80.49
Ethics	3	75.0	17	45.95	20	48.78
Law & Practice	3	75.0	17	45.95	20	48.78
Research Methods	2	50.0	12	32.43	14	34.15
Management	3	75.0	13	35.14	16	39.02
Economics of Care	2	50.0	23	62.16	25	60.98
Health Promotion	4	100.0	32	86.49	36	87.80
Study Skills	4	100.0	17	45.95	21	51.22
Quality Issues	4	100.0	13	35.14	17	41.46
Structural Organisation	4	100.0	21	56.76	25	60.98
Computing Skills	3	75.0	13	35.14	16	39.02

Because of the small number of teaching staff in the school it was not possible to statistically compare the results between them and the students.

The students were also asked to indicate their preferred learning styles in any shared learning initiative.

Table 5.86
Students preferred interdisciplinary learning methods

Learning Method	Yes	%	No	%	Undecided	%
Tutorials	24	64.86	3	8.11	10	27.03
Workshops	14	37.84	3	8.11	17	45.95
Case Studies	21	56.76	3	8.11	13	45.95
Seminars	23	62.16	3	8.11	11	29.73
Problem Based Learning	16	43.24	3	8.11	18	48.65
Role Play	11	29.73	15	40.54	11	29.73
Lectures	21	56.76	9	24.32	7	18.92
Visits to client areas	26	70.27	4	10.81	7	18.92

Visits to clinical areas was the option chosen most frequently (70.27%) by the DSA/DH students and role play was the least frequently chosen (29.73%). The rejection of role play was statistically significant ($\chi^2 = 23.06$, df = 2, p = < 0.1%)

Finally the teaching staff and students identified the other professions with whom they believed some shared learning could take place.

Table 5.87
Other professions suitable for interdisciplinary learning with dental hygienists and dental surgery assistants

Other Prof.	Teachers (N=4)	%	Students (N=37)	%	Total (N=41)	%
Dentists	2	50.00	28	75.68	30	73.17
Den. Tec.	0	0.00	12	32.43	12	29.27
Medicine	1	25.00	12	32.43	13	31.71
Nursing	4	100.00	22	59.46	26	63.41
Nut. & Diet.	3	75.00	20	54.05	23	56.10
Occ. Therapy	2	50.00	9	24.32	11	26.83
ODP	2	50.00	7	18.92	9	21.95
Physiotherapy	1	25.00	2	5.41	3	7.32
Podiatry	1	25.00	0	0.00	1	2.44
Radiography	3	75.00	14	37.84	17	41.46
Social Work	1	25.00	13	35.14	14	34.15
Sp. Therapy	1	25.00	5	13.51	6	14.63

Predictably the most frequently chosen other profession were the dentists (73.17% where N = 41). More respondents chose nurses (63.41%) than nutritionists and dietitians (56.10%). An unexpected number chose social workers (34.15%) where as very few chose speech therapists (14.63%).

5.5.3.3 The dental technologists

Six teaching staff and thirty students completed the questionnaires. The number of teaching staff was unexpected as the school of dental technology was listed as having only three teachers. The explanation was obtained when one completed questionnaire was returned with a note from the respondent. There are dental technologists employed within the Dental School who have a teaching remit. As these individuals had not received a questionnaire but wished to participate in the study a questionnaire received by a dental lecturer had been photocopied three times and then completed by the dental technologists !

Biographic data of the teaching staff
Of the six teaching staff, five were male and one female. Their ages ranged from 25-30 years (RS = 2), one was between 31-35 years, two were between 41-45 years and the other was between 56-60 years. Most had been in practice for 6-10 years before starting teaching (RS = 4) with one working between 1-5 years and the other between 11-15 years. Half of the respondents had been teaching for 1-5 years, with two teaching for 11-15 years and the other for more than 25 years.

Only one teacher identified other areas which he could teach and he listed these as "history of science, philosophy and sociology". This same respondent had taught sociology undergraduates and he and three others had taught dental students. Of the six respondents three had experienced shared learning, one before qualifying and one after with the third respondent indicating "Both". The other professions involved were listed as dental surgeons (RS = 2), nurses (RS = 1), podiatrists (RS = 1), social workers (RS = 1) and other professions (RS = 2).

Biographic data of the students

The biographic data obtained from the dental technology students (18 male and 10 female respondents) revealed that 17 were in the first year and 13 were in the second year. Their age distribution is presented in Table 5.88

Table 5.88
Age of the students

Age Group	N = 30	%
20 years or less	10	33.33
21-25 years	12	40.00
26-30 years	4	13.33
31-35 years	3	10.00
36-40 years	0	0.00
41-45 years	1	3.33
>46 years	0	0.00

Of the 30 respondents ten previously had undertaken relevant courses. These were variously described as "2 years dentistry in Rumania", "dental therapist in Australia", First Aid Certificates (RS = 3) and computing courses (RS = 4). A number had also gained relevant work experience (RS = 11). These experiences were described as "dental nursing" (RS = 1), voluntary work (RS = 4), work experience with physiotherapists (RS = 1), complementary health therapists (RS = 1), radiographers (RS = 1) and the respondent who had worked as a dental therapist. The 11 respondents who indicated that they had shared learning with other professions were those that had gained relevant work experience.

The sample's opinions regarding the concept of interdisciplinary learning

See tables and figure commencing on next page.

Table 5.89
Should there be interdisciplinary learning ?

Response	Teachers (N=6)	%	Students (N=30)	%	Total (N=36)	%
Yes	5	83.33	28	93.33	33	91.67
No	0	0.00	0	0.00	0	0.00
Undecided	1	16.67	2	6.67	3	8.33

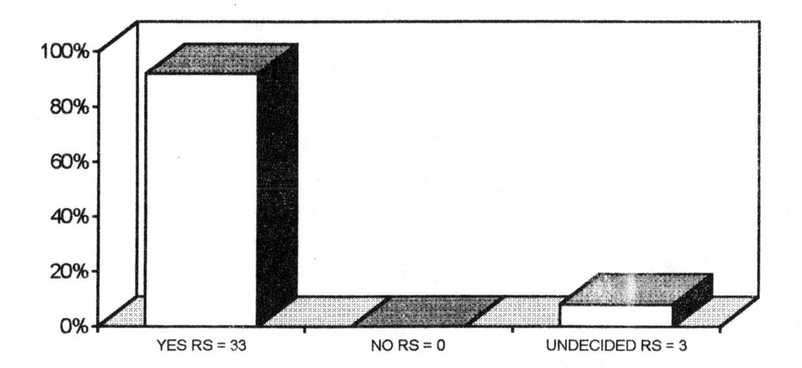

Figure 5.15 Should there be interdisciplinary learning ? All respondents, by percentage.

Table 5.90
At which stage should it take place ?

Response	Teachers (N = 6)	%	Students (N = 30)	%	Total (N = 36)	%
Beginning	0	0.00	2	6.67	2	5.56
Middle	0	0.00	9	30.00	9	25.00
End	0	0.00	4	13.33	4	13.33
Throughout	6	100.00	15	50.00	21	58.33
Post Qual	0	0.00	1	3.33	1	2.78

The rationale for their decisions was given by 24 of the 30 students and four of the teaching staff. One teacher (Resp. 1) commented , “a little and often would be of benefit as learning advances”. The second year student who chose the end of training believed however ,”It is essential to learn the tools of your own trade first”.

Table 5.91
Would there be advantages ?

Response	Teachers (N = 6)	%	Students (N = 30)	%	Total (N = 36)	%
Yes	4	66.67	26	86.67	30	83.33
No	0	0.00	1	3.33	1	2.78
Undecided	2	33.33	3	10.00	5	13.89

Only one student thought there would be no advantages and he was the one who was totally uninterested in the idea of interdisciplinary learning.

Table 5.92
Advantages of interdisciplinary learning

Response	Teachers (RS = 4)	Students (RS = 25)	Total (N = 36)
Increase understanding of each others role	2	8	10
Increase teamwork & collaboration	0	13	13
Broaden horizons, cross fertilise ideas	3	6	9
Make better use of scarce time & resources	0	0	0

Table 5.93
Disadvantages of interdisciplinary learning

Response	Teachers (RS =2)	Students (RS = 14)	Total (N = 36)
Time constraints	1	0	1
Organisation difficulties	0	0	0
Irrelevant material	1	3	4
Hierarchical domination & prejudice	0	9	9
Loss of professional identity	0	2	2
Different academic ability	0	0	0
Different knowledge base	0	1	1
Too many students in a class	0	0	0

Five students wrote “none at all” in response to this question.

Table 5.94
Level of interest in interdisciplinary learning

Response	Teachers (N = 6)	%	Students (N = 30)	%	Total (N = 36)	%
Very Interested	0	00.0	8	26.67	8	22.22
Interested	6	100.	16	53.33	24	66.67
Neutral	0	0.0	3	8.33	3	8.33
Uninterested	0	0.0	1	3.33	1	2.78
Totally Uninterested	0	0.0	1	3.33	1	2.78

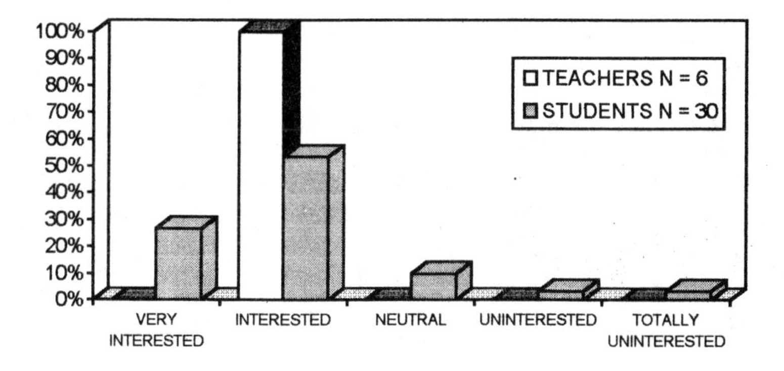

Figure 5.16 Level of interest in interdisciplinary learning : By percentage

Of the 36 respondents 32 (88.89%) were either "very interested" or "interested" in interdisciplinary learning.

The students opinions as to what constitutes the behavioural sciences are presented in Table 5.95

Table 5.95
Subjects students included in the behavioural sciences

Subject	Yes	%	No	%	Undecided	%
Psychology	28	93.33	1	3.33	1	3.33
Sociology	25	83.33	0	0.00	5	16.67
Ethics	15	50.00	7	23.33	8	26.67
Law & Prac.	13	43.33	5	16.67	12	40.00
Management	15	50.00	9	30.00	6	20.00
Health Prom.	23	76.67	4	13.33	3	10.00
Study Skills	17	56.67	5	16.67	8	26.67
Qual. Issues	8	26.67	8	26.67	14	46.67

Quality Issues were rejected by the majority of students as was Law and Practice. Apart from psychology and sociology, health promotion was the most frequently chosen subject. The teaching staff and students also selected from the list of core subjects those which would be suitable for some interdisciplinary learning.

Table 5.96
Subjects suitable for interdisciplinary learning

Core Subject	Teachers (N=6)	%	Students (N=30)	%	Total (N=36)	%
Psychology	6	100.0	23	76.67	29	80.56
Sociology	4	66.67	17	56.67	21	58.33
Ethics	6	100.0	18	60.00	24	66.67
Law & Prac.	6	100.0	15	50.00	21	58.33
Research Methods	5	83.33	22	73.33	27	75.00
Management	6	100.0	17	56.67	23	63.89
Economics	5	83.33	20	66.67	25	69.44
Health Prom.	6	100.0	27	90.00	33	91.67
Study Skills	6	100.0	19	63.33	25	69.44
Quality Issues	6	100.0	14	46.67	20	55.56
Structural Organisation	6	100.0	24	80.00	30	83.33
Computing Skills	6	100.0	25	83.33	31	86.11

Table 5.97
Students preferred interdisciplinary learning methods

Learning Method	Yes	%	No	%	Undecided	%
Tutorials	20	66.67	5	16.67	5	16.67
Workshops	19	63.33	4	13.33	7	23.33
Case Studies	22	73.33	2	6.67	6	20.00
Seminars	11	36.67	8	26.67	11	36.67
Problem Based Learning	16	53.33	4	13.33	10	33.33
Role Play	8	26.67	14	46.67	8	26.67
Lectures	16	53.33	8	26.67	6	20.00
Visits to Clinical Areas	28	93.33	0	0.00	2	6.67

The rejection of role play was highly significant ($\chi^2 = 18.12$, $df = 2$, $p = < 0.1\%$)

Of particular interest was the result of "visits to clinical areas" where 28 (93.33%) of the students selected this as an appropriate learning method. Currently dental technology students have no direct contact with clients, the dentist is the "middle man". This result may indicate the student's desire to make direct contact with the client.

Table 5.98
Other professions suitable for interdisciplinary learning with dental technologists

	Teachers (N=6)	%	Students (N=30)	%	Total (N=36)	%
Dentists	6	100.00	28	93.33	34	94.44
DSA/DH	4	66.67	25	75.00	29	80.55
Medicine	0	0.00	0	0.00	0	0.00
Nursing	1	16.67	4	13.33	5	13.89
N & D	0	0.00	10	33.33	10	27.78
Occ. Ther.	0	0.00	6	20.00	6	16.67
ODP	0	0.00	4	13.33	4	11.11
Physio.	0	0.00	3	10.00	3	8.33
Podiatry	1	16.67	1	3.33	2	5.56
Radio.	1	16.67	8	26.67	9	25.00
S.W	0	0.00	4	13.33	4	11.11
Sp. Ther.	2	33.33	18	60.00	20	55.56

The other professions most frequently chosen were the dentists, DSA/DH and the speech therapists. No respondent chose the medical profession.

5.5.3.4 The medical practitioners

In total 107 medical staff and 269 medical students completed the questionnaires. The response rate of the medical staff far exceeded expectations with some staff returning a completed questionnaire from other parts of the United Kingdom having moved to other jobs. Several of the staff identified themselves, specifically requesting that the results be made available to them at the earliest opportunity as they would like to be actively involved in any future developments. The biographic data of each set of respondents is presented separately.

Biographic data of the teaching staff
Of the 107 teaching staff who completed the questionnaire 80 were male and 27 were female.

Table 5.99
Age of the Teaching Staff

Age Group	N=107	%
Less than 25 years	0	0.00
25-30 years	0	0.00
31-35 years	11	10.28
36-40 years	21	19.63
41-45 years	19	17.75
46-50 years	21	19.63
51-55 years	19	17.75
56-60 years	12	11.21
Over 60 years	4	3.74

Table 5.100
Years in practice before commencing teaching

No. of years in practice	N=107	%
Less than 1 year	25	23.36
1-5 years	55	51.40
6-10 years	23	21.50
11-15 years	2	1.87
16-20 years	0	0.00
21-25 years	0	0.00
Over 25 years	1	0.93

Table 5.101
Years in teaching

No. of years in teaching	N =107	%
Less than 1 year	1	0.93
1-5 years	20	18.69
6-10 years	23	21.50
11-15 years	18	16.82
16-20 years	18	16.82
21-25 years	17	15.89
Over 25 years	9	8.41

Of the 107 teaching staff, 25 indicated that they could teach additional subjects to medicine. Some of the subjects identified could be categorised as extra curricular activities including "rugby coaching and swimming" (Resp 66) "sailing" (Resp 106), "classical music" (Resp 90) while others (RS = 13) could be broadly classified as the sciences (biology, chemistry, physics, pharmacology, anatomy, physiology, pure and applied mathematics, statistics, information technology). A further five members of staff identifed law and ethics as being areas of specialisation with three opting for management, industrial relations, business administration and auditing. Psychotherapy, counselling skills, staff support and the Social Services were listed by four teachers while another identified "international public health". The majority (RS = 96) of the teaching staff had taught members of the other professions (see Table 5.102).

Table 5.102
Experience of teaching other professions

Other professions	RS = 96	% (N=107)
Dentists	37	38.54
DSA/DH	2	2.08
Den. Tech.	3	3.12
Nursing	90	93.75
Nut. & Diet.	25	26.04
Occ. Therapy	22	22.92
ODP	12	12.50
Physiotherapy	37	38.54
Podiatry	18	18.75
Radiography	17	17.71
Social Work	22	22.92
Sp. Therapy	11	11.46
Other professions	35 *	36.46 *

* The category "other professions" produced a variety of responses. Environmental health officers (RS = 5), nursery nurses (RS = 1), biochemists (RS = 6), medical laboratory scientific officers (RS = 5), medical photographers (RS = 1), pharmacists (RS = 8), theology students (RS = 1), physicists (RS = 2), ambulance crew (RS = 2), psychology students (RS = 5) and members of the drug industry (RS = 2).

Of the 107 medical staff, 79 indicated that they had shared learning with other professions. Only 17 of these stated that this had occured at an undergraduate stage and all 17 identified dental students as those with whom they had shared learning. The 62 who had shared learning at a post graduate stage indicated a wide spectrum of other professions. This result must however be treated with caution as it is not known whether this post graduate shared learning took place on an interdisciplinary course or whether it indicates that the majority of respondents have included attendance at a multidisciplinary conference in their answers.

Table 5.103
Teachers shared learning experiences

Other Profession	No. of Resp. (RS = 79) *	% (N=107)
Dentists	17	15.89
DSA/Dental Hyg.	2	1.87
Dental Tech.	1	0.93
Nursing	27	25.23
Nutrition & Diet.	8	7.48
Occ. Therapy	6	5.61
ODP	4	3.74
Physiotherapy	8	7.48
Podiatry	3	2.80
Radiography	9	8.41
Social Work	18	16.82
Speech Therapy	5	4.67
"Other Professions" **	19	17.75

* Several respondents gave more than one response.
** The "other professions" category evoked a variety of responses. Administrators and managers (RS = 10), psychologists (RS = 6), basic scientists (RS = 5), teachers (RS = 1), police (RS = 1), environmental health officers (RS = 1), philosophers and ethicists (RS = 1), lawyers (RS = 1).

Biographic data of the medical students

Of the 269 respondents 120 (44.61%) were male and 149 (54.65%) were female.

Table 5.104
Age of the students

Age Group	N=269	%
20 years or less	5 *	1.86
21-25 years	239	88.85
26-30 years	16	5.95
31-35 years	7	2.60
>35 years	0	0.00

* As medical students, in conjunction with dental students, complete the first two years of pre-clinical training in another University College, this response was expected. It would seem that the majority of students commence their medical training straight from secondary school with only 2.60% of the sample being more than 30 years of age.

Table 5.105
Students year stage of training

Year of Training	N=269	%
1	0 *	0.00
2	0 *	0.00
3	78	29.00
4	119	44.24
5	65	24.16
6	7	2.60

* The first and second years of training are completed in another University College.

Previous courses relevant to the medical profession

Of the 269 respondents 41(17.10%) indicated that they had undertaken courses which they considered to be relevant to their medical training. Further analysis revealed that the majority of these courses tended to be science related degrees (RS = 29). These could be categorised into BSc Pharmacology (RS = 7), BSc Physics or Chemistry (RS = 9), BSc Medical Sciences (RS = 8), B.A. Biochemistry (RS = 2), BDS (Bachelor of Dental Surgery) (RS = 1), BSc Zoology (RS = 2). The remaining five respondents had completed first aid courses. No respondents had undertaken a behavioural science degree. All seven students who were over 30 years of age had previously completed a degree.

Work experience relevant to the medical profession

Of the 269 respondents 111 indicated that they had gained relevant work experience. The majority (RS = 88) had worked on a voluntary basis with physically or mentally handicapped children, in elderly peoples homes, nursing homes, with the Overseas Development Agency or in hospices. Of these 88 students 81 (92.05%) were female. Analysis for statistical probability produced a highly significant result (χ^2 = 38,87, df = 1, p = < 0.1%) indicating that similar to the female dental students, female medical students are more likely than their male colleagues to have gained relevant work experience.

The remaining 34 students from the 122 respondents included the dental surgeon, pharmacists (RS = 3) cardiology technicians (RS = 4), industrial experience (RS = 9), personnel and management experience (RS = 3), physicists (RS = 2), biochemists (RS = 4) and physiologists (RS = 3).

Previous experience of learning with other professions

In total 62 students indicated that they had experienced shared learning with professions other than their own. Predictably the most frequent group identified was the dental students (RS = 46). This occurs during the first two years of preclinical training undertaken in another University College. It is interesting to note that although 46 medical students acknowleged the shared learning which had taken place with the dental students 205 did not ! The results can be seen in Table 5.106

Table 5.106
Student's shared learning experiences (N = 269)

Professions Involved	RS = 62 *	% of N
Dentists	46	17.10
DSA/Dent. Hygienist	0	0.00
Den. Tech.	0	0.00
Nursing	4	1.49
Nutrition & Diet.	3	1.12
Occ. Therapy	7	2.60
ODP	1	0.41
Physiotherapy	11	4.09
Podiatry	0	0.00
Radiography	6	2.23
Social Work	5	1.86
Speech Therapy	5	1.86
Other Professions	9 **	3.35

* Several students indicated that they had shared learning with more than one profession.

** The responses for "other professions" were all related to those students who had gained previous relevant work experience. The other professions included probation officers, police, environmental health officers and psychologists. The overall response to this question reveals that medical students tend not to perceive themselves as sharing learning with the other health and social care professions. It is not known whether this is because they have not been given the opportunity or whether they do not recognise or acknowledge the teaching and learning which occurs in clinical practice such as multidisciplinary ward rounds and case conferences.

Opinions regarding the concept of interdisciplinary learning

The opinions of the 107 teaching staff and the 269 students are presented together wherever possible. The rationale for this being based on the recognition that both the opinions of the teaching staff and the students were of equal importance for any future developments. It also enables a comparison to be made more easily between the two groups.

Table 5.107
Should there be interdisciplinary learning ?

Response	Teachers (N=107)	%	Students (N=269)	%	Total (N=376)	%
Yes	83	77.57	177	65.80	260	69.15
No	5	4.67	42	15.61	47	12.50
Undecided	19	17.76	47	17.47	66	17.55

A significantly greater percentage of students than teachers rejected the idea of interdisciplinary learning ($\chi^2 = 8.82$, df = 2, $p < 5\%$).

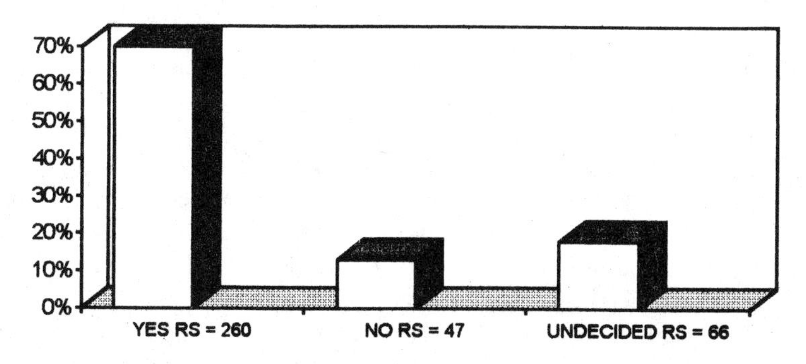

Figure 5.17 Should there be some shared learning : By percentage

Table 5.108
At which stage should it take place ?

Response	Teachers (N=107)	%	Students (N=269)	%	Total (N=376)	%
Beginning	21	19.63	37	13.75	58	15.42
Middle	9	8.41	69	23.31	78	20.74
End	2	1.87	33	12.27	35	9.31
Throughout	70	65.42	119	44.24	189	50.27
Post-Qual.	3	2.80	4	1.49	7	1.86

Only three lecturers and four students selected "post qualification" only. One lecturer (Resp. 30) replied "not at all".

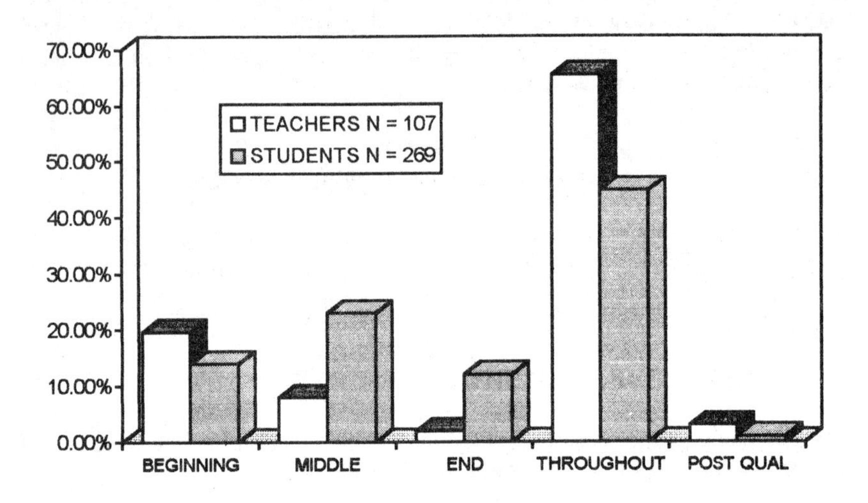

Figure 5. 18 At which stage of training should it take place ?

The majority of teachers thought that interdisciplinary learning should take place throughout training (RS = 70). A further 21 teachers suggested the beginning as the appropriate time. The medical students however were less certain with many choosing "the middle" of training (RS = 69). There was a significant difference between the teachers' and the students' responses. ($\chi^2 = 28.50$, df = 4, p = < 0.1% Yates correction applied). There may have been some confusion in the interpretation of this question however as it is not known whether the medical students included the preclinical years (completed elsewhere) as "the beginning" and therefore identified the commencement of clinical training as "the middle". What can be concluded however, is that the majority of teachers (RS = 103) and students (RS = 258) believed that some interdisciplinary learning should take place at the undergraduate stage. All respondents were asked to justify their choice. Comments included : -

1. *At the beginning*
" People become set in their ways as time goes on. New minds are generally more receptive to new ideas than minds that are already en route to specialisation." (Teacher resp. 6). "So it becomes as natural as breathing." (Student resp. 193).

2. *In the middle*
" Some experience is necessary." (Teacher resp. 29). "So we have the confidence to talk with the other professions." (Student resp. 107)

3. *At the end*
"It is vital to prepare medical students for team work." (Teacher resp. 41) "To prepare us for working as team leaders in the clinical areas." (Student resp. 205)

4. *Throughout*
"To allow continuing medical and professional education to keep pace with changing practice and trends." (Teacher resp. 1). "Achieving good healthy outcomes involves interplay of many health disciplines with social and environmental factors." (Teacher resp. 14). "So that these stupid jealousies and arguments stop and we can get on and do what I want to do which is care for the patients." (Student resp. 219)

5. *Post qualification*
"The undergraduate curriculum is too crowded." (Teacher resp. 42) "Too busy learning medicine before qualifying." (Teacher resp. 58). " I am struggling now to keep up. I am what is known as a weak student. I would love to be involved in such a programme though !" (Student resp. 94)

Table 5.109
Would there be advantages ?

Response	Teachers (N =107)	%	Students (N = 269)	%	Total (N = 3576)	%
Yes	84	78.50	177	65.80	261	69.41
No	4	3.74	42	15.61	46	12.23
Undecided	18	16.82	47	17.47	65	17.29

It would seem that the majority (78.50%) of qualified medical staff in this sample believed that there would be advantages in interdisciplinary learning. The students were less convinced with 17.47 % of the 269 respondents being uncertain. These differences may be due to the previous clinical experience of the teaching staff which has highlighted the need for closer collaboration with the other professions (χ^2 = 10.61, df = 2, p < 1%). Statistical analysis of the difference in the responses of the medical students when compared with all other students also revealed a highly significant result (χ^2 = 41.53, df = 2, p < 0.1%)

Table 5.110
Advantages of interdisciplinary learning?

Response	Teachers (RS = 65) *	Students (RS = 151) *	Totals (N =376)
Increase understanding of each others' role	41	123	164
Increase teamwork & collaboration	38	117	155
Broaden horizons, cross fertilise ideas	16	53	69
Make better use of time & scarce resources	13	3	16

* Many respondents listed more than one reason. The raw scores are therefore calculated against the total population (N = 376).

All respondents were also asked to list any disadvantages which they could identify. In total 51 teaching staff and 100 students listed disadvantages.

Table 5.111
What disadvantages would there be ?

Responses	Teachers (RS = 51)	Students (RS = 100)	Total (N = 376)
Time constraints	8	19	27
Organisational difficulties	6	3	9
Irrelevant material	19	22	41
Hierarchical domination & prejudice	6	14	20
Loss of prof. identity	0	3	3
Different academic ability	13	29	42
Different knowledge base	1	1	2
Too many students in a class	0	39	39

One student (Resp. 16), who had declared himself as "totally uninterested", commented "In real terms the process would be very hard to implement and a complete waste of time".

Table 5.112
Level of interest in interdisciplinary learning

Response	Teachers (N = 107)	%	Students (N = 269)	%	Total (N = 355)	%
Very Interested	23	21.50	25	9.29	48	12.77
Interested	46	43.00	118	43.87	164	43.62
Neutral	29	27.10	82	30.48	111	28.03
Uninterested	5	4.67	18	6.69	23	6.12
Totally Uninterested	5	4.67	18	6.69	23	6.12

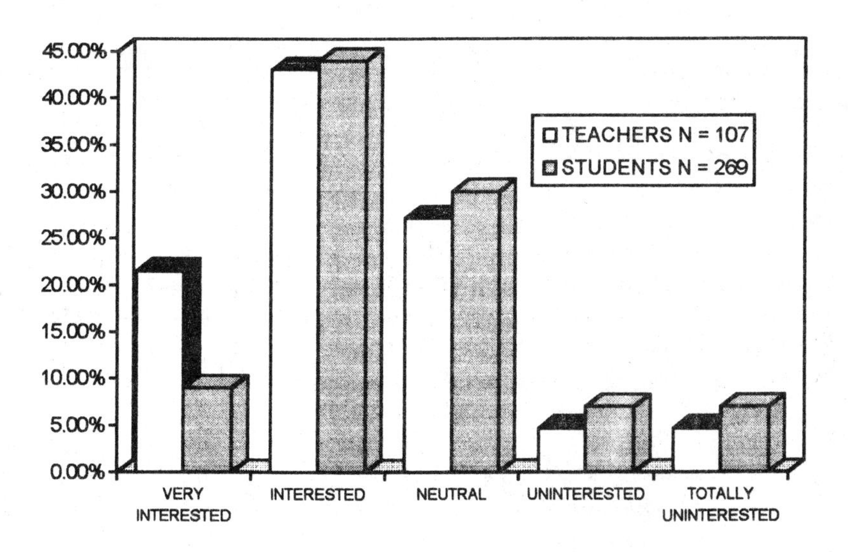

Figure 5. 19 The level of interest in interdisciplinary learning : By percentage

The results demonstrate that 69 (64.49% where N = 107) of the teaching staff and 143 (53.16% where N = 269) of the students were "interested" or "very interested" in interdisciplinary learning. A further 29 (27.10%) teachers and 82 (30.48%) students were neutral about the idea. Only 10 (9.35%) of the teaching staff and 36 (13.38%) of the students expressed little or no interest at all. Overall the teachers were more likely to express an interest in the concept than were the students ($\chi^2 = 9.97$, df = 4, p < 5%).

Table 5. 113
Subjects suitable for interdisciplinary learning

Subject	Teachers (N=107)	%	Students (N=269)	%	Total (N=376)	%
Psychology	99	92.52	185	68.77	284	75.53
Sociology	90	84.11	155	57.62	241	64.09
Ethics	103	96.26	192	71.38	295	78.46
Law & Practice	98	91.59	144	53.53	242	64.36
Research Methods	80	74.77	95	35.32	175	46.54
Management	100	93.46	129	47.95	229	60.90
Economics of Care	99	92.52	136	50.56	235	62.50
Health Promotion	101	94.39	205	76.21	306	81.38
Study Skills	86	80.37	104	38.66	190	50.53
Quality Issues	94	87.85	98	36.43	192	51.06
Structural Organisation	94	87.85	164	60.97	258	68.62
Computing Skills	95	88.78	178	66.17	273	72.61

The medical teachers were more positive than the medical students about suitable subjects for interdisciplinary learning in nearly every category. The students rejected "research methods" as a possible subject and were very uncertain about "study skills" and "quality issues". What is not known however is how relevant medical students believe these subjects are to their training anyway. What can be concluded is that the medical students returned a lower positive response rate for all categories when compared with all other student groups. Tests for significance between the teachers and students responses revealed the following findings :

Sociology : ($\chi2$ = 4.69, df = 1, $p < 5\%$)
Law & Practice : ($\chi2$ = 9.63, df = 1, $p < 0.1\%$)
Research Methods : (χ^2 = 15.86, df = 1, $p < 0.1\%$)
Management : (χ^2 = 14.63, df = 1, $p < 0.1\%$)
Economics of Care (χ^2 = 12.09, df = 1, $p < 0.1\%$)
Study Skills : (χ^2 = 15.86, df = 1, $p < 0.1\%$)
Quality Issues : (χ^2 = 22.48, df = 1, $p < 0.1\%$)
Structural Organisation: (χ^2 = 4.50, df = 1, $p < 5\%$)

The medical students had previously been asked to indicate from a list of eight subjects which ones they would include in the term "behavioural sciences" (see Table 5.114).

Table 5. 114
Subjects students included in the behavioural sciences

Subjects	Yes	%	No	%	Undecided	%
Psychology	262	97.40	2	0.74	2	0.74
Sociology	241	89.59	13	4.83	12	4.46
Ethics	147	54.65	56	20.82	63	23.42
Law & Practice	72	26.77	136	50.56	58	21.56
Management	71	26.39	149	55.39	46	17.10
Health Promotion	200	74.35	36	13.38	30	11.15
Study Skills	84	31.27	134	49.81	48	17.84
Quality Issues	60	22.30	110	40.89	96	35.69

The results demonstrate that there is a lot of indecision about what constitutes the behavioural sciences. Psychology (97.40%) and sociology (89.59%) were correctly identified by the majority of students. Health Promotion (74.35%) and ethics (54.65%) were also identified by a large number of students. Law and practice (50.56%) and management (55.39%) was rejected by more than half of the respondents. Many students were undecided about quality issues (35.69%), ethics (23.42%) and law and practice (21.56%).

The students were asked what would be appropriate learning methods in any future interdisciplinary initiatives (see Table 5.115).

Table 5.115
Students preferred interdisciplinary learning methods

Learning Method	Yes	%	No	%	Undecided	%
Tutorials	154	57.25	67	24.91	35	13.01
Workshops	123	45.72	75	27.88	58	21.56
Case Studies	119	44.24	86	31.97	50	18.59
Seminars	161	59.85	57	21.19	37	13.75
Problem Based Learning	132	49.07	57	21.19	66	24.54
Role Play	81	30.11	120	44.61	51	18.96
Lectures	90	33.46	120	44.61	45	16.73
Visits to Client Areas	182	67.66	38	14.13	35	13.01

Role play was rejected by a statistically significant number of medical students ($\chi^2 = 49.05$, df = 2, $p < 0.1\%$). Lectures on an interdisciplinary basis were also rejected by a significant number ($\chi^2 = 41.40$, df = 2, $p < 0.1\%$). There was also an unusually low response to "case studies" when compared with all other student groups.

The medical staff and students were asked to select which other professions they believed could undertake some interdisciplinary learning with their own. The results are presented as Table 5. 116 overleaf.

Table 5.116
Other professions suitable for interdisciplinary learning with the medical profession

Other Prof.	Teachers (N=107)	%	Student (N=269)	%	Total (N=376)	%
Dentists	52	48.60	93	33.57	145	38.56
DSA/DH	22	20.56	15	5.58	37	9.84
Den. Tec.	18	16.82	4	1.49	22	5.85
Nursing	87	81.31	171	63.57	258	68.62
Nut. & Diet.	55	51.40	148	55.02	203	53.99
Occ. Therapy	57	53.27	157	58.36	214	56.91
ODP	33	30.84	43	15.96	76	20.21
Physiotherapy	67	62.61	175	65.05	242	64.36
Podiatry	32	29.91	35	13.01	67	17.82
Radiography	53	49.53	150	55.76	203	53.99
Social Work	72	67.33	139	51.67	211	56.12
Sp. Therapy	46	42.99	91	33.83	137	36.44

The nursing profession was identified most frequently overall (68.62%). The medical students however selected the physiotherapists as their first choice with the nurses being second. Of particular interest is the result for potential interdisciplinary learning with social work students. More teachers (67.33%) than students (51.67%) selected this option. More teachers selected social work students (67.33%) than they did physiotherapy students (62.61%). In overall rank order, social work was the fourth most frequently selected profession suitable for interdisciplinary learning with the medical profession. This may indicate a desire to approach patient care from a truly biopsychosocial stance. While 84.21% of the dental profession in this study wanted to share some learning with the medical profession only 38.56% of the medical profession were of the same opinion.

5.5.3.5 The nurses

Ninety seven teaching staff completed the questionnaire all of whom were qualified nurses, midwives or health visitors. Twenty nine of the respondents were male and sixty eight female. Three hundred and ninety six students completed the questionnaire, sixty threee of whom were male and three hundred and thirty three were female. The respondents comprised teaching staff from a Department of Nursing Studies in a University College and also from an Institute of Nursing and Midwifery Education. The student respondents were either on the undergraduate Bachelor of Nursing four year degree programme or from the Project 2000 programmes which first commenced in the Institute in April 1992. Student nurses completing the traditional training were not included in this study as a decision had been made before the content analysis of the curricula began that courses which were not anticipated to continue after 1993 should be excluded. The biographic data of the teaching staff and students is presented separately.

Biographic data of the teaching staff

Table 5.117
Age of the teaching staff

Age Group	N = 97	%
Under 25 years	0	0.00
25 - 30 years	0	0.00
31 - 35 years	16	16.67
36 - 40 years	25	26.04
41 - 45 years	27	28.12
46 - 50 years	13	13.54
51 - 55 years	5	5.21
56 - 60 years	6	6.25
Over 60 years	0	0.00

Table 5.118
Years in practice before commencing teaching career

No. of years in practice	N = 97	%
Less than one year	0 *	0.00
1 - 5 years	26	27.08
6 - 10 years	42	43.75
11 - 15 years	18	18.75
16 - 20 years	10	10.42
21 25 years	0	0.00
Over 25 years	0	0.00

* This result was predictable as there are clearly prescribed criteria for entry into nurse teaching (UKCC /PS &D/ 88/03). The criteria include an advanced nursing qualification and a minimum of 3 years clinical practice.

Table 5.119
Years in teaching

No. of years in teaching	N = 97	%
Less than one year	2	2.08
1 - 5 years	27	28.12
6 - 10 years	23	23.96
11 - 15 years	28	29.17
16 - 20 years	10	10.42
21 - 25 years	4	4.17
Over 25 years	2	2.08

Fifty nine (61.46%) of the teachers identified additional areas which they could teach. One of the reasons for this high response rate could be due to the move over the recent years towards an all graduate profession for teachers of nurses, midwives and health visitors. In 1993 most new entrants to nurse teaching are graduates already but for those individuals who have been teaching some years the change to graduate status has been more gradual. The additional subject areas identified are displayed in Table 5.120.

Table 5.120
Additional related subjects

Subject	RS = 59
Psychology	10
Sociology	7
Ethics	7
Law, Criminology	3
Philosophy	4
Complementary Health Therapies	2
Counselling	7
Management	6
Education	9
Research Methods	5
Biological Sciences	5
Maths & Statistics	2

Additional subjects were described as Womens Health (RS = 1), Dental Health (RS = 1), Professional Development (RS = 1) and "Flower Arranging" (RS = 1). Sixty members of the teaching staff had taught professions other than their own. The professions identified are presented as Table 5.121.

Table 5.121
Experience of teaching other professions

Other Professions	RS = 60	% (N = 97)
Dentists	0	0.00
DSA/Dent. Hygienist	1	1.04
Den. Tech.	2	2.08
Medicine	18	18.56
Nut & Diet.	7	7.22
Occ. Therapy	17	17.53
ODP	11	11.34
Physiotherapy	26	26.80
Podiatry	1	1.04
Radiography	10	10.31
Social Work	17	17.53
Speech Therapy	2	2.08
"Other Professions"	22	22.68

The 22 respondent teachers who identified "other professions" described these as teachers (RS = 5), policemen (RS = 3), clergy (RS = 2), psychologists (RS = 3), managers & administrators (RS = 4), orthoptists (RS = 1), counsellors (RS = 2), environmental health officers (RS = 1), ambulance crew (RS = 1), medical photographers (RS = 2), sports trainers (RS = 1) and engineers (RS = 1).

Most respondents (RS =70) had experienced shared learning during their professional career. Only six indicated that they had done so at an undergraduate stage. The majority (RS = 64) had learned with other professions after qualification.

Of the 39 teachers who indicated "other professions" 28 identified their teaching training course as their interdisciplinary experience (Cert. Ed./PGCE). The other professions were identified as pharmacists (RS = 3), architects (RS = 4), NHS managers (RS = 5), prison officers (RS = 3), Armed Forces (RS = 2), librarians (RS = 1), economists (RS = 1), vetinerary students (RS = 1), housing association staff (RS = 2), environmental health officers (RS = 3), police (RS = 3), chaplains (RS = 2), psychologists (RS = 4), science students (RS = 1), medical illustrators (RS = 2).

Table 5.122
Teacher's experiences of shared learning

Other profession	(RS = 70)	% (N = 97)
Dentists	4	4.12
DSA/Den.Hygienist	1	1.06
Den. Tech.	2	2.06
Medicine	26	26.80
Nut. & Diet.	19	19.59
Occ. Therapy	20	20.8
ODP	2	2.06
Physiotherapy	21	21.65
Podiatry	7	7.22
Radiography	15	15.46
Social Work	31	31.96
Speech Therapy	7	7.22
"Other Profession"	39	40.21

Biographic data of the nursing students

Table 5.123
Age of the students

Age Group	N = 396	%
20 years or less	159	40.15
21 - 25 years	128	32.32
26 - 30 years	40	10.10
31 - 35 years	31	7.83
36 - 40 years	24	6.06
41 - 45 years	6	1.52
46 - 50 years	2	0.51
51 - 55 years	0	0.00
Over 55 years	0	0.00

The majority of nursing students (72.47%) of the sample were less than 25 years of age. Over 27% (RS = 95) however, were 26 years or older with two students declaring themselves to be more than 46 years old. It is likely therefore that many of the 396 students have had previous employment and have gained qualifications prior to commencing their nursing careers.

Table 5.124
Student's year stage of training

Year of Training	N = 396	%
1	234	59.09
2	125	31.57
3	22 *	5.56
4	8 *	2.02
5	0	0.00
Other	2 **	0.51

* The disproportionate number of students currently training can be explained. The undergraduate Bachelor of Nursing is a 4 year programme. Project 2000, (a 3 year programme) only commenced in April 1992. The students on this programme therefore are in either the first or second year of training. There are no third year Project 2000 nurses as yet. The 22 third year and eight fourth year respondents are therefore Bachelor of Nursing students.

** Two students indicated that they did not meet the criteria for years one to five. The reason for this is not known.

Of the 396 nursing students 119 had completed previous courses. These varied considerably from graduate programmes (RS = 29) to BTEC (RS = 36).

Table 5.125
Previous relevant courses

Relevant courses	N = 396
BSc (Hons) Psychology	7
BSc (Hons) Sociology	3
B. Ed (Hons)	5
BSc Life Sciences	4
BSc Biology	2
BSc Human Sciences	1
BSc Zoology	2
B.A. (Open Univ.)	5
BTEC Dip. Health Studies	24
BTEC Dip. Social Care	5
Access Life Science Course	7
NNEB (Nursery Nursing)	3
NVQ Level 1 - 3	9
Medical Tech. Courses	1
Pharmacy Tech. Courses	3
Pre Nursing Courses	14
Para medical training	6
Cert Ed./PGCE	9

These findings reveal that of the 396 nursing students in this sample at least 29 (7.32%) were graduate entrants. As the questionnaire requested information regarding relevant courses it may be that other nursing students were also graduates but with degrees that they did not consider relevant to health care.

Other courses completed by nursing students included veterinary nursing (RS = 1), first aid (N = 19), Mencap (N = 3) and NHS management (RS = 2).

Nearly two thirds of the respondents had gained relevant work experience (RS = 256, 64.5%). Many had had several jobs which they considered relevant. A large number of respondents had worked in different health and social care settings as part of their Access, NVQ and BTEC courses (RS = 44). Others had worked as auxilliary nurses (RS = 112) while waiting for their courses to commence. Voluntary work was frequently identified (RS = 63). Other relevant work experience was variously described as health and safety officer (RS = 2), environmental health officer (RS = 3), dispensing optician (RS =1), the police force (RS = 7), probation officer (RS = 2), counsellor (RS = 9), laboratory assistants (RS = 5), paramedic (RS = 6) and residential care officers (RS = 11).

A surprising number indicated that they had had the opportunity to learn with other professions (RS = 79). On further analysis of the responses however it seems most likely that this experience took place before the commencement of nurse training and occured during clinical placements on the Access, NVQ and BTEC courses or while working as auxilliary nurses and voluntary helpers. Of the 15 respondents who indicated "other professions" the professions identified reflected the job that the student had previously held. The probation officers and police, for example, had shared learning with each other, social workers and with residential care officers.

Table 5.126
Student's experiences of shared learning

Professions Involved	N = 396	%
Dentists	7	1.77
DSA/Den. Hygienists	8	2.02
Den. Tech.	3	0.76
Medicine	25	6.31
Nut. & Diet.	16	4.04
Occ. Therapy	25	6.31
ODP	4	1.01
Physiotherapy	29	7.32
Podiatry	4	1.01
Radiography	8	2.02
Social Work	21	5.30
Speech Therapy	12	3.03
"Other Professions"	15	3.78

Opinions regarding the concept of interdisciplinary learning

The opinions of the 97 teachers and the 396 students are displayed together wherever possible.

Table 5.127
Should there be interdisciplinary learning ?

Response	Teachers (N = 97)	%	Students (N=396)	%	Total (N=493)	%
Yes	84	86.60	344	86.87	428	86.82
No	5	5.15	9	2.34	14	2.84
Undecided	8	8.25	38	9.60	46	9.33

No significance was found between the opinions of the teachers and the students ($\chi^2 = 1.69$, df = 2, $p > 5\%$)

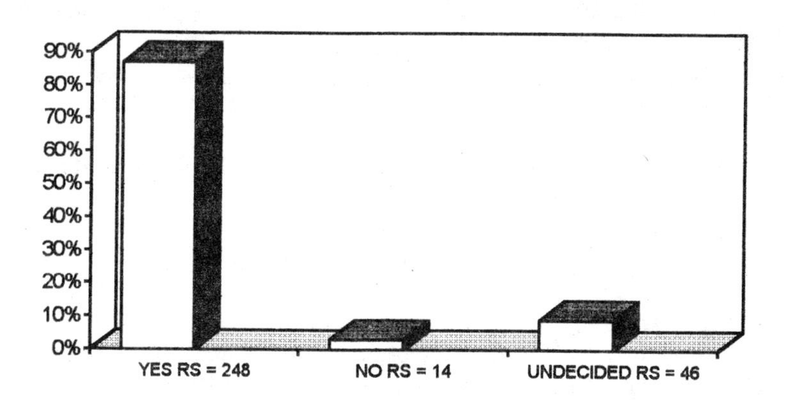

Figure 5. 20 Should there be interdisciplinary learning : By percentage

Table 5.128
At which stage should it take place ?

Response	Teachers (N = 97)	%	Students (N =396)	%	Total (N = 492)	%
Beginning	22	22.68	51	12.87	73	14.81
Middle	2	2.06	81	20.45	83	16.84
End	4	4.12	23	5.81	27	5.47
Throughout	69	71.13	239	60.35	308	62.47
Post. Qual.	0	0.00	7	1.77	7	0.20

The majority of teachers and students selected "throughout" as their preferred option. There was a statistically significant difference in the percentage of teachers (2.06%) and students (20.45%) who chose the "middle of training" ($\chi^2 = 23.64$, df = 4, $p < 0.1\%$)

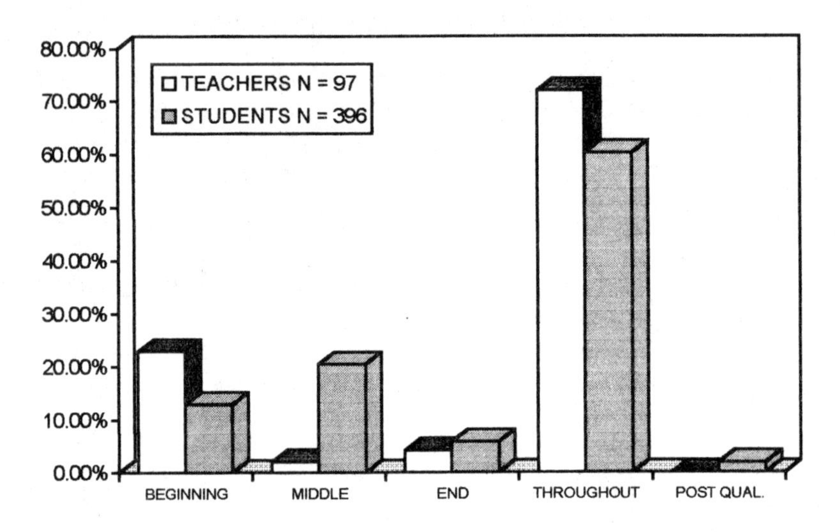

Figure 5.21 At which stage should it should take place? : By percentage

Comments from individual teachers and students were varied but nearly alwasupportive of the concept of some interdisciplinary learning.

1. *Beginning of training*

"The commonality of many of the subjects is best suited for an introductory approach. As the student progresses a more specific plan of study would be required to facilitate the application of the topic to their own area of practice." (Teacher resp. 40). "On going interaction is the key to sharing." (Student resp. 384)

2. *Middle of training*

"Professionals will/should have had enough insight into their course to appreciate the input of others." (Teacher resp. 95) "You would have some knowledge and so wouldn't feel so daunted by meeting so many different people." (Student Resp. 259)

3. *End of training*

"Students need to speak from the basis of some justified authority, experience enables theory to be explored. People would therefore be better placed, be confident to express themselves and have more to offer."(Teacher Resp. 13). "So you would have a firm knowledge of your own part of the professions first." (Student Resp. 176)

4. *Throughout training*
"......at the beginning of education and training it would help to sow the seeds of collaboration. At the end there would be sufficient understanding of ones' own profession to facilitate shared learning and after qualifying with the benefit of shared learning could be most fruitful. Perhaps by all this I mean throughout training"! (Teacher Resp. 21). "I think it is important to have continuity throughout the course so we are able to link what we have learned with what we practice." (Student Resp. 358).

The identified advantages and disadvantages of learning with other professions were similar to those described by the other professional groups.

Table 5.129
Would there be advantages ?

Response	Teachers (N = 97)	%	Students (N = 396)	%	Total (N = 492)	%
Yes	84	87.49	314	79.29	398	80.89
No	3	3.12	10	2.52	13	2.64
Undecided	8	8.33	67	16.92	75	15.24

The responses of the teachers and students were similar in that the majority believed that there would be advantages in interdisciplinary learning ($\chi^2 = 4.40$, $df = 2$, $p > 5\%$)

Table 5.130
Advantages of interdisciplinary learning

Response	Teachers (RS = 65)	Students (RS = 293)	Total (N = 492)
Increase understanding of each others role	61	121	182
Increase teamwork & collaboration	41	147	188
Broaden horizons, cross fertilise ideas	37	116	153
Make better use of time & scarce resources	15	4	19

One nursing student commented; "For the patient's sake I believe that it is absolutely essential that we all work as a team and the only way we will ever *really* do that is to learn together" (Resp. 248).

Table 5.131
Disadvantages of interdisciplinary learning

Responses	Teachers (RS = 64)	Students (RS = 134)	Total
Loss of teaching posts	23 *	0	23
Time constraints	4	7	11
Organisational difficulties	7	5	12
Irrelevant material	18	29	47
Hierarchical domination & prejudice	16	30	46
Loss of prof. identity	6	13	19
Different academic ability	5	6	11
Different knowledge base	0	9	9
Too many students in a class	0	11	11

* 23 nurse teachers mentioned the possibilty of job losses. No other group of teachers raised this issue. The possible reasons for this result are discussed in Chapter 6.

One nursing student observed; "I would want to be sure that nursing was favourably represented and not simply included as tokenism which is sometimes the case in multidisciplinary groups." (Resp. 226) Another student was concerned that; "It could deepen or confirm some professions' worst fears of others i.e. doctors/nurses, doctors/dentists, physios/occupational therapists if it is not structured properly." (Resp. 125)

Table 5.132
Level of interest in interdisciplinary learning

Level of Interest	Teachers (N = 97)	%	Students (N = 396)	%	Total (N = 492)	%
Very Interested	41	42.27	117	29.55	158	32.05
Interested	42	42.30	201	50.76	243	49.29
Neutral	8	8.25	56	14.14	64	12.98
Uninterested	3	3.09	5	1.26	8	1.62
Totally Uninterested	2	2.06	5	1.26	7	1.42

The teachers and students were similar in their level of interest in interdisciplinary learning. Although a greater percentage of teachers declared themselves to be "very interested" than did the students there was no statistical significance in this finding (χ^2 = 7.75, df = 4, p > 5%) with a significant Spearman Rank Coefficient of Rs = 0.97, n = 5, p < 5%.

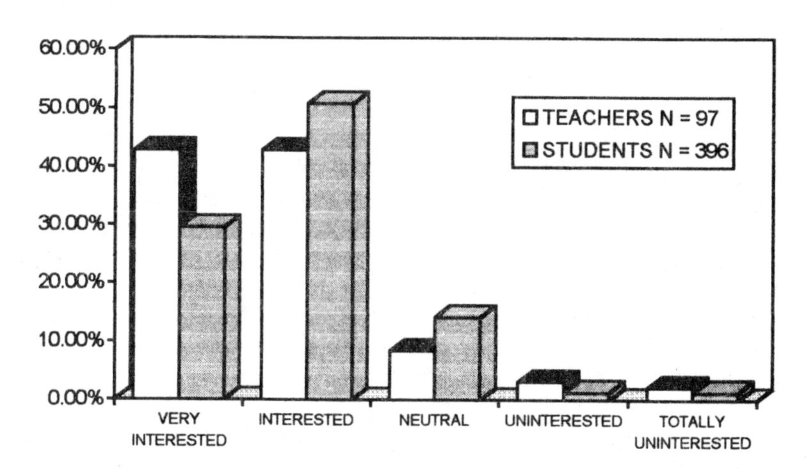

Figure 5.22 The level of interest in interdisciplinary learning : By percentage

Very few teachers expressed little or no interest in the idea of interdisciplinary teaching with 85.57% of the respondents declaring that they were "interested" or "very interested" in the idea. The response from the nursing students was similar with 80.30% of the sample expressing that they were "interested" or "very interested".

All respondents were asked to select from a given list what they thought were suitable topics for learning on an interdisciplinary learning basis. (See Table 5.133, next page))

The majority of teachers and students in the nursing profession believed that some of each of the core subjects identified as a behavioural science could be taught on an interdisciplinary basis. There was however significantly more support from the teachers in the following subjects ;

management (χ^2 = 4.02, df = 1, p < 5%),
study skills (χ^2 = 5.14, df = 1, p < 5%) and
quality issues (χ^2 = 4.71, df = 1, p < 5%).

Table 5.133
Subjects suitable for interdisciplinary learning

Subject	Teachers (N = 97)	%	Students (N = 396)	%	Total (N = 492)	%
Psychology	93	96.87	360	90.90	453	92.07
Sociology	94	97.92	357	90.15	451	91.67
Ethics	91	94.79	342	86.36	433	88.08
Law & Practice	87	90.62	257	64.89	344	69.92
Research Methods	88	91.67	264	66.67	352	71.54
Management	83	86.46	241	60.86	324	65.85
Economics of care	90	93.75	317	80.05	407	82.72
Health Promotion	94	97.91	369	93.18	463	94.10
Study Skills	92	95.83	258	65.15	350	71.14
Quality Issues	90	93.75	256	64.65	346	70.33
Structural Organisation	93	96.87	321	81.06	414	84.15
Computing Skills	93	96.87	304	76.77	397	80.69

The students were asked to choose which subjects they would include in the behavioural sciences.

Table 5.134
Subjects students included in the behavioural sciences

Subjects	Yes	%	No	%	Undecided	%
Psychology	381	96.21	3	0.76	7	1.77
Sociology	357	90.15	13	3.28	21	5.30
Ethics	176	44.44	91	22.98	124	31.31
Law & Practice	131	33.08	174	43.93	86	21.72
Management	121	30.55	166	41.92	92	23.23
Health Promotion	234	59.09	86	21.72	68	17.17
Study Skills	139	35.10	163	41.16	89	22.47
Quality Issues	113	28.54	108	27.27	170	42.93

Consistent with the responses from the other professions, nursing students seemed undecided about which subjects consitute the behavioural sciences.

Table 5.135
Preferred interdisciplinary learning methods: Students

Learning Method	Yes	%	No	%	Undecided	%
Tutorials	252	63.64	57	14.39	87	21.97
Workshops	291	73.48	44	11.11	47	11.87
Case Studies	266	67.17	39	9.85	91	22.98
Seminars	221	55.81	56	14.14	106	26.77
Problem Based Learning	254	64.14	35	8.84	107	27.02
Role Play	171	43.18	126	31.82	99	25.00
Lectures	210	53.03	82	20.71	104	26.26
Visits to Client Areas	307	77.53	37	9.34	52	13.13

The nurses were slightly more positive than most of the other student groups about role play as an acceptable learning method but more than half of the sample (56.82%) either rejected the idea completely or were undecided. Tests for significance still produced a highly significant result ($\chi^2 = 112.31$, df = 2, $p < 0.1\%$) All teaching staff and students were asked with which other professions they could share learning.

Table 5.136
Other professions suitable for interdisciplinary learning with nurses

Other Prof.	Teachers (N = 97)	%	Students (N = 396)	%	Total (N = 492)	%
Dentists	31	32.29	72	18.18	103	20.93
DSA/DH	28	29.17	164	41.41	192	39.02
Den. Tec.	21	21.87	51	12.88	72	14.63
Medicine	80	83.33	309	78.03	389	79.07
Nut. & Diet	66	68.75	340	85.86	406	82.52
Occ. Therapy	75	78.12	328	82.82	403	81.91
ODP	34	35.42	178	44.95	212	43.09
Physiotherapy	80	83.33	317	80.05	397	80.69
Podiatry	43	44.79	149	37.63	192	39.02
Radiography	39	40.62	137	34.60	176	35.77
Social Work	81	84.37	317	80.05	398	80.89
Sp. Therapy	60	62.50	254	64.14	314	63.82

Overall nurses thought that there was greater potential for interdisciplinary learning with nutritionists and dietitians, occupational therapists, social workers and physiotherapists than with the medical practitioners. The nurse teachers however were more supportive of learning with the medical practitioners than the students but this result was not statistically significant ($\chi^2 = 1.75$, df =1, $p > 5\%$). A possible explanation for the overall results may be the move away from the medical model to the holistic biopsychosocial model of care. A much greater emphasis has been placed on the holistic model of care in the Project 2000 programme than in the traditional training. It would have been interesting to compare these results with those of a sample of nurses who are completing their training on the old programme.

5.5.3.6 The nutritionists and dietitians

There are a relatively small number of teachers and students in this school. The questionnaire was distributed through the internal post to all four teachers with a 100% return. Direct access to three of the student year groups was obtained but the second year students were contacted with a postal questionnaire as they were away on clinical placements throughout the United Kingdom until the autumn of 1993. In total 45 nutrition and dietetics students completed the questionnaire.

Biographic data of the teaching staff

All four teachers were female with one aged between 36 and 40 years, four between 41 and 45 years and the other two aged between 46 and 50 years. The number of years in clinical practice before teaching varied from less than one year (RS = 1), 1 to 5 years (RS = 2) and 6 to 10 years (RS = 1). One lecturer had been teaching for more than 25 years, one between 21 and 25 years, another between 16 and 20 years and the youngest between 11 and 15 years. Three of the teachers identified additional subjects which they could teach. The subjects were research methods (RS = 2), computing skills, food science, educational methods and physiology. All four had taken the opportunity to teach professions other than their own. The others mentioned were medicine, nursing (RS = 3), social work, caterers (RS = 2), speech therapists and teachers. Two of the four respondents had participated in learning with professions other than their own. One of these had occured at the undergraduate stage with the dental profession and with home economists. The other respondent had shared learning after qualification with dental technicians, medics, nurses, podiatrists, social workers and speech therapists.

Biographic data of the nutrition and dietetics students

In total 45 students completed the questionnaire. Of these 41 were female and four were male. Fifteen were in the first year, five in the second year, ten in the third and 15 in the fourth year. The students were mainly less than 25 years of age.

Table 5.137
Age of the students

Age Group	(N = 45)	%
20 years or less	11	24.44
21 - 25 years	27	60.00
26 - 30 years	3	6.67
31 - 35 years	1	2.22
36 - 40 years	1	2.22
41 - 45 years	1	2.22
46 - 50 years	0	0.00
51 - 55 years	0	0.00
Over 55 years	0	0.00

Five of the students stated that they had completed previous relevant courses. One had completed an International Health Diploma, two had completed pre nursing Access courses and another had completed a food hygiene course. The fifth respondent did not identify the course. Twenty seven had gained relevant work experience. This was variously described as pharmacy assistant (RS = 3), voluntary work (RS = 7), health care assistant/nursing auxilliary (RS = 7), doctors receptionists (RS = 2), shadowing dietitians (RS = 3), health club (RS = 1), customer care relations officer (RS = 1), au pair (RS = 1), raising own family (RS = 1), physiotherapy assistant (RS = 1) work experience in dental hospital (RS = 1).

Only three students indicated that they had had the opportunity to learn with other professions. One with nurses, another with physiotherapists and the third with medical practitioners, social workers and psychologists. The respondent who had learned with nurses had been a nursing auxilliary and likewise the student who had assisted physiotherapists indicated physiotherapy. The response from the third student cannot be explained.

The opinions of the nutritionists and dietitians regarding the concept of shared learning

Table 5.138
Should there be interdisciplinary learning ?

Response	Teachers (N = 4)	%	Students (N = 45)	%	Total (N = 49)	%
Yes	4	100.00	42	93.33	46	93.88
No	0	0.00	1	2.22	1	2.04
Undecided	0	0.00	2	4.44	2	4.08

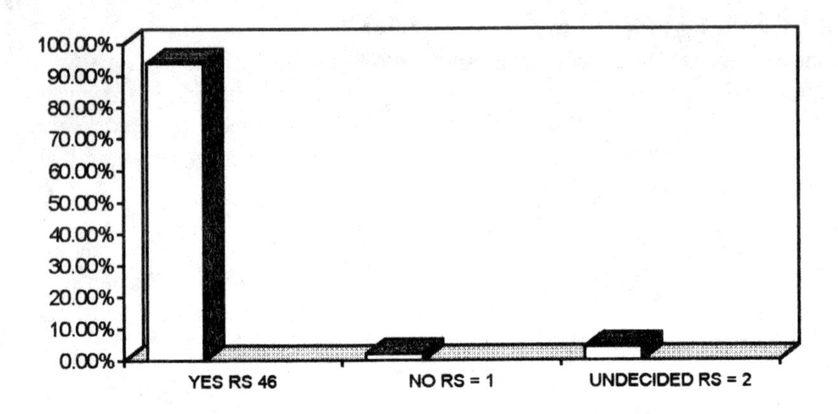

Figure 5.23 Should there be interdisciplinary learning ? : By percentage

Table 5.139
At which stage should it take place ?

Response	Teachers (N = 4)	%	Students (N = 45)	%	Total (N = 49)	%
Beginning	0	0.00	7	15.56	7	14.29
Middle	1	25.00	6	13.33	7	14.29
End	0	0.00	8	17.78	8	16.33
Throughout	3	75.00	22	48.89	25	51.02
Post Qual.	0	0.00	2	4.44	2	4.08

1. *Beginning of training*
"Because it prevents the genesis of prejudice." (Student Resp.18). "So that common subjects that apply to all can be shared and form a basis for all health professions." (Student Resp.5)

2. *Middle of training*
"Because a lot of knowledge about your own profession would be needed for this." (Student Resp. 9) "Some basic info. needed first and specialisation at the end therefore middle." (sic) (Teacher Resp. 4)

3. *End of training*
"At the end of training we have had some clinical experience of our own and have more to offer. Also we understand more about our own profession at this stage." (Student Resp. 14)

4. *Post Qualification*
One student selected 'post qualifying' justifying her decision by stating that, "after qualifying you should know what to do with the material." (Student Resp. 34) Interestingly this student did not list any advantages in interdisciplinary learning but identified several disadvantages. She also declared herself to be 'totally uninterested' in the idea.

5. *Throughout training*
"To give a better understanding of what other professionals do, to foster working together, being part of a team." (Teacher Resp.1) "We could build on each others experiences at every stage." (Student Resp. 10)

Table 5.140
Would there be advantages ?

Response	Teachers (N = 4)	%	Students (N = 45)	%	Total (N = 49)	%
Yes	4	100.0	41	91.11	45	91.84
No	0	0.00	4	8.89	4	8.16
Undecided	0	0.00	0	0.00	0	0.00

Table 5.141
Advantages of interdisciplinary learning

Response	Teachers (RS = 4)	Students (RS = 31)	Total (N = 49)
Increase understanding of each others role	3	19	22
Increase teamwork & collaboration	3	25	28
Broaden horizons, cross fertilise ideas	2	18	20
Make better use of time & scarce resources	1	1	2

Table 5.142
Disadvantages of interdisciplinary learning

Response	Teachers (RS = 3)	Students (RS = 15)	Total (N = 49)
Time constraints	0	2	2
Organisational difficulties	1	0	1
Irrelevant material	3	13	16
Hierarchical domination & prejudice	0	3	3
Loss of professional identity	0	3	3
Different academic ability	0	0	0
Different knowledge base	0	0	0
Too many students in a class	0	7	7

One student (Resp 33) raised the issue of how patient confidentiality could be maintained but then concluded; " Now I come to think of it, discussing this sort of problem with other members of the team would make it easier, not worse !"

Table 5.143
Level of interest in interdisciplinary learning

Level of interest	Teachers (N = 4)	%	Students (N = 45)	%	Total (N = 49)	%
Very interested	0	0.00	25	55.56	25	51.02
Interested	4	100.	18	40.00	22	44.90
Neutral	0	0.00	1	2.22	1	2.04
Uninterested	0	0.00	1	2.22	1	2.04
Totally uninterested	0	0.00	0	0.00	0	0.00

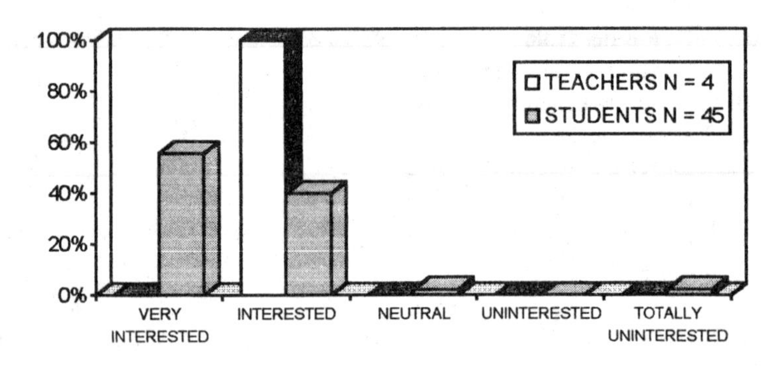

Figure 5.24 Level of interest in interdisciplinary learning

All four teachers expressed an interest in interdisciplinary learning with 43 students (95.6%) declaring themselves to be either "very interested" (RS = 25) or "interested" (RS = 18).

The respondents identified core subjects suitable, in their opinion, for interdisciplinary learning.

Table 5.144
Subjects suitable for interdisciplinary learning

Subject	Teachers (N = 4)	%	Students (N = 45)	%	Total (N = 49)	%
Psychology	4	100.0	43	95.56	47	95.92
Sociology	4	100.0	43	95.56	47	95.92
Ethics	4	100.0	39	86.67	43	87.76
Law & Practice	3	75.00	16	35.56	19	38.78
Research Methods	4	100.0	22	48.89	26	53.06
Management	4	100.0	31	68.89	35	71.43
Econ. of health care	4	100.0	36	80.00	40	81.63
Health Promotion	4	100.0	41	91.11	45	91.84
Study Skills	4	100.0	28	62.22	32	65.31
Quality Issues	4	100.0	27	60.00	31	63.27
Structural Organisation	4	100.0	34	75.56	38	77.55
Computing Skills	4	100.0	39	86.67	43	87.76

Consistent with the results from the other professions psychology, sociology and health promotion were chosen by more than 90% of the nutrition and dietetics respondents in this sample. Ethics, economics of health care and computing skills were also chosen by the majority of respondents.

The students had previously indicated which topics they would include in the behavioural sciences. The results are presented in Table 5. 145 (See next page)

The results demonstrate that nutrition and dietetics students accept psychology (100.00%) and sociology (95.56%) as the behavioural sciences but they are unsure about many of the other subjects. No subject was rejected outright with ethics, law and practice and quality issues causing the most indecision.

While most of the suggested learning strategies would be acceptable to the majority of students role play was accepted by only 5 students (11.11%). This was a highly significant finding ($\chi^2 = 56.95$, df = 2, p $< 0.1\%$)

Table 5.145
Subjects students included in the behavioural sciences

Subjects	Yes	%	No	%	Undecided	%
Psychology	45	100.00	0	0.00	0	0.00
Sociology	43	95.56	0	0.00	2	4.44
Ethics	24	53.33	2	4.44	19	42.22
Law & Prac.	6	13.33	19	42.22	20	44.44
Management	12	26.67	16	35.56	17	37.78
Health Promotion	35	77.78	4	8.89	6	13.33
Study Skills	19	42.22	11	24.44	15	33.33
Quality Issues	12	26.67	12	26.67	21	46.67

Table 5.146
Student's preferred interdisciplinary learning methods

Learning Methods	Yes	%	No	%	Undecided	%
Tutorials	36	80.00	5	11.11	4	8.89
Workshops	32	71.11	1	2.22	12	26.67
Case Studies	33	73.33	3	6.67	9	20.00
Seminars	25	55.56	7	15.56	13	28.89
Problem Based Learning	27	60.00	2	4.44	16	35.56
Role Play	5	11.11	19	42.22	21	46.67
Lectures	26	57.78	13	28.89	6	13.33
Visits to Client Areas	35	77.78	2	4.44	8	17.78

Finally, the teachers and students identified the other professions with which they believed interdisciplinary learning would be beneficial. (See Table 5.147 next page)

All 49 (100.00%) respondents identified nurses as an appropriate profession with which to share learning. The medical profession was also chosen by the majority of the respondents (87.76%). An unexpected finding was that 81.63% selected social workers in preference to speech therapists (69.39%) and the dental professions, dentists (48.98%) DSA/DH (32.65%) and dental technicians (8.16%). No teacher selected the dentists as opposed to 53.33% of the students .

Table 5.147
Other professions suitable for learning with nutritionists and dietitians

Other Prof.	Teachers (N = 4)	%	Students (N = 45)	%	Total (N = 49)	%
Dentists	0	0.00	24	53.33	24	48.98
DSA/DH	0	0.00	16	35.56	16	32.65
Den. Tec.	0	0.00	4	8.89	4	8.16
Medicine	2	50.00	41	91.11	43	87.76
Nursing	4	100.00	45	100.00	49	100.0
Occ. Ther.	3	75.00	30	66.67	33	67.35
ODP	0	0.00	8	17.78	8	16.33
Physio.	2	50.00	27	60.00	29	59.18
Podiatry	1	25.00	12	26.67	13	26.53
Radiog.	1	25.00	20	44.44	21	42.86
S.W.	3	75.00	37	82.22	40	81.63
Sp. Ther.	4	100.00	30	66.67	34	69.39

5.5.3.7 The occupational therapists

Seven teaching staff completed the questionnaire all of whom were qualified occupational therapists. Two were male and five were female. Eighty nine students completed the questionnaire of whom nine were male and eighty were female. Additional biographic data of each set of respondents is presented separately.

Biographic data of the teaching staff

The ages of the teaching staff ranged from 25-30 years (RS = 1), 31 - 35 years (RS = 2), 41 - 45 years (RS = 3) with one respondent being aged between 46-50 years. All teachers were in clinical practice for either 6 - 10 years (RS = 3) or 11 - 15 years (RS = 4) before they commenced their teaching careers. The majority (RS = 4) had been teaching for 1 - 5 years, two had been teaching for 6 - 10 years and the other for 16 - 20 years. Five of the seven teachers identified additional subjects that they could teach. These subjects comprised fieldwork education, health education, communication skills, health service management, legal aspects of mental health, education, "scuba diving", management and systems theory. All seven had taken the opportunity to teach students from other professions. The professions identified were medicine (RS = 3), nursing (RS = 3), physiotherapy (RS = 4), radiography (RS = 3), social work (RS = 2), speech therapy (RS = 2), pharmacists (RS = 1), psychologists (RS = 1), medical physicists (RS = 1), physiological measurement technicians (RS = 1) and hospital management trainees (RS = 1). All seven teachers had learned with professions other than their own, only two however had done so at an undergraduate level. Five of the respondents had shared learning with physiotherapists, with four of these indicating that they had also learned with a variety of other professions while undertaking teaching training. Two of the teachers had also completed management courses with a variety of other personnel in health care.

Biographic data of the occupational therapy students
Eighty nine occupational therapy students completed the questionnaire.

Table 5.148
Age of the students

Age Group	N = 89	%
20 years or less	21	23.59
21 - 25 years	36	40.45
26 - 30 years	13	14.61
31 - 35 years	6	6.74
36 - 40 years	2	2.25
41 - 45 years	7	7.87
46 - 50 years	3	3.79
> 5 years	0	0.00

The majority (64.04%) of occupational therapy students were less than 26 years of age. A significant number (35.96%) however were mature students.

Table 5.149
Students year stage of training

Year of training	N = 89	%
1	30	33.71
2	26	29.21
3	33	37.08
4	0	0.00
5	0	0.00
Other	0	0.00

Twenty one students indicated that they had completed relevant courses prior to commencing their training. These were variously described as B.Sc Social Sciences (RS = 4), B.A./B.Sc. Psychology (RS = 2), Counselling (RS = 2), B.Tec. Diploma in Social Care (RS = 3), B. Tec. Health Studies (RS = 2), Radiography

(RS = 1), Registered General Nurse (RS = 3), teacher training (RS = 4), managerial courses (RS = 3), British sign language course (RS = 1). Sixty three students (70.79%) had obtained relevant work experience. Much of this was on a voluntary basis (RS = 26) but 23 students had gained experience as occupational therapy helpers, 16 as nursing auxilliaries, one had worked as a policeman, three as registered nurses, two as probation officers, one as a medical laboratory scientific officer, one as a dental nurse, a teacher of children with special needs, radiography (RS = 1), physiotherapy assistant (RS = 1), podiatry assistant (RS = 1), social services (RS = 3).

Only eight students indicated that they had shared learning with any other health or social care profession. All eight had previously gained relevant work experience or undertaken other relevant courses. Six of the students had shared learning with social workers. This included the former policeman, the probation officer, the teacher of children with special needs and one of the respondents who had worked in social services. There was no evidence to suggest that any interdisciplinary learning had taken place during occupational therapy training.

The opinions of the occupational therapists regarding the concept of interdisciplinary learning

Table 5.150
Should there be interdisciplinary learning ?

Response	Teachers (N = 7)	%	Students (N = 89)	%	Total (N = 96)	%
Yes	5	71.43	84	94.38	89	92.71
No	0	0.00	0	0.00	0	0.00
Undecided	2	28.57	5	5.62	7	7.29

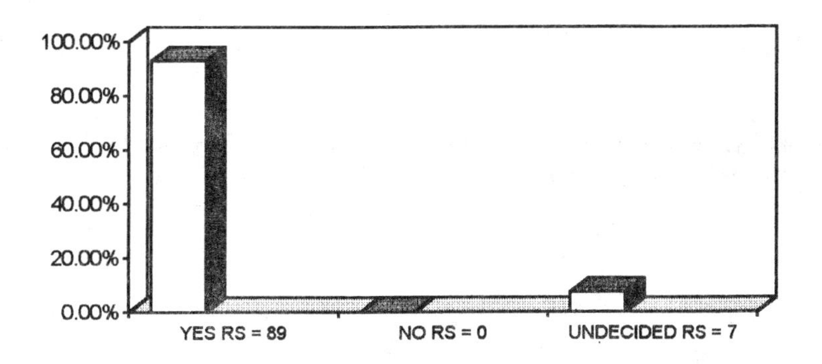

Figure 5.25 Should there be interdisciplinary learning ? : By percentage

Table 5. 151
At which stage should it take place ?

Response	Teachers (N = 7)	%	Students (N = 89)	%	Total (N = 96)	%
Beginning	0	0.00	17	19.10	17	17.71
Middle	1	14.29	11	12.36	12	12.50
End	2	28.57	2	2.25	4	4.17
Throughout	4	57.14	59	66.29	63	65.62
Post Qual.	0	0.00	0	0.00	0	0.00

The majority (66.29%) of students believed that interdisciplinary learning should take place throughout training. The teachers were more diverse in their opinions, with two of the seven opting for the end of training. "Professional identity should be reasonably well established by this stage and students could perhaps share knowledge and experience to promote further learning.....? may engage in shared research."(Teacher Resp. 3)

One teacher who selected "throughout" as his preferred option remarked :- "By careful planning and revisiting areas of common interest related to client centred, problem orientated process. Would help professionals clarify roles and discuss boundaries prior to doing the job." (Teacher Resp. 2)

Table 5. 152
Would there be advantages?

Response	Teachers (N = 7)	%	Students (N = 89)	%	Total (N = 96)	%
Yes	5	71.43	86	96.62	91	94.79
No	0	0.00	0	0.00	0	0.00
Undecided	2	28.57	3	3.37	5	5.21

Potential advantages were identified by 71.43% of the teachers and 96.63% of the students. These advantages are identified in Table 5. 153, next page.

Table 5.153
Advantages of interdisciplinary learning

Advantages	Teachers (RS = 6)	Students (RS = 83)	Total (N = 96)
Increase understanding of each others role	5	70	75
Increase teamwork and collaboration	2	45	47
Broaden horizons, cross fertilise ideas	3	23	26
Make better use of time and scarce resources	0	3	3

Table 5.154
Disadvantages of interdisciplinary learning

Disadvantages	Teachers (RS = 6)	Students (RS = 50)	Total (N = 96)
Time constraints	1	1	2
Organisational difficulties	1	0	1
Irrelevant material	2	10	12
Hierarchical domination & prejudice	1	11	12
Loss of professional identity	0	19	19
Different academic ability	1	1	2
Different knowledge base	0	5	5
Too many students in a class	0	1	1

Several of the students while identifying the potential disadvantages also commented that with careful planning from all the disciplines involved most of these problems could be overcome. One student suggested; "Why not involve us in the planning stage as we have not yet adopted the same suspicions and conflict that many of you teachers have. It is all of you that teach us to distrust all the others!" (Resp. 63)

Table 5.155
Level of interest in interdisciplinary learning

Response	Teachers (N = 7)	%	Students (N = 89)	%	Total (N = 96)	%
Very interested	2	28.57	37	41.57	39	40.62
Interested	4	57.14	49	55.06	53	55.21
Neutral	1	14.29	3	3.37	4	4.17
Uninterested	0	0.00	0	0.00	0	0.00
Totally Uninterested	0	0.00	0	0.00	0	0.00

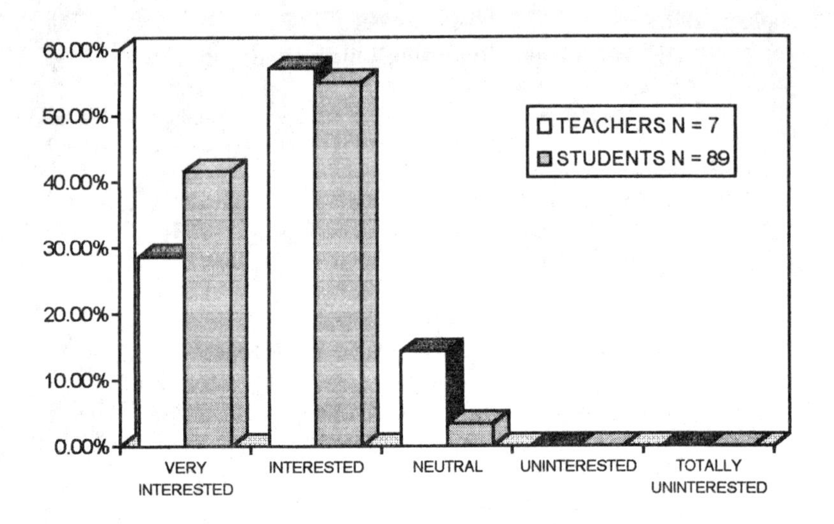

Figure 5.26 Level of interest in interdisciplinary learning : By percentage

One teacher and only three of the occupational therapy students were neutral in their level of interest regarding interdisciplinary learning. A substantial majority (95.83%) were either "very interested" or "interested" in the idea. No one in this professional group was uninterested in interdisciplinary learning. The respondents identified the core subjects which, in their opinion, would be suitable for interdisciplinary learning. The results are presented in Table 5.156

Table 5.156
Subjects suitable for interdisciplinary learning

Subject	Teachers (N = 7)	%	Students (N = 89)	%	Total (N = 96)	%
Psychology	5	71.43	83	93.26	88	91.67
Sociology	5	71.43	87	97.75	92	95.83
Ethics	6	85.71	79	88.76	85	88.54
Law & Practice	6	85.71	58	65.17	64	66.66
Research methods	6	85.71	63	70.79	69	71.87
Management	6	85.71	58	65.17	64	66.66
Econ. of health care	6	85.71	64	71.91	70	72.91
Health Promotion	6	85.71	76	85.39	82	81.42
Study skills	6	85.71	58	65.17	64	66.66
Quality Issues	6	85.71	64	71.91	70	72.91
Structural Organisation	6	85.71	80	89.89	86	89.6
Computing skills	6	85.71	78	87.64	84	87.50

Psychology and sociology were the most frequently chosen subjects although ethics, health promotion, computing skills and structural organisation were also selected by more than 80% of the respondents.

Table 5.157
Subjects students included in the behavioural sciences

Subjects	Yes	%	No	%	Undecided	%
Psychology	88	98.88	0	0.00	1	1.12
Sociology	79	88.76	4	4.49	6	6.74
Ethics	46	51.69	13	14.61	30	33.71
Law & Prac.	24	26.97	39	43.82	26	29.21
Management	27	30.34	40	44.94	22	24.72
Health Promotion	44	49.44	16	17.98	29	32.58
Study Skills	29	32.58	29	32.58	31	34.83
Quality Issues	25	28.09	24	26.97	40	44.94

This group of students were divided in their opinions. While psychology (98.88%) and sociology (88.76%) were widely accepted as behavioural sciences, less than half (49.44%) of the respondents included health promotion. There was indecision about several of the suggested subjects with quality issues raising the most uncertainty (44.94%).

Table 5.158
Student's preferred interdisciplinary learning methods

Learning Method	Yes	%	No	%	Undecided	%
Tutorials	60	67.42	11	12.36	18	20.22
Workshops	74	83.15	7	7.87	8	8.99
Case Studies	63	70.79	12	13.48	14	15.73
Seminars	47	52.81	17	19.10	25	28.09
Problem Based Learning	51	57.30	16	17.98	22	24.72
Role Play	36	40.45	34	38.20	19	21.35
Lectures	64	71.91	12	13.48	13	14.61
Visits to Client Areas	66	74.16	11	12.36	12	13.48

Role play was the least popular learning method with only 40.45% of the sample believing that this strategy could be used, another highly significant finding. ($\chi^2 = 38.64$, df = 2, $p < 0.1\%$).

Table 5.159
Other professions suitable for interdisciplinary learning with occupational therapists

Other Professions	Teachers (N = 7)	%	Students (N = 89)	%	Total (N = 96)	%
Dentists	0	0.00	5	5.62	5	5.21
DSA/DH	1	14.23	5	5.62	6	6.74
Den. Tec.	0	0.00	3	3.37	3	3.12
Medicine	3	42.86	70	78.65	73	76.04
Nursing	5	71.43	85	95.51	90	93.75
Nut & Diet	4	57.14	59	66.29	63	65.62
ODP	0	0.00	11	12.36	11	11.46
Physio.	4	57.14	86	96.63	90	93.75
Podiatry	1	14.23	20	22.47	21	21.87
Radio.	0	0.00	11	12.36	11	11.46
Social Work	7	100.00	86	96.63	93	96.87
Sp. Therapy	3	42.86	74	83.15	77	80.21

The occupational therapists identified social workers as the most suitable group with whom to learn (96.87%) with nursing and physiotherapy also selected by 93.75%.

5.5.3.8 The operating department practitioners

Biographic data of the teacher and student respondents
This group of respondents represented the smallest school participating in the study. Two teachers were employed and the students were less than thirty in number. Operating department practitioners are a relatively recent development with the first training programmes commencing in the United Kingdom in the mid seventies. Both teachers and 25 students completed the questionnaires. Both teachers were male and the student population (N = 25) comprised sixteen males and nine females. One of the teachers was less than 25 years of age, had been teaching less than five years and had less than five years clinical practice. The other teacher was aged between 41 and 45 and had been teaching between 21 - 25 years. He had also gained less than five years clinical practice before commencing his teaching career.

Eleven students were in the first year of training and fourteen in the second. Most of the students were aged between 21 and 25 years (RS = 14), with eight aged between 26 and 30 years, two between 31 and 35 years and the other aged between 36 and 40 years. Seven (28.00%) of the students had completed previous relevant courses. Two of the female respondents were Registered General Nurses whilst another had completed two years of her nurse training. One respondent had worked as an operating theatre orderly, one had completed a

BTEC Diploma in Life Sciences and another had completed various first aid courses.

Twenty students (80.00%) had gained previous relevant work experience. Of the sixteen male respondents ten had worked as operating theatre orderlies, the two female registered nurses had worked as staff nurses, two had worked as nursing auxilliaries, one as a part time hospital domestic, one in a vetinerary practice and another had completed a communications course while working in the retail business. Six of the students had shared learning with other professions. Interestingly both of the registered nurses gave a negative response. Four of the six had previously worked as theatre orderlies and the other two had worked as nursing auxilliaries.

The opinions of the operating department practitioners regarding the concept of interdisciplinary learning

Table 5.160
Should there be interdisciplinary learning ?

Response	Teachers (N = 2)	%	Students (N = 25)	%	Total (N = 27)	%
Yes	1	50.00	21	84.00	22	81.48
No	0	0.00	1	4.00	1	3.70
Undecided	1	50.00	3	12.00	4	14.81

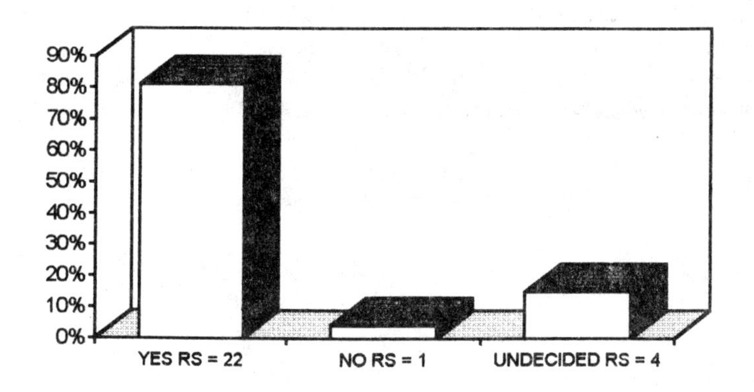

Figure 5. 27 Should there be shared learning ? : By percentage

Operating department practitioners while working with medical practitioners (surgeons and anaesthetists) and nurses in the operating theatres tend to work in isolation from most of the other professional groups. This point was reinforced by a number of respondents from the other professions who questioned who ODP's were. The number of positive responses received (81.48%) was therefore higher than expected for this group.

Table 5.161
At which stage should it take place ?

Response	Teachers (N = 2)	%	Students (N = 25)	%	Totals (N = 27)	%
Beginning	0	00.00	7	28.00	7	25.93
Middle	1	50.00	5	20.00	6	22.22
End	0	00.00	2	8.00	2	7.41
Throughout	1	50.00	7	28.00	8	29.63
Post Qual.	0	0.00	4	16.00	4	14.81

The operating practitioners were the most diverse group in response to this question. There was no clear consensus of opinion of when interdisciplinary learning should be introduced although it can be argued that more than 55% believed that it should start at the beginning or take place throughout training. Four students however, indicated that it should not take place until after qualifying. Of these, two declared themselves to be "very interested" in participating in interdisciplinary learning. One of these chose post qualification as the correct time because; "You are not competing in training with any other profession, you can concentrate on your own." (Resp. 9) Another student who was "neutral" about the concept declared; "Animosity is so high between us all it would be a disaster." (Resp. 5)

It could be argued that this is precisely why interdisciplinary learning should be introduced at the beginning of training !

Table 5.162
Would there be advantages ?

Response	Teachers (N = 2)	%	Students (N = 25)	%	Total (N = 27)	%
Yes	2	100.00	20	80.00	22	81.48
No	0	0.00	1	4.00	1	3.70
Undecided	0	0.00	4	16.00	4	14.82

Table 5.163
Advantages of interdisciplinary learning

Advantages	Teachers (RS = 1)	Students (RS = 12)	Totals (N = 27)
Increased understanding of each others role	1	5	6
Increase teamwork & collaboration	0	11	11
Broaden horizons, cross fertilise ideas	0	5	5
Make better use of scarce time & resources	0	3	3

Very few respondents identified any disadvantages although 12 of the respondents expressed anxiety about irrelevant material being introduced. The results are presented as Table 5.164

Table 5.164
Disadvantages of interdisciplinary learning

Disadvantages	Teachers (N = 2)	Students (N = 25)	Total (N = 27)
Time constraints	1	1	2
Organisational difficulties	0	0	0
Irrelevant material	2	10	12
Hierarchical domination & prejudice	0	4	4
Loss of professional identity	0	1	1
Different academic ability	0	0	0
Different knowledge base	0	1	1
Too many students in a class	0	1	1

Table 5.165
Level of interest in interdisciplinary learning

Response	Teachers (N = 2)	%	Students (N = 25)	%	Total (N = 27)	%
Very interested	0	0.00	7	28.00	7	25.93
Interested	1	50.00	13	52.00	14	51.85
Neutral	1	50.00	5	20.00	6	22.22
Uninterested	0	0.00	0	0.00	0	0.00
Totally uninterested	0	0.00	0	0.00	0	0.00

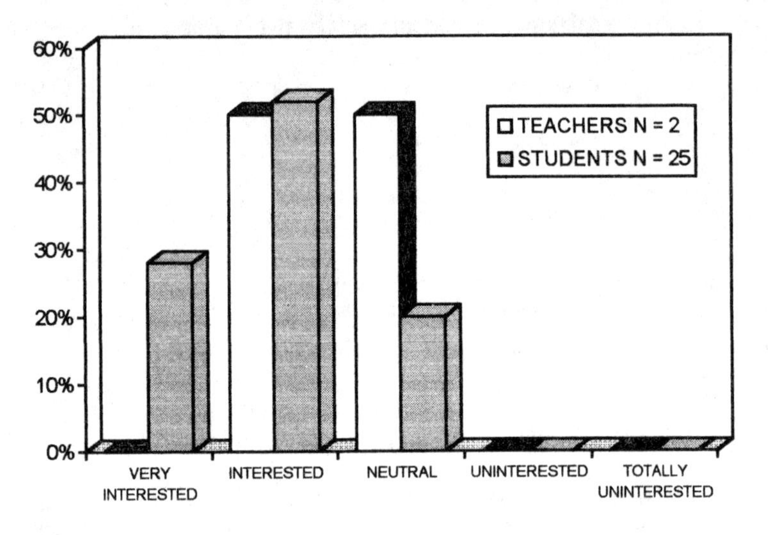

Figure 5.28 Level of interest in interdisciplinary learning : By percentage

Of the twenty seven operating department practitioners in this sample, 77.78% were "interested" or "very interested" in the concept of interdisciplinary learning. The core subjects which the operating department practitioners believed would be suitable for interdisciplinary learning are displayed as Table 5.166

Table 5.166
Subjects suitable for interdisciplinary learning

Subject	Teachers (N = 2)	%	Students (N = 25)	%	Total (N = 27)	%
Psychology	1	50.00	17	68.00	18	66.67
Sociology	1	50.00	13	52.00	14	51.85
Ethics	2	100.00	23	92.00	25	92.59
Law & Practice	2	100.00	14	56.00	16	59.26
Research methods	2	100.00	16	64.00	18	66.67
Management	1	50.00	16	64.00	17	62.96
Economics of care	1	50.00	16	64.00	17	62.96
Health promotion	2	100.00	21	84.00	23	85.19
Study skills	2	100.00	22	88.00	24	88.89
Quality issues	2	100.00	15	60.00	17	62.96
Structural organisation	2	100.00	13	52.00	15	55.56
Computing skills	2	100.00	18	72.00	20	74.07

The results are quite different from all other professional groups in that only 51.85% identify sociology as suitable while the learning of ethics on an interdisciplinary basis was deemed appropriate by 92.59% of the sample. The response to health promotion is consistent with other results in that more than 85% of the sample gave a positive response. The students were unsure which subjects comprised the behavioural sciences. While 80% of them correctly identified psychology and sociology, study skills (76%) and health promotion (72%) were also frequently identified.

Table 5.167
Subjects students included in the behavioural sciences

Subject	Yes	%	No	%	Undecided	%
Psychology	20	80.00	1	4.00	4	16.00
Sociology	20	80.00	1	4.00	4	16.00
Ethics	16	64.00	5	20.00	4	16.00
Law & Prac.	15	60.00	3	12.00	7	28.00
Management	12	48.00	6	24.00	7	28.00
Health Promotion	18	72.00	2	8.00	5	20.00
Study skills	19	76.00	4	16.00	2	8.00
Quality issues	13	52.00	3	12.00	9	36.00

Table 5.168
Students preferred interdisciplinary learning method

Learning Method	Yes	%	No	%	Undecided	%
Tutorials	17	68.00	5	20.00	3	12.00
Workshops	22	88.00	1	4.00	2	8.00
Case Studies	12	48.00	8	32.00	5	20.00
Seminars	18	72.00	4	16.00	3	12.00
Problem Based Learning	13	52.00	6	24.00	6	24.00
Role Play	10	40.00	12	48.00	3	12.00
Lectures	21	84.00	1	4.00	3	12.00
Visits to Client Areas	19	76.00	4	16.00	2	8.00

The most popular interdisciplinary learning style was workshops (88%) with lectures being identified by 84%. There was however no statistical significance in this finding ($\chi^2 = 5.61$, df =2, p >5%) While visits to the client areas were also deemed appropriate by 76% of the sample, a case study approach was only selcted by 48%. This finding differs from all the other professions. Consistent with the findings from the other students respondents, the operating department practitioners rejected role play ($\chi^2 = 13.45$, df = 2, p < 1%).

Table 5.169
Other professions suitable for interdisciplinary learning with operating department practitioners

Other Professions	Teachers (N = 2)	%	Students (N = 25)	%	Totals (N = 27)	%
Dentists	1	50.00	3	12.00	4	14.81
DSA/DH	0	00.00	1	4.00	1	3.70
Den. Tec.	0	00.00	4	16.00	4	14.81
Medicine	1	50.00	20	80.00	21	77.78
Nursing	2	100.00	23	92.00	25	92.59
Nut. & Diet.	0	00.00	3	12.00	3	11.11
Occ. Therapy	1	50.00	5	20.00	6	22.22
Physio.	2	100.00	10	40.00	12	44.44
Podiatry	0	00.00	1	4.00	1	3.70
Radiography	2	100.00	11	44.00	13	48.15
Social Work	0	00.00	5	20.00	5	18.52
Sp. Therapy	0	00.00	4	16.00	4	14.81

The most frequently selected profession was nursing (92.59%) with the medical practitioners chosen by (77.78%). In third place were the radiographers (48.15%). A possible explanation for this is that radiographers are frequently present in the operating theatres, thus as a profession they will work on a daily basis with ODP'S. It is interesting to note that 20% of the students perceived some value in sharing learning with social workers. Operating department practitioners frequently spend time with patients in anaesthetic rooms while awaiting surgery. Patients, at this time, are extremely vulnerable and it may be that they disclose problems of a personal or social nature.

5.5.3.9 The physiotherapists

Ten teachers and one hundred and one students from the School of Physiotherapy participated in the study. The biographic data is presented separately.

Biographic data of the teaching staff

Four male and six female physiotherapy teachers completed the questionnaire. One was aged between 25 and 30 years, three between 36 and 40 years, four between 41 and 45 years, one between 46 and 50 years and the other was more than 60 years of age.

Table 5.170
Years in practice before commencing teaching career

Years in Practice	N = 10	%
Less than 1 year	0	00.00
1 - 5 years	4	40.00
6 - 10 years	0	00.00
11 - 15 years	4	40.00
16 - 20 years	2	20.00
> 20 years	0	00.00

Table 5.171
Years in teaching

Years in teaching	N= 10	%
Less than 1 year	2	20.00
1 - 5 years	2	20.00
6 - 10 years	3	30.00
11 - 15 years	1	10.00
16 - 20 years	0	0.00
21 - 25 years	2	20.00
> 25 years	0	0.00

Five of the ten teachers could teach additional subjects. These were variously described as "the humanities", "sports injuries", "neurophysiology", "bioelectricity", "adult education", "problem solving skills" and "research methods."

Nine teachers had previously taught other professional groups. These groups were identified as nurses (RS = 7), radiographers (RS = 5), occupational therapists (RS = 3), MLSO, physiological measurement technicians (RS = 2), medics (RS = 1), remedial gymnasts and ODP's (RS = 1).

Seven had experienced interdisciplinary learning after they had qualified. Two of these however had also done so at an undergraduate level. Both of these had learned with occupational therapists. The other groups identified at the post graduate stage were nurses, dietitians, medics, radiographers, social workers, podiatrists, remedial gymnasts, occupational therapists, management personnel, speech therapists and teachers.

Biographic data of the physiotherapy students

Twenty three males and seventy eight females completed the questionnaire.

Table 5.172
Age of the students

Age Group	N = 101	%
20 years or less	43	42.57
21 - 25 years	29	28.71
26 - 30 years	18	17.82
31 - 35 years	6	5.94
36 - 40 years	4	3.96
41 - 45 years	1	0.99
> 45 years	0	0.00

Table 5.173
Students year stage of training

Year stage	N = 101	%
1	38	37.62
2	29	28.71
3	34	33.66

Twenty two of the students had completed previous courses which they believed relevant to their training. These courses were described as BA Psychology (RS = 2), BA Human Movement Studies (RS = 2), BSc Biochemistry, Life Sciences (RS = 2), BA/BSc Sports Sciences (RS = 3), HND Applied Biology (RS = 3), Medical student for 3 years (RS = 1), Remedial Therapist (RS = 1), HND Food Sciences (RS = 2), PGCE (RS = 2), Counselling Course (RS = 1).

Sixty students had relevant work experience. More than 50% had worked as physiotherapy helpers (RS = 32), with a further fourteen having worked as nursing auxilliaries, ten had worked on a voluntary basis in unspecified areas. Additional related work experience was described as dental nursing (RS = 1), occupational therapy helper (RS = 1), speech therapy helper (RS = 1), nanny (RS = 1), salesman for rehabilitation aids (RS = 1), BTEC clinical placements (RS = 1) and a hospital laboratory technician (RS = 1).

Only seven students had experienced any shared learning. They had done so whilst working as nursing auxilliaries (RS = 5) or as a dental nurse (RS = 1) or during the BTEC clinical placement (RS = 1). There was no evidence of any interdisciplinary learning having taken place as physiotherapy students.

The opinions of the physiotherapists regarding the concept of interdisciplinary learning

Table 5.174
Should there be interdisciplinary learning ?

Response	Teachers (N = 10)	%	Students (N = 101)	%	Total (N = 111)	%
Yes	6	60.00	72	71.29	78	70.27
No	0	00.00	5	4.95	5	4.50
Undecided	4	40.00	24	23.76	28	25.23

There was no statistical difference between the responses of the teachers and those of the students ($\chi^2 = 0.64$, df =2, $p > 5\%$).

While the majority of teachers and students indicated that there should be some interdisciplinary learning between the professions these results were less convincing than in most of the other professions. More than 25% of the physiotherapists were undecided.

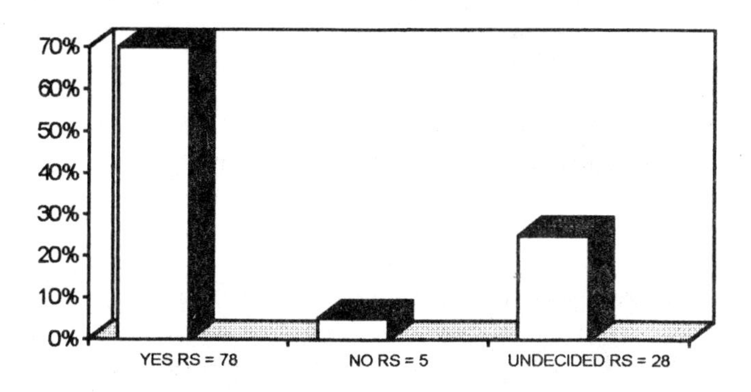

Figure 5.29 Should there be some shared learning : By percentage

Table 5.175
At which stage should it take place ?

Response	Teachers (N = 10)	%	Students (N = 101)	%	Totals (N = 111)	%
Beginning	0	00.00	19	18.81	19	17.12
Middle	0	00.00	20	19.80	20	18.02
End	4	40.00	5	4.95	9	8.11
Throughout	5	50.00	49	48.51	53	48.65
Post Qual.	1*	10.00	8*	7.92	9*	8.11

* This represents those nine respondents who chose "post qualification" only.

Although the number of teachers in this sample was small there was a statistical difference between the two sets of responses (χ^2 = 12.46,df = 4, p < 5%)

One teacher, who selected "throughout" remarked; "If only all the problems could be overcome it would not matter when." (Teacher Resp. 1) Another who chose "post qualification" had personally experienced shared learning both before and after qualification. She observed; "I have experienced both and think that once people are happy in their roles and have the experience of a few years working they can share a lot more valuable information and learn from each other" (Teacher Resp. 2)

Table 5.176
Would there be advantages ?

Response	Teachers (N = 10)	%	Students (N = 101)	%	Totals (N =111)	%
Yes	4	40.00	87	86.14	91	81.98
No	0	00.00	4	3.96	4	3.60
Undecided	6	60.00	10	9.90	16	15.84

The students were more convinced of the advantages than the teaching staff with 60% of the teachers being undecided ($\chi^2 = 15.28$, df = 2, p < 0.1%). This was a highly significant finding.

Table 5.177
Advantages of interdisciplinary learning

Advantages	Teachers (RS = 5)	Students (RS = 67)	Total (N =111)
Increase understanding of each others role	4	59	63
Increase teamwork & collaboration	5	55	60
Broaden horizons, cross fertilise ideas	5	34	39
Make better use of time & scarce resources	1	2	3

Table 5.178
Disadvantages of interdisciplinary learning

Disadvantages	Teachers (RS = 4)	Students (RS = 26)	Total (N = 111)
Time constraints	1	16	17
Organisational difficulties	0	4	4
Irrelevant material	3	23	26
Hierarchical domination & prejudice	0	7	7
Loss of professional identity	2	5	7
Different academic ability	0	0	0
Different knowledge base	0	8	8
Too many students in a class	0	9	9

Table 5.179
Level of interest in interdisciplinary learning

Response	Teachers (N = 10)	%	Students (N = 101)	%	Total (N = 111)	%
Very interested	1	10.0	20	19.80	21	18.92
Interested	3	30.0	54	53.46	57	51.35
Neutral	4	40.0	17	16.83	21	18.92
Uninterested	2	20.0	7	6.93	9	8.11
Totally uninterested	0	0.0	2	1.98	2	1.80

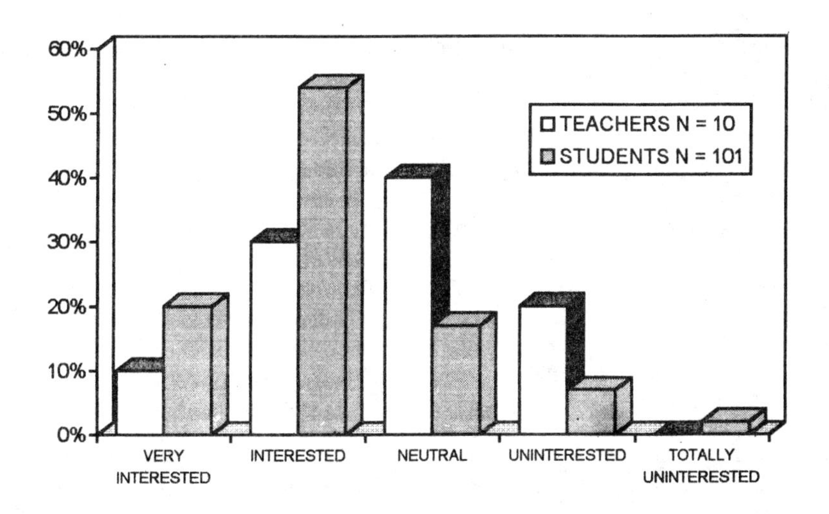

Figure 5.30 Level of interest in interdisciplinary learning : By percentage

More than 70% of the 101 students were "very interested" or "interested" in interdisciplinary learning. The 10 teachers were less convinced with 6 of them being "neutral" or "uninterested" in the idea although this was not a significant finding ($\chi^2 = 4.05$, df = 4, p > 5% Yates correction applied) This finding was reinforced by the results of the question which asked whether the physiotherapists believed there would be any advantages in introducing interdisciplinary learning.

Table 5.180
Subjects suitable for interdisciplinary learning

Subject	Teachers (N = 10)	%	Students (N = 101)	%	Total (N = 111)	%
Psychology	10	100.0	93	92.08	103	92.79
Sociology	9	90.0	89	88.12	98	88.29
Ethics	10	100.0	83	82.18	93	83.78
Law & prac.	9	90.0	64	63.37	73	65.77
Research Methods	7	70.0	60	59.41	67	60.36
Management	7	70.0	48	47.52	55	49.55
Economics of health care	7	70.0	77	76.24	84	75.68
Health promotion	9	90.0	75	74.26	84	75.68
Study skills	9	90.0	58	57.43	67	60.36
Quality Assurance	9	90.0	63	62.38	72	64.86
Structural Organisation	8	80.0	87	86.14	95	85.89
Computing Skills	10	100.0	94	93.07	104	93.69

The students had previously identified which subjects they believed constituted the behavioural sciences.

Table 5.181
Subjects students included in the behavioural sciences

Subjects	Yes	%	No	%	Undecided	%
Psychology	99	98.02	0	0.00	2	1.98
Sociology	99	98.02	0	0.00	2	1.98
Ethics	82	81.19	8	7.92	10	9.90
Law & Prac.	48	47.52	38	37.62	15	14.85
Management	49	48.51	33	32.67	19	18.81
Health Promotion	65	64.36	22	21.78	14	13.86
Study skills	54	53.47	32	31.68	15	14.85
Quality Issues	46	45.54	25	24.75	30	29.70

Table 5.182
Students preferred interdisciplinary learning methods

Learning Methods	Yes	%	No	%	Undecided	%
Tutorials	68	67.33	19	18.81	14	13.86
Workshops	61	60.40	21	20.79	19	18.81
Case Studies	59	58.42	20	19.80	22	21.78
Seminars	52	51.49	27	26.73	19	18.81
Problem Based Learning	62	61.39	22	21.78	17	16.83
Role Play	20	19.80	64	63.37	17	16.83
Lectures	56	55.45	26	25.74	19	18.81
Visits to Client Areas	74	73.27	16	15.84	11	10.89

Role play as a learning strategy was accepted by less than 20% of the sample. The majority rejected it completely (63.37%), ($\chi^2 = 83.26$, df = 2, $p < 0.1\%$) The most popular learning methods would be visits to the client areas.

Table 5.183
Other professions suitable for interdisciplinary learning with physiotherapists

Other Professions	Teachers (N = 10)	%	Students (N = 101)	%	Total (N = 111)	%
Dentists	1	10.0	8	7.92	9	8.11
DSA/DH	1	10.0	4	3.96	5	4.50
Den. Tec.	0	00.0	3	2.97	3	2.70
Medicine	8	80.0	88	87.13	96	86.49
Nursing	7	70.0	80	79.21	87	78.38
Nut. & Diet.	2	20.0	45	44.55	47	42.34
Occ. Therapy	8	80.0	93	92.08	101	90.99
ODP	1	10.0	18	17.82	19	17.12
Podiatry	4	40.0	39	38.61	43	38.74
Radiog.	4	40.0	50	49.50	54	48.65
Social Work	6	60.0	71	70.30	77	69.37
Sp. Therapy	6	60.0	69	68.32	75	67.57

Occupational therapists were the most frequently chosen group with whom physiotherapists would wish to learn. Social workers were identified by 69.37% of the sample. Less than 40% selected podiatry. This was an unexpected finding as both professions are implicitly concerned with rehabilitation and mobility.

5.5.3.10 The podiatrists

Eight teachers and sixty three students from the school of podiatry completed the questionnaire. The biographic data is presented separately.

Biographic data of the teaching staff
Four male and four female teachers completed the questionnaire. Of these five were aged between 41 and 45 years, two between 46 and 50 years and the other was more than 60 years. One had been in practice for less than one year before commencing his teaching career. Of the others three had practised between one and five years (N = 3) and the remaining four had done so for six to ten years. All eight had been teaching for at least 6 years, with one between 6 and 10 years, one between 11 and 15 years, three for 16 to 20 years, two between 21 and 25 years and the other for more than 25 years. Four of them indicated that they were able to teach subjects in addition to podiatry. These were described as health education, sociology, research methods, dermatology, histology and lower limb injuries. Three of them had experience of teaching other professions. Two had taught medical practitioners, one had taught nurses, two had taught physiotherapists, another had taught occupational therapists, and one had taught teachers and human movement study students. Three teachers had shared learning with other professional groups after they had qualified. The other professions were identified as nurses, occupational therapists and physiotherapists.

Biographic data of the podiatry students
Fifteen males and forty seven females completed the questionnaire.

Table 5.184
Age of the students

Age Group	N = 63	%
20 years or less	19	30.16
21 - 25 years	18	28.57
26 - 30 years	9	14.29
31 - 35 years	7	11.10
36 - 40 years	6	9.52
41 - 45 years	3	4.76
46 - 50 years	1	1.59
51 - 55 years	0	0.00
> 55 years	0	0.00

Table 5.185
Students year stage of training

Year of training	N = 63	%
1	31	49.21
2	16	25.40
3	16	25.40

Twenty of the students had completed relevant courses prior to commencing their podiatry training. Of these eight were Registered Nurses. Other courses were variously described as B.Sc Applied Biology (RS = 1), B.Sc. Behavioural Sciences (RS = 1), HNC. Pharmaceutical Scineces (RS = 1), HND Applied Biology (RS = 1), BTEC Diploma in Science (RS = 2), science access courses (RS = 2), and a paramedic (RS = 1). These results are reflected in the number of mature students in podiatry training. It is not known whether these individuals chose to make a career change or whether they were unemployed prior to commencing the course. The number of Registered Nurses was an unexpected finding.

Thirty eight students had obtained relevant work experience. Of these eight had worked as Registered Nurses, four as nursing auxilliaries, seven in voluntary work, three as physiotherapy helpers, four as podiatrist's assistants, one as a paramedic, two as medical secretaries, one as an unqualified social worker, one as a student nurse and one as a teacher.

Twelve had shared learning with other professions. All of these respondents had gained previous qualifications or relevant work experience and eight of them were Registered Nurses. A variety of shared learning experiences had taken place. These included with medics, dental hygienists, dietitians, social workers, speech therapists. The unqualified social worker had shared learning with the police and probation officers. There was no evidence that any learning with other professions had taken place as podiatry students.

The opinions of the podiatrists regarding the concept of interdisciplinary learning

Table 5.186
Should there be interdisciplinary learning ?

Response	Teachers (N = 8)	%	Students (N = 63)	%	Total (N = 71)	%
Yes	7	87.50	60	95.20	67	94.37
No	1	12.50	1	1.60	2	2.82
Undecided	0	0.00	2	3.20	2	2.82

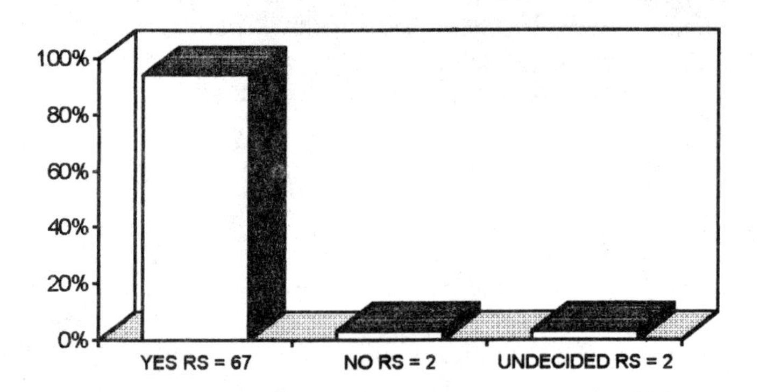

Figure 5.31 Should there be interdisciplinary learning? : By percentage

Table 5.187
At which stage should it take place ?

Response	Teachers (N = 8)	%	Students (N = 63)	%	Total (N = 71)	%
Beginning	3	37.50	8	12.70	11	15.49
Middle	1	12.50	15	23.81	16	22.54
End	1	12.50	5	7.94	6	8.45
Throughout	2	25.00	35	55.56	37	52.11
Post Qual.	1 *	12.50	0 *	00.00	1 *	1.41

* Only 1 podiatry teacher selected "post qualification" only.

No student selected this option. The teacher justified his response by commenting; " Whilst there is a need for the integration of professions, this should not be at the expense of deviation of specific bias. Shared learning can only occur when extra resources to follow up are provided, it is consequently inefficient since this is rarely the case." (Teacher Resp. 8)

This respondent was obviously convinced that additional resources would be needed. His responses throughout the questionnaire tended to be contradictory in that he specifically wrote that "none" of the other twelve professions would be suitable for shared learning with podiatrists, that no advantages would be evident, and yet he identified all twelve core subjects as potentially suitable for shared learning and declared himself to be "interested" in teaching on an interdisciplinary basis !

Many of the students justified their choices. Most of them made similar comments to those made by students from the other professions. One student (Resp 5) however, saw "an extremely limited relevance of psychology and sociology" and declared himself to be "uninterested" in any shared learning. Student Resp. 26 who selected "throughout training" observed; "The new advances and rapid pace of change make a continual association absolutely imperative." Student Resp. 19 chose 'the middle of training' because; "The basics need to be learnt before someone can even consider expressing their views.......you can't explain something if you haven't learnt it yet. But it shouldn't be left too late otherwise we will never get on."

Table 5.188
Would there be advantages?

Response	Teachers (N = 8)	%	Students (N = 63)	%	Total (N = 71)	%
Yes	7	87.50	59	93.65	66	92.96
No	1	12.50	1	1.59	2	2.82
Undecided	0	0.00	2	3.17	2	2.82

Table 5.189
Advantages of interdisciplinary learning

Advantages	Teachers (RS = 7)	Students (RS = 60)	Total (N = 71)
Increase understanding of each others role	6	37	43
Increase teamwork & collaboration	1	34	35
Broaden horizons, crosss fertilise ideas	3	27	30
Make better use of time & scarce resources	3	1	4

Table 5.190
Disadvantages of interdisciplinary learning

Disadvantages	Teachers (RS = 7)	Students (RS = 29)	Total (N = 71)
Time constraints	0	7	7
Organisational difficulties	0	0	0
Irrelevant material	3	11	14
Hierarchical domination & prejudice	2	4	6
Loss of professional identity	1	0	1
Different academic ability	1	0	1
Different knowledge base	0	2	2
Too many students in a class	0	0	0

Teacher Resp. 8 noted that; " It has been my experience in visits to other schools that this has been deemed unsuccessful by the recipients. That specific relevances are lost and preferences are often detected or 'suspected' (sic) to the professions and invariably there has been a need for extensive top up to repair the damage."

It would have been invaluable to be able to explore this statement in further detail with this respondent as no evidence has been found in the review of the literature of any interdisciplinary initiatives involving podiatry students and none of the literature reviewed mentioned remedial work in order to "repair the damage" in any of the professions. This respondent's observations must therefore be treated with caution as his observations are not substantiated by the literature review.

Table 5.191
Level of interest in participating in interdisciplinary learning

Response	Teachers (N = 8)	%	Students (N = 63)	%	Total (N = 71)	%
Very interested	2	25.0	33	52.38	35	49.30
Interested	6	75.0	23	36.51	29	40.85
Neutral	0	0.0	6	9.52	6	8.45
Uninterested	0	0.0	0	0	0	0.00
Totally uninterested	0	0.0	0	0	0	0.00

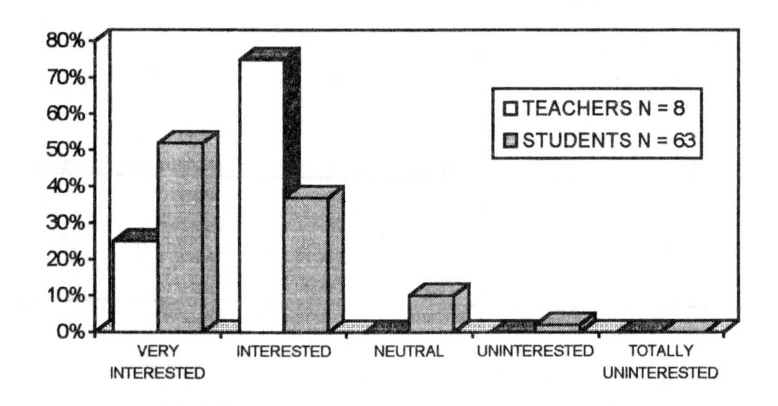

Figure 5.32 Level of interest in interdisciplinary learning : By percentage

More than 90% of the podiatry respondents were "very interested" or "interested" in the concept of interdisciplinary learning. Of the 71 respondents 67 (94.37%)

thought there would be advantages. Only one teacher (Resp. 8) and one student thought that no advantages would result. Two students were undecided.

Table 5.192
Subjects suitable for interdisciplinary learning

Subject	Teachers (N = 8)	%	Students (N = 63)	%	Total (N = 71)	%
Psychology	8	100.0	54	85.71	62	87.32
Sociology	8	100.0	54	85.71	62	87.32
Ethics	8	100.0	50	79.37	58	81.69
Law & Prac.	8	100.0	46	73.02	54	76.06
Research methods	8	100.0	40	63.49	48	67.61
Management	8	100.0	42	66.67	50	59.15
Econ. of health care	8	100.0	36	57.14	44	61.97
Health Prom.	8	100.0	46	73.02	54	76.06
Study skills	8	100.0	55	87.30	63	88.73
Qual. issues	8	100.0	39	61.90	47	66.20
Structural organisation	8	100.0	32	50.79	40	56.34
Computing skills	8	100.0	53	84.13	61	85.92

Table 5.193
Subjects students included in the behavioural sciences

Subjects	Yes	%	No	%	Undecided	%
Psychology	61	96.83	0	00.00	2	3.17
Sociology	55	87.30	2	3.17	6	9.52
Ethics	33	52.38	13	20.63	17	26.98
Law & Prac	23	36.51	21	33.33	19	30.16
Management	30	47.62	19	30.16	14	22.22
Health Promotion	51	80.95	2	3.17	10	15.87
Study Skills	28	44.44	21	33.33	13	20.63
Quality Issues	17	26.98	19	30.16	27	42.86

Apart from psychology and sociology the only core subject that the majority (80.95%)of the podiatry students included in the behavioural sciences was health promotion. Ethics was selected by 52.38% of the sample but all other subjects were rejected by the majority.

Table 5.194
Student's preferred interdisciplinary learning methods

Learning Method	Yes	%	No	%	Undecided	%
Tutorials	44	69.84	5	7.94	14	22.22
Workshops	43	68.25	5	7.94	15	23.81
Case Studies	38	60.32	10	15.87	15	23.81
Seminars	33	52.38	12	19.10	18	28.57
Problem Based Learning	38	60.32	7	11.11	18	28.57
Role Play	19	30.16	19	30.16	25	39.68
Lectures	40	63.49	6	9.52	17	26.98
Visits to Client Areas	58	92.06	1	1.59	4	6.35

The podiatry students rejected role play as an appropriate method ($\chi^2 = 40.54$, df = 2, $p < 0.\ 1\%$) but the majority accepted all other methods. The most popular method was to visit the clinical areas. Interestingly the use of case studies was selected by only 60% of the sample.

Table 5.195
Other professions suitable for interdisciplinary learning with podiatrists

Other Professions	Teachers (N = 8)	%	Students (N = 63)	%	Total (N = 71)	%
Dentists	3	37.50	6	9.52	9	12.68
DSA/DH	1	12.50	1	1.59	2	2.82
Den. Tec.	1	12.50	0	00.00	1	1.41
Medicine	7	87.50	61	96.83	68	95.77
Nursing	6	75.00	51	80.95	57	80.28
Nut & Diet	2	25.00	33	52.38	35	49.30
Occ. Therapy	4	50.00	46	73.02	50	70.42
ODP	2	25.00	38	60.32	40	56.34
Physiotherapy	5	62.50	59	93.65	64	90.14
Radiography	6	75.00	45	71.43	51	71.83
Social Work	3	37.50	38	60.32	41	57.75
Sp. Therapy	3	37.50	9	14.29	12	16.90

Whilst the podiatry teachers and students appeared to be broadly in agreement about the value of learning with medics and nurses, a greater percentage of students selected physiotherapists, occupational therapists, nutritionists and dietitians and social workers than did the teaching staff. Conversely a higher percentage of teachers selected speech therapists as appropriate. The reason for this is not clear although this may be due to the fact that both the School of

Speech Therapy and the School of Podiatry were in close geographical proximity on the same site !

The other point of interest was that 14% of the podiatry students specifically rejected learning with the dental profession. This was evident from their previous responses to Question 13 which had asked whether there were any specific topics which they would reject. Respondent 52 observed "they deal with mouths and we deal with feet." A holistic approach to client care would not seem to have been adopted by this student ! Interestingly the student was "very interested" in the concept of interdisciplinary learning and selected all other professions apart from dental technicans, dental hygienists, dental surgery assistants and speech therapy. It would seem that any profession who dealt with a client below the head and neck was acceptable.

5.5.3.11 The radiographers

Six teachers and fifty two students from the school of radiography completed the questionnaire. The biographic data is presented separately.

Biographic data of the teaching staff

Three male and three female teachers completed the questionnaire. Two were aged between 31 and 35 years, two between 36 and 40 years, one was between 46 and 50 years and the other between 51 and 55 years. Four of them had been in clinical practice for 6 to 10 years before commencing their teaching careers, one had practised for 1 to 5 years and the remaining respondent for 11 to 15 years. Three had been teaching for 1 to 5 years, one for 6 - 10 years, one for 16 - 20 years and the other for 21 - 25 years. Two of the respondents identified additional subjects which they could teach. These were as described by Respondent 3 as management, research methods and education and by Respondent 4 as sociology, ethics and first aid. Five of the six teachers had had the opportunity to teach other professions. The professions were identified variously as dental surgeons (RS = 1), DSA/DH (RS = 1), medical practitioners (RS = 1), nurses (RS = 1), ODP (RS = 2), podiatrists (RS = 2), physiotherapists (RS = 2), and medical photographers (RS = 1). Only one teacher indicated that she had experienced any shared learning before she qualified. This was with occupational therapists and physiotherapists. Four others had experience post qualification. The professions identified were dental surgeons (RS = 1), DSA/DH (RS = 2), dental technicians (RS = 1), nurses (RS = 3), occupational therapists (RS = 4), physiotherapists (RS = 4), podiatrists (RS = 2), social workers (RS = 1), speech therapists (RS = 1).

Biographic data of the radiography students

Ten male and forty two female students completed the questionnaire.

Table 5.196
Age of the students

Age Group	N = 52	%
20 years or less	29	55.77
21 - 25 years	16	30.77
26 - 30 years	5	9.62
31 - 35 years	1	1.92
36 - 40 years	1	1.92
41 - 45 years	0	00.00
46 - 50 years	0	00.00
51 - 55 years	0	00.00
Over 55 years	0	00.00

Table 5.197
Students year stage of training

Year of training	N = 52	%
1	20	38.46
2	18	34.62
3	14	26.92

There were very few students older than 25 years. The majority were less than 20 years old thus indicating that most individuals who commence radiography training are likely to be school leavers who enter the programme at 18 years of age. Nine of the students had completed relevant courses prior to commencing radiography training. These were described as BA Sociology (RS = 1), BSc Physics and Biology (RS = 1), physiological measurement technician (RS = 1), Diploma in Health Studies (RS = 1) and first aid courses (RS = 5).

Seventeen had gained relevant work experience. One had completed one year of nurse training, two had worked as auxilliaries, residential care officer (RS = 1), day centre worker for the mentally ill (RS = 1), working with children with special needs (RS = 1), work experience in health centres (RS = 3), work experience in radiography departments (RS = 3), physiotherapy assistant (RS = 1), social security clerk (RS = 1).

Nine students indicated that they had shared learning with another profession. All nine were in the third year of training and indicated that this experience had taken place with orthoptic students. This finding can be explained by the fact that a now closed school of orthoptics existed in the same institution as the school of radiography. What shared learning took place is unknown.

The opinions of the radiographers regarding the concept of interdisciplinary learning

Table 5.198
Should there be interdisciplinary learning ?

Response	Teachers (N = 6)	%	Students (N = 52)	%	Total (N = 58)	%
Yes	4	66.67	45	86.34	49	84.48
No	0	00.00	5	9.62	5	8.62
Undecided	2	33.33	2	3.85	4	6.90

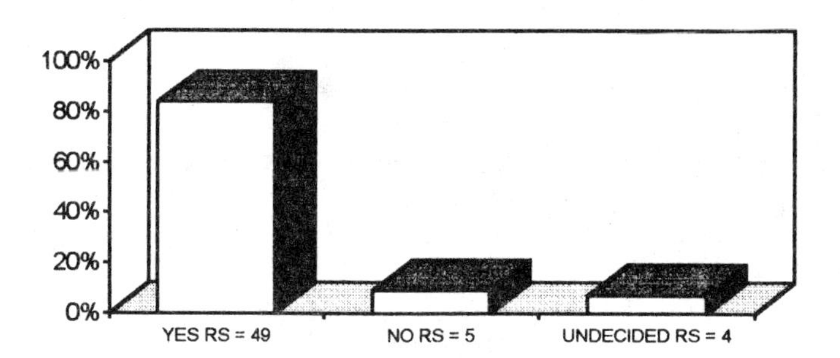

Figure 5.33 Should there be some shared learning? : By percentage

Table 5.199
At which stage should it take place ?

Response	Teachers (N = 6)	%	Students (N = 52)	%	Total (N = 58)	%
Beginning	2	33.33	19	36.54	21	36.21
Middle	0	00.00	7	13.46	7	12.07
End	0	00.00	5	9.62	5	8.62
Throughout	· 4	66.67	20	38.46	24	41.38
Post Qual.	0	00.00	1*	1.92	1	1.72

Only one male student selected "post qualification" only. His stated reason for his choice was; "Before qualifying the main objective should be to learn your own job as thoroughly as possible. The shared learning could be an important part of ongoing professional development after qualifying." (Student Resp 7) This student subsequently declared himself to be "uninterested" in interdisciplinary learning. One teacher who selected "throughout" training introduced a slightly different perspective; "It is unlikely that all topics suitable for shared learning would take place at the same time during education." (Teacher Resp. 1)

A third year student who chose "throughout training" commented; "New techniques need to be incorporated. Shared knowledge of this is essential. Health workers all have the same aim, namely the well being of the individual patient. This should be nurtured into a skill throughout training since contact with patients begins immediately training commmences." (Student Resp. 3)

Table 5.200
Would there be advantages ?

Response	Teachers (N = 6)	%	Students (N = 52)	%	Total (N = 56)	%
Yes	4	66.67	42	80.77	46	82.14
No	0	0.00	5	9.62	5	8.93
Undecided	2	33.33	5	9.62	7	12.50

One of the students observed; "There would be less snobbery and bickering between the professions." (Resp 42), while another wrote "we would learn to work as an interdisciplinary team" (Resp. 35). Nevertheless there were disadvantages as displayed in Table 5.202

Table 5.201
Advantages of interdisciplinary learning

Advantages	Teachers (RS = 4)	Students (RS = 43)	Total (N = 58)
Increase understanding of each others role	3	32	35
Increase teamwork & collaboration	4	22	26
Broaden horizons, cross fertilise ideas	2	18	20
Make better use of time/ scarce resources	2	0	2

Table 5.202
Disadvantages of interdisciplinary learning

Disadvantages	Teachers (RS = 5)	Students (RS = 32)	Total (N = 58)
Time constraints	0	1	1
Organisational difficulties	0	1	1
Irrelevant material	2	16	18
Hierarchical domination & prejudice	0	3	3
Loss of professional identity	0	3	3
Different academic ability	0	0	0
Different knowledge base	0	0	0
Too many students in a class	0	9	9

One student (Resp. 38) was concerned that; "medical and dental students would attempt to take over the forum." He also declared himself to be "uninterested" in the concept of interdisciplinary learning and believed there were no advantage.

Table 5.203
Level of interest in interdisciplinary learning

Response	Teachers (N = 6)	%	Students (N =52)	%	Total (N = 58)	%
Very interested	3	50.0	15	28.85	18	31.03
Interested	1	10.0	25	48.08	26	44.83
Neutral	2	20.0	9	17.31	11	18.97
Uninterested	0	0.0	2	3.85	2	3.45
Totally Uninterested	0	0.0	1	1.92	1	1.72

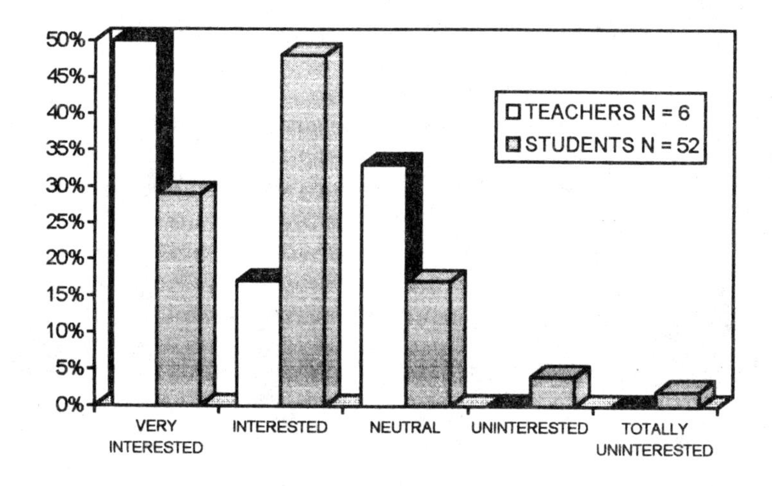

Figure 5.34 The level of interest in interdisciplinary learning: By percentage

More than 75% (RS = 44) of the radiography respondents were "very interested" or "interested" in the concept of interdisciplinary learning with 47 respondents believing that there would be advantages.

Table 5.204
Subjects suitable for interdisciplinary learning

Subject	Teachers (N = 6)	%	Students (N = 52)	%	Total (N = 58)	%
Psychology	5	83.33	44	84.62	49	84.48
Sociology	5	83.33	41	78.85	46	79.31
Ethics	6	100.0	42	80.78	48	82.76
Law & Prac.	6	100.0	27	51.92	33	56.90
Research methods	4	66.67	36	69.23	40	68.97
Management	6	100.0	23	44.23	29	50.00
Econ. of health care	6	100.0	28	53.85	34	58.62
Health Prom.	6	100.0	39	75.00	45	77.59
Study skills	6	100.0	32	61.54	38	66.52
Quality Issues	5	83.33	32	61.54	37	63.79
Structural Organisation	6	100.0	43	82.69	49	84.48
Computing skills	6	100.0	44	84.62	50	86.21

Table 5.205
Subjects students included in the behavioural sciences

Subject	Yes	%	No	%	Undecided	%
Psychology	51	98.08	0	00.00	1	1.92
Sociology	45	86.54	5	9.62	2	3.85
Ethics	30	57.69	8	15.38	14	26.92
Law & Prac.	23	44.23	23	44.23	6	11.54
Management	17	32.69	25	48.08	10	19.23
Health Prom.	36	69.23	13	25.00	3	5.77
Study skills	15	28.85	29	55.77	8	15.38
Qual. Issues	18	34.62	19	36.54	15	28.85

Although psychology and sociology were clearly identified by the students as behavioural sciences, health promotion and ethics were also selected by the majority of the sample.

Table 5.206
Student's preferred interdisciplinary learning methods

Learning Method	Yes	%	No	%	Undecided	%
Tutorials	41	78.85	8	15.38	3	5.77
Workshops	32	61.54	8	15.38	12	23.08
Case Studies	39	75.00	5	9.62	8	15.38
Seminars	30	57.69	7	13.46	15	28.85
Problem Based Learning	28	53.85	7	13.46	17	32.69
Role Play	16	30.77	20	38.46	16	30.77
Lectures	34	65.38	8	15.38	10	19.23
Visits to Client Areas	44	84.62	4	7.69	4	7.69

Only role play as a learning method was rejected by the student radiographers ($\chi^2 = 29.76$, df = 2, $p < 0.1\%$). Problem based learning and seminars were also less popular than the other options. The reason for this is not known. It may be that radiography students do not normally experience these learning strategies.

Table 5.207
Other professions suitable for interdisciplinary learning with radiographers

Other Professions	Teachers (N = 6)	%	Students (N = 52)	%	Total (N = 58)	%
Dentists	5	83.33	16	30.77	21	36.21
DSA/DH	3	50.00	4	7.69	7	12.07
Den. Tec.	1	16.67	4	7.69	5	8.62
Medicine	6	100.0	41	78.85	47	81.03
Nursing	5	83.33	48	92.31	53	91.38
Nut. & Diet.	3	50.00	9	17.31	12	20.69
Occ Therapy	3	50.00	16	30.77	19	32.76
ODP	2	33.33	17	32.69	19	32.76
Physiotherapy	5	83.33	33	63.46	38	65.52
Podiatry	4	66.67	4	7.69	8	13.79
Social Work	3	50.00	21	40.38	24	41.38
Sp. Therapy	4	66.67	11	21.15	15	25.86

An unexpected finding of interest was the 50% of the radiography teachers and 40% of the students in this sample who selected social workers as an appropriate group with whom to learn. It could be argued that radiographers and social workers are one of the least likely of all the professions to meet as radiographers are based within specialist departments in the acute hospital setting while social workers have their maximum client contact within a community social setting. Professions such as dentists, speech therapists, nutritionists and dietitians who have a client case load are more likely to collaborate with radiographers on a professional basis.

5.5.3.12 The social workers

Seven teachers and one hundred and thirty students comprised the social work population in this study. The biographic data is presented separately.

Biographic data of the teaching staff
Three males and four females completed the questionnaire. Two were aged between 25 and 30 years, one between 36 and 40 years, three between 41 and 45 years and the remaining respondent was aged between 46 and 50 years. Four of them had been in practice for 11 to 15 years before commencing their teaching careers, with the remaining three having practised for less than one year, 1 to 5 years and 6 to 10 years respectively. Three had been teaching for less than one year, two for 1 to 5 years, and two for 6 to10 years. The reason for the number of staff who had been in their teaching post for less than one year can be attributed to the development of the new Diploma course which commenced in 1992 and had a very large student intake. A number of teaching staff had therefore been appointed to resource this course. Five of the teachers identified additional subjects which they could teach. These subjects were variously identified as counselling (RS = 2), management (RS = 1), housing and the environment (RS = 1), problem solving skills, social psychology (RS = 1). All seven had taught professions other than their own. The professions involved were described as nursing (RS = 3), nutrition and dietetics (RS = 2), occupational therapy (RS = 1), housing departments (RS = 1), voluntary organisations (RS = 1), Local Authorities (RS = 1) and nursery nurses (RS = 1).

Only three of the social work teachers had experienced shared learning with other professional groups. Two had done so with medical practitioners and one with nurses and occupational therapists. Only one respondent indicated that this had occured before qualification.

Biographic data of the social work students
Thirty five male and ninety two female social work students completed the questionnaire. Seventy eight were in their first year of training and fifty one in the second year.

Table 5.208
Age of the students

Age Group	N = 130	%
20 years or less	0	0.00
21 - 25 years	1	0.77
26 - 30 years	35	26.92
31 - 35 years	34	26.15
36 - 40 years	17	13.08
41 - 45 years	20	15.38
46 - 50 years	8	6.15
51 - 55 years	2	1.54
Over 55 years	0	0.00

The absence of students less than twenty years of age has previously been explained in Section 5.5.2.2. The age distribution in this group however is the most diverse with more than 20% being more than 40 years of age. The two respondents who were more than 51 years of age were female. Of the 130 social work students 77 had completed relevant courses.

Table 5.209
Previous relevant courses

Relevant Courses	RS = 77
BSc (Hons) Behavioural Sciences	3
BA Humanities	1
B. Education	2
Registered Nurse (RGN,RMNH, RMN)	8
Teacher training (Cert. Ed)	5
C & G Inservice Community Course	15
BTEC Welfare Studies/Community Care	19
Management training	5
OU Courses	3
Counselling Courses	4
Access Courses	5
Police training	1
Diploma in Social Sciences	3
HNC Public Administration	1
Nursery nursing (NNEB)	3
Occupational therapy (12 months)	1
Richmond Fellowship training	1

More than 86% of the sample had gained relevant work experience. This finding was expected because as has previously been explained the social work students were older when they commenced their training and many have been working in an unqualified social worker capacity before they commenced training. The range and depth of experience was very varied but relevant to social work.

Table 5.210
Relevant work experience

Work Experience	RS = 113
Residential social worker (Unqualified)	22
Residential child care worker	15
Nursing auxilliary	11
Residential home for the elderly	20
Work with children with special needs	18
Day care assistants : physically /mentally disabled clients	17
Community work, substance abuse, rape crisis, womens aid, child protection,family support	25
Registered Nurse practice	12
Probation service	6
Occupational therapy helper	4
Play group assistant	5
Nursery nursing	2
Teaching in primary/secondary schools	3
Home care organisers	3
Art therapist	1

With this amount of work experience identified, it was not surprising that 61 respondents indicated that they had experienced shared learning with some of the other professions participating in this study. Nurses were the most frequently identified group (RS = 41) although occupational therapy (RS = 34), speech therapy (RS = 13) and medicine (RS = 15) were also identified. Further analysis of the questionnaires revealed that those working with physically and mentally disabled children and those working in residential homes for the elderly had the most experience of shared learning. One of the Registered Nurses had shared learning with operating department practitioners, radiographers, physiotherapists and dietitians. Twenty four "other professions" were identified. Again these tended to reflect the students previous job experiences. Several had learned with psychologists (RS = 11). These students had worked as residential workers in childrens homes. Probation Officers, prison officers, the police, solicitors, barristers and welfare rights officers were identified by thirteen respondents who had worked in childrens homes or as community workers with substance abusers, abused children, abused women and the homeless.

The samples opinions regarding the concept of interdisciplinary learning

Table 5.211
Should there be interdisciplinary learning ?

Response	Teachers (N = 7)	%	Students (N = 130)	%	Total (N = 137)	%
Yes	7	100.00	124	95.38	131	95.62
No	0	0.00	1	0.77	1	0.73
Undecided	0	0.00	5	3.85	5	3.65

This result clearly demonstrated the perceived needs of the social workers to enter into a more collaborative relationship with the health care professions. The desire for interdisciplinary learning is evidenced by the 95.62% of the sample who responded positively.

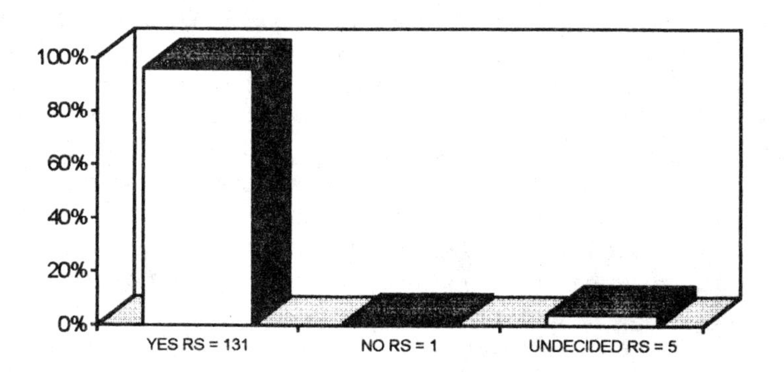

Figure 5.35 Should there be some shared learning ? : By percentage

Table 5.212
At which stage should it take place ?

Response	Teachers (N = 7)	%	Students (N = 130)	%	Total (N = 137)	%
Beginning	2	28.57	17	13.08	19	13.87
Middle	0	0.00	20	15.38	20	14.60
End	1	14.29	7	5.38	8	6.15
Throughout	5	71.43	85	65.38	90	65.69
Post Qual	0	0.00	0	0.00	0	0.00

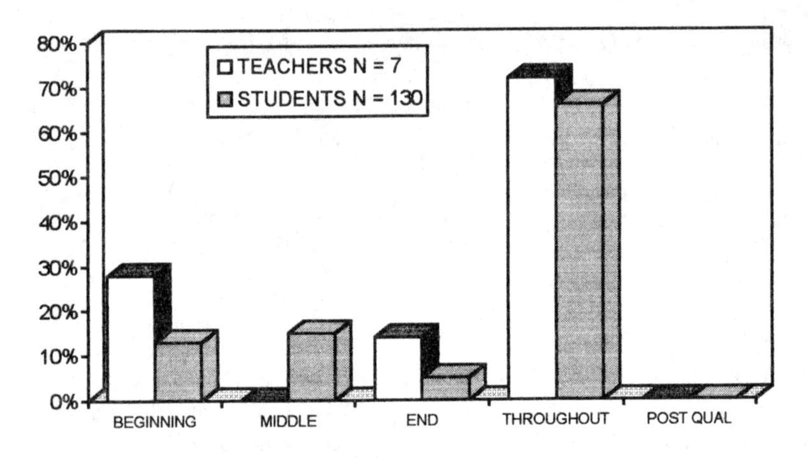

Figure 5.36 At which stage should it take place ? : By percentage

The rationale for including interdisciplinary learning at the beginning was given as; "The sooner the better." (Student Resp.88) and; "This is a difficult question. I think we need to work towards shared learning at 1-2-3 stage but need to start at the beginning first to see the context." (Teacher Resp. 1). Another student (Resp 106) commented; "I chose the middle as I feel that with having some knowledge of my chosen profession, I would be more equipped to share this with others." One student (Resp 76) had already considered this; "I have thought about this prior to receiving this questionnaire. We need to practice (sic) mutual respect in our professions if we are to demonstrate respect for our clients. It must, without question be throughout our training."

Table 5.213
Would there be advantages?

Response	Teachers (N =7)	%	Students (N = 130)	%	Total (N = 137)	%
Yes	7	100.0	123	94.62	130	94.89
No	0	0.0	1	0.77	1	0.73
Undecided	0	0.0	6	4.62	6	4.38

Only six students were undecided as to whether there would be advantages in interdisciplinary learning. All seven teachers and 123 students indicated that there would be advantages. One student gave a negative response. This student was the one who declared himself to be "totally uninterested" in the concept of interdisciplinary learning.

Table 5.214
Advantages of interdisciplinary learning

Response	Teachers (RS = 7)	Students (RS = 123)	Total (N = 137)
Increase understanding of each others role	6	64	70
Increase teamwork and collaboration	3	71	74
Broaden horizons, cross fertilise ideas	2	37	39
Make better use of scarce time & resources	1	0	1

The one student (Resp 11) who was "totally uninterested" in the idea commented; "there are NO advantages." He also rejected all topics stating; "social work is no longer regarded as a clinical approach or a process to "make better".

Table 5.215
Disadvantages of interdisciplinary learning

Response	Teachers (RS = 2)	Students (RS = 39)	Total (N = 137)
Time constraints	0	7	7
Organisational difficulties	1	11	12
Irrelevant material	2	36	38
Hierarchical domination & prejudice	0	23	23
Loss of professional identity	1	9	10
Different academic ability	0	0	0
Different knowledge base	0	3	3
Too many students in a class	0	0	0

One student (Resp 109) was more than concerned that a potential problem was the medical profession and emphatically wrote; "I believe that the medical profession is assumed to hold the most powerful position. It *must* be recognised that they *are not* GOD and hence must allow for sociological perspectives rather than just the medical model."

Table 5.216
Level of interest in interdisciplinary learning

Level of interest	Teachers (N = 7)	Students (N = 130)	Total (N = 137)	%
Very Interested	5	78	83	60.58
Interested	2	47	49	27.51
Neutral	0	2	2	1.46
Uninterested	0	1	1	0.73
Totally Uninterested	0	1	1	0.73

There was a significant level of interest expressed ($\chi^2 = 9.88$, df = 4, $p < 5\%$, Yates correction applied). More than 88% of the social workers in this study were "very interested" or "interested" in the concept of interdisciplinary learning.

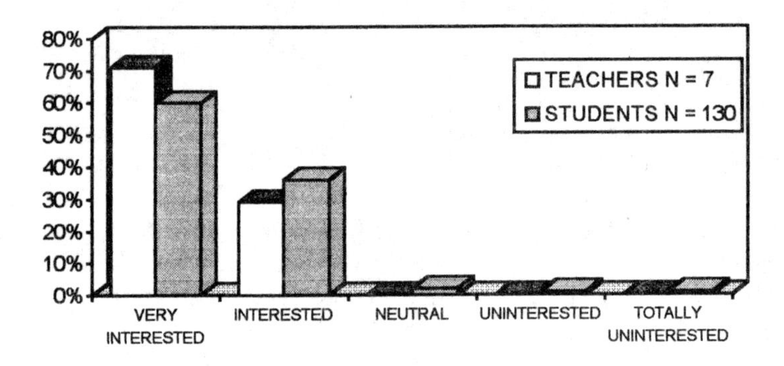

Figure 5.37 The level of interest in interdisciplinary learning : By percentage

The social workers were asked to select from the given list which subjects they thought suitable for interdisciplinary learning.

Table 5.217
Subjects suitable for interdisciplinary learning

Subject	Teachers (N = 7)	%	Students (N = 130)	%	Total (N = 137)	%
Psychology	7	100.0	127	97.69	134	97.81
Sociology	7	100.0	121	93.08	128	93.43
Ethics	6	85.71	116	89.23	122	89.05
Law & Prac.	5	71.43	117	90.00	123	89.78
Research Methods	6	85.71	98	75.38	104	75.91
Management	4	57.14	99	76.13	103	75.18
Economics of care	4	57.14	101	77.69	105	76.64
Health Promotion	3	42.86	110	84.62	113	82.48
Study skills	7	100.0	89	68.46	96	70.07
Quality Issues	6	85.71	106	81.54	112	81.75
Structural Organisation	6	85.71	113	86.92	119	86.86
Computing skills	6	85.71	115	88.46	121	88.32

All the suggested core topics were accepted by at least 75% of this sample from the social work profession. The students (84.62%) viewed health promotion as an interdisciplinary core subject more positively than did the teaching staff. Overall the students seemed to be more positive than were the teaching staff although because the teacher sample was small, this result should be treated with caution.

Table 5.218
Subjects students included in the behavioural sciences

Subject	Yes	%	No	%	Undecided	%
Psychology	128	98.46	0	00.00	1	0.33
Sociology	114	87.69	4	3.07	11	8.46
Ethics	78	60.00	5	3.85	46	35.38
Law & Practice	64	49.23	37	28.46	28	21.54
Management	78	60.00	21	16.15	30	23.08
Health Promotion	79	60.77	22	16.92	28	21.54
Study skills	59	45.38	33	25.38	37	28.46
Quality Issues	67	51.54	26	20.00	36	27.69

Apart from psychology and sociology there was a lot of indecision about which subjects comprise the behavioural sciences. None of the subjects were completely rejected.

Table 5.219
Preferred interdisciplinary learning methods: Students

Learning Method	Yes	%	No	%	Undecided	%
Tutorials	75	57.69	13	10.00	41	24.26
Workshops	119	91.34	2	1.54	8	6.15
Case Studies	112	86.15	3	2.31	14	10.77
Seminars	96	73.85	12	9.23	21	16.15
Problem Based Learning	100	76.92	6	4.62	23	17.69
Role Play	81	67.69	18	13.85	30	23.08
Lectures	73	56.15	20	15.38	36	26.69
Visits to Client Areas	98	75.38	7	5.38	24	18.46

The social work students were the only group who would accept role play as an appropriate interdisciplinary learning method. It was however, still ranked in only sixth place. It is not known whether role play is used more frequently in social work training than in the other programmes. There was no significant difference between role play and the other learning methods ($\chi^2 = 4.29$, df = 2, $p > 5\%$). Tests for significance for the "lecture" $\chi^2 = 28.15$, df = 2, $p < 1\%$) and the "tutorial" ($\chi^2 = 18.21$, df = 2, $p < 5\%$) categories did however identify a difference. Lectures were selected by 73 students and tutorials by 75 students. These were the lowest ranked learning methods.

Table 5.220
Other professions suitable for interdisciplinary learning with social workers

Other Profession	Teachers (N = 7)	%	Students (N = 130)	%	Total (N = 137)	%
Dentists	2	28.57	5	3.85	7	5.11
DSA/DH	2	28.57	13	10.00	15	11.54
Den. Tec.	1	14.29	3	2.31	4	3.08
Medicine	7	100.0	97	74.62	104	75.91
Nursing	7	100.0	114	87.69	121	88.32
Nut & Diet	4	57.14	77	59.23	81	59.12
Occ. Therapy	7	100.00	121	93.08	128	93.43
ODP	1	14.29	19	14.62	20	14.60
Physiotherapy	3	42.86	79	60.77	82	59.85
Podiatry	2	28.57	19	14.62	21	15.33
Radiography	2	28.57	9	6.92	11	8.03
Sp. Therapy	6	85.71	102	78.46	108	78.83

The most frequently chosen profession with whom the social workers would wish to learn are the occupational therapists (93.43%). Nurses were selected by 88.32% of the social workers. Speech therapists were also seen as appropriate by 78.83% of the sample. Speech therapists were selected more frequently than the medical profession (75.91%).

5.5.3.13 The speech therapists

Two teachers and fifty four students completed the questionnaire. Both teachers and fifty three of the students were female. The biographic data of each set of respondents is presented separately.

Biographic data of the teaching staff
One of the teachers was aged between 41 and 45 years and the other between 51 and 55 years. One had practised for 1 to 5 years before commencing her teaching career and had been in her teaching post for 21 to 25 years. The other had been

in practice for 11 to 15 years and had subsequently been teaching for 11 to 15 years. One teacher identified additional areas which she could teach and described these as "cerebral palsy, feeding disorders, alternative and augmentative communication." Both teachers had gained experience of teaching professions other than their own. Respondent 1 had taught dentists, medical practitioners, nurses, occupational therapists, physiotherapists, social workers and teachers. Respondent 2 had taught social workers, teachers and psychologists. Both teachers had participated in learning with other professions at the post qualification stage. Both had learned with medics and teachers and one had learned with occupational therapists and physiotherapists, social workers and bio-engineers.

Biographic data of the speech therapy students

Table 5.221
Age of the students

Age Group	N = 54	%
20 years or less	17	31.48
21 - 25 years	22	40.74
26 - 30 years	1	1.85
31 - 35 years	4	7.41
36 - 40 years	2	3.70
41 - 45 years	4	7.41
46 - 50 years	3	5.56
> 51 years	0	0.00

More than 22% of the speech therapy students were more than 25 years of age with 7 of these being more than 40 years of age.

Table 5.222
Students: Year stage of training

Year of training	N = 54	%
1	18	33.33
2	12	22.22
3	16	29.63
4	8	14.81
5	0	0.00
6	0	0.00

Ten of the students had completed relevant courses previously. These courses were described as Registered Nursing (RS = 3), BTEC Diploma in Social Care (RS = 1), BTEC Nursery Nursing (RS = 1), BTEC National Diploma in Science (RS = 1), BA Humanities (RS = 1) and adult literacy (RS = 1). Thirty four had gained relevant work experience. Of these nine had worked as speech therapy helpers, three had worked on a voluntary basis in schools, three had registered nurse experience, six had worked with children with special needs, six in elderly persons homes and nursing homes, three as voluntary workers in day centres for clients with learning difficulties, one had worked as a psychology research assistant, one had work experience with a social worker and the final respondent had experience as an occupational therapy assistant.

Fifteen students reported that they had experienced shared learning with professions other than their own. All fifteen were first year students. This response can be explained by the introduction of the new course introduced at one Institution where speech and language therapy students share the first year with psychology students.

The speech therapist's opinions regarding the concept of interdisciplinary learning.

Table 5.223
Should there be interdisciplinary learning ?

Response	Teachers (N = 2)	%	Students (N = 54)	%	Total (N = 56)	%
Yes	2	100.00	47	87.01	49	87.50
No	0	0.00	0	0.00	0	0.00
Undecided	0	0.00	7	12.96	7	12.49

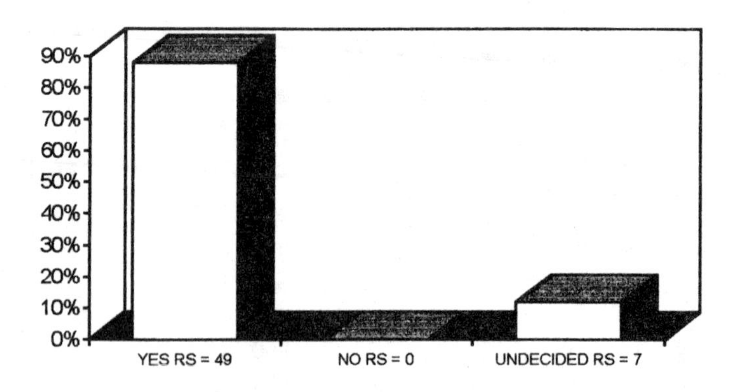

Figure 5.38 Should there be interdisciplinary learning ? By percentage

Table 5.224
At which stage should it take place ?

Response	Teachers (N = 2)	%	Students (N = 54)	%	Total (N = 56)	%
Beginning	0	0.00	3	5.56	3	5.36
Middle	0	0.00	11	20.37	11	19.64
End	0	0.00	5	9.26	5	8.93
Throughout	2	100.0	33	61.11	35	62.50
Post Qual.	0	0.00	2	3.70	2	3.57

Although the majority of students opted for "throughout training" nearly 20 % chose "the middle of training". One of the teachers (Resp 2), commented; "Communication is fundamental to our profession and should therefore be involved at all stages. An essential aspect is communication with related professions."

One student (Resp 44) who was "uninterested" in the concept selected "post qualification" as the stage when interdisciplinary learning should take place. Her rationale for this decision was; "One could feel that shared learning is merely a device by the college to increase numbers of students, cut down the number of lecturers and increase income." Another student (Resp. 42) was more positive; "If this is introduced right from the beginning students will be aware of the need to share knowledge and to work *with* other professionals. It will only go to improve multidisciplinary teams in the workplace." A third year student (Resp 20) selected the end of training because she believed; "You need to be sure of your own role, so that clear messages of expectations and knowledge base was transferred from one group to another." (Sic)

Table 5.225
Would there be advantages ?

Response	Teachers (N = 2)	%	Students (N = 54)	%	Total (N = 56)	%
Yes	2	100.0	51	94.44	53	94.64
No	0	0.00	0	0.00	0	0.00
Undecided	0	0.00	3	5.56	3	5.36

Table 5.226
Advantages of interdisciplinary learning

Advantages	Teachers (RS = 2)	Students (RS = 51)	Total (N = 56)
Increase understanding of each others role	2	33	35
Increase teamwork & collaboration	2	21	23
Broaden horizons, cross fertilise ideas	0	15	17
Make better use of scarce time & resources	0	0	0

Table 5.227
Disadvantages of interdisciplinary learning

Disadvantages	Teachers (RS = 2)	Students (RS = 19)	Total (N = 56)
Time constraints	1	3	4
Organisational difficulties	0	1	1
Irrelevant material	0	13	13
Hierarchical domination & prejudice	0	2	2
Loss of professional identity	1	7	8
Different academic ability	0	0	0
Different knowledge base	1	2	3
Too many students in a class	0	1	1

Table 5.228
Level of interest in interdisciplinary learning

Response	Teachers (N = 2)	%	Students (N = 54)	%	Total (N = 56)	%
Very interested	1	50.00	28	51.85	29	51.79
Interested	0	0.00	20	37.04	20	35.71
Neutral	1	50.00	3	5.56	4	7.14
Uninterested	0	0.00	3	5.56	3	5.36
Totally Uninterested	0	0.00	0	0.00	0	0.00

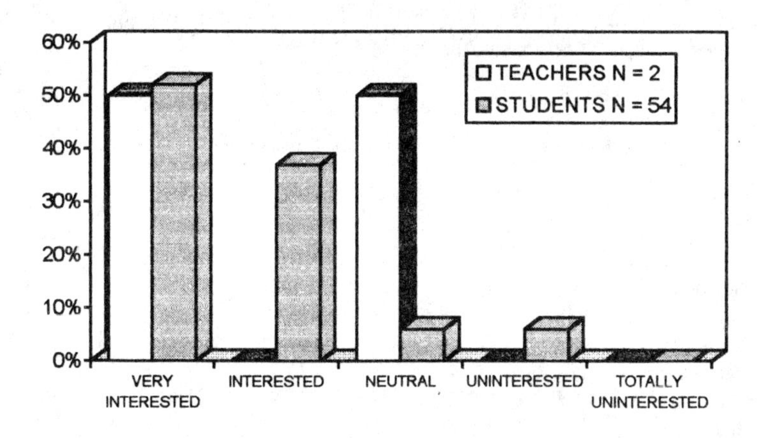

Figure 5.39 Level of interest in interdisciplinary learning : By percentage

More than 88% of the speech therapy students were "very interested" or "interested" in the concept of interdisciplinary learning. As there were only two teachers in this sample, conclusions cannot be drawn about the level of interest.

Table 5.229
Subjects suitable for interdisciplinary learning

Subject	Teachers (N = 2)	%	Students (N = 54)	%	Total (N = 56)	%
Psychology	2	100.0	51	94.44	53	94.62
Sociology	2	100.0	41	75.93	43	79.63
Ethics	2	100.0	48	88.89	50	89.29
Law & Prac.	2	100.0	25	46.30	27	48.21
Research methods	2	100.0	35	64.81	37	66.07
Management	2	100.0	30	55.56	32	57.14
Econ. of health care	2	100.0	39	72.22	41	73.21
Health Prom.	2	100.0	44	81.48	46	82.14
Study skills	2	100.0	34	62.96	36	64.29
Qual. Issues	2	100.0	29	53.70	31	55.36
Structural organisation	2	100.0	45	83.33	47	83.93
Computing skills	2	100.0	46	85.19	48	85.71

Less than 50% of the students believed that law and practice could be learned on an interdisciplinary basis. Although sociology was identified as potentially suitable by nearly 80% of the sample this response was lower than most other professional groups. The reason for this is not clear.

Table 5.230
Subjects students included in the behavioural sciences

Subject	Yes	%	No	%	Undecided	%
Psychology	54	100.00	0	0.00	0	0.00
Sociology	45	83.33	2	3.70	7	12.96
Ethics	33	61.11	5	9.26	16	29.63
Law & Prac.	13	24.07	26	48.15	16	29.63
Management	27	50.00	14	25.93	14	25.93
Health Prom.	35	64.81	9	16.67	10	18.52
Study skills	27	50.00	12	22.22	15	27.78
Qual. Issues	14	25.93	13	24.07	27	50.00

All speech therapy students accepted psychology as a behavioural science. Only 83% were sure that sociology should be included and 50% of the sample were unsure about quality assurance. Most of the options caused a number of students indecision.

Table 5.231
Preferred interdisciplinary learning methods: Students

Learning Method	Yes	%	No	%	Undecided	%
Tutorials	38	70.37	6	11.11	9	16.67
Workshops	45	83.33	3	5.56	5	9.26
Case Studies	44	81.48	3	5.56	5	9.26
Seminars	28	51.85	11	20.37	14	25.93
Problem Based Learning	24	44.44	7	12.96	23	42.59
Role Play	15	27.78	28	51.85	11	20.37
Lectures	27	50.00	13	24.07	13	24.07
Visits to Client Areas	43	79.63	3	5.56	7	12.96

As with all the other student groups apart from social work students, the speech therapists rejected role play. ($\chi^2 = 51.65$, df = 2, p $< 0.1\%$) The most popular learning style for the speech therapists would be interdisciplinary workshops.

Table 5.232
Other professions suitable for interdisciplinary learning with speech therapists

Other Professions	Teachers (N = 2)	%	Students (N = 54)	%	Total (N = 56)	%
Dentists	0	0.00	28	51.85	28	51.85
DSA/DH	0	0.00	11	20.37	11	20.37
Den. Tec.	0	0.00	15	27.78	15	27.78
Medicine	2	100.0	42	77.78	44	81.48
Nursing	1	50.00	45	83.33	46	82.14
Nut. & Diet.	1	50.00	20	37.04	21	37.50
Occ. Therapy	2	100.0	46	85.19	48	85.71
ODP	0	0.00	5	9.26	5	8.93
Physiotherapy	2	100.0	44	81.48	46	82.14
Podiatry	0	0.00	3	5.56	3	5.36
Radiography	1	50.00	12	22.22	13	23.21
Social Work	2	100.0	46	85.19	48	85.71

More than 50% of the students selected dentists as an appropriate profession with whom to share learning whereas neither teacher did. Both teachers and most students selected medicine, occupational therapy, physiotherapy and social work as appropriate. The students appeared to place more value on learning with nursing than did the teachers.

6 Interpretation and discussion of the results

6.1 Introduction

In January 1991 the first paragraph of the work from which this present book was derived, was written and the observation made that maintaining health, preventing disease and caring for the sick was so complex a problem that it was impossible for any health profession to deliver quality care in isolation. Five years later it would seem that this complex problem remains and in some instances has been exacerbated by the rapid and fundamental changes in the delivery of health and social care in the United Kingdom. Little empirical evidence could be found which specifically examined the concept of integrated interdisciplinary learning at an undergraduate stage. Spitzer (1975) argued that before any conclusive and definitive statement about interdisciplinary learning could be made, someone should attempt to determine the feasibility of its introduction into practice. In consequence this study was conceived in order to try and meet the challenge laid down by Spitzer. The study commenced with the following aims :

1. To analyse the behavioural science content specified within the current curricula for each health care profession in order to determine commonality.
2. To identify the behavioural science textbooks listed in the current curricula for each health care profession in order to determine replication.
3. To determine the opinions of a sample of teachers and students from each health care profession regarding :
    - 3.1 The concept of interdisciplinary learning.
    - 3.2 The perceived advantages/disadvantages of interdisciplinary learning.
    - 3.3 When interdisciplinary learning should take place, if at all.
    - 3.4 The favoured learning methods which should be adopted.
    - 3.5 The level of interest in interdisciplinary learning.

3.6 Which professions would be acceptable to each other on an interdisciplinary learning basis.

3.7 Which core subjects would be acceptable to the teachers and students on an interdisciplinary basis.

4. To determine :

4.1 The operational strategies required to implement integrated interdisciplinary learning.

4.2 The preparation needed by the teachers themselves prior to the implementation of an interdisciplinary programme.

5. To ascertain from the statutory and professional bodies :

5.1 Whether integrated interdisciplinary learning in the behavioural sciences would fulfil the statutory requirements of the individual professions.

5.2 Their level of support for any potential developments in interdisciplinary learning between the health and social care professions.

Due to the diversity and amount of data collected in this study, the discussion of the findings are presented in the same order as the data collection was undertaken. The presentation of this chapter therefore reflects that of Chapters 3, 4 and 5. Reference to the aims of the study are made where appropriate throughout the Chapter.

6.2 Content analysis of the curricula

Content analysis it is acknowledged, can be subjective and biased. (Holsti 1969, Kerlinger 1986, Polit & Hungler 1989, Judd et al 1991). Attempts were made to minimise this problem when undertaking this study, by inviting either the course director of each programme or a senior member of the teaching staff, to analyse the results of their own curricula and make amendments if they so wished. The rationale for their involvement at this stage was two fold. By involving the teachers at this crucial stage, it was hoped that their interest and commitment to the study would be maintained or even enhanced. This strategy seemed to be essential.

Stanford (1987) mentioned "empowerment" of people while Treece and Treece (1986) referred to the need for an orientation towards the consumer. Heron (1985) was certain that successful action research hinged on co-operation and succinctly concluded that it is a way of "doing research with people rather than on people" (p 128). The commitment and level of interest from the teachers seemed to be maintained throughout the study as evidenced by their willingness to complete yet another task and by the many subsequent informal enquiries received about the overall results and progress in completing the written report.

The second reason for involving the teachers at this stage was to try and minimise the subjectivity and bias that a content analysis undertaken by one individual may have invoked. The validity of the results would be enhanced by the fact that teachers who were very familiar with their own curriculum were able to moderate the results if they so chose. The adoption of this strategy also ensured that evidence of expert opinion was included as suggested by Moore (1983), Marshall & Rossman (1989), Tesch (1990). All fourteen content analyses were returned, most with no alterations and a few with one or two deletions or additions. As each of the fourteen teachers received the content analysis of his/her own curriculum only, this ensured that no comparisons could be made with the results of the other professions. This also enhanced the validity of the results by excluding any potential bias from the teachers themselves. Confidentiality was also maintained as it was unknown at this stage of the study how each teacher would react to the results. Absence of a particular concept in the results could have been interpreted as an implied criticism of a curriculum. As all 14 teachers returned the analysis without any negative comments, knowing that the final content analysis was to be included in this report, implicit approval has been given and these particular results of the content analysis are no longer confidential.

The content analysis of the fourteen curricula revealed 108 items or single words which were included in many of the course documents as part of the behavioural sciences component (see Chapter 5, Table 5.1). In some of the curricula however, some of these items were clearly identified as discrete subject areas such as "law and practice", "ethics" or "management". It was because of the different approaches to curriculum design and content that the original plan to examine the behavioural science component only was abandoned and the inclusion criteria extended to include the above elements along with "research methods", "economics of care", "health promotion", "study skills", "quality assurance issues" and the "structural organisation of health care". This decision (made in the early stages of this project) later proved to be entirely justified. The responses obtained during the structured interviews with the teaching staff (N = 29) and the students (N = 22) resulted in a question being asked in the main study student questionnaire which enabled students to select which subjects they would include in the behavioural sciences. The results indicated that there was confusion and uncertainty about their choices (see Chapter 5, Table 5.54).

No firm conclusions can be drawn from this study as to which subjects constitute the behavioural sciences. Many of the behavioural scientists cited in Section 2.8 of the literature review would appear to agree with this. Dervin and Harlock (1976) included ethics, law, health promotion, communication and management in their behavioural science modules. Northouse and Northouse (1985) included all aspects in their course on teamwork, while Crute, Hargie and Ellis (1989) in their micro skills communication component, adopted every subject when using role play. As a result of the finding that role play has been rejected overwhelmingly in this current study, perhaps Crute and Hargie should re-evaluate their chosen teaching methods and ask their students whether the use of role play is acceptable ! Dickens et al (1985) and Van Dalen et al (1989) also used a combination of academic disciplines when presenting patient vignettes to students who had to use problem solving strategies when planning care. Jameton and Todes (1982) were the most prescriptive in their recommendations when they concluded that the study of law, ethics, economics, health policies, and the philosophy of health care should be included in all behavioural science courses.

Their recommendations can be substantiated in this study. The 108 items in the content analysis were examined by a number of individual teachers who apart from their professional qualification held a degree in one of the following : psychology ; sociology ; law ; ethics ; management. Each teacher was asked to claim each item in his/her academic discipline. It is acknowledged that this was an entirely subjective exercise and indeed several individuals included this caveat with their response. The exercise demonstrated, nevertheless that many of the 108 items sit comfortably in several of the academic disciplines indicating that there is a great deal of blurring and overlap between subject areas (the results are presented as Table 6.1 overleaf).

The results emphasise the importance of regular meetings between any teaching team on any course where the content and presentation should be discussed. The rationale for this recommendation is justifed by the suspicion that in some instances there will be duplication in the material presented to students whilst in others the material may be omitted entirely by teachers who assume that one of their colleagues will be covering the topic.

It may be that this 108 item content analysis could be used as a checklist for future curriculum developers in the health and social care professions. This would encourage a more consistent approach in the theoretical preparation of students for practice but would also enable each professions autonomy and specific knowledge to flourish in that the concepts could be learned initially in a generalist way followed by application to profession specific needs.

The completion of the 108 item content analysis of the fourteen curricula in which many topics have proved to be common to many (and in some cases all) of the professions achieved the first stated aim of this study.

Table 6.1 Topics claimed by the different academic disciplines

TOPICS	PSYCHOLOGY	SOCIOLOGY	ETHICS	LAW & PRACTICE	RESEARCH METHODS	MANAGEMENT	HEALTH ECONOMICS	HEALTH PROMOTION
AGEING PROCESS	1	1	0	0	0	0	0	1
AGGRESSION	1	0	0	1	0	0	0	0
ANDRAGOGY / ADULT LEARNING	1	0	0	0	0	0	0	0
ASSERTIVENESS	1	0	0	0	0	1	1	0
ATTRACTION	1	0	0	0	0	0	0	0
ATTITUDES	1	1	0	1	0	1	0	1
BEHAVIOURIST APPROACH	1	0	0	0	0	0	0	1
BEREAVEMENT	1	1	1	1	0	0	0	1
BIOLOGIGAL APPROACH	1	0	0	0	0	0	0	1
BODY IMAGE	1	0	1	0	0	0	0	1
BUDGETING	0	0	0	0	0	1	0	0
CHILD HEALTH	1	1	1	1	0	0	1	1
CLIENT ASSESSMENT	1	1	0	0	0	1	1	1
COGNITIVE APPROACH	1	0	0	0	0	0	0	1
COGNITIVE DEVELOPMENT	1	0	0	0	0	0	0	0
COMP.HEALTH THERAPY	1	0	0	0	0	0	0	1
COMPETENCIES	0	1	0	1	1	1	0	1
COMPUTING SKILLS	0	0	0	0	1	1	0	0
CONCEPT FORMATION	1	0	0	0	0	0	0	1
CONCEPTS,HEALTH/ILLNESS	1	1	0	0	0	0	0	1
CONFIDENTIALITY	1	1	1	1	0	0	0	1
CONFLICT RESOLUTION	1	0	0	0	0	1	0	0
COPING MECHANISMS	1	0	1	0	0	0	0	1
COUNSELLING	1	0	1	1	0	0	1	1
CULTURAL VALUES	1	1	1	1	0	0	0	1
DECISION MAKING	1	1	0	1	0	1	1	1
DIFFERING GROUPS	0	1	0	1	0	0	1	1
DISABILITY	1	1	1	1	0	0	0	1
ECON OF HEALTH CARE	0	0	1	1	0	1	1	1
EMPLOYMENT	0	1	0	1	0	1	1	0
ETHICS	1	1	1	1	0	0	0	0
ETHNICITY	1	1	1	1	0	1	0	1

	PSYCHOLOGY	SOCIOLOGY	ETHICS	LAW & PRACTICE	RESEARCH METHODS	MANAGEMENT	ECONOMICS OF CARE	HEALTH PROMOTION
EVALUATION OF CHANGE	0	1	0	0	0	1	0	1
FAMILY GROUPS	1	1	0	0	0	0	0	1
FAMILY NEEDS	1	1	1	1	0	0	0	1
FAMILY THERAPY	1	1	0	0	0	0	0	0
FIRST AID	0	0	0	0	0	0	0	1
GENDER	1	1	0	1	0	1	0	0
GRIEF	1	1	1	0	0	0	0	1
GRIEVANCES	0	0	0	0	0	1	0	0
GROUP DYNAMICS	1	1	0	0	0	1	0	0
GROUP THERAPY	1	1	0	0	0	0	0	0
HEALTH BEHAVIOURS	1	0	0	0	0	0	0	1
HEALTH BELIEFS	1	0	1	0	0	0	0	1
HEALTH PROMOTION	1	1	0	0	0	0	0	1
HEALTH/SAFETY AT WORK	0	0	0	1	0	1	0	1
HOLISTIC CARE	1	0	0	1	0	0	1	1
HUMANIST APPROACH	1	1	0	0	0	0	0	0
I.Q.TEST	1	0	0	0	0	0	0	0
ILLNESS PERCEPTION	1	0	0	0	0	0	0	1
IMAGERY	1	0	0	0	0	0	0	0
IMPLEMENTING CHANGE	0	1	0	1	0	1	1	1
INDIVIDUALITY	1	0	1	1	0	0	0	1
INFORMATION TECHNOLOGY	0	0	0	0	1	1	1	0
INFORMED CONSENT	0	0	1	1	0	0	0	0
INTELLIGENCE	1	0	0	0	0	0	0	0
INTERDISCIPLINARY	1	1	1	1	0	1	1	1
INTERPERSON PERCEPTIONS	1	0	0	0	0	0	0	0
INTERVIEWING	0	0	0	1	0	1	0	0
KELLY'S CONSTRUCT THEORY	1	0	0	0	0	0	0	0
LAW & PRACTICE	0	0	0	1	0	1	0	0
LEADERSHIP	1	0	0	1	0	1	0	0
LEARNING DIFFICULTIES	1	0	1	1	0	0	0	1
LEARNING STYLES	1	0	0	0	0	0	0	0
LISTENING	1	0	0	0	0	0	0	1
LISTENING SKILLS	1	0	0	0	0	0	0	0

	PSYCHOLOGY	SOCIOLOGY	ETHICS	LAW & PRACTICE	RESEARCH METHODS	MANAGEMENT	ECONOMICS OF CARE	HEALTH PROMOTION
LITERATURE REVIEWS	0	0	0	0	1	0	0	0
MANAGING CHANGE	0	1	0	1	0	1	0	0
MEMORY	1	0	0	0	0	0	0	0
MINORITY GROUPS	1	1	0	1	0	0	0	1
MORAL DEVELOPMENT	1	0	0	0	0	0	0	0
MOTIVATION	1	0	0	0	0	1	0	1
NATURE/NURTURE	1	0	0	0	0	0	0	0
NON-VERBAL COMMUNICATION	1	0	0	0	0	0	0	0
ORGANISATION THEORY	0	1	0	0	0	1	0	0
PARTNERSHIP	0	0	0	1	0	1	0	0
PATIENT CHOICE	1	0	1	1	0	0	0	1
PATIENT DIGNITY	1	0	1	1	0	0	0	1
PATIENT & ENVIRONMENT	1	1	0	1	0	1	1	1
PATIENT RIGHTS	1	0	1	1	0	1	0	1
PEDAGOGY	1	0	0	0	0	0	0	0
PERCEPTION	1	0	0	0	0	0	0	1
PERSONAL ORGANISATION	1	0	0	0	0	1	0	1
POWER	1	0	0	1	0	1	0	0
PRESENTATION SKILLS	0	0	0	0	1	1	0	0
PROBLEM SOLVING	1	0	0	0	1	1	0	0
PROFESSIONAL BODIES	0	1	0	1	0	1	0	0
PROFESSIONALISM	0	1	0	1	0	1	0	0
PSYCHOLOGY & AGEING	1	0	0	0	0	0	0	1
PSYCHOANALYTIC APPROACH	1	0	0	0	0	0	0	0
PSYCHOLOGY OF PAIN	1	0	1	1	0	0	0	1
QUALITY ASSURANCE	0	0	0	1	1	1	1	0
QUESTIONNAIRE DESIGN	0	0	1	0	1	0	0	0
QUESTIONS CLOSED	0	0	0	0	1	0	0	0
QUESTIONS OPEN	0	0	0	0	1	0	0	0
REFLECTIVE QUESTIONING	0	0	0	0	1	1	0	1
RESEARCH METHODS	0	0	0	0	1	0	0	0
RESEARCH SAMPLING	0	0	0	0	1	0	0	0
RISK TAKING	1	0	1	1	0	1	1	1
ROLE	1	1	0	1	0	1	0	1

	PSYCHOLOGY	SOCIOLOGY	ETHICS	LAW & PRACTICE	RESEARCH METHODS	MANAGEMENT	ECONOMICS OF CARE	HEALTH PROMOTION
SEXUALITY	1	0	0	0	0	0	0	1
SOCIAL DEVELOPMENT	1	1	0	0	0	0	0	1
SOCIAL SKILLS	1	1	0	0	0	0	0	0
STAFF.DEVEL.TRAINING	1	1	0	1	0	1	1	0
STATISTICS	0	0	0	0	1	1	1	0
STEREOTYPING	1	1	0	0	0	0	0	1
STRESS	1	0	0	0	0	1	0	1
STUDY SKILLS	0	0	0	0	1	0	0	0
SUBSTANCE ABUSE	1	0	0	1	0	1	0	1
TASK & FUNCTION	0	1	0	1	0	1	1	0
TEAM WORK	1	1	0	1	0	1	1	1
THEORY & PRACTICE	0	0	0	0	0	0	0	0
VERBAL COMMUNICATION	1	0	0	0	0	0	0	0
WORK RELATED STRESS	1	1	0	1	0	1	0	1
WRITING REPORTS	0	0	0	1	1	1	0	1

6.3 The indicative reading lists

These results were the least satisfactory in the whole study. Content analysis of each of the fourteen curricula yielded very different amounts of information about the reading material recommended to students on each course (see Chapter 5, Table 5.2). One of the reasons for these differences it is suggested, may be due to some curriculum planning teams including only minimal examples of the available reading materials in the course documents while others include a comprehensive list of references. It is presumed that in many instances, reading lists are distributed at each year stage of a course and are updated on a regular basis. What was of interest was that the course documents of newly validated degree courses were extremely comprehensive whereas those that had been established for a number of years tended to be sparse in some areas. Quality assurance and validation procedures and the concommitant expectations would seem to have improved beyond all recognition over the past five years. As courses are subject to quinquennial reviews it can be anticipated that a consequent improvement in the quality of documentation will continue.

The information obtained from the reading lists (however incomplete) did enable some general observations to be made. Approximately 440 textbooks were identified from the documents. Very few were adopted by more than one course. Where there was evidence of several courses using the same textbooks, the common factor tended to be a teacher who taught on more than one course and who tended to use the same textbook for all teaching sessions. Several issues are raised by this finding. If, as some claim, it is essential for each profession to learn in isolation in order to concentrate on specific knowledge how can this claim be justified when in psychology and sociology in particular the key texts are the same ? Surely this adds to the argument that basic theory can be taught to all and then subsequent consideration of those theories can be given in profession specific tutorials. The cost of education is such that a rationalisation of library services should be an important area of concern. This is not to suggest that the breadth of textbooks should in any way be reduced but that because of the need to purchase multiple copies of essential reading texts for each course, many of these texts will be under utilised for many months of each year. Interdisciplinary discussion and negotiation between all teaching staff and the librarians may enable substantial savings to be made. Rationalisation of some of the multiple copy purchases most certainly would ensure optimum use of these texts. The cost of many academic books is often high and in the field of health and social care they tend to be outdated almost as soon as they are in print. By ensuring the maximum useage of these books would represent the best value for money.

These findings have addressed the second aim of the study by identifying some of the textbooks adopted in each course. The content analysis indicated that there is very little replication of books between the courses but that this problem could be partly resolved through increased debate and negotiation on an interdisciplinary basis. These results could be utilised in an initial discussion document.

6.4 The overall picture

Three hundred teachers and 1383 students representing thirteen professions in health and social care completed the questionnaires (see Chapter 5, Section 5.1) The response rate for the postal questionnaire distributed to the teachers was 86.96% indicating a very high level of interest in the study (Oppenheim 1992). In some of the smaller schools a response rate of 100% was achieved. Since the commencement of this study in January 1991 there has been a substantial increase in the number of publications which refer to the need for shared learning, teamwork and collaborative care (Welsh Office 1991,1992, 1993, Dept. Of Health 1991, 1993, Audit Commission 1992) Many of these documents have been in the form of government directives which have placed the onus on the health care professions to examine both the current levels of collaborative practice and the content of the educational programmes which prepare students to become qualified practitioners in a health team. It is believed that these directives have had a positive effect on the response rate in this study as the questionnaire enabled the teachers to address the issues surrounding interdisciplinary learning and to express their opinions anonymously with regard to any potential changes in the curricula. The response rate of 86.96% seemed to indicate that in South East Wales the teachers were committed to exploring the concept of interdisciplinary learning. A further impetus may have been that in the absence of many empirical studies a possible outcome would be some definitive answers which could be assimilated into any future discussions, developments and innovations. The opinons and level of interest expressed by the teaching staff from the thirteen professions was therefore fundamental to any conclusions and recommendations that subsequently would be made.

Of equal consequence were the opinions of the student population who will be the qualified practitioners in the next millenium. The majority of students in this sample had experienced a limited amount of client contact and also had the opportunity to work with qualified practitioners from their own professions. This means that they may have observed some of the other professions at work in a variety of clinical settings. Their initial impressions of the health team at work would have been likely therefore to influence their opinions and their level of interest in interdisciplinary learning.

The method of distributing and collecting the student questionnaires differed from that of the teacher questionnaire in that time was negotiated within each programme for each year stage of training for all thirteen professions. In essence this meant that large numbers of students were present on many occasions and were potential recruits to the study. The ethical issue relating to the potential coercion of these students was minimised by withdrawing for a period of time following the distribution of the questionnaires. This enabled the students to complete the questionnaire, if they so wished without being scrutinised. It is acknowledged however, that some individual students may have felt under peer pressure to complete the questionnaire and may have discussed the responses with their peers.

The number of students who completed the questionnaire was still extremely high with 1359 being completed as previously described and a further 24 being returned through the post. The overall response rate was 96.26% (see Chapter 5, Section 5.2). It should be remembered however, that the population represents only those students who were present on a particular date at a particular time. No attempt was made to contact any individuals who were absent on that date.

Although it was less likely that many of the students had access to the documents advocating increased interdisciplinary learning and collaborative care it is suggested that the concept was being introduced regularly by the teaching staff in both the clinical areas and within the educational institutions. The students responses suggested that they fully understood the concept and the implications of what they were writing.

The biographic data of the respondents

Overall there were more male (RS = 159) than female (RS = 139) teachers in this sample There were however substantial differences between the professions (see Table 5.31). In both the dental and medical professions the ratio of male teachers exceeded the female teachers by 29 : 11 and 80 : 27 respectively. Conversely in the nursing profession the male teachers were exceeded by the female teachers by a ratio of 29 : 68. The student populations from these three professions however, presented a different picture. The male dental students outnumber the female dental students but the ratio differential was much smaller at 53 : 40. The medical students comprised more females than males (149 : 120). The nursing students were predominantly female (RS = 333) with only 63 male students (see Table 5.49).

There are several interesting questions which arose from these results which were outside the remit of this study to resolve. In the dental and medical professions the results indicated that more males than females had been appointed into academic posts. It may be that previously more men than women entered these professions and that the gender ratio reflected the gender ratios of undergraduate dental and medical students a few years ago. This assumption was justified by noting that the traditional entry criteria into dental and medical schools had been science related Advanced Levels. More males than females completed science Advanced Levels, therefore more males than females met the entry criteria. Another possibility was that there had been a deliberate policy to recruit more females into the dental and medical professions. The King's Fund Report (Towle 1991) advocated the need for a greater number of females to be recruited into the medical profession. The nursing profession as a whole has always been predominantly female. Within the profession itself however, there have been exceptions. One exception was in the field of psychiatric nursing where in some instances there were more male nurses than females (HMSO 1980) and another was in mental handicap (HMSO 1979). The number of male nurse teachers in this sample (RS = 29, 30.21%) (Table 5.31) is representative of nurse teachers (HMSO 1972, GNC 1975, RCN 1964, RCN 1985a, Nolan 1987) but is not representative of the number of men in the nursing profession as a whole where the percentage continues to be between 10 and 15% (UKCC 1993). It is not known whether these results are representative of the gender distribution amongst teachers in the health and social professions in general.

The other professions sample sizes were too small to enable any in depth analysis. The trend however seemed to suggest that where the student population was predominantly female so was the teaching population. Examples of these being nutrition and dietetics, dental surgery assistants/dental hygienists and speech therapists. Paradoxically where there were more male students then the teachers were also male as was evident in the dental technology and operating practitioner samples.

The student population (N = 1383) was predominantly female (RS = 1018, 73.61%) with only 364 males. The results by profession demonstrated wide variations however, with the dental surgery assistants/dental hygienists comprising only females (N = 37, 100.00%). There was only one male in the nutrition and dietetics sample (N = 45) and one in speech therapy (N = 54). In other professions there were more male than female students (see Table 5.49). As previously suggested in Chapter 5, this may be due to the high technological content in training programmes such as dental technology and operating department practice. There was a significant difference between the number of males who were training as physiotherapists (RS = 23, 22.77% where N = 101) and occupational therapists (RS = 9, 10.11% where N = 89) (see Table 5.49). The reason for this was unclear. One possible attraction of physiotherapy as a career for men may be the close links that this profession has with many types of physical sports and is a service which is frequently prescribed for young healthy individuals who have been temporarily disabled by trauma. Conversely occupational therapy has the lay persons reputation as dealing with long term disabled individuals who tend to be in the older age group.

The overall results confirm that most of the health and social care professions continue to attract females in significantly greater numbers than males. Whether this is due to the traditional picture of caring as "women's work" is not known. In this decade with the high level of unemployment, the reasons for the failure to recruit more men into the professions allied to medicine and nursing would be an interesting area of research to pursue.

The number of teaching respondents who were less than 30 years of age was very small (RS = 9) (see Table 5.32 and Figure 5.4). This can be explained by the fact that an individual's teaching career (in any of the professions which participated in this study) normally commences after a few years of gaining credibility and expertise in clinical practice. Of the 30 respondents who were aged 56 years or more, only four were female. Many women retire after 40 years service in the NHS and nearly all leave by the age of 60 years. As 20 of the respondents who were over 56 years belonged to either the dental or medical professions, which the results showed were predominantly male, this finding was not surprising. It would be interesting to compare these findings in a few years time with future teachers age distributions. It may be that there will be a noticeable change as the increasing numbers of mature student entrants progress through their professional careers. They will not complete 40 years service and it may be that they would wish to continue in employment as long as possible. Another factor which may influence any future results would be the increasing number of women entering the dental and medical professions.

More than 70% of the 1383 students were less than 25 years of age (RS = 982) (Table 5.50). Seventeen students did not disclose their age. Of the 384 students who were more than 25 years of age, 116 (30.29%) were training to be social workers. Indeed, of the 130 social work students 81 (62.31%) were more than 31 years of age. There are several explanations for this finding. The social work programme is essentially a non graduate entry and prospective students therefore have to be able to demonstrate that they have undertaken previous relevant courses or gained appropriate work experience. Many of the students in this sample, had been working in an unqualified capacity and had been seconded by their employers. They were therefore more likely to be in the older age categories. Finally, in 1991 CCETSW published a document entitled "Dip. SW Rules and Requirements for the Diploma in Social Work" (sic) which stated that social work students must be a minimum of 22 years before they can be awarded the Diploma. This meant, in effect, that in order to complete the two year programme they could not commence training until they were at least 20 years of age. It was not known whether the adoption of the 22 year rule was an arbitary choice or whether there was a legal reason for this.

The second profession with a noticeable number of mature students was nursing with 103 students (26.01% where N = 396) being more than 25 years of age (Table 5.50). As was demonstrated in a subsequent question many of these students had previously worked in either a voluntary capacity or as nursing auxilliaries prior to commencing training (Table 5.52). A large number (RS = 119) had completed related courses previously, and of these at least 29 were graduates in related subjects (Table 5.51). It could be argued that one effect of the current high levels of unemployment has been to attract graduate entrants into nursing, who have brought a wealth of related knowledge with them which can only benefit the profession as a whole.

The other professions tended to recruit younger students thus confirming that many of the health professions continue to train individuals who have met the required academic qualifications at school but have little or no life experiences.

This was particularly true of the medical profession with only 23 students who were more than 25 years of age (8.55% where N = 269) and the dental profession who had only 7 students who were more than 25 years of age (7.53% where N = 93) (Table 5.50). If the age of the students in the preclinical years who did not participate in this study had also been included, the percentages overall for both of these professions may well have been still lower. It is suggested that while, without doubt there are advantages in recruiting teenagers into the professions such as getting the maximum financial return for the investment made in expensive training programmes, there is also a negative aspect in that the emotional demands made upon individuals who may be only just maturing into adulthood could be detrimental to those individuals themselves and also to the patient/client for whom they care.

Of the 1383 students, 358 (25.89%) had previously undertaken courses which they considered relevant to their current training (Table 5.51). Many of the courses described were directly related to the students current training. Examples of these included the medical students who had completed science degrees, podiatry and operating department practitioner students who were Registered Nurses and social work students who had trained as probation officers or police officers. A limitation within the design of the questionnaire became evident when analysing this question. The question (Number 5) asked the students whether they had previously undertaken any courses which they considered relevant to their current training. Most of the 29 medical students who had science degrees had in fact completed these as an option at the end of their pre - clinical course and were therefore medical students at the time of graduation. This conclusion can be justified by referring to the ages of these respondents which indicate quite clearly that they must have commenced their pre - clinical training at the age of 18 years. On reflection, it would have been more appropriate to include the word "before" they commenced their current training as the ambiguity of the wording inadvertently caused this confusion.

Nearly 60% of the students had gained relevant work experience (Table 5.52). This result was higher than expected (RS = 820 where N = 1383). There were however wide variations between the professions with as many as 94.62% of the social work students and as few as 26.88% of the dental students. The high percentage of social work students has been explained by the entry criteria requisites for the social work programme. Predictably the more mature students had more relevant work experience than the younger students. The work experience described varied considerably although most could be directly attributed to either voluntary work or paid employment in health or social care. Examples of this included "nursing auxilliary" ; "occupational therapy helper" ; "working with mentally handicapped children" ; "work in a childrens home". Interpretation of the results by profession is subsequently discussed in this chapter however it seemed that most students had gained work experience which was directly relevant to their own profession. An occupational therapy student, for example would have worked as an occupational therapy helper whereas a radiography student would have worked in a radiography department. What is not known however, is whether students, by chance gain experience in a field of health or social care and as a result of this experience subsequently apply for formal training or whether they apply to work in a specific area having already chosen the profession which they wish to join. These findings may have implications for future manpower planning within the NHS and the Social Services. If more opportunities were made available for work experience in a variety of clinical and social settings, then prospective students would be able to make an informed choice regarding their future careers. It would enable them to discuss with practitioners the strengths and weaknesses, the opportunities and threats which exist within each profession. If individuals were able to consider the options available to them and then select the profession which best reflected their own values, needs and aspirations, the attrition rate may well be reduced.

Although 231 teachers reported that they had taught professions other than their own, many of the responses indicated that these "other professions" related closely to their own (Table 5.36). The clustering of responses from the dental surgeons, dental surgery assistants, dental technologists, nutritionists and dietitians and the speech therapists illustrate the point. While there is no doubt that the need for 'regional' specialism and sharing of knowledge should continue and indeed expand there would seem to be a lamentable lack of imagination into the possibilities for promoting health as a holistic concept. The promotion of dental and oral health would seem to be a fundamental principle that all the health and social professions should adopt in their dealings with clients. The most appropriate way in which to approach this would be to involve teachers from the above professions in leading interdisciplinary discussions on oral health, appropriate prostheses and healthy eating. A heightened awareness amongst nurses, social workers and general practitioners would enable for example, a more informed assessment of the clients who are supported in the community.

A further point of interest was that whilst it was likely that the dentists had taught the other related professions, it was unlikely that the other professions had taught dentists. The same trend could be observed in the percentage of medical practitioners (93.75%) who had taught for example, nurses (18.56%), podiatrists (25.00%), physiotherapists (10.00%) and occupational therapists (42.86%) whereas very few of those professions had taught medical practitioners (The percentages in brackets after the professions other than medicine indicate the numbers from those professions who had taught medical practitioners). The reason for the unequal exchange of information and expertise cannot be positively concluded. It is suggested however, that this may be due to the perceived hierarchical structure in which dentists and medical practitioners are seen as the dominating professions who therefore share their superior knowledge (Swift and MacDougall 1964, Martin 1969, Shortell 1974, Gomes 1985, Brunning and Huffington 1985, Hancock 1990). The emergence of the biopsychosocial model of care may well redress the balance in that the specific expertise within each profession will be acknowledged.

The results from this study have revealed that generally, hierarchical dominance is not perceived in reality and that references to professional domination may well be a self perpetuating myth. What is evident however from both the teachers and students results is the lack of insight into the other professions roles and contribution to care. It is therefore not surprising that podiatrists have not contributed to the medical curriculum. The inclusion of such an innovation should improve medical practitioners insight into the invaluable contribution that the podiatrists can make towards maintaining an elderly or disabled persons mobility for example. Addressing the issues surrounding the contributions of each profession on an interdisciplinary basis at the beginning of each professions training would help to alleviate this problem.

Of the 300 teacher respondents 186 (61.99%) had experienced some shared learning with other professions (Table 5.37). However of these only 42 (13.99%) had done so prior to qualifying (11 were dentists and 17 were medical practitioners who indicated that this had occured during their pre - clinical years). There was no evidence that the dental and medical professions had experienced undergraduate interdisciplinary learning other than with each other. The six nurse teachers who indicated that they had experienced shared learning at an undergraduate level indicated subjects such as "liberal studies". The results of this question confirm that the majority of learning between the professions had taken place after individuals qualify. Even then clustering of the professions tended to occur as a result of attending conferences of shared professional interest. This confirms the conclusions drawn in the literature review (Shakespeare 1989, Team Care Valleys 1990).

The students results were no more encouraging. It would seem that no progress has been made as far as any interdisciplinary learning is concerned since the teachers were students themselves. Of the 1383 respondents 336 (24.30%) had experienced interdisciplinary learning (Table 5.53). Some of these were first year speech therapy students (N = 15) who had commenced the new degree course where speech therapy and psychology students share teaching sessions for the first year. Another easily identifiable group were the 68 dental students (73.12% where N = 93) and 62 medical students (23.05% where N = 269) who had shared learning during their preclinical years. What was more interesting was the number of dental and medical students who did not seem to have shared learning! There was a substantial difference between the two groups. Medical students were less likely to remember (or admit) that this shared learning had taken place in that 205 (76.21%) indicated that they had not whereas only 25 (26.88%) of the dental students did not acknowledge the experience.

In-depth analysis of the remaining respondents from the other professions revealed that all had gained a previous qualification (such as the eight podiatry students who were Registered Nurses) or had previously worked in the health and social professions. No evidence was found to suggest that any other interdiscplinary learning at an undergraduate stage is taking place between the health and social care professions in any of the educational institutions which participated in this study. It would appear that in spite of the numerous publications reviewed in the literature, that have appeared over the last three decades which have recommended shared learning, the professions continue to learn in isolation.

The breadth and depth of expertise amongst the teaching staff was revealed in their response to the question of whether they considered that they possessed additional areas of expertise which they could teach. Of the 300 respondents 112 (37.33%) indicated additional expertise. Of these 112 respondents 78 (69.64%) were teachers of nursing or from the professions allied to medicine. The explanation for this finding is thought to be due to the move towards an all graduate status for teachers of nursing and the professions allied to medicine. Consequently during the last few years many of the teachers have completed degree courses in subjects which have a direct relevance to their own professions and indeed many are now teaching these subjects to their students. Examples of these degree subjects were listed as psychology, sociology, health promotion, ethics and law, education, management, physiology. As both the dental and medical professions have had an all graduate training for many years, implicitly all teaching staff were already graduates when they commenced their teaching careers. Recently papers published by the UKCC (1993) and the WNB (1993) have highlighted the need to recruit future teachers of nursing from the increasing number of graduate nurses with a nursing degree. If this directive is achieved it is probable that for the nursing profession at least, fewer teachers will have related degrees such as in the behavioural or life sciences. It is not unreasonable to predict that the same trend will occur in the professions allied to medicine. Most training is now taught as an undergraduate degree course. In the last few years there has been a rapid move in South East Wales towards an all graduate status in nutrition and dietetics, occuaptional therapy, physiotherapy, podiatry, radiography and speech therapy. A degree course in dental technology will commence in the near future and it is possible that as the number of nurses in training reduces there will be a move towards an all graduate profession. Individuals who are appointed into teaching posts in five years time are likely to be graduates with a vocational degree representing every profession. This is a development which must be supported. It would be a pity however to discourage those individual practitioners who wished to study a related subject in greater depth to degree level as their acquired knowledge could be invaluable in the linking of theory to practice.

6.5 Should there be integrated interdisciplinary learning ?

The 300 teachers and 1383 students who completed the main study questionnaires represented the majority of a local population of thirteen health and social care professions. Whilst the total number of teachers and students involved in similar programmes throughout the United Kingdom is not available, the number of training programmes in evidence in South East Wales surely represents one of the largest clusterings in the United Kingdom. It can be argued that the sample obtained is a reasonable representation of other centres in the United Kingdom. It is acknowledged however, that the results obtained from these respondents may not be reflected throughout the United Kingdom as a whole and most certainly not on an international basis. The only way in which the validity of the findings could be substantiated would be through replication studies. There would be inherent difficulties nevertheless in achieving this. As each curriculum is unique to each degree programme, a content analysis of the curriculum of the same thirteen professions in a different geographical location may yield substantially different results. It should be possible to use the content analysis developed in this study as a framework in any further studies which may be undertaken. Moore 1983, Marshall and Rossman 1989 and Tesch 1990 would certainly advocate testing the validity of the analysis in a replication study. The evidence obtained from the results of the questionnaires should prove a useful starting point for any future debates regarding the feasibility and desirability of interdisciplinary learning. Since this study commenced in January 1991, various Institutions in South East Wales have undergone further organisation and rationalisation. Implicitly this means that there are now further degree programmes which have been assimilated into the three organisations which have participated in this study. The opportunity may now be available to involve for example, medical laboratory scientific officers and environmental health officers. There is no reason why the content analysis checklist should not be used to analyse the curriculum of these courses and the questionnaires (with some modifications) distributed to the teaching staff and students on these courses in order to ascertain their opinions about the potential for interdisciplinary learning. It would seem reasonable to conclude that any profession contributing to health and social care could be subjected to the same analysis if this was requested.

Without a level of interest in the concept of interdisciplinary learning by the teachers and students, this study may not have been completed as the participation of the respondents was vital to its success. As has already been discussed the response rate from both the teachers and students was excellent. This acted as a motivator for the next stage of the study and an impatience to view the overall results in order to compare them with the anecdotal evidence found in the review of the literature. The crucial questions seemed to be, should there be some interdisciplinary learning, at which stage of training should it take place (if at all) and how interested were the respondents in the concept ?

The results of the first question demonstrated that 82.99% of the teachers (N = 300) and 83.14% (N = 1383) of the students believed that some interdisciplinary learning should take place (Table 5.25). This finding therefore challenges previous authors who have stated that most people do not believe that it is necessary (Howard & Byl 1971, Mason & Parascandola 1972, Infante et al 1976, Williams & Williams 1982,Darling & Ogg 1984). The majority (83.30% where N = 1683) of the respondents in this sample believed that there should be some interdisciplinary learning. There were variations between each professional group and these have been presented in Chapter 5. Section 5.5.3. Table 6. 2 presents the overall support in percentages by profession in rank order.

Table 6.2
The overall support for interdisciplinary learning: (N = 1683)

Profession	N =	%	Rank Order
Social Work	137	95.62	1
Podiatry	71	94.37	2
Nutrition & Dietetics	49	93.88	3
Occupational Therapy	96	92.71	4
Dental Technology	36	91.67	5
Speech Therapy	56	90.74	6
Nursing	493	86.82	7
Radiography	58	84.48	8
Op. Dept. Practitioners	27	81.48	9
DSA/Dental Hygienist	41	80.49	10
Dentistry	107	80.45	11
Physiotherapy	111	70.27	12
Medicine	376	69.15	13

In summary the medical profession were the least sure about whether interdisciplinary learning should take place. Nonetheless 69.15% (where N = 376) believed that some interdisciplinary learning should take place. Only 12.50% of the medical practitioners rejected the idea (Table 5.107). The medical teachers (77.57% where N = 107) were much more positive about the idea than the medical students (65.80% where N = 269). This refutes the findings of previous authors who have stated that medical practitioners are very resistant to learning with other professions (Christman 1965, Bates 1969, 1970, Kalisch & Kalisch 1977, Hoeklemann 1978, Steel 1981, Mechanic & Aitken 1982, Ferguson Johnston 1983, Coluccio & Maguire 1983, Webster 1985, Keddy et al 1986, Brooking 1991). It does indicate however, that they are less keen than most of the other professions in participating but there is ample evidence to demonstrate that many would take a positive attitude towards any firm proposals. The number of medical teachers who identifed themselves in their questionnaires asking to be involved in the future adds weight to this claim.

The 111 physiotherapy respondents were also less sure than most of the other professions about whether there should be some interdisciplinary learning with the teachers being less positive (60%) than the students (71.29%). Only five of the respondents (4.50%) rejected the idea completely (Table 5.174). The reasons for the physiotherapists comparatively low response rate is not known. The literature review did not identify physiotherapists as being a particularly cloistered group. It may be that in this sample the percentage of teachers who were undecided (40%) have influenced the student group. It should be remembered nonetheless that a substantial majority believed that shared learning should take place.

The group who were most certain that there should be some interdisciplinary learning were the social workers. Of the 137 social work respondents 95.62% responded positively (Table 5.211). The conclusions that have been drawn previously and perpetuated amongst the health care professions that social workers do not view themselves as involved in health care must be challenged as a result of this finding (Butrym 1967, Hooper 1970, Hirschon 1976, Quataro & Hutchinson 1976, Hawker 1977, Kendall 1977, Williams et al 1978, Bywaters 1986, Brooks 1987, Henk 1989, Allen 1991, Peryer 1991). It is suggested that while this may have been the case whilst the medical model of care was at its zenith but with the move towards a holistic model of health care, the philosphy of the health professions now complements that of the social care professions. It would seem opportune to grasp this spirit of collaboration and move forward into a new era of client centred care which can be achieved in part through interdisciplinary learning. These results meet Aim 3.1 of this study.

6.6 When should interdisciplinary learning be introduced ?

The question of when interdisciplinary learning should be introduced also produced results which challenge the traditionally held ideas about multidisciplinary learning. Of the 1683 respondents in this study only 2.26% (N = 38) thought that interdisciplinary learning should commence after individuals have qualified. The majority (57.34%) indicated that it should take place throughout undergraduate training with the rest indicating at the beginning (15.27%), the middle (17.64%) or at the end of training (7.37%) (Table 5.29). In the literature review several authors were cited who had differing ideas on the appropriate time to introduce interdisciplinary learning. Tanner et al (1972), Furnham et al (1981), Owen (1982) Dickens et al (1985) and Knox and Thompson (1989) all concluded that interdisciplinary learning should take place throughout undergraduate training. It would appear from the results that they are supported by the majority of teachers and students in this study (and as such meet Aim 3.3) Snodgrass (1966) and Mazur et al (1979) advocated the middle of training as the correct time. No empirical evidence has been found in this current study which supports their suggestion, indeed the middle of training would appear to be the least favoured option. Nonetheless there was a significant difference between the teachers (6.99%) and the students (19.96%) responses about the middle of training. Analysis of the qualitative responses which accompanied this question revealed that students seemed keen to find their professional identity and learn their role within the health team before they undertake any interdisciplinary learning. This need for security is understandable but it could be argued that individuals will not understand their role and contribution to a team if they have not the slightest idea what the other team members do.

The idea of being immersed into an isolated professional identity also suggests that the learning environment will be ripe for the introduction of stereotyping, interprofessional jealousies and negative attitudes between the professions so widely documented in the literature (Berkowitz and Malone 1968, Dana and Sheps 1968, Johson et al 1968, Martin 1969, Kenneth 1969, Pluckhan 1970, Banta and Fox 1972, Rosenaur and Fuller 1973, Lloyd 1973, Bendall 1973, Beckhard 1974, Ratoff et al 1974, Kendall 1977, Alaszewski 1977, Parkes 1977, Westbrook 1978, Challela 1979, Kuenssberg 1980, Lonsdale et al 1980, Beales 1980, Pritchard 1981, Turnbull 1981, Lishmann 1983, Williams and Williams 1982, Webster 1985, Osborne and Wakeling 1985, Wright 1985, Linsk et al 1986, Guy 1986, Webster 1988, Iles and Auluck 1990, Brooking 1991, Fawcett-Henesy 1991, Mocellin 1992). The interdisciplinary cone model described by Leninger (1971) would seem to be the most appropriate way in which interdisciplinary learning could take place throughout undergraduate training (see Chapter 2. Figure 2.5). The adoption of such a model would encourage a level of interdisciplinary learning throughout whilst at the same time enabling students to find their own identity and spend time in their own professional groups. The experience of the Faculty of Health Sciences in the University of Linkoping, Sweden has proved that once a programme is established in which interdisciplinary learning is a fundamental element the students start to request more shared learning experiences rather than less (see Chapter 4, Section 4.4.2).

The need for post graduate interdisciplinary courses is not in doubt. Interprofessional collaboration is a greater necessity than ever before. Many of the Magister degrees are now interdisciplinary and these should continue. A question should be asked however, regarding the teachers' and students' knowledge of each others' real contribution to health and social care at the commencement of these courses. Could it be that each student recognises for the first time the contribution of other professions ?. Could it be that this is the first time that a student has ever really considered the question ? If this is the case then it could be argued that this is a sad reflection of the health care teams that currently exist. For all those qualified personnel currently practising, these sort of opportunities would seem to be essential. It is exciting to envisage the quality of debate at a post graduate level if interdisciplinary learning was seen as an implicit part of undergraduate training. There would be no need for titles of degrees to include such nomenclature as "interprofessional" or "multidisciplinary" in order to advertise their uniqueness. Such degrees would be accepted as the norm and it may mean that profession specific degrees would be the ones to advertise their uniqueness. It is acknowledged that changes of this size and importance could not happen immediately as it would require a fundamental change in philosophy but taking the example of the Linkoping programme anything is possible providing there is motivation and a desire for change.

6.7 What would the level of interest be ?

The level of interest in the concept expressed by the teachers and the students give grounds for optimism that at least some change could take place over the next few years. In this study 1297 (77.06%) of the 1683 respondents were either "interested" or "very interested" in the idea (Tables 5.26, 5.27, 5.28 and Figure 5.2). The differences between the opinions of the teachers and the students overall were minimal. Direct comparison between the teachers and the students by individual profession was inappropriate in many instances as the number of teachers was so small and the percentages were therefore meaningless. There were substantial differences between the levels of interest of the medical teachers and those of the medical students in that 64.50% of the teachers were either interested or very interested in the concept against the 53.16% of the students who selected those same categories (see Table 5.112) It could be argued that one of the reasons for this anomaly is that the link between theory and practice has not yet been fully forged for the medical students because of the cloistered nature of medical student training. Webster (1985) came to a similar conclusion in a study which found a significant difference between the conceptual understanding of first and fourth year medical students when they were questionned about health care teams. Webster observed that the fourth year students related the health team specifically to patient centred care whereas the first year students related it to other professional groups.

It would be very interesting to question a number of medical practitioners after they had completed their pre registration year as house officers, in order to measure whether attitudes differed between these two groups as a result of the reality shock of working in clinical practice and the concommitant accountability that results which was so aptly described by Kramer and Schmalenberg (1977).

The physiotherapists results were interesting in that only 40% of the 10 teachers selected these two categories of "very interested" and "interested" against 73.27% of the 101 students who did (Table 5.179 and Figure 5.30). As there were only

10 teachers in the sample no firm conclusions can be drawn but it would appear that most physiotherapy students would be interested in any further developments but there could be more of a problem with involving many of the teachers.

The level of interest expressed in interdisciplinary learning was very encouraging and gives reason to believe that progress and change may be possible. It is perhaps just as well that there is now evidence of the level of interest as the trend towards shared learning would seem to be gathering pace in the number of Government publications which have appeared over the last few years which have been reviewed in the literature.

It would appear that there could be a conflict here between the altruistic desire for interdisciplinary learning in order to enhance the quality of teamwork in health and social care (which could in turn enhance the quality of client care) against the entirely reasonable suspicion that the move towards interdisciplinary learning has been advocated in order to dilute the power of the individual professions and to save money on expensive individual training programmes. It would seem important to remember that the World Health Organisation's Alma Ata declaration in 1978 had no political agenda and indeed was signed and ratified by all the participants at this conference and the need for closer collaboration and shared learning was identified quite clearly. Indeed the subsequent publication of "Targets for Health for All" (WHO 1985) refers on several occasions to the need for interdisciplinary training and research opportunities for all health personnel (Targets 29, 31, 32 and 37). Any directives which are delivered in Government White Papers are likely to continue to be met with resistance and cynicism from the health professionals who see only the negative aspects of new strategies. It would appear vital that the rewards and opportunities that the introduction of interdisciplinary learning could bring are not lost in a wave of apathy or suspicion.

6.8 The advantages and disadvantages of interdisciplinary learning

Of the 1683 respondents, 81.34% (248 teachers (Table 5.39) and 1121 students (Table 5.55)) indicated that there would be advantages in interdisciplinary learning. Only 86 (5.11%) of the sample did not believe there would be advantages. The remaining 216 (12.83%) were undecided. The percentage responses from the teachers and students were very similar for each category. Of the 78 students who thought there would be no advantages 42 (53.85% where N = 78) were medical students (Table 5.55). Closer examination of the results revealed a most interesting finding. Most of these medical students were male (RS = 36 where N = 42) and all 42 were in their third year of training (the first year of clinical training). The reason for this finding is unknown but it is postulated that it may be linked with the previous finding that male medical students tend not to have gained previous relevant work experience whereas as the female students have (see Chapter 5, Section 5.5.3.4). The amount of direct clinical practice that these students had gained was therefore minimal to date and it may be that as yet there was no real insight into the teamwork necessary to achieve client centred care. The female students all indicated that there would be advantages. Another possible explanation which cannot be discounted is that these students collaborated when completing the questionnaires. As each student group was left alone to complete the questionnaire it was not possible to ensure that collaboration did not occur.

All respondents were asked to identify the advantages and disadvantages of interdisciplinary learning. The questions were open ended thus encouraging as many different responses as possible. One of the problems with qualitative data collecting is that the response rate tends to decrease (Youngman 1978, Marshall and Rossman 1989, Leedy 1989, Judd et al 1991, Oppenheim 1992, Cohen and Mannion 1992). It was therefore no surprise that the response rates for these questions were lower. Nevertheless, 177 teachers (Table 5.40) and 1089 students (Table 5.56) listed advantages and 61 teachers (Table 5.41) and 485 students (Table 5.57) listed the disadvantages. An encouraging finding was that although more disadvantages were identified than advantages far fewer respondents identified them. The amount of data collected for these two questions was immense and no content analysis could ever do justice to the richness of some of the responses. A decision had to be made however which most accurately portrayed the responses. It is therefore acknowledged that some of the respondents who were assigned into one or other of the categories may have been misrepresented.

The advantages could be broadly classified into four main categories (see Chapter 5. Table 5.40 and Table 5. 56) :

1. An increased understanding of each other's roles and contribution.
2. Increase teamwork and collaboration.
3. Broaden horizons and cross fertilise ideas.
4. More efficient use of scarce time and resources.

In category one, 157 teachers and 699 students indicated that there should be greater understanding and insight into the roles of the other professions and their contribution to health care. In category two 113 teachers and 704 students indicated that an advantage would be an increase in teamwork and collaboration.

These findings confirm that there is an awareness amongst the professions that there is an ignorance about each other and a lack of understanding about what contributions the other professional groups make to client care. They also implicitly acknowledged that the current levels of teamwork and collaboration were not good. More than half of the 1383 students (50.90%) obviously believed that interdisciplinary learning may help address this problem (Table 5.56). What is particularly alarming is that 52.33% of the teachers in this sample (all of whom are qualified in their own professional field) acknowledged their lack of understanding about the other professions (Table 5.40). This means that whilst in clinical practice they were not fully aware of the potential contributions that the other professions, with whom they were working side by side, were making.

The implications of this for the patient/client are enormous. If a truly holistic model of care is to be adopted then it is imperative that as a client's needs are assessed, a problem solving approach is adopted to meet those needs and the professions which can best help the client to meet those needs should be utilised. It is suggested that without a fundamental consideration of this issue that practitioners (from any of the professions) could be accused of lacking accountability in order to protect professional territory. This means in essence that the interdisciplinary team should not be a rigid, inflexible organisation. Client centred care by its very nature, calls for an adaptable and versatile interdisciplinary team which is both proactive and reactive to a constantly changing situation. There would seem to be an infinite number of combinations of professions whom could constitute an interdisciplinary team. The structure of a client centred team must always depend on the needs of the client at any given moment in time. The adoption of the model described by Pritchard (1984) in which an intrinsic team responds to a given situation and then devolves as the clients problem resolves would appear to be the solution here.

In Chapter 2, Section 2.7, a detailed review was undertaken which examined all aspects of teamwork in health and social care. Simon (1961) concluded that communication was the central tenet for successful interdisciplinary collaboration while Harding et al (1981) identified four basic requisites if teamwork was to be achieved. One of these was a clear understanding by each team member of his/her own role and responsibilities. A second, which was perceived to be equally important to the first was a clear understanding of the roles and responsibilities of other team members with a constituent mutual respect for each other's contributions. This according to Harding et al "is a fundamental prerequisite" (p 63). Based on the results obtained in this study it would appear that whilst great emphasis is placed on encouraging students to identify their own professional roles (and consequently their own little niche) in health and social care, very little emphasis is placed on trying to understand the roles and contributions of the other professions.

The completed content analysis substantiates this claim as there is no mention of "collaboration" at all. Beckhard (1974), Kinston (1983) and Iles and Auluck (1990) would have blamed this lack of collaboration on the hierarchical domination which they noted to exist, while other authors attribute it to the protection of professional territory (Berkowitz and Mallone 1968, Dana and Sheps 1968, Johnston et al 1968, Martin1969, Kenneth 1969, Pluckhan 1970, Banta and Fox 1972, Rosenaur and Fuller 1973, Lloyd 1973, Bendall 1973, Ratoff et al 1974, Kendall 1977, Alaszewski 1977, Parkes 1977, Westbrook 1978, Challela 1979, Kuenssberg 1980, Lonsdale et al 1980, Beales 1980, Pritchard 1981, Turnbull 1981, Williams and Williams 1982, Lishman 1983, Webster 1985, Osbourne and Wakeling 1985, Wright 1985, Linsk et al 1986, Guy 1986,

Webster 1988, Brooking 1991, Fawcett-Henesy 1991, Mocellin 1992). Although the word "teamwork" was included in all fourteen curricula, its meaning was unclear. It is suspected that in many instances this referred to one of Ovretveits (1986d) "managed teams" which he described as consisting of individuals of different seniority from the same profession. The nursing and medical professions seem to excel at these with a now well established grading system for nurses evident on acute and community units and the historical "firms" for the medical profession in which the consultant is the managing director and then his/her firm comprises senior registrars, registrars, senior house officers, house officers and has a clutch of medical students attached to it.

While there is no doubt that managed teams comprising a single professional group ensure cohesiveness and a sense of identity these teams should not be mutually exclusive and operate at the expense of an interdisciplinary team, the two types of team should work in tandem. Ovretveits definition of a "joint accountability" team would enable this to happen. A democratic team where shared accountability is the accepted norm but where each team member emphasises their independence and autonomy, if adopted as an interdisciplinary philosophy would encompass both approaches to client care. This democratic team should be the one that is flexible and versatile in its inclusion of members and should vary according to the needs of the client with whom it is dealing. Fulop (1976) would have strongly endorsed this conclusion as he wrote "There can of course be no universally acceptable composition for a health team."

The implications for the future are clear. Flexible collaborative interdisciplinary teams should be an integral part of health and social care. Policy makers are developing strategies to achieve this, the professions in the sample want this and the client needs this. Immediate steps should be taken to implement this through a re-examination of the curricula for undergraduates from every health and social care profession and increased efforts to resource and implement programmes at a postgraduate level should be made. An immediate strategy that could be adopted would be one of interdisciplinary teaching where teachers from the professions contributing to health and social care are invited to speak to groups of students from the existing specific professions. An examination of teamwork and its contribution to care could be therefore undertaken from a multidisciplinary perspective.

The third advantage that was categorised was that interdisciplinary learning would enable the professions to broaden their horizons and cross fertilise their ideas. This was mentioned by 92 teachers and 387 students. Rowbottom and Hey (1978) maintained that to achieve this a change in attitude would be required from the professions concerned. They argued that a cross fertilisation of ideas would ensure a better continuity of care. One of the perceived problems in adopting this approach would seem to be the continuing debate on whom should be the leader of the interdisciplinary team. As has been identified in Chapter 2, Section 2.7.2 this subject is perhaps the most sensitive area of all with many medical practitioners resisting the possibility that they may lose control of the reins (British Medical Association 1974, Hodkinson 1975, Appleyard and Madden 1979 Mitchell 1984, Webster 1985).

Other medical practitioners (Ferguson and Carney 1970) found to their surprise that when patients were asked whom should be the team leader the response was different. Their sample of patients chose nurses as their preferred option, their rationale being that nurses were around twenty four hours a day and therefore would ensure continuity of care. Many authors advocated the changing nature of team leadership and suggested that the leader should be identified from the profession who had the most to contribute to a client and his/her family at a specific time (Abercrombie 1966, George 1971, Kindig 1975, Ward 1979, Nodder 1980, Salkind and Norrell 1980, Macfarlane 1980, Parker 1982, Von Schilling 1982, Kinston 1983, Wright 1985, Ovretveit 1986d, Campbell Heider and Pollock 1987, Newman 1987). The changing nature of health care with its emphasis on primary health and the community certainly mitigates against the medical model of care that used to be adopted.

Many of the authors who questionned the automatic ascension of a medical practitioner to the role of team leader, were medical practitioners themselves but recognised that it was not always in the patients best interests to have the "doctor" as the team leader. Wright (1985) believed that "in theory .....the most appropriate leader emerges according to the patients needs" (p 36). These conclusions nevertheless would have been strongly contested by several medical practitioners who fiercely defended their position to remain as team leader (Hodkinson 1975, Appleyard and Madden 1979, Mitchell 1984 and Webster 1985)

In 1993 the emphasis has been placed on patient empowerment, patient choice and consumer satisfaction. This change in health care philosophy is perhaps best illustrated by the introduction of "Patients Charters", and is epitomised by Winterton (1992) who on behalf of the British Government examined the contribution of obstetricians and midwives towards maternal and child health. His conclusion that a midwife could and should take responsibility for a woman throughout her pregnancy and delivery, providing both mother and child were fit and well has raised a storm of debate and dire warnings of recriminations if anything untoward happens. The focus of the Winterton Report would seem to be that pregnancy and childbirth is a healthy thing to do and that it is precisely for this purpose that a midwife trains. The midwife will take total responsibility for the mother and child in a normal pregnancy and delivery and will therefore be accountable and autonomous. In this situation Tolliday (1978) would have described the midwife as a "fully fledged practitioner" (p 47) acting in a state of primacy. This has fundamental implications for the future in all areas of health and social care. If the move towards biopsychosocial model of care is to be maintained then perhaps the answer is to place the client (wherever possible) in the position of team leader as Challela (1979) and Brandt and Magyary (1989) have already suggested. In situations where this is not possible, such as in the case of a child of less than sixteen years of age then perhaps the parent or legal guardian could take on this responsibility. In certain circumstances it may be that the principal co-ordinator of care should be a social worker whilst in others it should be a medical general practitioner.

Primary Health Care Centres have had a significant impact on health care and it is interesting to note that this term has generally superseded "the doctor's surgery". There would seem to be an ideal opportunity to extend the remit that these centres have. The employment of a social worker, podiatrist, physiotherapist, occupational therapist and a nutritionist within these health centres would go a long way towards promoting health in the community. Dental surgeons, dental hygienists and dental technologists would also fit very well into a primary health centre. The whole emphasis on care could then become one of health with the possibility of opportunistic health promotion, education and primary intervention from all these professions being tantamount to the success of "Health for All by the Year 2000" (WHO 1985). If such a dream is to be attained then it would seem absolutely essential that a true spirit of cross fertilisation of ideas and collaborative care should be achieved in part through interdisciplinary learning.

One of the anxieties expressed in the literature and by one or two people in this study, has been that of the issue of maintaining confidentiality (Batchelor and McFarlane 1980, Dimond 1989).

Teamwork, collaboration and a cross fertilisation of ideas would seem at first glance to mitigate against this ethos. A dilemma already exists for an accountable practitioner (of any profession) when a client shares information of a highly confidential nature. Information such as this is not normally recorded without a client's permission. The debate must therefore centre on what should be recorded and by whom. However in view of the findings by Stimson and Webb (1975), Horder 1977, and Gray (1980) that patients receive, on average five to six minutes consultation time with their medical practitioner it is debatable whether the client has the opportunity to share confidential information anyway.

Perhaps the most simple answer would be for the client to record in writing what he/she chooses ! If the client is to be the team leader then this would not pose an ethical problem. If a situation arises where a practitioner is in possession of confidential information that may be shared either verbally or in writing with colleagues within their own profession then this implies that the information is no longer confidential and that the practitioner has made the decision to trust individuals in his/her own profession but not those in others. The urgent introduction of Codes of Conduct for all practitioners in health and social care such as the one in force in nursing, midwifery and health visiting (UKCC 1992) and clear directives on confidentiality (UKCC 1987) may clarify the situation for everyone.

The fourth advantage classified was the more efficient use of scarce time and resources. Comparatively few respondents seem to consider this as only 42 teachers (14.00% where N = 300) and 14 students (1.01% where N = 1383) mentioned it (Tables 5.40 and 5.56). Interestingly very few respondents mentioned "time constraints" as a disadvantage either. No evidence has been found in the review of the literature that suggests that time or resources can be saved in monetary terms as the number of students learning would remain the same as would the number of teachers needed to facilitate their learning. In addition, Statutory Bodies prescribe the number of theoretical and practical hours that a student must study in order to complete a statutory training. What may occur though is a more appropriate use of quality time.

The Concise Oxford Dictionary (1985) describes efficiency as "productive of effect" and "the ratio of useful work done to total energy expended." It may be that the teachers who identified the more efficient use of scarce time in this study were implicitly recognising that a lot of time and energy is spent undertaking repetitive teaching with different groups of students. Certainly the tendency to professionally isolate teachers as well as students adds to this problem. Great emphasis is made on the need for teachers to spend more time in clinical practice in order to maintain their professional credibility and over the past few years there has been an increasing demand for teachers to undertake more research and publish more papers by including this criteria on job descriptions and appraisal forms. Theoretically few teachers seem to disagree with this and indeed many would positively welcome the opportunity. In practice however, this is usually impossible because of the current and increasing demands made upon a teachers time. This state of affairs can be resolved only by a fundamental restructuring of the existing course programmes.

Efforts are being made to address the problem with the development of modular undergraduate degree programmes in the form of "Health Care Studies" (CIHE 1993). The introduction of generic courses such as these in which students study aspects of health care to degree level before undertaking a profession specific training would without doubt increase the efficiency of student/teacher interaction. There is also the implication that the length of the profession specific training could be reduced as the students would have already studied core subjects such as the behavioural sciences applied to health care for a given number of hours. Graduates with a degree in Health Studies should be able to fast track any profession specific training. It is acknowledged that such a development would be seen as controversial and is likely to be resisted by many individuals from the different professions who would wish to protect their territory and professional exclusivity. However the data collected in this study has indicated that the majority of teachers and students believe that there should be some interdisciplinary learning. The introduction of a common core programme such as this would ensure integration on an interdisciplinary basis even before profession specific training commenced. In addition, the adoption of the interdisciplinary cone model described by Leninger (1971) during profession specific training would ensure integration continued.

The number of disadvantages of interdisciplinary learning which were identified were greater in number than the advantages. What was encouraging, none the less was that only 61 teachers and 405 students identified these (Tables 5.41 and 5.57). The most frequently identified disadvantage was that "some of the material may be irrelevant" (teachers RS = 58, students RS = 143). Without careful planning, discussion and negotiation between a planning team the possibility of this happening is immense. It would be most unsatisfactory for all concerned if this was to happen and would certainly not help the interdisciplinary cause. Any material perceived as not relevant by all professions should be addressed in profession specific training. It should be remembered however that such material may be relevant to a cluster of professions and consequently could be taught to several groups of students. It is obvious for example, that much of the course content that dental students study will not be relevant to podiatrists or social workers. It is suspected however, that there is much in common between the dentists, dental hygienists and dental technologists curricula. Speech therapists may also discover more commonalities with these professions. The content analysis completed in this study has proved that many of the curricula are similar in places (see Chapter 5, Section 5.2).

Some of the respondents identified "time constraints" (teachers RS = 18, students RS = 60) and "organisational difficulties" (teachers RS = 22, students RS = 3) as disadvantages. This, it is believed may be the result of individuals thinking that any interdisciplinary learning would be in *addition* to the existing teaching commitment rather than instead of the traditional method of programme delivery. It would be essential that this point was publicised loudly and clearly if any changes are to be made to the existing programmes.

It is interesting to speculate that the "hierarchical domination and prejudice" identifed as a disadvantage by 26 teachers and 65 students would be overcome by the "increased understanding of each other's roles" and "increased teamwork and collaboration" which so many teachers and students believe are the advantages of interdisciplinary learning. The hierarchical domination and prejudice occurs precisely because of the lack of understanding and collaboration between the professions. The teachers and students who are fearful of being dominated are doing so from a position of inside knowledge and experience. The need to explore interprofessional conflict and introduce team building exercises on postgraduate interdisciplinary courses even before the course content begins is well documented (Beloff and Willett 1968, Aradine and Hansen 1970, Orem 1971, Parker 1972, Mason and Parascandola 1972, Rosenaur and Fuller 1973, Engstrom 1986, Snyder 1981).

Closer examination of the respondents by profession who had identified "hierarchical domination and prejudice" as a potential problem raised several interesting points. Nurses (traditionally dominated by the medical profession) were twice as likely to identify this as a problem (RS = 46 (9.33%) where N = 493) than the medical profession (RS = 20 (5.63%) where N = 376) ($\chi^2 = 4.22$, df = 1, p < 5%) Even closer analysis of this finding revealed that of the 46 nurse respondents, 16 (where N = 97) were nurse teachers while only 30 (where N = 396) were nursing students. In essence this means that 16.49% of the nurse teacher respondents believed that hierarchical domination would occur while only 7.57% of the nursing students did ($\chi^2 = 5.80$, df =1, p < 5%) (Tables 5.131 and 5.111).

This finding could be interpreted in several ways and raises still more unanswered questions. Assuming the nurse teachers responses reflect not only their teaching experience but also their clinical experience, the question arises of whether their opinions are representative of the nursing profession as a whole or whether this was one of the reasons that they disappeared into the "ivory tower of learning" described in a paper by Kramer and Schmalenberg (1977). Could it be that nurse teachers prejudice their students against the medical profession but initially nursing students do not feel dominated by the medical profession ? In other words is this a learned response ? Or could it be that because of the many uncertainties that nurse teachers are facing regarding their professional futures that their responses tend to be rather negative anyway ? Justification for this possibility has already been raised in Chapter 5 Section 5.5.1 where the reasons for the 23 nurse teachers (23.71% where N = 97) identifying as a disadvantage the "threat of redundancy" were considered. If low self esteem and vulnerability is a major problem for the nurse teachers, then they should be reassured by the fact that they are *the* most frequently chosen profession with whom the other twelve professions in this study would wish to share learning on an interdisciplinary basis.

Loss of professional identity was an anxiety expressed by 11 teachers (3.67% where N = 300) and 71 students (5.13% where N = 1383). Whilst this is a realistic worry, it could be argued that interdisciplinary learning would give each student the opportunity to examine in detail, their own role and contribution to health and social care. If professions learn in complete isolation from each other and are denied the chance to discuss with other professional groups what comprises holistic care, how can they possibly find their own professional identity? The need to incorporate profession specific learning into any interdisciplinary learning experience is highlighted here. The application of interdisciplinary concepts of care to specific professions is paramount.

Few teachers (RS = 21, 7.00% where N = 300) and very few students (RS = 23, 1.66% where N = 1383) mentioned differing academic ability as a potential problem. These responses appeared to be randomly distributed amongst the thirteen professions. This response was also interesting in that it raises the question of different levels of academic entry criteria for courses. The results of this study show that there is a significant difference between the ages of the students who commence medical and dental training from those who commence nurse and social work training for example. There is also a significant difference between the life and previous relevent work experience that these different groups of students can offer. While medical and dental students are much younger, they are also implicitly much less "street wise". They therefore have to depend on theoretical concepts at the beginning of their training whereas the nursing and social work students are more likely to be able to bridge the theory and practice gap. Any deficiencies in academic terms such as Advanced Level qualifications should therefore be offset by life experience. Core skills such as effective communication are learned through a combination of theory and practice.

It is true of course, that as students commence their training they will have and indeed need a different knowledge base. An in-depth knowledge of the life sciences features more strongly in some of the professions than others and this will always continue to be the case. The social sciences will remain the central tenet for social work while the life sciences will remain the central tenet for medicine and dentistry. Quite rightly, these three professions are contributing to client care from three entirely different perspectives. These differing perspectives are the central thesis for arguing that profession specific training should always continue. It is interesting to note however that even within the medical profession there is an increased awareness that a greater emphasis should be placed during undergraduate training on a biopsychosocial model of care (Towle 1991).

The number of students in a class was not seen to be a problem by any of the teachers in this sample. It was an anxiety expressed by 74 students (5.35% where N = 1383) however. No mention was made in the questionnaire or introductory letter of the numbers of students that would be learning on an interdisciplinary basis. The number of students has increased on many of the traditional training courses over the past few years (Audit Commission 1992, Annual Course Reports CIHE, SEWINME 1993) and this has put additional demands on the teachers and students in that there is a need to develop effective ways of teaching large groups. The amount of student centred learning has also expanded to cope with the increased numbers. It is not anticipated that the size of the student groups would increase apart from the possibility of the number of students attending a formal lecture. As it is now common practice for more than a hundred students to attend a lecture it could be argued that the inclusion of fifty more would make no difference. With large numbers such as these, personal interaction between a lecturer and a student in this scenario has already disappeared.

Finally it was most encouraging to observe that where the students were asked to identify the disadvantages, 173 (12.51% where N = 1383) wrote down that there were "none at all". It seems reasonable to assume that they wished to emphasise this point as otherwise they would not have commented. This can be interpreted therefore as a positive mandate for interdisciplinary learning.

In summary the advantages would seem to far outweigh the disadvantages. Some of the disadvantages could be, it is suggested minimised or even ameliorated by the introduction of interdisciplinary learning. Discussion, negotiation and planning must be executed in fine detail before any interdisciplinary learning should commence. These findings have determined the opinions of the teachers and students regarding the advantages and disadvantages of interdisciplinary learning and so fulfils another of the study aims (Aim 3.2).

6.9 Which professions could learn with which ?

One of the aims of this study was to ascertain which professions would be acceptable to each other on an interdisciplinary learning basis. It was recognised at an early stage that whilst many of the core topics were common to most if not all of the thirteen professions, there was also likely to be specific areas of knowledge related to patient/client care that should be addressed by clusters of professions. An obvious example of this would be interdisciplinary learning between dental students, dental hygiene and dental surgery assistants students, dental technology students and perhaps speech therapy and nutrition and dietetics students. A healthy mouth and the ability to eat and drink a healthy diet would appear to be mutually interdependent.

The results obtained from the 300 teachers and 1383 students reveal some very interesting findings. The overall results can be seen in Chapter 5, Tables 5.43 and Table 5.59 and the results by individual profession are displayed in Sections 5.5.3.1 to 5.5.3.13. Many of the respondents did indeed select professions which are closely related to their own but the overall ranking of the most suitable professions are presented in two tables.

Table 6.3
Rank order most chosen professions : All respondents

Profession	Rank Order
Nursing	1
Medicine	2
Social Work	3
Occupational Therapy	3
Physiotherapy	5
Nutrition & Dietetics	6
Speech Therapy	7
Radiography	8
Dentists	9
DSA/Dental Hygienists	10
Operating Department Practitoners	10
Podiatrists	12
Dental Technologists	13

Table 6. 4
Rank order choices : By profession

Prof.	Den	DSA	D.T	Med	Nur	Diet.	Oc.T	ODP	Phys	Pod	Rad	Soc	Sp.T	Totals	R.O
Den	-	1	1	8	11	7	11	7	10	10	5	11	6	88	9
DSA	1	-	2	11	8	9	10	11	11	11	11	9	10	104	10
D.T	4	7	-	12	12	12	12	7	12	12	12	12	8	122	13
Med	1	6	12	-	5	2	5	2	2	1	2	4	5	47	2
Nur	7	2	7	1	-	1	2	1	3	3	1	2	3	33	1
Diet	3	3	4	5	1	-	6	10	7	8	9	6	7	69	6
Oc.T	9	8	6	3	2	5	-	5	1	5	6	1	1	52	3
ODP	11	9	8	9	7	11	8	-	9	7	6	8	11	104	10
Phys	10	11	10	2	4	6	2	4	-	2	3	5	3	62	5
Pod	12	12	11	10	8	10	7	11	8	-	10	7	12	118	12
Rad	5	4	5	6	10	8	8	3	6	4	-	10	9	78	8
Soc	8	5	8	3	3	3	1	6	4	6	4	-	1	52	3
Sp.T	6	10	3	7	6	4	4	7	5	9	8	3	-	72	7

KEY R.O = Rank Order Den = Dentists, DSA = DSA/DH, D.T = Dental Technologists, Med = Medical Practitioners, Nur = Nurses, Diet = Nutritionists & Dietitians, Oc.T = Occupational Therapists, ODP = Operating Department Practitioners, Phys = Physiotherapists, Pod = Podiatrists, Rad = Radiographers, Soc = Social Workers, Sp.T = Speech Therapists.

The Rank Order by Profession is presented in the vertical columns with the overall rank order in the last vertical column.

The nursing profession was chosen most frequently by the other professions. Nursing was the first choice for the medical profession, the nutritionists and dietitians, the operating department practitioners and the radiographers. Nursing was the second choice of the DSA/dental hygienists, the occupational therapists, and the social workers and the third choice of the physiotherapists, the podiatrists and the speech therapists. Only two professions ranked nurses lower than third and these were the dentists and the dental technologists both of whom ranked nurses in seventh position. The question arises of why the nurses were so frequently chosen by the other professions ? Could it be that they are perceived as being central to the continuity of patient care ? It has been argued that as nurses care for patients on a twenty four hour basis that they should undertake the central coordinating role in care as they are in the best position to have an overview of the clients total needs.

In section 6.8 it was suggested that the team leader wherever possible should be the patient/client. The fact that nurses have been identified as the most frequently chosen profession with whom the other professions would wish to share learning may help this to evolve. As one of the few professions which are currently bound by mandatory codes of conduct, nurses are in an ideal position to act as a patient's mentor and advocate (UKCC 1992) (see Appendix 2.4). Essentially this means that nurses should be able to facilitate patient choice and patient empowerment. The introduction of primary nursing in many areas of practice has further promoted this concept.

The second overall choice of medical practitioners was also interesting. Only two professions (the dentists and podiatrists) selected the medical practitioners as a first choice. The nutritionists and dietitians, the operating department practitioners and the radiographers rank ordered them second while the nurses, occupational therapists, social workers and speech therapists rank ordered them fifth. These results were unexpected in that it seems to suggest that the move away from the medical model towards a more holistic model of care is occurring more rapidly than previously thought. Further evidence to substantiate this assumption can be made by the overall rank ordering of the social workers and the occupational therapists. Both were ranked in third position. Another possible explanation for the move away from medical domination is that as the other professions have developed their own research based practice they have become increasingly autonomous and consequently less dependent on and less subservient to the medical profession.

Closer analysis of the results related to the social workers also revealed some interesting anomalies. The speech therapists and the occupational therapists selected social workers in first place while the physiotherapists ranked social workers fourth. The similarities and empathy between the social workers and the occupational therapists has been discussed already but no convincing explanation can be offered for the speech therapists choice. The medical profession, overall ranked social workers in third place. The lecturers however placed the social workers in second place while the medical students placed them in sixth place (see Chapter 5, Table 5.116). This may be an indication that from experience, the medical lecturers know that patient's social problems and needs play a crucial role in health and illness, while the medical students are still focused on the reactive interventionist medical model of care. It would be interesting to revisit the students to test this hypothesis once these students are qualified and determine whether their opinions had altered.

The infrequency with which podiatrists were chosen was unexpected. Currently the podiatrists would appear to be in a position where they are unvalued and therefore under utilised by the rest of the health care team. This may be due to ignorance on the part of the other professions as to what podiatrists actually do or a level of elitism by the longer established professions. The old adage of the chiropodist as a "corn remover" no longer holds true as in 1993 a podiatrist can undertake diagnostic investigations, prescribe treatment, execute minor surgical procedures and administer local anaesthesia. (BSc Podiatry Course Document 1992). A podiatrist makes a crucial contribution towards the health of the nation, most particularly in helping to maintain the mobility of the elderly and the disabled. Physiotherapists rank ordered podiatrists as tenth whilst the medical profession ordered the podiatrists in tenth place. In direct contrast the podiatrists themselves rank ordered medical practitioners in first place and physiotherapists in second place. Nurses were the third most frequently chosen profession with whom podiatrists would wish to learn yet nurses placed podiatrists in eighth place. One immediate solution which would help raise the profile of the podiatrists would be for a podiatry lecturer to speak to students in the other professions in order to outline the role of a podiatrist and also to make explicit what skills a qualified podiatrist can contribute to patient care.

There was a high level of consensus amongst several of the professions. The nutritionists and dietitians were most keen to learn with the nurses while the nurses also selected the nutritionists and dietitians as their first choice. The reasons for this are not clear but it is suggested that since the introduction of a "cook chill" method of serving meals in hospitals which are distributed (to the patients) and collected by ward orderlies, nurses are no longer aware of their patients dietary habits and nutritional intake. The introduction of the Project 2000 curriculum has addressed this omission and there is now a much greater emphasis on healthy eating. Evidence was found in the literature review of dietitians and nurses learning together but the rationale for selecting these two particular groups was not given (Caliendo and Pulaski 1979, Wessell 1981, Dickens et al 1985, Bersky et al 1987).

There was also complete agreement between the social workers and the occupational therapists, both groups choosing each other as the first choice. The psychosocial model of care adopted by the occupational therapists may be the explanation for this finding. The two professions obviously perceive a close relationship and recognise the contribution that each makes to client care. The results of the content analysis from each professions course documents, also emphasises the similarities between the two groups. There would appear to be a very good case for exploring the possibilities of introducing some shared learning between these two groups immediately. A potential problem however would be encountered in that these two training programmes are undertaken in different training institutions which would mean that difficulties would be encountered in the financing and management of the initiative. It is not believed that this problem would be insurmountable if adequate time was allowed to negotiate at a strategic level. No evidence was found in the literature review of social workers and occupational therapists learning together on a specific course. Clear indications of which professions could learn together have been obtained and these fulfil Aim 3.6 of the study.

6.10 The learning methods which should be adopted

The way in which an adult student effectively learns is well documented. Various authors have recommended a student centred, interactive approach where problem solving and integrating theory and practice is adopted (Pask 1976, Renzulli & Smith 1978, Claxton & Ralston 1978, Entwistle 1981, Huck 1981, Brown 1983, Knowles 1984, Child 1986, Clark 1986, Conti & Welborn 1986, Lovell 1986, Shakespeare 1989). Shakespeare (1989), in one of the most comprehensive surveys found on interprofessional education in primary health care, discovered that 7% of the courses surveyed used formal teaching methods only. She identified 505 instances in which lectures were used but tutorials in only five instances. Shakespeare found 97 instances where role play was used. Nearly all these learning experiences were for qualified staff. Shakespeare questioned whether the aim of promoting interprofessional teamwork could be possibly achieved through a non interactive course. In Chapter 2 of this book, stereotyping, prejudice, interprofessional conflict and teamwork has been discussed at length. The students that Shakespeare reviewed in her study were, on the whole, qualified practitioners and it is therefore presumed that they displayed all these attributes. In this current study which focused on undergraduate students from thirteen health and social care professions it was hoped that these attributes would not be evident or if they were that they would not be so fixed.

The results of this study have demonstrated that some interdisciplinary learning is wanted and needed throughout undergraduate training by a substantial majority of teachers (82.99%) and students (83.14%) (Table 5.25). In view of this finding it would seem imperative that the views of the students regarding which learning methods they would prefer to use are taken into consideration, if any interdisciplinary initiative is to have any chance of a successful evaluation. An early decision was taken to question the students about their preferred learning methods. Unfortuntely the decision was taken to omit a similar question from the teacher's questionnaire. The rationale for this decision being that the teachers already had other questions which lengthened their questionnaire and remembering the advice given by Oppenheim (1992) to keep a questionnaire as short possible it was feared that the response rate would decrease.

On reflection this omission was a mistake. If the teachers had been questionned about their preferred interdisciplinary teaching methods this may have contrasted entirely with the students views. The justification for this conclusion is made on the basis of the result of the students preferred learning methods in this study and comparing those with the learning methods which were being imposed by teachers to the students on the different courses studied by Shakespeare (1989).

Table 6.5
Rank order of the students's preferred interdisciplinary learning methods

Learning Method	Rank Order	Yes Responses	% of N =1383
Visits to patients/clients	1	1045	75.56
Workshops	2	911	65.87
Case studies	3	891	64.43
Mixed Tutorials	4	888	64.21
Seminars	5	801	57.92
Problem Based Learning	6	795	57.48
Lectures	7	712	51.48
Role Play	8	456	32.97

The student's responses indicate quite clearly their preferences. The most popular method is that which is patient/client centred. This has huge implications for future curriculum planners as there is clearly a limit on the number of students who can be accommodated in the clinical areas and even more significantly in a client's home. Previous American studies have shown however that students representing the different disciplines can and do work well together when in direct contact with clients (McPherson and Sachs 1982, Brazeau et al 1987, Ramos and Moore 1987c). Clients have also indicated that within reason this approach is perfectly acceptable and indeed in some studies have shown that they positively welcome the development (Ferguson and Carney 1970, Costello 1977, Day 1979, Ley 1982, Kreps and Thornton 1984, Mosley 1988) The students second choice of learning method is the workshop. Again this is an interesting and encouraging finding for two reasons. The students have chosen a method which encourages maximum interaction between the students themselves and also one in which, providing they are adequately briefed, they spend a lot of time in preparation and group work without any direct teacher input unless requested.

Table 6.6
Rank order of the preferred interdisciplinary learning methods : By profession.

Profession ⇒ Learning Method	Den	DSA	D.T	Med	Nur	Diet	Oc.T	ODP	Phys	Pod	Rad	Soc	Sp.T
Tutorial	3	2	3	3	5	1	5	5	2	2	2	7	4
Workshop	5	7	4	5	2	4	1	1	4	3	5	1	1
Case Study	2	4	2	6	3	3	4	7	5	5	3	2	2
Seminar	4	3	7	2	6	7	7	4	7	7	6	5	5
Problem Based L.	6	6	5	4	4	5	6	6	3	5	7	3	7
Role Play	8	8	8	8	8	8	8	8	8	8	8	6	8
Lectures	6	4	5	7	7	6	3	2	6	4	4	8	6
Client Visits	1	1	1	1	1	2	2	3	1	1	1	4	3

Key
Den = Dentists, DSA = DSA/DH, D.T = Dental technologists,
Med = Medical Practitioners, Nur = Nurses, Diet = Nutritionists & Dietitians,
Oc.T = Occupational Therapists, ODP = Operating Dept. Practitioners,
Phys = Physiotherapists, Pod = Podiatrists, Rad = Radiographers,
Soc = Social Workers, Sp.T = Speech Therapists.

Their third, fourth and fifth choices also reflect maximum student interaction and minimal teacher intervention unless invited. It would seem that for interdisciplinary learning at least, students would prefer minimal teacher intervention. Only 51.48% of the 1383 students voted for lectures where there is little or no interaction between the students and a didactic approach is frequently adopted by a lecturer.

The most significant result was the rejection of role play ($p < 0.1\%$). Only 456 (32.97%) of the 1383 students accepted role play as an appropriate learning method. In all professions (with the exception of social work) the use of role play was not acceptable and was placed last in the rank order. The implications of this finding may not necessarily be confined to interdisciplinary learning. It is suspected that many students gave their instinctive responses to the options from a stance of preferred learning within their own professional training. Hence they projected their likes and dislikes of a learning method into interdisciplinary learning. The question must be asked whether some of the formal teaching is so bad and perceived by the students as so irrelevant to their needs, that the students would prefer to do it themselves? From the role play perspective, could it be that students are inadequately briefed and most importantly inadequately debriefed by teachers who are inexperienced themselves in using this as a teaching method? Role play is often used in a situation where sensitive issues are explored and when it would be totally inappropriate to involve a "real" patient or "client". If students inadvertently reveal information of a very sensitive nature based on their own life experiences the results can be catastrophic, not only for the student concerned but also for the rest of the participants. Group dynamics can be altered permenantly. It takes a very skilled facilitator to deal with such a situation (Bergevin et al 1963, Nichol 1971) It would seem likely that the social work students who accept role play as appropriate, have experienced the strengths of this method in the hands of experienced social work teachers. It would be wise for inexperienced teachers in many of the professions to consider the recruitment of social work teachers to facilitate role play sessions if students are to be persuaded that it is a valid method.

It would have been sensible to ascertain the learning methods that students currently experience as what is not known is whether students rejected some of the methods because they did not know their meaning. Alternatively a brief explantion of what each method was may have been helpful on the student questionnaire. The justification for this decision is based on the response related to "problem based learning". Several of the different student professions recorded a high level of indecision. This is suggestive of uncertainty of what would be required of them and indicates that the term at least was unfamiliar. An explanation of what problem based learning modelled on the Canadian McMaster University programme described by Walsh (1978) and the University of Linkoping, Sweden described by Areskog (1988b, 1992) may have improved the response to this question. An understanding of the fact that problem based learning in health care emanates from patient problems and that the onus is on the students to identify the causal factors and plan the interventions according to those needs would seem to fit the philosophy that the students adopted in this study that of maximum interaction between the patient/client and the students.

What would seem patently clear is that in any interdisciplinary programme the learning methods must be chosen with extreme care and should reflect the opinions of the student population. Teachers cannot ensure the success of a programme it is the students who evaluate whether a course meets their needs and the reputation of a course is based upon the value that previous students place upon it. The learning methods acceptable to the student population in this study (N = 1383) have been clearly identified and as such meet one of the aims (Aim 3.4) of this study.

6.11 What could be learned on an interdisciplinary basis ?

The thirteen professions who participated in this study could and should be able to learn together in any interdisciplinary initiative. The results demonstrate that each profession believes that there should be some interdisciplinary learning and the advantages identified by each profession were very similar. There was also a broad consensus of agreement that any such initiative should take place throughout undergraduate training. It was of the utmost importance therefore, to decide which professions should learn together and what they should learn. The 300 teachers and 1383 students completed two questions which were exactly the same on both questionnaires. They were asked to decide, from a list of topics which would be suitable for interdisciplinary learning. This list of topics had been generated from the analysis of the fourteen curricula and comprised psychology ; sociology ; ethics ; law and practice ; research methods ; management ; economics of health care ; health promotion ; study skills ; quality assurance ; the organisation of health and social care ; computing skills. Table 6.7 shows the teacher and students responses by percentage and in rank order of choice.

The teachers recorded a higher percentage than the students in every category. The reason for this is not clear although it may be due to a lack of experience and insight on the part of the student population. There were clear differences between the student groups with the medical students returning a lesser percentage than any of the others (see Chapter 5, Table 5.113). A further interesting point was noted in that the more senior students in every profession scored a higher percentage than the students in their first year of training. It would be interesting to repeat this part of the study with these first year students at a later stage in their training in order to see if these results would be replicated or if the percentage responses were higher.

Table 6.7
Rank ordered selection of suitable interdisciplinary topics : By percentage

Topics	Teachers (N = 299)	Rank Order Teachers	Students (N = 1383)	Rank Order Students	Overall Rank Order
Psychology	92.64%	2	84.82%	1	1
Sociology	88.63%	6	79.39%	2	4
Ethics	93.98%	1	78.60%	3	2
Law & Practice	88.96%	5	60.09%	7	6
Research Methods	81.60%	11	58.25%	8	10
Management	86.62%	10	55.97%	11	11
Economics	87.62%	8	68.55%	6	7
Health Promotion	92.64%	2	76.21%	4	3
Study Skills	86.96%	9	56.62%	9	9
Quality Issues	88.29%	7	56.11%	10	8
Organisation of care	90.30%	4	75.70%	5	5

There was a clear agreement between the teachers and the students that psychology, health promotion, ethics, sociology and the organisation of health and social care could be undertaken on a shared learning basis. The response for "law and practice" is interesting. The teachers (88.96%) strongly supported this but the students (60.09%) were less sure. Much of the content of this component comprises topics such as confidentiality, accountability, competency, documentation, informed consent, equal opportunities, patient rights. Many of these, by their very nature imply an interdisciplinary perspective as each individual health professional is dependent on both his/her own professional conduct and that of the other members of a multidisciplinary team. The literature review has revealed that issues related to law and practice frequently cause the most animosity and distrust between the professions. If students were given the opportunity to explore these issues on an interdisciplinary basis during their undergraduate training this may help them clarify some of the current confusion and misunderstanding that occurs.

Ethics as an interdisciplinary topic was considered in a more positive light by the students (78.60%). This again is interesting when considered with the level of support for law and practice. Ethics and law and practice would seem to be inextricably linked in many instances. In Table 6.1 (at the beginning of this Chapter) it can be seen that many of the topics such as confidentiality, informed consent, patient rights are claimed within both the academic discipline of ethics and that of law and practice. It is difficult to see how these two subjects can be taught in isolation from each other.

The final observation pertaining to this section is that it is most encouraging to note that the topics which are rank ordered the highest are those which have essentially a client focus. It could be argued that many of the topics on the list are not at the sharp end of care. Study skills are essential for students but the patient/client will not take those into consideration when evaluating the quality of care received. What will matter is the level of interaction and communication between the health team and the patients and their families, the quality of individualised care received, the level of privacy and dignity maintained and a continued sense of empowerment and control experienced by the patient/client. These essential human needs can be aimed for by the health and social care professions only if they have a fundamental understanding of psychology, sociology, ethics, health promotion, law and practice and organisation of health and social care.

The results obtained indicate quite clearly that many topics would be acceptable on an interdisciplinary basis and as such could constitute the broad concepts for a core curriculum. These findings meet Aim 3.7 in this study.

6.12 Profiles of the individual professions

In this section a brief summary of the results from each of the thirteen participating professions is undertaken.

6.12.1 The dentists

In total 40 teaching staff and 93 students completed the questionnaire (Chapter 5, Section 5.3.1). The teaching staff were predominantly male (29 males, 11 females) but there was a more even gender distribution among the student population (53 males, 40 females). It is not known whether this is because more men than women choose or are appointed to teach in the Dental School or whether there is a greater number of females entering the dental profession in 1993 than there was twenty years ago. More than 70% of the teaching staff had commenced their teaching career within ten years of qualifying, with 60% having worked in clinical practice for less than five years (Table 5.64). Of the 30 teaching staff who had taught different professions, 27 had done so with dental surgery assistants and dental hygienists. More had taught nurses (RS = 13) than dental technologists (RS = 12). Only three had taught nutritionists and dietitians (Table 5.66). This finding is of interest as 75.00% of the dental lecturers and 66.67% of the dental students indicated that it would be useful to learn with nutritionists and dietitians (Table 5. 80).

Conversely, none of the nutrition and dietetics lecturers selected the dentists as an appropriate profession with which to learn, but 53.33% of the nutrition and dietetics students did (Table 5.147). As more than half of the students from both professions believed it would be valuable, attempts should be made to implement some shared learning on a trial basis. Similarly only two dental lecturers had taught speech therapists, yet 55.00% of the dental lecturers and 48.39 % of the students selected speech therapists (Table 5.80). Again neither speech therapy teacher selected the dentists whereas 51.85% of the students did (Table 5.232). If the students opinions are taken into consideration interdisciplinary learning between these three groups should be introduced forthwith.

The majority of dental students (91.40%) were less than 25 years of age (Table 5.68). If the sample can be assumed to be typical, it would appear that dental students tend to commence their training immediately after completing secondary school. Consequently very few had obtained any work related experience and those that had were female. Apart from learning with medical students (in pre-clinical training) few of the dental students had been given the opportunity to learn with other professions which confirms that dental students tend to learn in isolation from all other professions. Most dental students (76.34%) would prefer to experience some interdisciplinary learning and the concept would be supported by 90.00% of the teaching staff (Figure 5.11 and Table 5.71).

The majority of the dental profession (68.42%) believed that interdisciplinary learning should take place throughout training (Table 5.72) and 74.44% of the sample would be interested or very interested in participating in any further developments (Table 5.76 and Figure 5.13). The professions with which they mainly would chose to learn apart from nutrition and dietetics and speech therapy were the dental hygienists/DSAs' (84.21%), dental technology (66.17%), medicine (84.21%) and radiography (59.40%) (Table 5.80). The teachers and students were very similar in their opinions regarding which of the core subjects could be adopted in interdisciplinary learning with the exception of the research category (Table 5.85). No explanation can be offered for this finding.

Craig (1970) was the only author identified in the literature review who attempted to analyse the effectiveness of teamwork in dental care. He found in that in a team of four individuals, the dentist was the team leader in that he was the employer of a dental hygienist, a dental nurse and a dental technician. Craig observed a hierarchical system in which there was no mutual decision making between the four individuals. The dentist made the decisions and communicated these to the others. In 1993, without doubt there has been progress in the concept of teamwork in dental care. Nonetheless there would appear to be room for increased collaboration and co-operation and the respondents in this sample are willing to participate with a variety of other professions particularly those that are implicitly involved with the head and neck, thus indicating that there is still a tendency to categorise the client into regions rather than treat them holistically.

6.12.2 The dental surgery assistants/dental hygienists

All four teachers and 37 students were female. The results obtained from these respondents were diverse and interesting. The four teachers had all experienced teaching other professional groups including nurses, occupational therapists and physiotherapists. The students tended to be very young with nearly half of the sample being less than 20 years of age. There was however, a surprisingly varied response to relevant work experience and previous courses from the older students. The 15 students who had experienced learning with other professions had done so in their previous work experience prior to commencing their training. The majority of the respondents in this school believed that there should be some interdisciplinary learing (80.49%) (Table 5.81 and Figure 5.14) however there were divided opinions about when it should take place. While 41.46% selected throughout training, 26.83% chose the beginning and 21.95% chose the middle of training (Table 5.82). The rationale for the middle of training was based on the need to get to grasp their own subject and role first. As the literature review has indicated, this professionalisation is not desirable from the teamwork point of view as cloistering, isolation and stereotyping will have taken place by the time these students integrate with the other professional groups. More than 70% (RS = 29) of the sample were interested in the idea of interdisciplinary learning with nine of the students expressing themselves as "very interested" (Table 5.83).

The dentists were the most frequently chosen profession with whom this group would wish to learn (73.17% of the sample). What was very interesting however, was that the dentists (both teachers (75%) and students (88.17%)) were more positive about learning with the DSA/DH than conversely. Could it be that the DSA/DH lack in self esteem and believe that the dental profession views them as very inferior ? If so this adds credence to the claim made earlier in this chapter (see section 6.4) that perceived professional hierarchical domination may be a self perpetuating myth which continues only because those professions who perceive themselves as the underdogs repeat the myth to junior members of the profession while those that are perceived as the dominating professions are quite happy to let this state of affairs continue. Apart from the occasional comment on an individual basis no qualitative evidence has been found in this study which indicates that the professional hierarchy even exists in 1993, except in health service mythology.

Apart from Craig (1970), no articles were found that specifically examined the roles of dental hygienists and dental surgery assistants in the dental health team. There appears to be many unanswered questions that have arisen from these results and it would be useful to commence a study which specifically examines the existing level of teamwork and the perceived hierarchical system in dental care.

6.12.3 The dental technologists

The dental technologists were the only respondents in this sample, who did not have any direct patient/client contact. The responses of these individuals were therefore of particular interest as understandably they must have a very limited experience of the concept of holistic care. Six teaching staff and 30 students completed the questionnaire (the discrepancy in the number of teachers has already been explained in Chapter 5, Section 5.5.3.3). The students tended to be in the younger age groups and were predominantly male (Table 5.88). Five of the teachers were male. A substantial majority (91.67%) believed that there should be some interdisciplinary learning with no respondents giving a negative response (Table 5.89). The majority (58.33%) selected "throughout training" as the appropriate time to undertake this although 30.00% of the student population selected the middle of training (Table 5.90). The level of interest expressed by this group was also unexpectedly high with 88.89% being interested or very interested (Table 5.94 and Figure 5.16). These results suggest that the dental technologists are well aware of their isolation and would welcome any developments that would redress the balance. Their choice of other professions with which to learn was more predictable (Table 5.98). Dentists were selected by 94.44% of the sample, DSA/dental hygienists by 80.55%, and speech therapists by 55.56%. The other professions which featured in the results were nutrition and dietetics, chosen by 27.78% and radiography by 25.00%. If the recommendations made in the Nuffield Report (1993) where dental technologists would have direct client contact are implemented it would be interesting to repeat this question as other professions such as social work or occupational therapy much take on a greater significance. It was interesting to note that no respondent in this sample, selected the medical profession.

6.12.4 The medical practitioners

The respondents in this group represented the second largest sample (N = 376). The excellent response rate far exceeded expectations and calls into question the observations made by authors in their anecdotal reports of medical practitioners not wishing to be involved in any joint initiatives with other professions (Akester and McPhail 1964, Pelligrino 1966, Bates 1969, 1970, Hoekleman 1975, Singleton 1981, Copp 1987, Garvin and Kennedy 1988). If this was the case, then the response rate would have been much lower and most certainly individuals would not have bothered to identify themselves.

As has been noted in Chapter 5 Section 5.5.3.4. and discussed in Section 4 of this chapter, while the medical teachers were predominantly male (80 male, 27 female), the medical students revealed a different picture (120 male, 149 female). The recommendations of the Towle Report (1991) are therefore being met in this medical school. There was a highly significant difference between the number of male and female medical students who had gained relevant work experience ($p < 0.1\%$). The female students tended to be slightly older than their male counterparts. The majority of medical students, nonetheless in this sample are less than 25 years of age with only 23 (where N = 269) being 26 years or more (Table 5.104). Most medical students commence their training at eighteen years of age on completion of their secondary schooling.

The teachers had very wide experience in teaching professions other than their own with 96 (89.72%) of the 107 respondents having taught at least one other health care profession (Table 5.102). A substantial majority of them (RS = 76) had also experienced learning with other professions but only 16 had done so at an undergraduate level. The length of the experience is not known but it is suspected that few medical practitioners will have undertaken shared learning for more than a few hours or days.

The medical teachers were more convinced of the need for, and more interested in, the concept of interdisciplinary learning than were the medical students (Tables 5.107 and 5.112, Figures 5.17 and 5.19). The senior medical students however were more positive and interested than the junior ones. There was a significant difference between the responses of the male and female third year students. The explanation for this may be due to the significantly greater number of female medical students who had gained relevant work experience and had in most instances, worked in a health or social care team thus giving them a greater insight into the concept of holistic care. The finding that the more senior students (of both sexes) were more interested and more convinced of the need for interdisciplinary learning was a very encouraging finding and would suggest that as a student becomes more experienced they are able to link theory to practice in client centred care.

The teachers also responded more positively to the suggested subjects for interdisciplinary learning and to the number of professions with whom medical students could usefully learn (Table 5.116). Medical students were less likely to select the professions who emphasise a psychosocial model of care rather than a medical model. The medical students for example, ranked social workers in sixth position whereas the teachers placed them second. The medical students were less keen to learn with the dental students than vice versa. Although many of these statements are seemingly negative this is not the case. It should be remembered that the majority of medical students believed that there should be some interdisciplinary learning throughout training bringing the advantages of increased collaboration, teamwork and cross fertilisation of ideas and reducing the interprofessional conflict. Kirkland (1970) would have been delighted with these results as he had complained so bitterly of the professional isolation that medical students suffer. It is interesting to note however that the problem for Kirkland and his colleagues was the entrenchment of the teaching staff in the Faculty of Medicine. The results of this current study would appear to indicate the complete antithesis of this with some of the medical students being more entrenched than most of the teaching staff !

Mention has already been made of a possible self perpetuating myth regarding the professional elitism within the dominating hierarchical professions. Whilst there is some evidence that this still occurs amongst some of the medical students in this study, the majority of the teachers and most of the students do not display this trait. It would appear that much of the responsibility for this myth should be taken by the nursing and paramedical professions. The medical practitioner (Respondent 23, see Section 5.5.1) who observed that one of the disadvantages of interdisciplinary learning was that "everyone will gang up on the dotors" may well have been right !

6.12.5 The nurses

The 493 teachers and students in this group comprised the largest population in the study. This was no surprise as the nursing profession is the largest single group of health care workers. As nurses traditionally have a twenty four hour commitment to caring for patients in the acute sector of health care and an increasing time commitment to caring for clients in the community, it is this group who are in regular contact with the other health and social care professions, frequently on a daily basis. It was therefore expected that this group would give a generally positive response to interdisciplinary learning. The results demonstrate that this is the case. The student population consisted of Project 2000 and the four year Bachelor of Nursing undergraduate students. As the traditional three year training is due to finish in 1994, the students on this programmed were excluded from the study. The student population tended to be older than the other groups with the exception of social work, with many of them having previously completed relevant courses and/or gained relevant work experience. Nearly 7.00% of the students were graduate entrants (Table 5.125).

The move towards an all graduate status for teachers of nursing explains the number (RS =59) of teachers who were graduates in related subjects (Table 5.120). The depth and breadth of knowledge of these individuals, along with the fact that they have mandatorily completed a teacher training course can only add to the quality of teaching that nursing students receive. The 23 nurse teachers who mentioned redundancy as a possible disadvantage of interdisciplinary learning, highlighted the insecurity and vulnerability of this group in 1994. The fact that no teacher from any of the other professions seemed to consider this, was an indication of the level of stress being experienced by nurse teachers. The issues surrounding the rationalisation and amalgamation of Colleges of Nursing and Midwifery and the associated issues of affiliation or integration into the higher education sector should be resolved with the greatest urgency.

The teacher's and student's responses were on the whole, very similar regarding the concept of interdisciplinary learning, with more than 86% of both groups indicating that it should be introduced (Table 5.127). There was however, a difference of opinion about when such learning should be introduced (Table 5.128 and Figure 5.21). Although the majority of students indicated that it should be throughout training, a significant minority selected the middle of training as their preferred option. This trend could also be seen in several of the other professions. Their rationale was that they wanted to find their professional identity before mixing with the other professions. This is understandable but as the literature review has revealed professional identity rapidly becomes professional territorialism and isolation with the concomitant interprofessional conflict, jealousies and entrenched attitudes that this brings. For this reason it is essential that interdisciplinary learning is introduced from the beginning of undergraduate training. As all students are given notice of their tutorial groups (on a profession specific basis) from the beginning of training, it would be very simple to also include notice of their tutorial groups on an interdisciplinary basis.

The teachers and students were also in agreement in most instances, on the subjects which would be suitable for interdisciplinary learning, although there was significantly more support for management, study skills and quality issues by the teachers. Nevertheless all subjects were deemed suitable by the majority of respondents from both samples (Table 5.133).

Consistent with the other student respondents, the nursing students selected visiting client areas as the most appropriate learning method with workshops being their second choice. A statistically significant number rejected role play ($p < 0.1\%$) although their response was more positive than all other student groups with the exception of social work (Table 5.135).

The nursing profession would appear to have made a fundamental change in their philosophy away from the medical model towards the biopsychosocial model of client care. This is evidenced from their selection of the professions with whom they would choose to share interdisciplinary learning. Although the medical profession was chosen by approximately 80% of the teachers and the students, the nutritionists and dietitians, physiotherapists, occupational therapists and social workers were selected by more respondents overall (Table 5.136). The results suggest that the nursing professions dependence on the medical profession, which has been noted by so many authors (MacGregor 1960, Akester and McPhail 1964, Schlotfeldt 1965, Rosinski 1965, Peeligrino 1966, Peeples and Francis 1968, Berkowitz and Malone 1968, Hoekleman 1975, Kalisch and Kalisch 1977, Burkett et al 1978, Steele 1981, Singleton 1981, Mechanic and Aiken 1982, Ahmedazai 1982, Goodwin 1982, Collucio and Maquire 1983, Ferguson-Johnston 1983, McClure 1984, Kurtzman et al 1985, Webster 1985, Whitehouse 1986, Keddy et al 1986, Copp 1987, Garvin and Kennedy 1988, Brooking 1991) is lessening and consequently the opportunity for a true partnership in collaborative care may now be presenting itself.

6.12.6 The nutritionists and dietitians

As the number of teachers in this school was small (N = 4) it was not possible to undertake a statistical analysis between the results of the teachers and students. Nevertheless some general observations can be made and comparisons with the results overall attempted. There was a broad consensus of agreement that there should be some interdisciplinary learning (teachers 100% and students 93.33% where N = 45) with a similar percentage believing that advantages would accrue (Tables 5.138 and 5.140). There were differences in opinion however, of when it should take place. Three of the four teachers believed that it should occur throughout training. Their opinions reflected those of most of the teachers from the other professions. The nutrition and dietetics students responses were more divided with a proportionate number choosing the beginning, middle and the end of training. Less than 50% selected throughout training. This result was lower than the other student groups. The reason for this finding is not known (Table 5.139).

The level of interest in the concept was very high with the 4 teachers stating that they were interested and 55.56% of the students being very interested (where N = 45) and 40.00% being interested (Table 5.143 and Figure 5.24). This result makes these respondents the third most interested group overall with the social workers and the podiatrists being in first and second places respectively.

There was a difference in opinion regarding the subjects which would be suitable for interdisciplinary learning. With the exception of law and practice (RS = 3) the four teachers indicated that all subjects were acceptable. Most students however rejected law and practice and also research methods (Table 5.144). All other subjects were thought to be suitable, with psychology, sociology and health promotion being particularly favoured. The students correctly identified psychology and sociology as the behavioural sciences but were very undecided about the other subjects (Table 5.145).

There was a 100% response to the question of whether nurses were a suitable profession with which to learn (Table 5.147). This result was the only one which returned a 100% positive response in the whole study. It can be concluded therefore that the nutritionists and dietitians in this study would like the opportunity to learn with the nursing profession. As the nursing professions response was also very high (82.52% where N = 492) it would appear reasonable to suggest that ways of organising some shared learning between these two groups should be explored as a matter of urgency (Table 5.136). The concept is not new as similar programmes have already been described by Caliendo and Pulaski (1979), Wessell (1981), Dickens et al (1985) and Bersky et al (1987). Medicine and social work was also selected by a substantial majority of the respondents. There were differences between the opinions of the teachers and students in their choice of some of the professions. An obvious example was that of dentistry. No teacher selected the dental profession whereas 53.33% of the students did. The zero response by the teachers was unexpected and does not reflect the opinions of the dental profession where 75% of the teachers (where N = 40) and 66.67% (where N = 93) of the dental students identifed nutritionists and dietitians as a suitable profession with which to learn. Similarly the nutrition and dietetics teachers rejected the dental hygienists and the dental technologists where 35.56% of the students identified dental hygienists and 8.89% of them identified dental technologists as appropriate (Table 5.147). Three (75%) of the dental hygiene lecturers and 20 (54.05%) of the students selected the nutritionists and dietitians (Table 5.87). Interestingly no dental technology lecturer selected nutrition and dietetics but 10 (33.33% where N = 30) students did (Table 5.98). As the numbers of teaching staff are so small in these professions it was not possible to test for the significance of these findings. It is not unreasonable to conclude however, that there is a diversity of opinions between the teachers and students in several of these professions. This adds substance to the claim that one of the advantages of interdisciplinary learning (identified by 157 teachers and 699 students in this study) would be to gain insight into what the other professions contribute to client care. If everybody was given the opportunity to gain this insight it would enable individuals to make an informed choice about the professions with which they would wish to learn !

6.12.7 The occupational therapists

Although 96 representatives of the occupational therapy profession participated in this study the small number of teachers (N = 7) made statistical analysis between the two groups questionable. The sample was predominantly female. An interesting finding was the number of mature students in the sample with 10 (where N = 89) being more than 41 years of age (Table 5.148). The reason for this is not known although analysis of the qualitative data revealed that several of these mature students had obtained other qualifications (ie Registered Nurses, teacher training). It may be that these students had opted for a career change or that they were returning to employment after a career break (Chapter 5, Section 5.3.7).

There was no evidence that any interdisciplinary learning had taken place as occupational therapy students, although eight students indicated that they had done so on previous occasions. Five of the teachers (71.43%) and 84 (94.38%) of the students believed that there should be some interdisciplinary learning and no respondent in this sample rejected it completely (Table 5.150). The majority selected throughout training as the appropriate time for it to take place and 100% of the sample (where N = 96) believed that it should take place before qualifying. One student in this sample (the only one in the study where N = 1383) suggested that students should be involved in the planning stages of such an event as students "have not yet adopted the same suspicions and conflict...." that many of the teachers had. The students are taught by the teachers she suggested, to distrust all the other professions. Judging by the overall results it would seem that she may be right. With the exception of the medical profession where the teachers expressed a higher level of interest than the students, the students in general were more keen than the teaching staff, although the difference was so small as to be non significant.

In some instances a higher percentage of students identified subjects as suitable for interdisciplinary learning. Examples of this can be cited as psychology and sociology. One teacher however, did not complete this whole question and subsequently these results while interesting are in no way conclusive and should be treated with caution. What can be concluded however, is that all the suggested subject areas were accepted as suitable for interdisciplinary learning by the majority of respondents.

The favoured learning method by these students was a workshop, with visits to client areas as their second choice (Table 5.158). The selection of the lecture as the third choice was surprising as the occupational therapy curriculum has an integrative, problem based philosophy. It is not known whether the lecture is a common teaching strategy on this course but the course document suggests that this would not be the case. Perhaps there is an element of the novelty factor here. More than 96% (where N = 96) of the sample selected social work as an appropriate profession with whom to share learning (Table 5.159). Their allegiance to the social work profession was reciprocated in that the social workers also selected the occupational therapists as their first choice. The nurses (93.75%) and the physiotherapists (93.75%) also featured strongly with the speech therapists being identifed by 80.21%. The medical profession was selected by 76.04% but was in fifth place. This contrasts with the medical practitioners who selected the occupational therapists in third place (Table 5.116), it should be remembered though that the overall percentage response rate of the occupational therapists was much higher than the medical practitioners.

6.12.8 The operating department practitioners

This group was not only the smallest in the study, but also by the very nature of their work, likely to be comparatively isolated from many of the professions who were also participating. This set of respondents was one of the two that was predominantly male. Twenty had worked previously in a related occupation, with two of the females having worked as qualifed nurses. It was outside the remit of this study to ascertain who was a qualified nurse and why they had changed careers but it would certainly be an interesting area of study to pursue in the future. The presence of only two teachers militates against specific comment as any of the responses could have occured by chance, but suffice it to say that the two sets of responses were diverse suggesting that there was no collaboration ! Their results can be seen in Chapter 5, Section 5.5.3.8.

Of the 25 students, 21 (84.00%) believed that there should some interdisciplinary learning with only one rejecting the concept entirely. There was a very diverse set of responses regarding the stage at which it should be introduced with 4 students recommending post qualification (in spite of two of these being very interested in the idea). The remaining students proportionately selected all three categories in undergraduate training (Table 5.161). Both teachers and 20 of the students thought there would be advantages in interdisciplinary learning with 20 (80.00%) of the students being interested or very interested in the idea (Table 5.165).

The subject which was most favoured by this group of respondents for interdisciplinary learning was ethics with 92.59% giving a positive response (Table 5.166). Although the reason for this is not clear it is suggested that one reason for this finding is that in operating departments where patients are frequently unable to make their own decisions or take any responsibility for their own care, ethical issues and dilemmas are frequent encountered and cause on occasions, extreme tension and conflict between the professions. It is acknowledged that this statement is unsubstantiated but personal experience demonstrates this to be the case. It is therefore surprising that only 56% of the students supported the idea of law and practice as a subject suitable for interdisciplinary learning as the two are inextricably linked.

The favourite learning method was lectures (Table 5.168). The operating department practitioners were the only students who selected this method in first place and indeed the majority of professions ranked lectures in the lower categories. Again no explanation for this finding can be offered except to suggest that this group may be choosing a method which is very familiar to them. As has been previously discussed lectures while having their place in any educational programme can only be used to good effect on an interdisciplinary basis if they are supported by tutorials or any method which achieves integration between the students. Lectures where students do not interact do not constitute interdisciplinary learning in themselves.

The professions with which the operating department practitioners would wish to learn were the nurses (92.59%) followed by the medical practitioners (77.78%). The radiographers were selected by 48.15% of the sample with the physiotherapists in fourth place (44.44%). After this the percentage of respondents who identifed any other professions dropped considerably (Table 5.169). There is a perfectly logical explanation for this finding. Within the operating department itself, operating department practitioners, nurses and medical practitioners are to be found. Radiographers are frequently called to the department to take "on table" X Rays and the physiotherapists make their first therapeutic intervention to patients following major surgery in the recovery unit, which is an integral part of the operating department. These four professions therefore, come into frequent contact with the operating department practitioners.

It would be unusual for there to be any professional interaction with any of the other groups.

6.12.9 The physiotherapists

The physiotherapists produced a most interesting set of results with the 10 teachers and 101 students frequently producing very similar responses. Apart from the medical profession, the physiotherapists were the least supportive of the concept of interdisciplinary learning. Nevertheless 60.00% of the teachers and 71.29% of the students believed that some should take place (Table 5.174). The other teachers and the majority of the remaining students would appear to be open to persuasion as they were undecided. There was a significant difference ($p < 5\%$) between the teacher and student's responses regarding when interdisciplinary learning should be introduced although 50.00% of the teachers and 48.51% of the students selected throughout the other responses were very different with 40.00% of the teachers but only 4.95% of the students choosing the end of training (Table 5.175).

A highly significant finding ($p < 0.1\%$) was that the students were more convinced than the teachers of the advantages which would result with 60.00% of the teachers being undecided (Table 5.176). The teachers were also very neutral in their support of the concept with two being uninterested whereas the students were much more positive in their approach with 74 (73.27% where $N = 101$) being interested or very interested (Table 5.179, Figure 5.30). The teachers results reveal that they were the least interested respondents amongst the teachers. This was an unexpected finding as the literature had suggested that the medical profession would be the least supportive but this did not turn out to be the case with 69 (64.49% where $N = 107$) of the medical staff selecting the interested or very interested categories. The question arises therefore of whether these physiotherapy teachers are representative of teachers of physiotherapy as a whole or whether they are an isolated group who have differing ideas and are more entrenched than their colleagues in other schools of physiotherapy ? It is impossible to reach a conclusion, but it would be of value to replicate the study by distributing the questionnaires to teachers and students in other schools of physiotherapy to explore whether the results would be similar.

In spite of the lower level of support from the teachers, the majority indicated that most of the subjects suggested would be suitable for interdisciplinary learning. The students were also very positive in their selection with the exception of management where only 47.52% of the sample thought this would be acceptable (Table 5.180). Consistent with the majority of the other professions the students selected visits to client areas as the most popular interdisciplinary learning method and rejected role play by a significant majority ($p < 0.1\%$) (Table 5.182).

Occupational therapists, medical practitioners and nurses were the most frequently selected profession with whom physiotherapists would wish to learn (Table 5.183). A substantial majority (69.37%) also identifed social workers. This was an interesting finding which appeared to suggest that physiotherapists in the course of their work, may encounter many clients with social problems. It was interesting to note the low response rate to learning with the podiatrists. As has been previously discussed in Section 6.9 the podiatrists selected the physiotherapists in second place after the medical profession. More than 44% of the physiotherapy students identified nutritionists and dietitians as appropriate. This is encouraging as it indicates an awareness of the need for an appropriate, healthy diet in order to maintain or regain mobility and healing.

The results obtained from the physiotherapists indicate a diverse group with the students demonstrating a more collaborative philosophy than the teaching staff. It is interesting to speculate whether these students will be as supportive of interdisciplinary learning after they qualify or whether they will have become more professionally isolated.

6.12.10 The podiatrists

These respondents were on the whole very supportive of the concept of interdisciplinary learning with 87.50% of the teachers and 95.20% of the students believing that it should take place (Table 5.186). There were fairly diverse results regarding when it should be introduced but again all the respondents (with the exception of one teacher) indicated that it should occur prior to qualification (Table 5.187). There was an unexpected finding of eight Registered Nurses in the student population which comprised 12.70% of the sample. An explanation for this has already been offered although it is admitted that it is entirely speculative. There was a very high level of interest expressed by this group with only six students being neutral about the concept (Table 5.191 and Figure 5.32). The teachers gave a 100% positive response to the subjects which could be taught on an interdisciplinary basis whereas the students appeared to be less sure. Because of the small number of teachers (N = 8) however this disparity may have occurred by chance (Table 5.192).

The students preferred learning methods concentrated on visits to the client areas (92.06%) with all the other methods being selected by upwards of 60.00% with the exception of role play which was rejected by a significant majority ($p < 1\%$) (Table 5.194). The podiatrists were very positive about learning with most of the other professions but their preferred choices of medicine and physiotherapy did not return the same responses (Table 5.194). As the overall ranking indicated that the podiatrists came in twelth position as an appropriate profession with whom to learn it would appear that they have been marginalised along with the dentists, dental hygienists and the dental technologists (Table 6.4). This is an interesting but alarming finding as it is suggestive that in the opinions of some of the professions, the professions who deal with regional parts of the human body are believed to do just that. This does not support the concept of holism and sits much more comfortably with the medical model rather than the biopsychosocial model care. Comparisons between the dentists and podiatrists results however reveal a similar picture. Whilst both groups would wish to learn with the professions who have an input into caring for a client as a whole, they reject each other as suitable interdiscplinary learning partners. This was a highly significant finding ($\chi^2 = 57.89$, df = 4, $p < 0.1\%$). It is suggested that the podiatrists should attempt to raise their profile in order to highlight the contribution they are able to make to maintaining the populations mobility.

6.12.11 The radiographers

The student population in this profession tended to be younger than many of the other professions allied to medicine with more than 55% being less than 20 years of age. Nine of the students had experienced shared learning with another profession, all of whom were in the third year of training. The shared experience had been with orthoptic students from the now closed school of orthoptics.

Overall 84.48% (where N = 58) of this profession believed that there should be some interdisciplinary learning (Table 5.198 and Figure 5.33) with all but one student indicating that it should take place at the undergraduate stage (Table 5.199). There was a difference in opinion however between the teachers and the students as to when it should be introduced. While 66.67% of the teachers selected throughout training only 38.46% of the students did. Nearly as many students selected the beginning of training (36.54%) which is still an encouraging finding as they are implicitly recognising the importance of early interaction with the other professions. The majority of the teachers and the students expressed an interest in interdisciplinary learning with only three students (where N = 52) being uninterested or totally uninterested (Table 5.203). Many of the subjects suggested as potentially suitable for interdisciplinary learning were accepted by all six teachers. There was also a high positive response from the students in many of the categories (Table 5.204). Management however was rejected by the majority. This is an interesting finding as it was this category that was also rejected by the physiotherapy students. No explanation can be offered for this finding and it may be that it has occurred by chance. Visits to client areas was seen as the most appropriate learning method by the radiography students with role play being significantly rejected (Table 5.206).

The professions which were identifed as appropriate for learning with the radiographers revealed some interesting responses (Table 5.207). Nursing and medicine were the most frequently selected with the professions who deal with the head and neck and the feet being the least popular. It is very interesting to note that social work was chosen by 41.38% of the respondents but only 36.21% of these same respondents selected the dental profession, 25.86% the speech therapists, 8.62% the dental technologists and 13.79% the podiatrists. The dentists and podiatrists in particular frequently require X rays of the head and feet respectively in order to assess the needs of the client and plan the appropriate care. It would appear that these two professions do not feature highly in a radiographers perception of teamwork and yet 59.40% of the dental profession (Table 5.80) and 71.83% of the podiatrists (Table 5.195) selected the radiographers. Could it be that the radiographers do not understand the roles of these other professions and consequently have not had the opportunity to appreciate the contribution that their own profession makes to the others ? The answer is not known but it is very encouraging to see the commitment to learning with social workers particularly as unlike many of the professions, radiographers do not have an identifed case load on a long term basis which may necessitate social service involvement.

6.12.12 The social workers

The 137 respondents who comprised this sample are the only group who are not classified as a health care profession. However, as was discussed in Chapter 1, social workers make an essential contribution to the maintenance of a patient's biopsychosocial equilibrium and are without doubt, a crucial member of the team as they are inextricably linked with health care. In the literature review the question of collaboration between the health and social services was examined. Several Government Reports highlighted the inadequacies of the working relationships between the two and concluded that this was due on the whole, to resistance and conflict within the professions involved (HMSO 1959, HMSO 1968, HMSO 1974a, HMSO 1978, HMSO 1979, HMSO 1981, HMSO 1986b). Cypher (1979) however had concluded that the two services were going to have to work together whether they liked it or not ! Within the past decade, the emphasis on health, the move from hospital to community care, the issue of patient choice and empowerment, and the recognition that a biopsychosocial model of care is the appropriate way forward have made Cypher's observations even more pertinent. In 1993, the opinions of the social workers and the opinions of the other professions about the social workers regarding interdisciplinary learning were therefore of the upmost importance as the results would give an indication of the level of resistance and conflict that has been noted to exist.

The results obtained in this study have demonstrated that the other professions recognise the invaluable contribution that social workers make to caring. The justification for this conclusion is based on the overall rank order in which the social workers were placed. Against all expectations, and most certainly not supported by the literature (Nunally and Kitross 1958, Shortell 1974, Furnham et al 1981), the social workers were ranked in third place by the health professions (see Table 6.3). The lowest ranking they were given was eighth by the dentists

(Table 5.80). There were several unexpected results. The medical profession ranked social workers in third place (Table 5.116), as did the nurses (Table 5.136) and the nutritionists and dietitians (Table 5.147) while the speech therapists (Table 5.232) and the occupational therapists (Table 5.159) ranked them first. It would appear that even the medical practitioners are moving away from the traditional medical model towards a biopsychosocial model of care. It can be concluded that without doubt, social workers are viewed as essential members of the team. From the health care professions' perspective, closer collaboration is wanted.

The social workers themselves were the most positive of all thirteen professions about the need for interdisciplinary learning with 131 (95.62% where N = 137) believing that it should take place (Table 5.211 and Figure 5.35). The social work students presented a different picture from most of the other student groups. They were older with only one (0.77% where N = 130) being less than 25 years of age (Table 5.208), with 77 (59.23%) having completed previous relevant courses (Table 5.209) and 113 (86.92%) having gained relevant work experience (Table 5.210). There were eight Registered Nurses in the sample, but the majority of students had worked for the social services in some capacity. There were a large number of students (RS = 61) therefore, who had experienced shared learning at some stage. Most of this would appear to be at case conferences, study days and conferences. There was no evidence that any of the students had completed an interdisciplinary course of any duration. Nonetheless, the insight gained into the advantages of interdisciplinary learning may well have influenced their opinions and hence explains the results. The respondents did not seem to have experienced any interdisciplinary learning as social work students.

The majority of teachers (71.43%) and students (65.38%) were in agreement that interdisciplinary learning should take place throughout training (Table 5.212 and Figure 5.36). No respondent chose post qualification as their option. This finding is encouraging as several authors who had specifically examined the collaboration between social workers and other groups had recommended this (Tanner et al 1972, Ratoff et al 1974, Kendall 1977, Furnham et al 1981, Owen 1982, Dickens et al 1985, Knox and Thompson 1989). All seven teachers and 123 (94.62%) of the students believed there would be advantages with only one student rejecting the idea completely (Table 5.213). The level of interest expressed by this profession was significant ($p < 5\%$) with 60.58% of the sample stating that they were very interested. Of the total sample of 137, only four students indicated that they were neutral, uninterested, or totally uninterested in the concept (Table 5.216 and Figure 5.37)

The suggested core subjects for interdisciplinary learning were accepted by at least 75.00% of the overall sample in every category (Table 5.217). There was, however a difference between the opinions of the teachers and the students. The students were more positive than the teachers about law and practice, management, economics of care, and health promotion but the teachers were more positive than the students about study skills. Because of the small number of teachers in the social work school it was not possible to test for any significance and consequently these results should be treated with caution. Nevertheless the inference was that social work students in 1993 would welcome the opportunity to learn with the health professions and would participate positively if any of the suggested subjects were introduced.

It may be that the 117 students (90.00% where N = 130) who identifed law and practice as a suitable subject are aware of the potential conflict that arises between the health and social services over professional accountability, confidentiality, informed consent and clients rights. The opportunity to explore these issues on an interdisciplinary basis may do much to clarify the situation and resolve some of the conflict between the professions. The comparatively low response rate by the teachers (42.86%) for health promotion, although this may have occurred by chance, may be an indication that social workers do not see health promotion as their responsibility. The social work students appear to think differently as 110 (84.62% where N = 130) included it as an acceptable subject.

The preferred learning strategies expressed by the students presented a similar picture to that of most of the other student respondents (Table 5.219). The most frequently chosen response was workshops followed by case studies and visits to client areas. This means that the students have implicitly chosen those methods which involve maximum interaction with other students with the teacher in a facilitative role. These students were the only ones to accept role play (67.69%). It should be noted however that it was still ranked in sixth position although there was no significant difference between the result of the role play category and the majority of the others ($p > 5\%$) There was a significant difference however, between the results of the lecture ($p < 1\%$) and tutorial categories ($p < 5\%$) and the remaining ones. The unpopularity of the lecture as a learning strategy can perhaps be explained by the fact that a lecture tends to be didactic and does not involve much interaction between the students. As these respondents are mature students then it is likely that they would wish to actively participate rather than passively learn (Schein 1972, Barrows and Tamlyn 1980, Boud et al 1985, Boud and Griffin 1987, Boud 1988).

The social workers indicated that most of the professions would be suitable for sharing learning on an interdisciplinary basis (Table 5.220). Closer analysis of the results however, reveals some interesting points. Social workers also tend to marginalise the professions who specialise in the areas of the head and feet of clients. The dentists were chosen by only 7 (5.11% where N = 137) of the social workers the dental hygienists by only 15 (11.08%) and the podiatrists by only 21 (15.33%). As 57 dentists (42.86% where N = 133), 14 (34.15% where N = 41) of the dental hygienists and 41 (57.75% where N = 71) of the podiatrists selected social workers it would appear that as a profession, social workers might not always recognise where they are needed and valued (Tables 5.80, 5.87, 5.195).

The high percentage responses identifed in the other professions seem to indicate that some of the clients who are undergoing treatment to their feet or mouth have social problems as well! Many of the dentists, dental hygienists and podiatrists need to be given the opportunity to learn with social workers.

6.12.13 The speech therapists

The results obtained from this school represent only two teachers but 54 students. Although percentages for the teacher responses have been included in Chapter 5 for the sake of consistency, it is recognised that they are meaningless. The students however consitute a sizeable sample and therefore the findings may be taken to be representative of speech therapy students. There was a high level of support for interdisciplinary learning with 90.74% (where N = 56) indicating that some should take place (Table 5.223). The majority (62.50%) thought that it should occur throughout training although nearly 20.00% of the students thought it should not commence until the middle of training (Table 5.224). More than 90.00% of the sample thought there would be advantages with very few identifying disadvantages (Tables 5.225, 5.226, and 5.227). The level of interest was very high with 49 (87.50%) of the sample being interested or very interested (Table 5.228 and Figure 5.38).

Both teachers indicated that all the suggested subjects would be acceptable on an interdisciplinary basis but the students whilst taking a positive approach to the majority of the subjects rejected law and practice with only 46.30% indicating that this would be acceptable. Management and quality issues, consistent with many of the other students results, again tended to register a lower positive response (Table 5.229). The preferred learning methods would be workshops, case studies and visits to client areas. Role play was rejected by a highly significant number with only 15 (27.78%) giving a positive response ($p < 0.1\%$), but problem based learning was also rejected by the majority of students with only 44.44% giving a positive response. The reason for this is not known but it is suggested that this may be because problem based learning is not an identified learning strategy in the speech and language therapy programme and consequently the students may not fully understand its implications (Table 5.231).

The question which ascertained the professions with whom speech therapists believed they should share learning, yielded some interesting results (Table 5.232). It was anticipated that the dentists, dental hygienists, the dental technologists and the nutritionists and dietitians would feature strongly in their choice. The results were the complete antithesis. Medicine, nursing, occupational therapy and social work were the favoured professions with neither teacher selecting the dentists, the dental hygienists or the dental technologists. The students also gave a low response rate for the dental hygienists and dental technologists although 28 (51.85%) of them selected the dentists. The nutritionists and dietitians also recorded a low response (37.50% where N = 56). More than 50% of the dentists (50.38% where N = 133), and 55.56% (where N = 36) of the dental technologists selected the speech therapists although the dental hygienists returned a low response (14.63% where N = 41) (Tables 5.80, 5.98, and 5.87). The majority of nutritionists and dietitians indicated that it would be useful to learn with speech therapists (69.39% where N = 49) (Table 5.147). These contrasting results again raise the issue of whether each profession has any real insight into what the other professions contribute to health and social care. If each profession understood the role of the others then it would be reasonable to expect that the results would reflect each other, (ie the speech therapists and the nutritionists and dietitians would agree that it would be either appropriate or inappropriate to learn together). With such diverse findings the recommendation must be made that students from the different professional groups should be introduced to the roles of the other professions at the earliest stage of training.

6.13 Does the nomenclature matter ?

In Chapter 1 the various nomenclature for shared learning was debated and the decision made that "interdisciplinary learning" should be the term adopted, at least for the purposes of this study as it suggests a meaningful level of interaction between the participants. The 300 teachers who completed the main study questionnaire gave no clear indication of what shared learning should really be called although nearly 50% of the sample (RS = 144) used the term "multidisciplinary" (Table 5.38). It is suggested that this finding is not particularly significant as this word is the one that has tended to be used most frequently (and very often incorrectly) in many of the publications identifed in the literature review and as such has been adopted by the professions without due consideration to its real meaning.

In the autumn edition of the Journal of Interprofessional Care (published December 1993) Clark raised the issue of the nomenclature and asked "are we doing what we say we are?" (p 217). In a very comprehensive paper Clark suggested ways of differentiating between the various terms and called for them to be standardised. Unidisciplinary he described as "the traditional university level of instruction" ie a single profession learning in isolation from others. Multidisciplinary he described as "bringing various disciplines together to understand a particular problem or experience." Crucially he continued; "Importantly though, there is often very little interaction or collaboration among these disciplines : while they may acknowledge each others existence, there is little interest in forging linkages which could spawn collaborative or co-operative endeavours, such as joint research projects or team taught courses."(Clark 1993 : 220) Interdisciplinary learning however, Clark believed was :

> the level at which real integration of perspectives occurs. Instead of parallel lines of communication among different disciplines, intersecting lines of communication and collaboration are the norm. ....The hallmark of this level is the kind of cognitive and behavioral change that occurs : participants understand the core principles and concepts of each contributing discipline........
>
> (Ibid : 220)

Clark (an associate professor of gerontology) related each of these definitions to caring for the elderly. He concluded that interdisciplinary learning was what should be aimed for and that in order to achieve this a fundamental cognitive change would have to occur. He believed that :

> our level of sophistication in understanding and supporting cognitive change must be substantially improved if we are to move interdisciplinary education forward to meet the challenges facing it's proponents in the future
>
> (Ibid :224)

It is encouraging to read an established author concluding that the overall aim should be one of interdisciplinarity and it is concluded that the adoption of the nomenclature "interdisciplinary learning" in this current study was entirely justified and that the term should be adopted when interactive learning occurs between the health and social care professions. It is recommended that Clark's typology should be used to reclassify the nomenclature of existing courses so that the type of learning that occurs is absolutely clear. In this way further confusion as to the correct nomenclature should be avoided.

6.14 What preparation would the teachers require ?

In the main study teacher questionnaire there was a clear indication that at least 159 of the teachers believed that there should be the opportunity for special preparation for interdisciplinary teaching (Table 5.47). All but five of the 159 respondents who completed this question had declared themselves to be either "very interested" or "interested" in interdisciplinary teaching. A supposition that can be made therefore from these two reponses is that these teachers are indeed the ones who would be prepared to be involved in any future initiatives. The preparation that they were given therefore would be absolutely crucial. Many of them (RS = 92) indicated that a clear identification of objectives, the expected outcomes and the expected assessment strategies would be essential (see Chapter 5, Table 5.47).

It would seem imperative however, to address the other issues that were raised by the respondents before even considering the ramifications of interdisciplinary teaching. These included "gaining insight into each others work" (RS = 65), "breaking down existing barriers" (RS = 26), "the opportunity to clearly identify areas of responsibility" (RS = 8), "the opportunity to experience interdisciplinary learning" (RS = 23) and finally the "opportunity to practice interdisciplinary teaching" (RS = 31). It would seem eminently sensible in any preparatory programme to start by gaining insight into each professions contribution to care and to attempt to breakdown the acknowledged barriers which continue to contribute to interprofessional conflict.

At the commencement of any preparatory workshops for teachers it is recommended that a lecturer from each of the participating professions presents a short profile of the profession to which he/she belongs, giving a broad outline of its philosophy and aims and the contribution that the profession makes to holistic care both on a strategic level and on an individual client basis. On the completion of all the presentations the opportunity should be given for the teachers to describe the positive and negative attributes that each has about each other specific profession. This may allow for any misconceptions about each other to be addressed. A possible benefit of this strategy may be that following the presentations many of the negative stereotypical perceptions will have been corrected already. The traditional team building exercises should not be utilised at the beginning of any workshop where teachers obviously view each other with a level of misunderstanding and ignorance.

If these two objectives could be met, at least in part, the identification of clear areas of responsibility may start to emerge or the participants may decide that some of the areas that they had traditionally jealously guarded in their professional territory could indeed be shared !

An additional advantage of leaving the question of responsibility until later in any programme would be that following the presentation of each professions profiles participants may change their minds about the appropriateness of a particular profession undertaking a specific responsibility.

The most frequent response to the preparation required was the need to have the objectives, the expected outcomes and the assessment strategy clearly identifed for any interdisciplinary learning programme (RS = 92). This would appear to indicate that the teachers assume that an interdisciplinary programme would be thrust upon them. This was never intended to be the case. It would be crucial for all teachers involved in such an initiative to have ownership of the programme by being involved from the first day of planning and as such they should be members of a curriculum development team which negotiates and mutually identifies and agrees its own objectives, expected outcomes and assessment strategies. This would ensure that each profession was represented and that the demands of each Statutory Body were not forgotten. The content analysis completed in this study and the results of the question which indicates the broad topic areas which could be taught on an interdisciplinary basis, could be utilised as a framework for the curriculum development as it would enable the teachers to start with a reference point.

It is suggested that the objectives, outcomes and assessment strategies would evolve over a period of time and confirms previous authors recommendations that if there are any plans regarding the introduction of interdisciplinary programmes, the planning team should be formulated at least one year in advance (Areskog 1994) The teachers indicated clearly what preparation they would expect prior to commencing interdisciplinary teaching. This answers the question set by Aim 4.2 in Chapter 1.

6.15. How much support can be expected from the statutory and professional bodies?

A written response was received from each of the organisations contacted (see Chapter 4, Section 3). All expressed a high level of interest in the study and indeed several of the organisations have remained in regular contact by sending additional information as it is published. All have requested that they be contacted as soon as the results of this study are available as they would like to incorporate some of the findings into their strategic planning. Verbal anecdotal evidence was obtained at the commencement of this study from individuals who warned that most of the Statutory Bodies would not support the concept of interdisciplinary learning, and indeed may positively obstruct any developments. This has not proved to be the case at all and the written evidence obtained indicates on the whole, that the Statutory and Professional Bodies welcome this initiative and would be very willing to give advice and support if requested so to do (see Chapter 4, Section 4.3). Each indicated their desire to be involved in any further developments.

There were several issues which must be considered if any further progress is to be made. The Statutory and Professional Bodies, whilst giving their support to the concept of interdisciplinary learning, emphasised the necessity of maintaining profession specific training and "providing it would not be at the cost of lowering standards or of weakening the provision and approach necessary to each specific profession" (CPSM 1992). Several of the responses referred to the need to work in tandem with the Statutory Bodies from the earliest possible stage. The General Medical Council although it "does not generally have in mind an approach of the kind you envisage" (GMC 1992) observed that it was not "prescriptive in its approach and seeks to encourage innovation on the part of medical schools in the design and implementation of their curricula" (GMC 1992). The implication here would seem to be that the GMC while not anticipating such a radical change in their traditional approach to curriculum design, through their Education Committee would certainly welcome any approach from a medical school who submitted an innovative curriculum.

The time is opportune to do just that. The Towle Report (1991) recommended a radical overhaul of the medical curriculum in order to more appropriately meet the needs of the population the medical profession serves. The results obtained in this current study demonstrate the level of interest and the perceived need for interdisciplinary learning by the medical profession. The number of questionnaires (N = 107) returned from the medical teachers indicate a high level of awareness and the number of these teachers who identified themselves and requested personal contact on the completion of this study also indicates that there is an intention that the results obtained should be utilised.

It is imperative that all Statutory Bodies are invited to participate in any future interdisciplinary developments from their inception. With their guidance and approval at each stage of planning any problems or anomalies should be resolved before any documentation is submitted for a validation event. A sensitive approach towards negotiation must be adopted as it should be remembered that all Statutory and Professional Bodies comprise individuals who are highly qualified senior members of a specific profession and as such are likely to have experienced their undergraduate training in isolation from the other professions. These individuals may have been exposed therefore, to the same prejudices, stereotyping and interprofessional conflicts described in the literature review and evidenced from the results obtained in this current study.

From the encouraging responses received from the Statutory and Professional Bodies in this study it is concluded that there is the potential for them all to work together in a spirit of co-operation and collaboration towards interdisciplinary learning in the health and social care professions. (Aims 5.1 and 5.2)

6.16 What operational strategies should be adopted ?

During the review of the literature it became evident that in most instances, shared learning at an undergraduate stage was practically non existent. Where evidence was found it usually comprised two or three professions learning together for a very limited period during training. Centres of excellence were identifed, (the Faculty of Health Sciences, University of Linkoping, Sweden being the obvious example) where educators had identifed the need to address undergraduate training and had consequently fundamentally changed their approach to curriculum development for the health and social care professions. Nils-Holger Areskog and the other staff in Linkoping can only be described as visionaries and pioneers as far as interdisciplinary learning is concerned. The courage to introduce a core programme at the beginning of training should not be underestimated and the fact that the Linkoping programme has not only continued but expanded is a testimony to the commitment of most of the staff and students in the Faculty of Health Sciences.

Hawkins (1972) argued that a core curriculum had distinct advantages when compared with the traditional isolated training programmes. It could "help provide the horizontal mobility that is desperately needed in education in the health field" (p 167), that the efficiency of a Faculty would increase, that as far as the teachers themselves were concerned a core curriculum would be a constant reminder of the need to work as a team in the delivery of health and social care. In 1972, Hawkins argued that that "what is sorely needed is one central source of information on what has been done, what problems have been overcome and what problems have yet to be solved" (p 171). Weil and Parrish (1967) identified a similarity in the requirements for sociology and psychology between eleven health professions and suggested that these could be learned together.

The reasons why there have not been more interdisciplinary programmes developed should therefore be discussed. It is suggested, that in the absence of empirical data indicating the desirability and the feasibility of interdisciplinary learning between the health and social care professions, it has been easy to ignore the issue. In this current study, evidence has been collected which clearly indicates that there is a much higher level of interest than was previously suspected. It appears that the majority of the teacher and student populations in South East Wales would be willing to participate in interdisciplinary teaching and learning should such a development commence (Table 5.24, 5.26 and Figures 5.1 and 5.2)

In 1994 global progress has been made in that organisations such as CAIPE, HCPEF, EMPE, NCOEIHS have evolved and are making sterling efforts to co-operate and collaborate in an exchange of information and ideas. "Learning together to work together for health" as the World Health Organisation described in 1988 (WHO 1988b) does seem to have gained some credence but the suggested operational strategies described in this core document (see Appendix 2.1) seem to have been largely ignored to date at a local level. South East Wales would be in an ideal position to put these WHO operational strategies to the test.

What has become increasingly clear from the review of the literature is that organisations such as EMPE, NCOEIHS, CAIPE and HCPEF are rapidly gaining expertise, credibility, political power and perhaps most importantly increasing commitment and enthusiasm for interdisciplinary education. Whilst operating independently and in different countries, an interdependent network has emerged in which each organisation mutually recognises and supports the others. Membership of these organisations is growing rapidly. It is interesting to note however, that both institutions and individuals committed to the philosophy have joined several, if not all of the organisations. Paradoxically other institutions which purport to be contributing to interdisciplinary learning and state that their aim is to enhance the concept of teamwork in health care, do not subscribe to any of these organisations. They do not benefit therefore from the numerous publications, newsletters and correspondence which describe innovatory interdisciplinary programmes and the reported successes and failures. Much can be learned from the experiences described. It would appear essential that any educational establishment considering the introduction of interdisciplinary learning should invest in joining all these organisations when in the initial planning stage.

This study has justified the need to introduce interdisciplinary education and has already addressed many of the WHO suggested strategies. The empirical evidence called for by previous authors is now available and the obvious next stage would be to form a "nucleus of colleagues" (WHO 1988b : 54) who would act as the steering team for introducing interdisciplinary learning. It would be essential to recruit this team from each of the professions involved and to invite representatives from each of the Statutory Bodies to participate. The need for adequate time to plan is not in doubt and it would be necessary to obtain appropriate funding to release this "nucleus of colleagues" from their usual responsibilities as in this time of constant change and unprecedented work schedules, additional tasks such as the enormity of introducing interdisciplinary learning could not be contemplated.

Each stage of development should be subjected to extensive critical evaluation and the views of the general teaching and student populations should be sought before any final decisions are made. This would involve a commitment from the participating institutions to include regular agenda items on academic boards, faculty boards, joint boards of studies, student representative committees and any other formally recorded means of communication.

A further suggestion which may be more difficult to achieve would be to involve the people who are central to all health and social care training ; the patient/client. The consumers views on the issues of confidentiality and informed consent for example, should take precedence over professional wrangles over territorial rights. The World Health Organisation (1977) in a Technical Report entitled "The criteria for the evaluation of learning objectives in the education of health personnel" asked "what mechanism has been used to ensure that society's real health needs are reflected in the objectives?" (p 19). Unless society is invited to contribute their views and opinions the curriculum planners will never know. Steps should be taken to ensure that representatives from all members of the society which the training institutions serve are involved in planning. This would then help redress the problem of specialisation and fragmentation of knowledge within higher education establishments and link the education of health and social care professions with the real world, that was described in Chapter 1 of this book in which the WHO was acknowledged as observing "communities have problems, universities have departments" (WHO 1984a : 13). The WHO (1977) had no time for "special interest group pressures" (p 18) and posed the question of whether objectives within a programme are biased by these groups. The WHO suggested that this question should form a criterion for evaluation and concluded that "if so, please explain." They continued "are the objectives biased by narrow speciality or disciplinary interests? If so, please explain." It seems quite clear that the WHO envisages courses which are developed to meet the needs of the society in which they are based. Hawkins (1972) ruefully had observed that; "while this knowledge is helpful, it would further aid core development if the accrediting bodies would state their objectives and requirements in behavioural terms rather than in clock hours of instruction." (Ibid : 168)

In 1996, many curriculum do indeed contain learning outcomes in behavioural terms whilst still prescribing the number of hours that a student should study a particular topic. It is suspected that this is unlikely to change in the immediate future. With the advent of accumulated credit and transfer systems however, there is the possibility that this more flexible approach to learning will play a much more significant part in accreditation.

Several interdisciplinary learning models have been considered in this book, (see Chapter 2, Section 2.9) and Leninger's Interdisciplinary Cone Model (see Figure 2.5) was identified as the one which could most appropriately meet the needs of all the professions involved in this study in spite of the potential administrative problems. The adoption of this model would ensure that all the advantages of interdisciplinary learning could be gained, whilst minimising the disadvantages and ensuring that each professions specific knowledge and competency could be maintained. The acceptance of an appropriate interdisciplinary model would seem to be a fundamental consideration for a planning team to adopt as an operational strategy.

Areskog (1994) in an as yet unpublished document entitled "Multiprofessional education (MPE) and team training of health students and personnel" gives some practical guidelines for planning and implementation. He outlines the goals and the reasons for multiprofessional education and then describes the pre-requisites needed. He categorises these as at a political level, at an education institutional level, didactic and educational principles and structures and finally teacher education and training. At a political level he observed; "There must be a positive political will with legal, organisational and monetary incentives in order to create good conditions for successful MPE. Thus MPE and team approach should be an established part of the government policy." (Areskog 1994 : 9)

This aspect of interdisciplinary learning has not been addressed directly in this current study, apart from the observations made in Chapter 2, Sections 2,3,4 and 5. It would seem reasonable to conclude nonetheless, that because of the number of White and Green Papers published by the British Government that interdisciplinary learning between the health and social care professions is very much on the political agenda. Indeed the Caring for People Joint Training Project (1991) commissioned by the NHS Training Directorate and the Social Services Inspectorate adds weight to this claim. Although it examined the possibilities of joint inservice training for qualified personnel in order to enhance the quality of client care from a management perspective it is perhaps an indicator of the Government's future plans. While undergraduate interdisciplinary learning is not yet Government policy it is suspected, in view of the increased number of official documents which refer to the need for shared learning, that it may well become so. If this is indeed the case it is absolutely vital that educational insititutions are prepared at an operational level. Broome

(1990) has argued that perceived and identified change from within is always preferable to imposed change from external agencies. The results obtained in this study indicate that both the teaching and student populations perceive the need for interdisciplinary learning. The three Institutions in South East Wales could be pro-active in their approach as they now have the empirical evidence required to justify the introduction of interdisciplinary learning.

7 Conclusions and recommendations

7.1 Introduction

In the past decade the issues of collaborative care, teamwork and the need for interdisciplinary learning have been the topics of much discussion and debate. An increasing number of publications have appeared which both explicitly and implicitly identify the need for a more cohesive approach to the education of the health and social care professions in order to enhance the concept of holistic client care. In 1991, when this study was commenced, it soon became evident that many authors had written extensively about the need for interdisciplinary learning but whilst others reported on existing shared learning initiatives very few of them had attempted to undertake empirical research on a large scale.

This study attempted to redress the absence of empirical evidence related to interdisciplinary learning through an examination of a total population of thirteen health and social care professions in South East Wales. An early decision was taken to concentrate on the undergraduate/pre-registration training programmes as the literature suggested that it was at this stage that students attitudes, values and core knowledge were fixed and interprofessional conflict begins to emerge. Interdisciplinary training at a post graduate stage is without doubt essential, but based on the results of this study, it is suggested that it should be viewed as a continuation of a process which commences from the beginning of undergraduate training. The literature has revealed that interdisciplinary learning at a post graduate level frequently involves remedial work through the examination of existing interprofessional conflict, stereotyping, the lack of insight into the contributions all professions make to holistic client care and the reasons for the absence of collaborative teamwork. The perceived advantages of interdisciplinary learning identifed by the 1683 respondents in this study substantiate this conclusion (Tables 5.39, 5.40, 5.55 and 5.56).

The level of interest in this study, which has been expressed by organisations and individuals on both an international (The WHO, NOEIHCS, EMPE) and national basis (The Department of Health, The Welsh Office, CAIPE) justifies the decision to examine the concept of interdisciplinary learning in depth. It would seem that the results obtained in this study could be pertinent to the education of the health and social care professions throughout this decade and into the next millenium. The results require to be disseminated as widely as possible in order that the information is shared and utilised if required, by both organisations and individuals. Several publishers have requested submissions for professional journals (representing many of the professions which have participated in this study) and it hoped that this book which summarises the findings of this study and suggests ways in which interdisciplinary learning could be introduced, will reach a large national and international readership. The opportunity has already been taken to present the findings in Finland and Greece and arrangements made to return to Sweden (Chapter 4, Section 4). On a national level, the Welsh Office and the Department of Health and The World Health Organisation and each Statutory and Professional Body have all been sent an abstract as requested.

The overall aims of the study, which were described in Chapter One, Section 1.6, were to analyse the behavioural science component of the current curricula of fourteen undergraduate programmes to identify commonalities between them ; to ascertain the opinions of the teachers and students of the thirteen professions about the feasibility and desirability of interdisciplinary learning ; and to identify what, when and how interdisciplinary learning should be introduced. The behavioural science component was quickly extended to encompass other subjects which many purists would/may not consider a behavioural science. The overall aims of the study have been achieved although it is acknowledged that the results have raised many more questions and potential areas for further research than the study may have answered.

As the study took place in a limited geographical area and involved the total population of the thirteen health and social care professions, the adoption of modified action research as the methodology was the only feasible procedure. The opportunity to reflect on the results obtained at each stage was invaluable as it limited the potential number of mistakes which may otherwise have been made. The flow chart (see Chapter 3, Figure 3.1) was an essential focus as the breadth of quantitative and qualitative data obtained frequently distracted from the main aims of the study. The level of interest, support and advice obtained from many of the senior teaching staff within the two participating Institutions facilitated the collection of data and enabled open access to all members of staff and the students. The literature search was enriched through the loan of unpublished pertinent documents and papers which otherwise would have been unobtainable and as further documents and discussion papers were received at a senior level these were also offered for consideration and for possible inclusion in the literature review.

The most crucial question pertaining to the study was the level of interest which would be expressed by the potential teacher and student respondents from the thirteen professions which participated. This could be measured in the first instance, only by the number of individuals who were prepared to be interviewed and complete the questionnaires (Appendix 4.8 and 4.10). It can be stated categorically that the response rate from both the teachers and students was outstanding and certainly way beyond expectations at the onset of the data collection. The level of interest into the aims of the study itself was therefore extraordinarily high and increased the reliability of the results as a substantial majority of the total teacher and student populations gave their opinions.

The seemingly disproportionate numbers (Chapter 5, Table 5.23) between the different professional groups is a true representation of the ratios within health and social care. The opinions of the smaller groups of respondents are therefore just as valid as those of the larger groups although the small sample sizes meant that statistical analysis was inappropriate in many instances. The variables were difficult to control. As the sample comprised a total population it was decided that the inclusion criteria for the potential teacher respondents should be that they were employed within one of the two Institutions on a given date, that they held a relevant professional qualification and that they had a specified teaching remit which included teaching undergraduate/pre-registration students who were training for entry into the teacher's own profession. All 300 teacher respondents met these criteria and no respondent was therefore excluded from the analysis. Although every attempt was made to ascertain any extraneous expertise and knowledge it cannot be assumed that the information obtained is a totally accurate reflection of the teaching population. During the questionnaire development stage (see Chapter 4), the decision was taken that although an indication of specialisation within each profession would have yielded very useful information, it was not practical to do this in view of the sample size involved. Within the medical and nursing sample it would have been easy to identify individuals who had specialised in mental health, primary care or care of the elderly for example. In the other professions however, it would have been more difficult to categorise as there are no specific mandatory post graduate training programmes. Because of these inherent difficulties it was believed that attempting to do this may have invited criticism as there is no doubt that many individuals in the professions allied to medicine have a high level of expertise in specialist areas. The level of support from the specialities within each profession therefore, is not known but as the overall response rate was so high it could be argued that representatives of each speciality have contributed to the results.

The inclusion criteria for the student population was that the individual was indexed on one of the undergraduate/pre-registration training programmes on a given date and was intending to qualify in one of the thirteen health or social professions. The results subsequently revealed that some of these students already held a professional qualification, the most frequently identifed being Registered Nurses who were training as podiatrists, operating department practitioners or social workers (Chapter 5, Table 5.51 and Section 5.5.3). It was outside the remit of this study to discover the reasons why these students had decided to retrain, although it is suggested that one possible reason to train as a podiatrist may be the opportunity to commence private practice. No such explanation can be offered to account for those nurses who were training to be operating department practitioners. The career structure for operating department practitioners is less well defined and the salary scales are lower. What can be concluded however is that these student's previous nurse training will not have been wasted as the knowledge and competency they have acquired will be utilised in their new careers. However, as Registered Nurses the UKCC Code of Conduct would presumably still apply even in a non-nursing post.

The majority of the 1683 respondents indicated that some interdisciplinary learning should take place between the health and social care professions throughout undergraduate training (Figure 5.6 and Table 5.42) and that the advantages of introducing such a strategy would outweigh the disadvantages. Although many of the respondents were selective in regard to the other professions with whom they would wish to learn there was evidence of a wide acceptance of all the professions learning the core subjects together (Tables 5.44 and 5.61). Nurses, medical practitioners and social workers were the most frequently chosen professions deemed suitable for learning with others. There were significant similarities between the professions' choices with many of the rank ordered choices correlating (Tables 6.3 and 6.4). The core subjects identifed extended beyond the original concept of the behavioural sciences and the respondents indicated that in addition to psychology and sociology the following subjects would be acceptable for interdisciplinary learning : ethics, law and practice, research methods, organisation of health and social care, management, health promotion, quality assurance and study skills (Table 6.7).

More than 80% of the 1683 teachers and students would be interested or very interested in participating in interdisciplinary learning (Figure 5.2, Tables 5.26, 5.27 and 5.28). The students were prepared to utilise most learning methods with the exception of role play which was rejected by a significant majority. The favoured learning methods involved interaction with patients and with other students. Didactic methods such as lectures were less popular than the other suggested strategies (Table 5.97).

The results indicate that in the thirteen professions which participated in this study, the belief in the need for and the level of interest in interdisciplinary learning is higher than was previously suspected by many of the authors reviewed in the literature. The health and social care professions in these two Institutions do wish to undertake some interdisciplinary learning (Figure 5.2 and Table 5.26).

7.2 Limitations of the study

7.2.1 Re-organisation of the participating institutions

In September 1993 a further re-organisation took place within one of the institutions which participated in this study. Two Faculties merged and within the new larger Faculty, established related courses have been accommodated. These include the degree courses for medical laboratory scientific officers and also the environmental health officers. These courses it is suspected, would have been entirely suitable for inclusion in this study. As the questionnaire collection had been completed by April 1993 and transcribed for data analysis by July 1993 however, it was regretfully decided that it was too late to include these professions. The results of this study do not therefore reflect the current Faculty portfolio. It would be reasonably easy however, to analyse the relevant curriculum and distribute the questionnaires to the teachers and students in these professions.

At the time of writing (1996), an announcement is still awaited from the Welsh Office on the future organisation of the participating institutions. This announcement could influence the future of interdisciplinary learning in South East Wales in one of two ways. It may facilitate or constrain future developments. This must be regarded therefore, as a potential limitation or enhancement to any implementation of the results.

7.2.2 The content analysis of the fourteen curricula

Every attempt was made to minimise subjectivity and bias with in the content analysis, by involving course directors in decision making by requesting that they confirmed that the analysis was an accurate interpretation of their own programmes. The few suggested amendments made by the course directors were incorporated into the analysis. Nevertheless, the analysis may not be a totally accurate interpretation of each course curriculum as it is presented in 1996. Course documents quickly become outdated as student evaluations are collated and subsequent changes to course content are common on an annual basis. In addition, the pace of change within health and social care within the last five years has meant that some of the issues related to law and practice for example, are now obselete and new topic areas have been introduced. This will remain a problem for all educationalists involved with curriculum development regardless of the profession. Whilst the adoption of this content analysis may be of value as a framework for future developments, it must be treated with the same caution and should itself, be regularly reviewed.

7.2.3 Content analysis of the reading lists

It is acknowledged that the reading lists are not a true reflection of the breadth and depth of literature that students are recommended to read. With a number of new publications each year, reading lists need to be updated on an annual basis and the indicative reading lists in course documents may have been superceded even before the new programme commences. The number of books identified in the content analysis, which could not be described as profession specific and which would appear to be used by only one or two of the professions has raised the issue of appropriate use of limited financial resources. The content analysis, upon which the study was based, would seem to have raised more questions than it has answered but it is suggested that the issues surrounding shared resources should be examined urgently and for this reason alone the content analysis can be justifed as a basis for further discussion and debate.

7.2.4 The structured interviews

The results obtained in the structured interviews if compared with the main study questionnaires, reveal a higher level of interest and a greater number of professions selected to share interdisciplinary learning. As the respondents were identifed through random stratified sampling and as the number of agreements to be interviewed was high, it could be argued that they should have been representative of most of the professions as a whole. Nevertheless it is suspected that the reason for the results obtained from these interviews can be attributed to the respondents wanting to please the interviewer by giving the appropriate responses. Another possibility was that the interviewer, in spite of using a structured interview schedule, inadvertently biased the respondents by using nonverbal cues which positively or negatively re-inforced the respondents answers. As the purpose of the structured interviews was to generate questions for the teacher and student questionnaires, it was not felt that the possibility of interviewer bias detracted from the validity of the overall results.

7.2.5 The questionnaires

The overall design of the questionnaires (Appendices 4.4 and 4.5) on reflection, seem to have obtained all of the information which was anticipated at the outset of the study. The opportunity to pilot the questionnaires in other institutions was invaluable as was the high number of respondents who completed the pilot study. Minor amendments were made after the pilot study results were analysed and the information obtained from the teacher's questionnaire meant that the student pilot study was amended before the first draft was distributed and no further alterations had to be made. The overall format of the questionnaires could be used in a replication study but the questions which identify the thirteen specific professions who participating in this study would need to be adjusted to reflect the professions which were going to participate in any subsequent study.

There was one major omission which should be addressed if the teacher questionnaire was to be used again. A question should have been included which asked teachers which teaching methods they thought would be suitable for interdisciplinary learning. A similar question was included on the student questionnaire and the results yielded some highly significant findings. Role play was rejected by a significant number of all the student groups with the exception of social work (Table 5.219). The 1383 students indicated a clear preference for patient centred, student interactive learning strategies (Table 5.60). Unfortunately the opinions of the teachers are not known. It would have been extremely useful to compare the two sets of opinions.

A question which would need clarifying before the student questionnaire was used again was the one which asked students to identify any courses which they had completed which they considered relevant to their current training. The insertion of the phrase "before you commenced your current training" should discourage respondents from including qualifications such as the science degrees obtained by the medical students during their medical training. Additionally, a question to exactly determine what the students were doing prior to commencing their current studies and in the case of non school leavers, why they were now undertaking their current training, would have yielded some useful information and obviated the speculation that has had to made.

7.3 Recommendations

The results obtained in this study enable the following recommendations to be made some of which can be generalised and others of which are specific to the Institutions which participated in the study.

7.3.1 Overall recommendations

1 The term "interdisciplinary" should be adopted only when there is interaction between two or more health and social care professions. The typology described by Clark (1993) and also identified in this study, should be adopted as the correct nomenclature for future course developments.

2 Interdisciplinary learning should be an integral part throughout undergraduate training for all health and social care professions and should continue throughout each individual's career.

3 Interdisciplinary learning should not be considered as an alternative to profession specific training, rather it should be viewed as an enhancement within the existing programmes.

4. All institutions who are contemplating the introduction of interdisciplinary learning should become members of established organisations such as NOECIHS, EMPE and CAIPE. This will ensure that the institutions receive appropriate advice and support from others which have already established interdisciplinary programmes.

5 All Statutory and Professional Bodies should be invited to participate in an advisory capacity before any planning for interdisciplinary learning commences.

6 With the modifications outlined in the limitations of the study (Chapter 7, Section 2) the study should be replicated in other institutions where similar undergraduate courses exist.

7 Greater efforts should be made to incorporate the expertise of some of the professions allied to medicine into primary health care. The skills of professions such as podiatry, physiotherapy, occupational therapy, nutrition and dietetics and speech therapists are under utlised in the community sector.

The feasibility of any or all of these recommendations being implemented will depend on future directives from the British Government and from within the Statutory Bodies which regulate the professions.

7.3.2. Specific recommendations for the participating Institutions.

1 The interdisciplinary cone model described by Leninger (1971) would be the most appropriate framework to adopt if interdisciplinary learning is introduced within existing profession specific programmes in South East Wales, even though there would be many administrative problems.

2 Initial discussions should take place between the two Institutions in order to consider the strategic implications of the results obtained as a matter of urgency. The level of commitment to interdisciplinary learning should be decided. A corporate approach should be planned, if further developments are desired.

3 The issues regarding the funding and resourcing of any interdisciplinary initiatives should be addressed and where possible resolved.

4 An interdisciplinary working group should be convened. Interested volunteers should be identifed from the teaching staff within each profession from each of the two Institutions. Adequate funding should be made available to this group which would enable additional resources to be made available in the form of administrative and secretarial support. Arrangements should be made to release teaching staff from some of their usual responsibilities. Membership of this group should not place additional demands on teachers.

5 The working group should begin discussions based on the content analysis of the fourteen curricula, using the core interdisciplinary concepts identified by the 1383 respondents as a preliminary basis for negotiation.

6 Core modules should be developed which are undertaken by all the professions. These should include psychology, sociology, ethics, law and practice, health promotion, management of health and social care, quality assurance. The core modules should be linked with profession specific modules where the students can apply the core knowledge to their profession specific practice.

7 The undergraduate programmes which were not included in this study should be subjected to the same content analysis. If sufficient similarities are identified, the teaching staff and students should be invited to complete the main study questionnaires. If the results are encouraging then these professions should participate in all future developments.

8 An inter -library committee comprising staff from the two Institutions should be convened in order to discuss the results of the content analysis of the reading lists. A more comprehensive approach to resourcing these libraries should be explored.

9 The lack of insight into other professions' contributions to patient care which was implicitly suggested by the teaching staff suggests that the opportunity for qualified practitioners to explore the roles of professions other than their own should be addressed as a matter of urgency. Interdisciplinary study days should be planned for both the teaching staff and clinical practitioners from all health care professions. The social workers should also be invited to participate. Traditional team building exercises should be preceded by presentations of professional profiles to each group of participants thus enabling positive and negative stereotypes to be identifed and addressed.

10 Existing undergraduate curricula should be modified in order that the contributions made by each profession towards collaborative care are explored. An interdisciplinary teaching strategy in which students in each profession spend even one day exploring these issues with teachers from the other professions could help increase understanding and collaboration.

11 Where there has been a high level of agreement regarding interdisciplinary learning between different professions, efforts should be made to introduce this as soon as possible. Examples of this include ; dentists, dental technologists, dental surgery assistants, dental hygienists, nutrionists and dietitians and speech therapists ; nurses and nutritionists and dietitians ; occupational therapists and social workers.

12 In future years first year students should be allocated into interdisciplinary tutorial groups as well as profession specific tutorial groups. Urgent consideration should be given to ways of increasing interdisciplinary learning which involves direct client contact in both the community and acute hospital sectors.

13 Any interdisciplinary learning strategies which are introduced must be subjected to formal evaluation on a regular basis. The results of the evaluations should be made available for general scrutiny and should be shared with organisations such as NOECIHS, EMPE and CAIPE.

7.3.3 Potential research topics for future consideration.

1 A longitudinal study should be undertaken which measures whether interdisciplinary learning increases collaboration and teamwork and decreases interprofessional conflict.

2 The entry criteria for each undergraduate programme should be examined. With the increase in mature students and with the evidence obtained in this study regarding students who have previously worked in related occupations, there is reason to question the traditional entry of an eighteen year old with appropriate school leaving qualifications but little life experience.

3 In a time of recession and high unemployment, the reasons for the continuing failure to recruit men into the professions allied to medicine and nursing should be explored.

4 Using the results obtained from the first year medical students, a follow up study should be completed when these students are working as house officers in their pre- registration year. Their level of interest in interdisciplinary learning and their opinions regarding the need for collaboration may have increased. It would also be interesting to measure whether they had moved towards a more biopsychosocial model of care.

5 The career pathways of teachers and the gender distribution of teachers would be of interest as the evidence obtained in this study indicates that greater numbers of females are entering the medical profession than previously. The expectation would be therefore that a greater number of women will be teaching the medical students in the next decade.

6 The results obtained from the physiotherapists suggest that other schools of physiotherapy should be approached and permission obtained to distribute the questionnaires to the teachers and students. This may confirm that the physiotherapists as a whole are less keen on interdisciplinary learning than the other professions allied to edicine, or it may indicate that the physiotherapists who participated in this study do not reflect the opinions of the profession overall.

7 The results revealed a number of Registered Nurses undertaking other professional training programmes. The reasons why Registered Nurses choose to migrate to other professions would be of great interest.

References

Abbatt. F. McMahon. R. (1985) *Teaching health care workers.* Macmillan, Basingstoke.

Abercrombie. M.L.J. (1966) Small Groups, in Foss. B. *New horizons in psychology.* Penguin, Harmondsworth.

Abramson. M. (1984) Collective responsibility in interdisciplinary collaboration : An ethical perspective for social workers. *Social work in health care* Vol 10, No. 1, pp 35-43.

Abrahamson. S. (ed.) (1985) *Evaluation of continuing education in the health professions.* Kluwer : Nijhoff, Boston.

Adair. J. (1987) *Effective team building,* Gower, Aldershot.

Adcock.M. Craig. D Gardiner.G. Jaques. D Woodhall. C. Lindsey. A. (1977) Experiment of much binding in the Plumstead Marshes, *Health and social science journal* Vol. 6, No.10, p 1428

Agatstein. F. (1980) Attitude change and death education : a consideration of goals. *Death education* Vol 3, No 4, pp 323-332

Ahmedzai. S. (1982) Dying in hospital : The residents viewpoint. *British medical journal* Vol 3, No. 285, pp 712-714

Akester. J. M. McPhail A.N. (1964) Health visiting and general practice. *The lancet* Vol 11, No 7356, pp 405-408

Alaszewski. A. (1977) Doctors and paramedical workers - the changing pattern of interprofessional relations. *Health and social services journal* Vol CLXXXVIII No 4562, pp B1- B4

Allen. I. (ed.) (1991) *Health and social services - the new relationship* Policy Studies Institute, London.

Allen. D. (1992) With one voice. *Nursing Standard* Vol 6, No 34, p 23

Allibone. A. (1981) It does work *British medical journal* Vol 2, No 283, pp 1581-1582.

Appleyard. J. Madden. J.G. (1979) Multidisciplinary teams. *British medical journa*l Vol 2, No 70, pp 1305-1307

Aradine. C.R. Hansen. M.F. (1970) Interdisciplinary teamwork in family healthcare. *Nursing clinics of North America* Vol 5, No 2, pp 211- 222

Archer. S.E. (1987) Political involvement by nurses.*Recent advances in nursing* . No 18, pp 25-45

Areskog. N.H. (1984) Multidisciplinary undergraduate education for the health professions - some aspects of how and. why.*W.H.O Report ICP/ HMC 103M02/6/4323E* Copenhagen.

Areskog. N.H. (1986) Multiprofessional team training within the health care sector. *W.H.O. Report ICP/HMD/136/7* Copenhagen.

Areskog N.H .(ed.) (1988a) Need for multiprofessional health education in undergraduate studies. *Medical education* No 28, pp 251-252

Areskog. N.H. (1988b) Learning together to work together for health. *W.H.O. Technical Report Series 769* Geneva.

Areskog. N.H. (1992) The new medical education at the Faculty of Health Sciences, Linkoping University - A challenge for both students and teachers *Scandinavian Journal of Social Medicine* Vol 20, No 1, pp 1-4

Areskog N.H. (1992) *Multiprofessional education and team training of health students and personnel* WHO Geneva

Arlton. D. (1984) The rural nursing practicum project. *Nursing outlook* Vol 34 No 4 pp 204-206

Armitage. P. (1983) Joint working in primary health care. *Nursing times : Occasional paper* Vol 79, No 28 pp 75-78

Ash. E. (1992) The personal professional interface in learning : towards reflective education *Journal of interprofessional care* Vol 6 No 3 pp 261-272

Ashley Miller M (1990) Community Care *British Medical Journal* Vol 300 No 6723 pp487

Audit Commission (1992) *Homeward Bound : A new course for community health* HMSO, London

Ausubel. D.P. (1968) *Educational psychology : a cognitive view* Holt Rhinehart Winston, New York

Authier. J. Gustafson. K. (1975) Application of supervised and non supervised micro counseling in the training of para professionals *Journal of counseling psychology* Vol 22, No 1, pp 74-78

Bakemeier. R.F. (1984) The teaching of cancer medicine by objectives. *Journal of medical education* Vol 59, No 1, pp 24-32

Balassone. P.D. (1981) Territorial issues in an interdisciplinary experience. *Nursing outlook* Vol 29, No 4, pp 229-232

Baldwin. L.J. (1988) Performance based management of troubled nurses. *Nursing management* Vol 19, No 11, pp 64n-64p

Bair. J. (1983) Nationally speaking. *American journal of occupational therapy* Vol 37, No 9, pp 11-13

Banta. H.D. Fox. R.C. (1972) Role strains of a health care team in a poverty community. *Social science and medicine* Vol 6, No 11, pp 697-722
Barber. J.H. Kratz. C.R.(eds) (1980) *Towards team care* Churchill Livingstone Edinburgh.
Barbou. J. (1975) The dying persons bill of rights. *American journal of nursing* Vol 85, No 6, pp 75-79
Barker. J.C. (1964) Team work in the service of the mentally ill. *Nursing mirror* Vol 119, No 52, pp 285-287
Barnes. J.A. (1979) *The ethics of inquiry in social science* Oxford university press.
Bass. R.L. Paulman. P. (1983) The rural preceptorship as a factor in the residency selection : The Nebraska experience. *Journal of family practice* Vol 17, No 11, pp 716-719
Bassett. P. (1989) Team care at work. *Journal of district nursing* Vol 7, No 8, 4-6
Batchelor I. McFarlane. J. (1980) *Multidisciplinary clinical teams* Kings Fund project paper. London
Bates. B. (1965) Comprehensive medicine : A conference approach with inpatient emphasis. *Journal of medical education* Vol 40, pp 778-784
Bates. B. (1966) Nurse-physician teamwork. *Medical care* Vol 4,No 4, pp 69-73
Bates. B. (1970) Doctor and nurse : Changing roles and relations. *New England journal of medicine* Vol 283, No 3, pp 129-133
Beachey W. (1988) Multicompetent health professionals : needs combinations & curriculum development *Journal of allied health* Nov. pp 319-329
Beales. J.G. (1980) Stresses in the primary health care team *Journal of the Royal College of General Practitioners.* Occasional Paper No 14, pp 5-7
Beckhard. R. (1974) Applied behavioural science in health care systems : Who needs it ? *Journal of applied behavioural science* No 10, pp 93-107
Beloff. J.S. Weinerman. E.R (1967) Yale studies in family health care - part 1. *J.A.M.A.* Vol 199, No 6, pp 133-139
Beloff. J.S. Snoke. P.S. Weinerman. E.R (1968) Organisationof a comprehensive health care program.part 2, *J.A.M.A.* Vol 204, No 5, pp 63-68
Beloff. J.S. Willet. M. (1968) Part 3 : The health care team. *J.A.M.A* Vol 205, No 10, pp 73-79
Beloff J.S. Korper. M. (1972) The health team model and medical care utilisation. *J.A.M.A.* Vol 219, No 3, pp 359-366
Bendall. E. (1973) Nursing attitudes in the health care team. *Nursing times* occasional paper Vol 2, No 15 pp 25-27
Bennet. G. (1987) *The wound and the doctor* Secker & Warburg. London.

Bennet. G. (1988) *Multidisciplinary teamwork issues in community drug teams.* Paper presented to conference on Community drug teams : clinical and organisational issues. University of London.

Bennett. P. Dawar. A. Dick. A (1972) Interprofessional co-operation. *Journal of the Royal College of General Practitioners* No 22, pp 603-609

Bennett. P. Blackall.M. Clapham. M. Little. S. Player. D. (1988) A multidisciplinary approach to the prevention of coronary heart disease. *Health education journal* Vol 47, No 4, pp 164-166

Benor. D.E. (1982) Interdisciplinary integration in medical education : Theory and method. *Medical education* No 16, pp 355-361

Bergevin P. Morris D. Smith RM (1963) *Adult education procedures* Seabury Press, USA

Berkowitz. N. Malone. M.F. (1968) Intraprofessional conflict *Nursing forum* No 1, pp 50-71

Bersky. A.K. Keys. E.J. Dickens. R.N. (1987) Learning interdisciplinary and assessment skills through videotaped client interviews and collaborative planning. *Journal of nursing education* Vol 26, No 5, pp 202-204

Beynon. G.P.J. Wedgewood. J Newman. J. Hutt. A (1978) Multidisciplinary education in geriatrics : An experimental course at the Middlesex Hospital. *Age and ageing* Vol 7, No 4, pp 193-200

Biggs S. (1993) User participation & interprofessional collaboration in community care *Journal of interprofessional care* Vol 7, No 2, pp 151 -160

Birkinshaw. W. Darby. P. Strasser. S. (1991) The parents group : A multidisciplinary project. *Health visitor* Vol 64, No 8, pp 259-261

Blackett. M.E. Maybin. R.P. Dudgeon. Y. (1957) Medical social work in general practice. *The lancet* No 1, p 37

Bligh. D. (1980) Some principles for interprofessional teaching and learning. *Journal of Royal College of General Practitioners* Occasional Paper No 14, pp 8-11

Bloch. D. (1975) Evaluation of nursing care in terms of process and outcome. *Nursing research* Vol 24, No 4, pp 256- 263

Bloom. S. (1959) The role of the sociologist in medical education. *Journal of medical education* Vol 34, No 7, pp 667-673

Bloom. S. (1964) Growth of the behavioural sciences in medical education. Some implications for social workers. *Journal of medical education* Vol 39, No 9, pp 820-827

Boelen C. (1992) Medical education reform : the need for global action *Academic medicine* Vol 67, No 11, pp 745-749

Boelen C. (1993) The challenge of changing medical education & medical practice *World Health Forum* Vol 14, pp 213- 216

Bolles. R.C. (1979) *Learning theory* Holt, Rhinehart & Winston U.S.A.

Bond. J. Cartlidge. A.M. Gregson. B.A. Barton. A.G Philips. P.R. Armitage. P Brown. A.M. Reedy. B.L.E.C. (1985) *Professional collaboration in primary health care organisations.* Report No 27, Health Care Research Unit. University of Newcastle Upon Tyne. U.K.

Bond. J. Cartlidge. A.M.Gregson. B.A. Barton. A.G Philips. P.R Armitage P Brown. A.M. Reedy. B.L.E.C. (1987) Interprofessional collaboration in primary health care. *Journal of the Royal College of General Practitioners* Vol 37, Original paper, pp 158-161

Boss. W.R. (1983) Organisational development in the health care field A confrontational team building design. *Journal of health and human resources administration* Summer 1983, pp 73-91

Boud. D. Keogh. R. Walker. D. (1985) *Reflection : Turning experience into learning* Kogan Page, London.

Boud.D. Griffin. V. (1987) *Appreciating adult learning form the learners perspective.* Kogan Page, London

Boud. D. (ed.) (1988) *Developing student autonomy in learning* Kogan Page, London

Bouhuijs. P.A.J. Schmidt. H.G. Snow. R.E. Wijnen. W.H.F.W (1978) *Development of medical education* The Riksuniversiteit Limburg, Maastricht The Netherlands

Bowling. A. (1980a) To do or not to do ? *Nursing Mirror* Vol 42, No 29, pp 30-32

Bowling. A. (1980b) Nurses in the primary care team. *The lancet* Vol 11, No 8194 pp 590

Bowling. A. (1981) *Delegation in general practice* Tavistock Press, London

Boyer.L. Lee. D. Kirchner. C. (1977) A student run course in interprofessional relations *Journal of medical education* Vol 52, No 3, pp 183- 190

Bracht. N.F. Anderson. I. (1975) Community fieldwork collaboration between medical and social work students. *Social work and health care* No 1, pp 7-17

Braithwaite D Stark S. (1992) Who should teach nurses ? The debate. *Nursing standard* Vol 6, No 46, pp 25-27

Brazeau. N. Jones. J.W. Hickner. J.M. Vantassel. J.L. (1987) The upper peninsula medical education program and the problem based clinical alternative. Michegan State University, in WHO (1987) *Innovative Tracks* Geneva.

Brill. N.I. (1976) *Teamwork- Working together in the human services* Lippincott, Philadelphia.

British Association of Social Workers (?) *Teamwork for and against. An appraisal of multidisciplinary practice* B.A.S.W. Publications. Birmingham.

British Geriatric Society & The Royal College of Nursing (1975) *Improving geriatric care in hospital* Royal College of Nursing, London

Britsh Medical Students Association (BMSA) (1965) *Reports on medical education. Suggestions for the future.* B.M.S.A. Tavistock House, London

British Psychological Society (BPS) (1990) *Responsibility issues in clinical psychology and multidisciplinary teamwork* B.P.S. Leicester

Broad. J. (1985) Marrying the team. *Community Outlook* Vol 5, No 1, pp 37-39

Brocklehurst. J.C. (1966) Co-ordination in the care of the aged. *The lancet* Vol 1, No 7451, p 1363

Brooking. J. (1991) Doctors and nurses : A personal view *Nursing standard* Vol 6, No 12, pp 24-28

Brooks. M.B. (1973) Management of the team in general practice *Journal of the Royal College of General Practitioners* Vol 23, pp 239-252

Brooks. S. (1987) Nursing and the social service. Collaboration or conflict ? *Social work today* Vol 6 No 23 pp 12-13

Brooks. D. Hendy. A Ponsonage.A. (1981) Towards the reality of the primary health care team : An educational approach. *Journal of the Royal College of General Practitioners* Vol 31, No 29, pp 491-495

Broome.A. (1990) *Managing change : Essentials of nursing management* Macmillan, London

Brotherston. J.H.F. (1971) *Doctors in an integrated health service* Scottish Health and Home Department, Edinburgh

Brown G (1983) Studies of student learning implications for medical teaching. *Medical Teacher* Vol 5, pp 52 -56

Brown. J.D. Brown. M.I. Jones. E.(1979) Evaluation of a nurse practitioner - staffed preventive medicine program in a fee for service multi speciality clinic. *Preventive medicine* Vol 8 pp 53-63

Bruce. N. (1980) *Teamwork for preventive care* Research Studies Press, Chichester

Bruner. J. Goodnow. J. Austin. G. (1956) *A study of thinking* Wiley, New York

Bruner. J.S. (1963) *The process of education* Vintage Brooke, New York

Brunning. H. Huffington. C. (1985) Altered images. *Nursing times* Vol 8 No 30, pp 24-27

Bryant. J.H. (1993) Educating tomorrows doctors *World Health Forum* Vol 14, pp 217

Bryar. R. (1991) *Primary health care teamwork education in Wales : An exploratory study.* Team Care Valleys, Cardiff

Bumphrey. E.E. (1989) Occupational therapy within the primary health care team. *British journal of occupational therapy* Vol 52, No 7, pp 252-255

Burgess. R.G. (ed.) (1985) *Issues in educational research : Qualitative Methods* Falmer Press, Lewes, Lewes, Sussex

Burgess. R.G. (ed.) (1989) *The ethics of educational research* Falmer Press, Lewes, Sussex

Buri. R. Katz. F.M. (1978) *Teaching community health care* Faculty of Medicine, Ramathibodi Hospital, Bankok, in WHO (1978), Personnel for health care, Geneva

Burke. J.W. (ed.) (1990) *Competency based educaton and training* Falmer Press, Lewes, Sussex

Burkett. G. Parker Harris. M. Kuhn. J. Escovitz. G. (1978) A comparative study of physicians and nurses conceptions of the role of the nurse practitioner *American journal of public health* No 68, p 1090-1096

Burnard. P (1988) Developing counselling skills in health visitors : An experiential approach. *Health visitor* Vol 61, pp 147-148

Burns. N. Groves. S. (1987) *The practice of nursing research* W.B. Saunders, Philadelphia, USA

Burr. M. (1975) Multidisciplinary health teams *The medical journal of Australia* Vol 2, pp 833-834

Business & Technician Education Council (BTEC) (1987) *BTEC National Diploma Awards in Science Dental technology course guidelines* BTEC, England & Wales, UK.

Butrym. Z. (1967) *Social work in medical care* Routledge, Kegan & Paul, London

Butrym. Z. Horder. J.(1983) *Health, doctors and social worker* Routledge, Kegan & Paul, London

Buttery. C.M.G. Moser. D.L. (1980) A combined family and community medicine clerkship. *Journal of family practice* No 11, pp 237-244

Bywaters. P. (1986) Social workers and the medical professions Arguments against unconditional collaboration. *British journal of social work* Vol 16, No 6, pp 661-667

Caliendo. M.A. Pulaski. M.A. (1979) Teaching the health care team concept to dietetic and nursing students : simulated team conferences. *Journal of the American Dietetics Association* No 74, pp 571-573

Campbell D. (1993) Talk about teaming up *Nursing standard* Vol 7, No 41, pp 12-13

Campbell. E.J.M. (1972) McMaster University and Medicine *Journal of the Royal College of Physicians* No 2, pp 331 -358

Campbell-Heider. N. Pollock. D. (1987) Barriers to physician/nurse collegiality An anthropological perspective. *Social science and medicine* Vol 13a, No 5, pp 515-521

Canham.J. (1982) Towards professionalism - Time to speak our minds *Nursing Mirror* Vol 155, No 3, pp 50-51

Carlaw. R.W. Callan. L.B. (1973) Team training, an experiment with promise. *Health services report* Vol 88, No 4, pp 328-336

Carpenter J. (1989) Interprofessional education *Primary health care* July p. 21

Carpenter. K.F. Kroth. J.A. (1976) Effects of videotaped role playing on nurses therapeutic communication skills. *Journal of continuing education in nursing* Vol 7, No 4, pp 47-53

Carr. W. Kemmis.S. (1986) *Becoming critical : Education, knowledge and action research.* The Falmer Press, Lewes, Sussex.

Carroll. J.G. Monroe. J. (1980) Teaching clinical interviewing in the health professions: A review of empirical research. *Evaluation and the health professions* No 3, pp 21-40

Cassata. D. (1980) Health communication theory and research : a definitional overview. *Communication Yearbook* No 4, pp 583-589

Cartlidge. A.M. Bond.J. (1986) *Collaboration among professionals in the delivery of primary health care.* Report No. 30. Health Care Research Unit University of Newcastle upon Tyne, U.K.

Cartlidge.A.M. (1987) *Collaboration : A study among primary health care professionals in 4 London and 16 Non London Health Authorities.* Report No 32, Health Care Research Unit, University of Newcastle upon Tyne

Cartlidge. A.M. Bond. J. Gregson. B.A. (1987a) Interprofessional collaboration in primary health care organisations. *Nursing times* Occasional Paper No 83.

Cartlidge. A.M. Gregson. B.A Bond J . (1987b) Interprofessional collaboration in primary health care *The family practitioner services* Vol 14 pp 327-332

Cartwright. A. (1964) *Human relations and hospital care* Routledge, Kegan & Paul, London

Cassata. D. (1978) Health communication theory and research, an overview of the communication interface. *Communication yearbook* No 2, pp 495-496, 498-503

Castles.M. (1987) *Primer of nursing research* W.B. Saunders, Philadelphia,

Central Council for the Education and Training of Social Workers (1989) *Multidisciplinary teamwork : Models of good practice* CCETSW, London

CCETSW (1991) Dip. SW : Rules & Requirements for the Diploma in Social Work *Paper 30 (2nd Ed)* CCETSW, London

CCETSW (1992) *Personal communication*

Challela. M. (1979) The interdisciplinary team : A role definition for nursing. *Image* No 11, 9-15

Chartered Society of Physiotherapy (1992) *Personal communication*

Child. D. (1986) *Psychology and the Teacher* Holt, Rhinehart & Winston, London

Christensen. K. Lingle, J.A, (1972) Evaluation of effectiveness of team and non team public health nurses in health outcomes of patients with strokes and fractures *American journal of public health* Vol 62, No 3, pp 483-489

Christman. L. (1970) Education of the health team. *J.A.M.A.* Vol 213, No 2 pp 284-285
Church. G.M. (1956) Understanding each other to achieve a common goal. *American journal of nursing* Vol 21, No 5, pp 201-204
Clare. A.W. Corney R.H. (1982) *Social work and primary health care* Academic Press, London
Clark. K. (1986) Recent developments in self directed learning *Journal of continuing education in nursing* Vol 17, No 3, pp 76-80
Clark P.G. (1993) A typology of interdisciplinary education in gerontology and geriatrics : Are we really doing what we say we are ? *Journal of interprofessional care* Vol 7, No 3, pp 217-227
Claxton C. Ralston Y. (1978) *Learning styles : Their impact on teaching and administration* American Association for Higher Education. ERIC clearing house on higher education Research Report No 10, Washington DC
Cohen. L. (1958) The physicians debt to radiology *British journal of radiology* No 31, pp 170-173
Cohen.L Manion. L. (1980) *Research methods in education* Croom Helm, London
Cohen. L. Manion. L. (1992) *Research methods in education (3rd Edition)* Routledge, London
Collee. J. (1992) Schools for scandal *Observer Newspaper Supplement* 16/8/92
College of Occupational Therapists (1992) *Personal communication*
College of Radiographers (1992) *Personal communication*
Collins. J. (1983) *Education for the paramedical professions in Cardiff and the possibility of rationalising some of the courses.* Unpublished M.Ed Thesis, University College Cardiff
Collier. G. Clarke. R. (1986) Syndicate methods : Two styles compared. *Higher education* No 15, pp 609-618
Coluccio. M. Maquire. P. (1983) Collaborative practice : becoming a reality through primary nursing. *Nursing Administration Quarterly* Summer 1983
CTI (1989) *Review of the C.T.I.* The Roberts Report Cardiff
Comite Pedagogique (1978) *Preparing health personnel for Algeria* The Institute Technologique de la sante publique Constantine, Algeria. (in WHO 1978, Personnel for health care)
Commission of the European Communities (CEC) (1989) *Health care and nursing in the 21st century* Report EUR 12040 EN , Brussels
C.E.C. (1990a) *Interim report on the primary health care content in the training of nurses responsible for general care* Advisory Committe on Training in Nursing, Doc 111/D/5011/6/89 EN, Brussels

C.E.C. (1990b) *Reports and recommendations adopted by the committee during the first 3 terms of office (1979-1990)* Advisory Committee on Training in Nursing Doc 111/D/5084/90 EN, Brussels

C.E.C. (1991a) *Education and Training* European File Series Office for Official Publications of the E.C.L 2985, Luxemborg

C.E.C. (1991b) *Europes Parliament and the Single Act* U.K. Office of the European Parliament,London

C.E.C. (1991c) *The Institutions of the E.C.* Office for Official Publications of the E.C.L 2985, Luxemborg

C.E.C. (1991d) *A Community of Twelve : Key Figures* Office for Official Publications of the E.C.L2985, Luxemborg

C.E.C. (1991d) *The European Community in the 1990's* Office for Official Publications of the E.C. L2985, Luxemborg

C.E.C. (1991e) *Life sciences and technologies for developing countries* (S.T.D.3) Directorate General XII for Science, Research and Development, Brussels

Connelly T. (1978) Basic organisational considerations for interdisciplinary education development in the health sciences *Journal of Allied Health* Vol 4, pp 274-280

Conti G S Welborn R B (1986) Teaching/Learning styles and the adult learner *Lifelong Learner* Vol 9, No 8, pp 20 -24

Copp. L. A. (1987) Patterns of interdisciplinary liaison *Recent advances in nursing* No 18, pp 90-108

Cormack. D.F.S. (ed.) (1987) *The research process in nursing* Blackwell, Oxford

Corney. R.H. (1980) Health visitors and social workers *Health Visitor* Vol 53, pp 409-413

Coser. L.A. (1956) *The functions of social conflict* The Free Press, New York

Costello. D. (1977) Health communication theory and research : An overview. *Communication Yearbook* No 1, pp 555-567

Council for the Professions Supplementary to Medicine (!973) *Report of the remedial professions committee* (The Burt Report) CPSM, London

CPSM (1979) *The next decade* CPSM, London

CPSM (1980) *Future requirements and opportunities* (The Lindop Report) CPSM, London

CPSM (1992) *Personal communication*

Craft. A. Brown. C. (1985) Getting a team to pull together. *Health and social services journal* Vol XCV, No 10, pp1168

Craig. J.W. (1970) Teamwork in dentistry. *British dental journal* Feb pp 198-202

Cramond. W.A. (1973a) The psychological care of patients with terminal illness(Part 1) *New Zealand nursing journal* Vol 66, No 9 pp 27-29

Cramond.W.A. (1973b) The psychological care of patients with terminal illness(Part 2) *New Zealand nursing journal* Vol 66, No 10 pp 23-25

Crews. B. (1990) A physiotherapists contribution to the formation of an acute mental health team. *Physiotherapy* Vol 76, No 5, pp 296-298

Cricton. A. Crawford. M.P. (1963) *Disappointed expectations* Welsh Hospital Board, Welsh Staff Advisory Committee, Cardiff.

Croen. L. Hamerman. D. Goetzel. R.Z. (1984) Interdisciplinary training for medical and nursing students : learning to collaborate in the care of geriatric patients. *Journal of American Geriatrics Society* Vol 32, No 1, pp 56-61

Crute. V.C. Hargie.O.D.W. Ellis. R.A.F. (1989) An evaluation of a communication skills course for health visitor students *Journal of advanced nursing* Vol 14, 546-552

Cypher. J. (ed.) (1979) *Seebohm across 3 decades* BASW, Birmingham, UK

Dana. B. Sheps. C. (1968) Trends and issues in interprofessional education : Pride, prejudice and progress. *Journal of education for social work* Vol 4, No 3, pp 41-42

Danish Nurses Association (1981) *Basic nursing education of nurses responsible for general care in the countries of the European Communities*, Copenhagen

Darling. L.A. Ogg.H.L. (1984) Basic requirements for initiating an interdisciplinary process. *Physical therapist* Vol 64, pp 1684-1686

Dartington.T.(1986) *The limits of altruism : Elderly mentally infirm people as a test case for collaboration.* King Edwards Hospital Fund, London

Day.S.B. (1979) *Health communications*, International Foundation for Biosocial Development and Human Health.New York

Degner. L. Beaton. J.I. (1987) *Life-death decisions in health care* Hemisphere, Washington, D.C.

Department of Education (1989) *A survey of collaboration in nurse education* & Science *in four polytechnics and colleges* Ref : 6/91/NS, London

Department of Education & Science, Department of Health and Social Security & The Welsh Office (1974) *Child Guidance* Circulars 3/74, HSC (IS)9, London WHSC (IS)5, Welsh Office, Cardiff

Department of Health & Social Security (1974) *Report of the working party on social work support for the health service* DHSS, Elephant & Castle, London

Department of Health & Social Security (1981) *Report of joint working group of Standing Medical Advisory Committee & Standing Nursing and Midwifery Committee : The PrimaryHealth Care Team* DHSS, London

Department of Health Nursing Division (1989) *A Strategy for Nursing* Department of Health, London

Department of Health (1991) *Caring for People :Joint Training Project Report* NHSTA Bristol

Department of Health (1992) *The Patients Charter* HMSO, London

Dervin. B. Harlock. S. (1976) *Health communication research : The state of the art* Portland, Oregon
De Vaus. D.A. (1986) *Surveys in social research* George Allen & Unwin, London
Devereaux. P.M. (1981a) Does joint practice work? *Journal of nursing administration* Vol 11, No 4, pp 39-43
Devereaux. P.M. (1981b) Essential elements of nurse-physician collaboration *Journal of nursing administration* Vol 11, No 5, pp 19-23
Dickinson. G.E. Pearson. A.A. (1980) Death education and physicians attitudes towards dying patients *Journal of family practice* Vol 11, pp 167
Dickson. D.A. Maxwell. M. (1985) The interpersonal dimension of physiotherapy : Implications for training *Physiotherapy* Vol 71, No 7 pp 306-310
Discher. M. (1974) Building a health team with participation training *Journal of continuing education,* Vol 5, pp14-18
Dimond. B. (1987) Your disobedient servant *Nursing times* Vol 8 No 6 pp 26-31
Dingwall. R. (1976) Health visiting and social work -Where are the boundaries? *Health and social science journal* (22 November 1976)
Dingwall. R. (1980) Problems of teamwork in primary care (in Lonsdale, Webb & Briggs Eds) *Teamwork in the personal social services and health care* Croom Helm, London
Dingwall.R. McIntosh J. (eds) (1978) *Readings in the sociology of nursing* Churchill Livingstone, Edinburgh
Dingwall. R. Eekelaar. J.Murray. T (1983) *The protection of children* Basil Blackwell, Oxford
Donnison. J. (1977) *Midwives and medical men* Heinemann, London
Ducanis. A.J. Golin. A.K. (1979) *The interdisciplinary health care team : A Handbook* Aspen publishers, USA
Duncan. B. Kempe. C.H. (1968) Joint education of medical students and allied health personnel. *American journal of the disabled child* Vol 116, pp 449-453
Duncan. A. McLachlan. G. (1984) *Hospital medicine and nursing in the 1980's Interaction between the professions of medicine and nursing* Nuffield Provincial Hospitals Trust, Oxford
Dunlop. R.J. Hockley. J.M. (1990) *Terminal care support team* Oxford Medical Publications, Oxford
Durlak.J.A. (1978) Comparison between experiential and didactic methods of health education *Journal of death and dying* Vol 9, pp 57-66
Eaton. G. Webb.B. (1979) Boundary encroachment- pharmacists in the clinical setting *Sociology of health and illness* Vol 3 pp 69-84
Eichenberger. R.W. Gloor. R.F.(1969) A team approach to learning community health *Journal of medical education* Vol 44, No 8, pp 655-662

Engler. C.M. Saltzman.G.A. Walker.M.L. Wolf.F.M (1981) Medical student acquisition and retention of.communication and interviewing skills . *Journal of medical education* Vol 56, No 7, pp 572-578

English National Board for Nursing, Midwifery& Health Visiting (1987) *Employment of non nurse specialist teachers in schools of nursing* E.N.B., Sheffield, UK

Engstrom. B. (1986) Communication and decision making in a study of a multidisciplinary team conference with the registered nurse as conference chairman *International journal of nursing studies* Vol 23, No 4, pp 299-314

Entwistle N (1981) *Styles of learning and teaching* John Wiley & Sons, N. York

Eraut. M. (1984) *Institution based curriculum evaluation* Hodder & Stoughton, London

Eron. L.D. (1985) The effect of medical education on medical students attitudes. *Journal of medical education* Vol 60, No 7, pp 559-565

Eskin.F. (1974) The reality of health care planning teams *Health and social services journal* Vol ?, No ?, pp 2596-2597 (9 11 74)

Eskin. F. (1975) Planning teams -A progress report *Health & social services journal* 1 November 1975, pp 2449

Evers. H.K. (1977) The patient care team in the hospital ward : The place of the nursing student. *Journal of advanced nursing* No 2, pp 589-596

Evers. H.K. (1981) Multidisciplinary teams in geriatric wards : myth or reality ? *Journal of advanced nursing* No 6, pp 205-214

Fairwater.M. Law.K. (1978) Mutidisciplinary traing in family planning *Medical education* No 12, pp 205-208

Fawcett-Henesy. A. (1991) Partners in time *Nursing times* Vol 6, No 45, pp 43

Feiger. S.M. Schmitt. M.H. (1979) Collegiality in interdisciplinary health teams : Its measurements and its effects. *Social science and medicine* Vol 13a, pp 217-229

Fenwick. A.M. (1979) An interdisciplinary tool for assessing patients readiness for discharge in the rehabilitation setting. *Journal of advanced nursing* No 4, pp 9-21

Ferguson. R.S. Carney. M.W.P. (1970) Interpersonal considerations and judgement in a day hospital *British journal of psychiatry* No 117, pp 397-403

Ferguson-Johnston. P. (1983) Why argue ? Collaborative practice works. *Nursing administration quarterly* Summer 1983, pp 64-71

Field. D. (1984) Formal instruction in United Kingdom medical schools about death and dying *Medical education* Vol 18, pp 429-434

Field.D. Howells.K (1985) Medical students self reported worries about aspects of death and dying. *Death studies* Vol 10, No 2, pp 147-154

Fielding.P. (1987) *Research in the nursing care of elderly people* John Wiley & Sons Ltd, London

Fisek. N.H. (1978) *Fitting medical education to the needs of the community* School of medicine, Hacettepe University, Ankara, Turkey.in WHO (1978) Personnel for health care, Geneva

Fitton. F. Acheson. D. (1979) *The doctor/patient relationship : A study in general practice* HMSO, London

Flack G. (1976) Team training to bring the professionals to the people *Health & social services journal* pp 2194-2195

Flack G. (1977) Looking for dividends from the cooperative movement *Health & social services journal* pp 432-435

Flaherty. J.A. Sharf. B.F. (1981) Using communication specialists in the teaching of interview skills. *Journal of medical ed.* Vol 56, No 12, p 1021

Fraser-Holland. E.N. (1989) The participation of occupational therapists in the education of other professions about occupational therapy. *British journal of occupational therapy* Vol 52, No 9, pp 538

French. P. (1983) *Social skills for nursing practice* Croom Helm, London

Fried. R.J. Leatt. P. (1986) Role perceptions among occupational groups in an ambulatory care setting. *Human relations* Vol 39. No 12, pp 1155-1174

Friedman B.D. (1980) Coping with cancer, a guide for health care professionals. *Cancer nursing* Vol 3, No 2, pp 105-110

Fulop. T. (1976) New approaches to a permanent problem *WHO Chronicle* No 30 pp 433-441

Fulop. T. (1987) *Community based education of health personnel* WHO, Geneva

Furnham. A.Pendleton.D. Manicom.C (1981) The perception of different occupations within the medical profession *Social science and medicine* Vol 15, pp 289-300

Garvin.B.J. Kennedy.C.W. (1988) Confirming communication of nurses in interaction with physicians.*Journal of nursing education* Vol 27, No 4 pp 161-166

Geiger. D.L. (1978) How future professionals view the elderly : A comparative analysis of social work, law and medical students perceptions. *The Gerontologist* No 18, pp 591-594

General Nursing Council for England and Wales (1982) *Training syllabus register of nurses: Mental nursing* General Nursing Council, London.

General Medical Council (1977) *Professional conduct and discipline* General Medical Council, London

General Medical Council (1980) *Recommendations on basic medical education* Spottiswoode Ballantyne, London

General Medical Council (1991) *Undergraduate medical education* Unpublished discussion document
General Medical Council (1992) *Personal communication*
George. M. (1971) The comprehensive health team : A conceptual model. *Journal of nursing administration* Vol 1, No 4, pp 9-13
Germain. C.B. (1980) Nursing the dying : Implications of Kubler-Ross stage theory.*The annals of the American Academy of political and social science* No 447, pp 89-99
Germain. C.B. (1984) Social work practice in health care *The Free Press:* New York
Gill.D.G. (1975) Reflections on the behavioral sciences and medical education.*Journal of operational psychiatry* No 6, pp 123-125
Gilmore. M. Bruce.N. Hunt.M (1974) The work of the nursing team in general practice *Council for the education and training of health visitors* London
Given. B. Simmons. S. (1979) The interdisciplinary health care team : fact of fiction. *Nursing forum* Vol 2, No 2, pp 165-184
Glaser. B.G. Strauss. A.L. (1968) *Time for Dying* Aldine, Chicago
Goble. R. (1991) Keeping alive intellectually *Nursing* Vol 4, No 33, pp 19-22
Goldberg. E.M. Neill. J.E. (1972) *Social work in general practice* Allen & Unwin, London
Goldie. N. (1977) *The division of labour among the mental health professions-negotiated or imposed ?* in Stacey M. (ed.) (1977) Health and the division of Labour. Croom Helm, London
Gomes. J. (1985) Co-operation through core courses *Community outlook* No 1, pp 31-35
Gomez. L. (1986) *Liaison Psychiatry* Croom Helm, London
Goodlad.S. Hirst. B. (1989) *Peer tutoring* Kogan Page, London
Goodwin. S. (1982) The name of the team game *Nursing mirror* Vol 154, No 8,
Gotterer. G.S. Blumberg. P. Paul. H.A (1987) *The alternative pre clinical curriculum* Rush Medical School USA in WHO (1987) Innovative Tracks, Geneva
Gregson. B. Cartlidge. A. Bond. J. (1991) *Interprofessional collaboration in primary health care organisations* Occasional Paper 52 The Royal College of General Practitioners London
Griffith. C.J. (1990) *Modular courses and the faculty of science* Unpublished paper. South Glamorgan Institute of Higher Education.
Guck. T.P. Skultety. F.M. :Meilman. P.W. Dowd. E.T. (1985) Mutidisciplinary pain center follow up study Evaluation with a no treatment control group *Pain* No 21, pp 295-306
Guilbert. J.J. (1981) *Education handbook for health personnel* WHO Offset Publication No 35, Geneva

Guilbert. J.J. (1984) *Nurses and physicians of tomorrow : A world wide survey on professional roles and their use as a basis for educational programmes* Unpublished document. WHO/EDUC/84/183

Haggard. L. (1990) Making the team work *The health service journal* 12.4.90

Hamad. B. (1982) Interdisciplinary field training. Research and rural development *Medical education* No 16, pp105-107

Hamburg. J. (1969) Core curriculum in allied health education *J.A.M.A.* Vol 210, No 111, pp 61-69

Hamel-Cooke. C.K. Cope. D.H.P. (1983) Not an alternative medicine *British medical journal* Vol 287, No 6409, pp 1934-1936

Hamric. A.B. Spross. J.S. (1984) *The clinical nurse specialist in theory and practice* Grune & Stratton, New York

Hancock. C. (1990) A new partnership for a new century *Physiotherapy* Vol 76, No 11, pp 669-671

Hancock. C. (1991) Multidisciplinary clinical audit *Nursing standard* Vol 5, No 18, pp 37 -38

Hannay. D.R. (1980) Teaching interviewing with simulated patients *Medical education* Vol 14, No 4, pp 246-250

Hannay. D.R. (1980) Problems in role identification and conflict in multidisciplinary teams in Barber & Kratz (eds) *Towards team care*, Churchill Livingstone, Edinburgh

Harding. G. Taylor K.M.G. (1988) Pharmacies in health centres *Journal of the Royal College of General Practitioners* pp 566-567

Harding. G. Taylor. K.M. (1990) Interprofessional issues - professional relationships between general practitioners and pharmacists in health centres. *British journal of general practitioners* Vol 40, No 340, pp 464-466

Hargie. O. Bamford. D. (1984) A comparison of the reactions of pre-service and in- service social workers to micro training. *Vocational aspects of education* Vol 36, No 95, pp 87-91

Hargreaves. R. (1979) *Social services for the mentally ill* in Cypher. J. (ed.) Seebohm across 3 decades BASW publications, Birmingham

Harlem. O. (1977) *Communication in medicine : A challenge to the profession* Kager Press, Basel.

Hartings. M.F. Counte. M.A. (1977) An administrative and curricular model for behavioural science teaching *Journal of medical education* Vol 52, No 10, pp 824-833

Hasler. J.C. Klinger. M. (1976) Common ground in general practice and health visitor training : An experimental course *Journal of the Royal College of General Practitioners* Vol 26, pp 266-276

Hawker. M. (1977) Co-operation/co-ordination = Professional disaster *Social work today* Vol 8, No 17, pp 18

Hawkins. R.O (1972) *Core curriculum* in McTernan & Hawkins (eds) Educating personnel for the allied health professions and services C V Mosby, St Louis, USA

Hay. A. Minty.B. Trowell. J. (1991) *Right or privilege ? Post qualifying training social workers with special refence to child care* CCETSW, London

Hendy. A. (1978) The primary health care team : what you told us. *Nursing times- Community outlook* Vol , pp 254-8, 270

Henk.M.L. (ed.) (1989) *Social work in primary care* Sage publications, California

HMSO (1920) *Interim report on the future provision of medical and allied services (The Dawson Report)* Consultative Council on Medical and Allied Services London

HMSO (1950) *Reports of the Committees on Medical Auxilliaries (The Cope Reports) Cmnd 8188* HMSO, London

HMSO (1959) *Report of the working party on social workers in the local authority, health and welfare services (The Younghusband Report)* Dept. of Health for Scotland, Edinburgh

HMSO (1968a) *Royal Commission on Medical Education (The Todd Report)* HMSO, London

HMSO (1968b) *Report of the Committee on local authority and allied personal social services Cmnd. 3703* HMSO, London

HMSO (1969) *Communication between doctors, nurses and patients. Cmnd. 51583* HMSO, London

HMSO (1971) *Doctors in an integrated health service* Scottish Home and Health Department. Edinburgh

HMSO (1972) *Nurses in an integrated health service* Scottish Home and Health Department Edinburgh

HMSO (1972) *Report of the Committee on Nursing (The Briggs Report) Cmnd 5515* HMSO, London

HMSO (1973) *The Remedial Professions (The McMillan Report)* HMSO, London

HMSO (1974a) *Social Work support for the Health Service* HMSO, London. The Welsh Office, Cardiff

HMSO (1974b) *Report of the Committee of Inquiry into the pay and related conditions of service of the Professions Supplementary to Medicine and Speech Therapists (The Halsbury Report)* HMSO, London

HMSO (1975) *Report of the Committee of Inquiry into the Regulation of the Medical Profession (The Merrison Report) Cmnd 6018* HMSO London

HMSO (1976) *Fit for the Future : Report of the Committe on Child Health Services (The Court Report) Cmnd. 6684, Volumes 1 & 2*, HMSO, London

HMSO (1976) *Prevention and Health : Everybody's Business* HMSO, London

HMSO (1977) *The Way Forward* HMSO, London

HMSO (1978) *Collaboration in Community Care : A Discussion Document* Personal Social Services Council HMSO, London

HMSO (1979) *The Role of Psychologists in the Health Service*

HMSO (1981) *The Primary Health Care Team : Report of a Joint Working Group. (The Harding Report)* The Standing Medical Advisory Committe & The Standing Nursing & Midwifery Advisory Committee HMSO, London

HMSO (1985) *The Development of Higher Education into the 1990's Cmnd. 9524*, HMSO, London

HMSO (1986) *Neighbourhood Nursing : A Focus for Care (The Cumberledge Report)* Community Nursing Review, HMSO, London

HMSO (1986) *Primary Health Care : An Agenda for Discussion Cmnd 9771*, HMSO, London

HMSO (1987) *Promoting Better Health(The Trethowan Report)* Standing Mental Health Advisory Committee HMSO,London

HMSO (1979) *The Royal Commission on the NHS (The Merrison Report) Cmnd 7615,* HMSO, London

HMSO (1979) *Report of the Committee of Enquiry into Mental Handicap Nursing and Care (The Jay Report)Cmnd. 7468, Volumes 1 & 2,* HMSO, London

HMSO (1979) *The Doctor/Patient Relationship : A Study in General Practice* HMSO, London

HMSO (1980) *Organisation and management problems of mental illness hospitals. Report of a Working Group (The Nodder Report)* HMSO, London

HMSO (1987) *Promoting better health : The Governments Proposals for Improving Primary Health Care Cmnd. 249*, HMSO, London

HMSO (1989) *Working for Patients Cmnd. 555*, HMSO, London

HMSO (1989) *Working for Patients Education and Training : Working Paper 10* HMSO, London

HMSO (1989) *Caring for People : Community Care in the Next Decade and Beyond Cmnd. 849*, HMSO, London

HMSO (1992) *Health Committee Second Report on Maternity Services Vol 1. (The Winterton Report)* HMSO, London

Hicks. D. (1976) *Primary Health Care* HMSO, London

Hicks. C.M. (1990) *Research and Statistics* Prentice Hall, New York

Hirschon. R. (1976) Nurses and social workers can learn together *American journal of nursing* Vol 76, No 12, pp 1972-1973

Hockey. L. (1977) The nurses contribution to care in a changing setting. *Journal of advanced nursing* Vol 2, No 2, pp 147-156

Hodes. C. (1972) Education of nurses and health visitors in group practice. *Journal of the Royal College of General Practitioners* Vol ?, No 22, pp 477-479

Hodkinson. H.M.(1975) *An outline of geriatrics* Academic Press, London
Hoekleman. R.A.(1975) Nurse/physician relationships
American journal of nursing Vol 75, No 11 pp 1150-1152
Holm .K. Llewellyn. J.G. (1986) *Nursing research for nursing practice*
W.B.Saunders, Philadelphia
Holsti. O.R. (1969) *Content analysis for the social sciences and humanities*
Addison -Wesley, Massachussetts
Honeycutt. J.M. (1987) Impressions about communication styles and competence in nursing relationships *Communication education* Vol 36, No 3
pp 217-227
Hooper. D. (1970) Conflict and co-operation in hospital care *Medical social work* No 4, pp 53-58
Hooyman. N.R. Asuman-Kiyak. H. (1988) *Social gerontology - a multidisciplinary perspective* Allyn & Bacon Inc. London
Horder. J. (1977) Physicians and family doctors : A new relationship
Journal of the Royal College of General Practitioners Vol 27 pp 391-397
Horder. J. (1988) Education and training for general practice.
(in Jarman. B. (1988) *Student reviews : primary care* Heinemann, Oxford)
Horder. J. (1991) CAIPE : Striving for collaboration.
Nursing Vol 4, No 33, pp 16-18
Hòule. C. (1980) *Continuing learning in the professions*
Jossey -Bass, San Francisco
Howard. J. Byl. N. (1971) Pitfalls in interdisciplinary teaching
Journal of medical education Vol 46, No 9, pp 772-781
Hoy. A.M. Saunders.B.M. Kearney.M . (1984) Breaking bad news
British medical journal Vol 288, pp1833
Hoy.A.M. (1985) Breaking bad news to patients
British journal of hospital medicine Vol 34, No 2, pp 96-99
Huck M (1981) Adult students locus of control learning styles and satisfaction with the baccalureate nursing program.
Journal of advanced nursing Vol 11, pp 289-294
Hudson. B. (1991) A question of teamwork : Community interprofessional mental handicap teams *Health service journal* No 4, pp 18-19
Hughes.E. Thorne.B. De Baggis. A. Gurin. A Williams. D .(1973)
Education for the professons of medicine law, theology and social welfare
McGraw Hill, New York
Hughes. P. (1991) Who should teach nurses ?
Nursing standard Vol 6, No 4, pp 30-31
Hunt. M. (1972a) The dilemma of identity in health visiting -(1)
Nursing times Occasional paper Vol 68, No 5, pp 17-20
Hunt. M. (1972b) The dilemma of identity in health visiting (2)
Nursing times occasional paper Vol 68, No 6, pp 23-24

Hunt. M. (1974) *An analysis of factors influencing teamwork in general medical practice* Unpublished M.Phil.Thesis, Faculty of social sciences, University of Edinburgh.

Hunter D. (1991) Relief through teamwork*Nursing times* Vol 87, No 17, pp 35-38

Hutchinson.A. Gordon. S. (1992) Primary care teamwork - making it a reality *Journal of interprofessional care* Vol 6, No 1, pp 31-42

Hutt. A. (1980) Shared learning for shared care. A multidisciplinary course at the Middlesex Hospital *Journal of advanced nursing* Vol 5, No 4, pp 389-394

Hutt. A. (1986) What exactly is the team approach ? *Midwife, health visitor and community nurse* Vol 22, No 10, pp 340-342

Irwin. W.G. Bamber. J.H. (1984) An evaluation of medical students behaviour in communication. *Medical education* Vol 18, pp 90-95

Iles. P.A. Auluck. R. (1990) From organizational to interorganisational development in nursing practice : improving the effectiveness of interdisciplinary teamwork and interagency collaboration. *Journal of advanced nursing* Vol 15, pp 50-58

Infante. M. Speranza. K. Gillespie. P (1976) An interdisciplinary approach to the education of health professional students *Journal of allied health* Vol 5, No 1, pp 13-22

Ivey. S.L. Brown. K.S. Teske. Y. Silverman. D (1988) A model for teaching about interdisciplinary practice in health care settings. *Journal of allied health* Vol 3, No 2, pp 189-195

Janetakos. J. Schissel. C. (1979) Partners : Nurse practitioner and social worker *American journal of nursing* Vol 79, pp 1434-1435

Jameton. A. Todes. D. (1982) Humanities teaching and research at the University of California, San Francisco. *Journal of continuing education professionals in health sciences* Vol 2, No 3, pp105-114

Jaques. E. (ed.) (1978) *Health services, their nature, organisation and the role of patients and doctors and health professions* Heinemann, London

Jarman. B. (ed.) (1988) *Student reviews : Primary care* Heinemann, Oxford

Jarrold. K. (1990) Working together *Physiotherapy* Vol 76, No 11, pp 668-669

Jayawickramarajah. P.T. (1992) How to evaluate programmes in the health professions *Medical teacher* Vol 14, No 2/3, pp 159-166

Jeffreys M. (1980) The role of the behavioural & social sciences in medical education *Medical education & primary health care* Croom Helm, London

Johnston. A. Cummings. V. Pooler. L. (1968) Team mates are equal partners *Canadian Nurse* No 9, pp 36-41

Joice. A. (1989) A discussion of the skills of the occupational therapist working within a multidisciplinary team *British journal of occupational therapy* Vol 52, No 12, pp 466-468

Jones. R.V.H. (1986) *Working together- Learning together Occasional Paper 33*, The Royal College of General Practitioners.

Jones. R.V.H. (1992) Team work in primary care : How much do we know about it ? *Journal of interprofessional care* Vol 6, No 1, pp 25-29

Judd. C.M. Smith. E.R. Kidder. L.H. (1991) *Research methods in social relations* Holt, Rhinehart & Winston Inc, Fort Worth

Kalisch. B.J. Kalisch P.A. (1977) An analysis of the sources of nurse physician conflicts *Journal of nursing administration* No 7, pp 50-57

Kane. R. Kane.R (1969) Physicians attitudes of omnipotence in a University Hospital. *Journal of medical education* No 44, pp 684

Kane. A. (1983) *Interprofessional teamwork* Syracuse, New York

Kahn. G.S. Cohen. B.Jason. H (1979) Teaching of interpersonal skills in medical schools Journal of medical education No 54, pp 29-35

Kantrowitz. M. Kaufman. A. Mennin.S, Fulop. T, Guilbert. J.J. (1987) *Innovative tracks at established institution for the education of health personnel : An experimental approach to change relevant health needs* Offset Publications No 101, WHO, Geneva

Kaprio. L.A. (1979) *Primary health care in Europe* WHO, Geneva

Katz. F.M. (1978) *Guidelines for evaluating a training programme for health personnel* WHO, Geneva

Katz. F.M. Fulop. T. (1978) *Personnel for health care : Case studies of educational programmes* Public Health Paper Vol 1, No 70 WHO, Geneva

Keddy. B. Jones Gillis. M. Jacobs. P. Burton.H. Rogers. M. (1986) The doctor/nurse relationship : An historical perspective. *Journal of advanced nursing* Vol 11, No 6, pp 745-753

Kendall. P. (1977) The role relationship dilemma of health visitor and social worker. *Health Visitor* Vol 50, No 8, pp 261-264

Kenneth. H. (1969) Medical and nursing students learn together *Nursing outlook* Vol 17, No 11, pp 46-49

Kerlinger. F.N. (1986) *Foundations of educational research (3rd Ed)* Holt, Rhinehart & Winston Inc, Fort Worth

Kiereini. E.M. (1985) Whats happened since Alma Ata ? *International nursing review* Vol 32, No 1, p 85

Kindig. D.A. (1975) Interdisciplinary education for primary health care team delivery. *Journal of medical education* Vol 50, No 2, pp 97-110

King Edwards Hospital Fund (1968) *Working together. A study of co-operation and co-ordination between general practitioner public health and hospital services.* Kings Fund, London

Kingdon. D.G. (1992) Interprofessional collaboration in mental health *Journal of interprofessional care* Vol 6, No 2, pp 141-147

Kinston. W. (1983) Hospital organisation and structure and its effect on interpersonal behaviour and the delivery of care. *Social science and medicine* Vol 17, No 16, pp 1159-1170

Kirkland. D. (1970) The medical student as a loner.
J.A.M.A. Vol 213, No 2, pp 278-279

Klein. C.A. (1984) Informed consent. *Nurse practitioner* No 5, pp 56-62

Klein. C.A. (1985) Invasion of privacy. *Nurse practitioner* No 1, pp 50-52

Knight. M. Field. D. (1981) A silent conspiracy : Coping with dying cancer patients on an acute surgical ward. *Journal of advanced nursing* Vol 6, pp 221-229

Knowles. M. (1990) *Andragogy in action (3rd Ed)* Jossey Bass, California

Knowles. M. (1990) *The adult learner : A neglected species (4th Ed)* Gulf, Houston

Knox. J.D.E. Alexander. D.W. Morrison. A.T. Bennet. A(1979) Communication skills and undergraduate medical education. *Medical education_* Vol 13, No 5, pp 345-348

Knox. J.D.E. Bouchier. I.A.D. (1985)Communication skills teaching, learning and assessment. *Medical education* Vol 19, No 3, pp 285-289

Knox. J.D.E. (1989) Breaking bad news, medical undergraduate communication skills, teaching and learning. *Medical education* Vol 23, No 3, pp 258-261

Kogan. M. Pope. M. (eds) (1972) *The challenge of change* NFER, Berks

Korsch. B.M. Gozzi. E. K. Francis. V.(1968) Gaps in doctor/patient communication *Paediatrics* No 42, pp 855-871

Kosberg. J.J. (1983) The importance of attitudes on the interaction between health care providers and geriatric populations. *Interdisciplinary topics in Gerontology* No 17, pp 132-143

Kreps. G.L. Thornton. B. (1984) *Health communication : Theory and Practice* Longman, New York

Krippendorf. K. (1980) *Content analysis; An introduction to its methodology* Sage Pub., Beverly Hills

Kuenssberg. E. (1980) Introduction to education for co-operation in health and social work symposium. (in England. H. (ed.) *Education for co-operation in health and social work Occasional Paper 14*, The Royal College of General Practitioners.

Kurtzman. C. Block. D. (1985) Nursing and medical students attitudes towards the rights of hospitalised patients. *Journal of nursing education* Vol 24, No 6, pp 237-241

Lambert. H. Muras. H. (1967) *The medical social workers participation in medical student teaching* Written report of a conference proceedings held at the London Hospital Medical Centre (10/3/67)

Lambert. H. Riphagen. F.E. (1975) Working together in a team for primary health care : A guide to dangerous country. *Journal of the Royal College of General Practitioners* Vol 3, No 25 pp 435-438

Larkin. G. (1983) *Occupational monopoly and modern medicine* Tavistock, London

Leathard. A. (1990) Backing a united front
The health service journal 29/11/90, pp 1776
Leathard. A. (1992) Interprofessional developments at South Bank Polytechnic. *Journal of interprofessional care* Vol 6, No 1, pp 17-23
Leedy. P.D. (1989) *Practical research : Planning and design* Macmillan, New York
Leninger.M. (1971) This I believe.....About interdisciplinary health education for the future. *Nursing outlook* Vol 19, No 12, pp 787-791
Lenz. E.R. (1985) Disciplinary boundary maintenance in nursing education *Journal of nursing* education Vol 24, No 8, pp 326-332
Lewis. C.E. (1965) Home care revisited : An experiment in medical and nursing education. *Journal of medical education* Vol 40, No 2, pp 84-91
Lewis. C.E. Resnick. B.A. (1964) Relative orientations of students of medicine and nursing to ambulatory patient care. *Journal of medical education* Vol 39, No 3, pp 162-166
Lewis. C.E. Resnick. B.A. (1966) A study of the effects of a multidisciplinary home care teaching program on the attitudes of first year students *Journal of medical education* Vol 41, No3, pp 195-200
Ley. P. (1982) Satisfaction, compliance and communication : A review. *British journal of clinical psychology* Vol 21, No 4, pp 241-254
Ley. P. (1988) *Communicating with patients : Improving communication, satisfaction and compliance* Croom Helm, London
Ley. P. Whitworth. M.A. Skilbeck. C.E. Woodward. R Pinsent.R.J.F.H.Pike. L.A.Clarkson. M.E. Clark. P.B. (1979) Improving doctor/patient compliance *Journal of the Royal College of General Practitioners* No 26, pp 720-724
Light. D.W. (1988) Toward a new sociology of medical education *Journal of health and social behaviour* Vol 29, pp 307-322
Light. I. (1969) Development and growth of new medical allied health fields. *J.A.M.A* No 210, pp 114-120
Ling. J. Funnell. P Gill. J.(1990) Shared learning. *Nursing times* Vol 86, No 1, pp 65-66
Lishman. J. (1983) *Collaboration and conflict : Working with others* University of Aberdeen, Scotland
Llewellyn N. (1993) APS : A multidisciplinary team *Nursing standard* Vol 7, No 25, pp 7
Lloyd. G. (1973) An interdisciplinary workshop. *Journal of the Royal College of General Practitioners* No 23, pp 463-473
Lonsdale. S. Webb.A. Briggs. T.L. (eds) (1980) *Teamwork in the personal social services and health care.* Croom Helm, London
Lorenz. R.A. (1987) Teaching health profession students to be effective patient teachers. *Medical teacher* Vol 9, No 4, pp 403-408

Lorenz. R.A. Pichert. J.W. (1986) Impact of interprofessional training on medical students willingness to accept clinical responsibility *Medical education* No 20, pp 195-200

Lovell RB (1986) *Adult learning* Croom Helm, Beckenham

Lunt.B. Hillier. R. (1981) Terminal care, present services and future priorities. *British medical journal* Vol 283, No 6291, pp 595-598

McCally. M. Sorem. K. Silverman. M. (1977) Interprofessional education of the new health practitioner. *Journal of medical education* Vol 52, No 3, pp 177-182

McClure. L.M. (1984) Teamwork, myth or reality : community nurses experience with general practice attachment. *Journal of epidemiology and community health* No 38, pp 68-74

McCreary. J.F. (1968) The health team approach to medical education *J.A.M.A.* Vol 206, No 7, pp 1554-1557

McCue. J.D. (1982) The effects of stress on physicians and their medical practice. *New England journal of medicine* No 306, pp 458-463

McElhinney. T. (ed.) (1981) *Human values teaching programmes for health professionals.* Whitmore, USA

McFarlane. J. (1980) *The multidisciplinary team (Project Paper 12)* Kings Fund, London

McGaghie. W.C (1978) *Competency based curriculum development in medical education* WHO, Geneva

McGarvey.M. Mullan. F. Sharfstein. S.A. (1968) A study in medical action : The student health organisations. *The New England journal of medicine* No 279, pp 74-80

McIntosh. J.B. (1974) Communication in team work : A lesson from the district. *Nursing times* Vol 10, No 35, pp 85-88

McIntosh. J.B. (1974) *Communication and awareness on a cancer ward* Croom Helm, London

McPherson. C. Sachs. L.A. (1982) Health care team training in U.S. and Canadian medical schools. *Journal of medical education* Vol 57, No 4, pp 282-287

McTernan. E.J. Hawkins. R.O. (1972) *Educating personnel for the allied health professions and services* C.V. Mosby, St Louis, USA

MacDonald. I. (undated) *Working together : Professional expectations and understanding.* B.I.O.S.S. Brunel University, U.K.

MacDonald. I. (1988) Getting on with the real work *Mental Handicap* Vol 16, No 6, pp 65-67

MacDougall. M.G. Elahi. V.K. (1974) The comprehensive health care project : A multidisciplinary learning experience. *Journal of medical education* Vol 49, No 10, pp 752-755

MacGregor. F.C. (1960) *Social science in nursing* Russell Sage, New York.

Mager. R.F. (1961) On the sequencing of instructional content
Psychological reports No 9, pp 405-413

Maguire. G.P. Rutter. D.R. in Bennett. A.E. (1976) Training medical students to communicate *Communication between doctors and patients.*
Oxford University Press, London

Maguire. P.in Argyle. M. (ed.) (1981) Doctor/Patient skills
Social skills and health Methuen, London

Maguire. P. (1985a) Barriers to psychological care of the dying
British medical journal Vol 291, No 6510, pp 1711-1713

Maguire. P (1985b) The psychological impact of cancer.
British journal of hospital medicine Vol 34, No 2, pp 100-103

Manpower Consultancy (1989) *Review of the Combined Training Institute Service* MCS Commissioned by the Welsh Office, Cardiff

Marcer. D. Deighton. S. (1988) Intractable pain : A neglected area of medical education in the UK.*Journal of the Royal Society of Medicine Vol 81, pp 698-700*

Margolis. H.Fiorelli. J.S. (1984) An applied approach to facilitating interdisciplinary teamwork. *Journal of rehabilitation* No 50, pp 13-17

Mariano. C. (1989) The case for interdisciplinary collaboration
Nursing outlook Vol 37, No 6, pp 285-288

Marshall. M. (1991) Advocacy within the multidisciplinary team
Nursing standard Vol 6, No 10, pp 28-31

Marshall. C. Rossman. G.B. (1989) *Designing qualitative research*
Sage Publications, London

Martin. C. (1990) Opportunities now knocking.
Nursing standard Vol 4, No 35, pp 22-23

Martin. M. (1969) *Colleagues or competitors ?* Bell, London

Mase. D.J. (1967) The role of the medical center in the education of health personnel. *British journal of medical education* No 42 pp 489-493

Mason. E.J. Parascandola. J. (1972) Preparing tomorrows health care team
Nursing outlook Vol 20, No 11, pp 728-731

Mazur. H. Beeston. J.J. Yerxa. E.J. (1979) Clinical interdisciplinary health team care : An educational experiment. *Journal of medical education*
Vol 54, No 9, pp 703-713

Mechanic. D. Newton. M. (1965) Social considerations in medical education : points of convergence between medicine and behavioural science. *Journal of chronic diseases* No 18, pp 291-301

Mechanic. D. Aiken. L. (1982) A co-operative agenda for medicine and nursing
New England journal of medicine No 307, pp 747-750

Mehlomakhulu. M.N. (1991) *Report on review of health related curricula*
Ministry of Health, Zimbabwe

Mennin. S.P. Woodside. W.F. Bernstein.E. Kantrowitz. M Kaufman. A (1987) Primary care curriculum : University of New.Mexico USA In WHO (1987) *Innovative tracks at established institutions for the education of health personnel*

Milio. N. (1979) Health professions education and the nature of modern health problems : A basis for a multidisciplinary core. *Health values* No 3, pp 152- 160

Miller. G.E. (1980) *Educating medical teachers* Harvard University Press, Massachusetts

Milne. M.A. (1980a) Training for team care *Journal of advanced nursing* No 5, pp 579-589

Milne. M.A. (1980b) Student role perception of the primary health care team (1) *Nursing times* Occasional Paper Vol 76, No 14.

Milne. M.A. (1986c) Student role perception of the primary health care team (2) *Nursing times* Occasional Paper Vol 76, No 15.

Mitchell. J.R.A. (1984) Is nursing any business of doctors ? *British medical journal* Vol 288, pp 216-219

Mocellin. G. (1992) An overview of occupational therapy in the context of the American influence on the profession.*British journal of occupational therapy* Vol 55, No 2, pp 55-60

Monekosso. G.L. Quenum. C.A.A. (1978) Training the health team. The University centre for health sciences, Yaounde, United Republic of Cameroon in WHO (1978) *Personnel for health care,* Geneva

Moore. D.L. (1989) An interdisciplinary seminar on legal issues in medicine. *Journal of legal education* Vol 39, No 1, pp 113-120

Moore. G. (1983) *Developing and evaluating educational research* Little, Brown and Co. USA

Moreland. J.R. (1971) Videotaped programmed instructions in elementary psychotherapeutic and related clinical skills *Dissertation Abstracts International* 31.2404B

Morris-Thompson. P. (1992) Consumers, continuity and control *Nursing times* Vol 88, No 26, pp 29-30

Mosley. P. (1988) Communication and the education of health professionals. *Medical teacher* Vol 10, No 3, pp 323-332

Mullaney. J.W. Fox. R.A. Liston. M.F. (1974) Clinical nurse specialist and social worker clarifying the roles.*Nursing outlook* No 22, pp 712-718

Naidoo. P (1983) The microtraining approach in the training of school counsellors. *International journal for the advancement of counselling* Vol 6, No 1, pp 61-67

Nash. T.P. (1984) Breaking bad news.*British medical journal* No 288, pp 1996

Nason. F. (1981) Team tension as a vital sign *General hospital psychiatry* No 3, pp 32-36

Navarro. V. (1976) *Medicine under capitalism* Croom Helm, London

Navarro. V. (1978) *Class struggle, the state and medicine* Martin Robertson, London

Nchinda. T.C. (1974) Integrated approach to health personnel for developing countries : The Cameroon experiment. *Tropical doctor* Vol 4, No 1, pp 41-45

Nelson. M.J. (1989) *Managing health professionals* Chapman & Hall, London

Newman. J. (1987) Multidisciplinary education : A way for the future ? in Fielding. P. (1987) *Research in the care of elderly people* John Wiley & Sons Ltd., London

Newman. L.T. (1978) Working together : Multidisciplinary course for the primary health care team. *Medical digest* Vol 23, No 1, pp 38-45

National Health Service Training Authority (1990) *A first degree in health care in the NHS: A feasibility study on a collaborative scheme for post basic awards in the NHS.* NHSTA, Bristol

NHSTA (1990) *Effective teamworking in the community* Health Pickup module,Macmillan/Intek, London

NHSTA (1990) *National occupational standards for operating department practice Vol 1 & 2* NHSTA, Bristol

Nicklin. P.J. (1987) Attitudes towards death and dying among doctors and nurses. *Nursing times* Vol 83, No 44, pp 58

Nicol B.N.(ed.) (1971) *Training Techniques* Makerere University, Kampala, Uganda

Nitsun. M. Gledhill. R. Shanley. R. (1981) Multidisciplinary training groups in a psychiatric hospital. *Bulletin of the Royal College of Psychiatrists* No 5, pp 89-91

Noack M. (ed.) (1980) *Medical education in primary health care* Croom Helm, London

Nolan R.J. (1987) *Nurse Teachers at Work : An Analysis of Function* Unpublished PhD Thesis, University of Wales

Northouse. P. Northouse.L. (1985) *Health communication : A handbook for health professionals.* Prentice Hall, New Jersey

Nuffield Group for Research and Innovation in Higher Education. (1974) *Interdisciplinarity* Nuffield Group, Oxford

Nunally. J. Kittross. J. (1958) Public attitudes towards mental health professions *American psychologist* No 13, pp 589-591

Nursing Standard (un-named author) (1987) Joint training for nurses and social workers *Nursing standard* , pp 5 19/9/87

Nursing Standard(un-named author) (1992) World News *Nursing standard* Vol 6, No 19, pp 11

Nursing Times (un-named author) (1986) Welsh H.V.'s in bid to split from G.P.'s *Nursing times* Vol 82, No 6, pp 7

Nutter. D.O. (1983) Medical education in The Peoples Republic of China. *Journal of medical education* Vol 58, No 7, pp 555-561

Oken. D. (1961) What to tell cancer patients *J.A.M.A.* No 175, pp 1120-1128
Opoku. D. (1992) Does interprofessional co-operation matter in the care of birthing women ? *Journal of interprofessional care* Vol 6, No 2, pp 119-125
Oppenheim. A.N. (1966) *Questionnaire design and attitude measurement* Heinemann, London
Oppenheim. A.N. (1992) *Questionnaire design, interviewing and attitude measurement* Pinter Publishers, London
Orem. D. (1971) *Nursing : Concepts of practice* McGraw Hill, New York
Osborne. A. Wakeling. C. (1985) Co-operation in training. *Senior nurse* Vol 3, No 6, pp 21-23
Ovretveit. J. (1984) *Organising psychology in the NHS* Health Services Centre Working Party BIOSS. Brunel University. Uxbridge
Ovretveit. J. (1985a) *Organising multidisciplinary teams : Problems pitfalls and possibilities* Professional Organisation and Practice Programme BIOSS, Brunel University, Uxbridge
Ovretveit. J. (1985b) *Multidisciplinary team organisation and management* BIOSS, Brunel University, Uxbridge
Ovretveit. J. (1985c) *The social analytic research method* P.O.P.P Paper, BIOSS, Brunel University Uxbridge
Ovretveit. J. (1985d) Medical dominance and the development of autonomy in physiotherapy. *Sociology of health and illness* Vol 7, No 1, pp 76-93 Also referenced (by Ovretveit himself in 1986d) as
Ovretveit. J. (1985e) Professional autonomy and medical dominance. *Sociology of health and illness* Vol 7, No 1, pp 76-93
Ovretveit. J. (1986a) *Case responsibility in multidisciplinary teams* P.O.P.P Paper, BIOSS, Brunel University Uxbridge
Ovretveit. J. (1986b) *Aspects of community multidisciplinary team management and organisation* P.O.P.P. Paper, BIOSS, Brunel University Uxbridge
Ovretveit. J. (1986c) *Improving social work records and practice* BASW Publications, Birmingham,UK
Ovretveit. J. (1986d) *Organisation of multidisciplinary community teams* BIOSS, Brunel University, Uxbridge
Owen. J. (1982) Learning from each other. *Community outlook,* No 2, pp 15-18
Owen. N. (1982) How to organise and conduct joint and integrated teaching. *Medical teacher* Vol 4, No 2, pp 47-55
Pacoe. L.V. Maar.R. (1976) Training medical students in interpersonal relationship skills. *Journal of medical education* No 51, pp 743-750
Parahoo. K. (1991) Politics and ethics in nursing research *Nursing standard* Vol 6, No 6, pp 35-39

Parker. A.(1972) *The team approach to primary health care* Neighborhood Health Center Studies Seminar Program. Monograph Series No. 3 Berkely, University of California, USA

Parkes. M.E. (1977) The importance of seeing the whole picture *Australian nursing journal* Vol 11, No 6, pp 20-23

Pascasio. A. (1970) Relation of allied health education to medical education. *J.A.M.A.* Vol 213, No 2, pp 281- 285

Pask G. (1976) Styles and strategies of learning *British journal of educational psychology* Vol. 46 pp 128-148

Pathik.B. Goon.E. (1978) From medical assistants to physicians. Fiji school of medicine, Suva, Fiji in WHO (1978) *Personnel for health care*, Geneva

Pattishall. E.G. (1970) Concepts in the teaching of behavioural science *Social science and medicine* No 4, pp 157-160

Pattison. E.M. (1975) The behavioural sciences in medical education *Journal of operational psychiatry* No 6, pp 113-122

Pelligrino. E.D. (1966) The communication crisis in nursing and medical education. *Nursing forum* No 5, pp 45-53

Pelligrino. E.D. (1966) Closing the profession gap : Some notes on unity of purpose in the health professions.in McTernan E.J. Hawkins.R.O.(1972) *Educating personnel for the allied health professions and services* C V Mosby, St Louis, USA

Peeples. E. Francis. G.M. (1972) Social psychological obstacles to effective health team practices. *Nursing forum* Vol 11, No 3, pp 301-310

Pereira - Gray. D.J. (1980) Just a G.P. *Journal of the Royal College of General Practitioners* No 30, pp231-239

Peryer. D. (1991) Collaboration or conflict in community care planning : A social services perspective. In Allen. D. (ed.) *Health and social services the new relationship* Policy Studies Institute, London

Phillips. W.R. (1982) Clinical content of the WAMI community clerkship in family medicine *Journal of medical education*, No 57, pp 615-620

Pluckhan. M. (1972) Professional territoriality : A problem affecting the delivery of health care. *Nursing forum* Vol 11, No 3, pp 301-310

Polgar. S. (1961) Health and human behavior : Areas of interest common to the social and medical sciences. *Current anthropology* No 11, pp 122-162

Polit. D.F. Hungler. B.P. (1989) *Essentials of nursing research* J.B.Lippincott, Pensylvania

Poulton. B.C. (1993) Effective multidisciplinary teamwork in primary health care. *Journal of advanced nursing* Vol 18, pp 918-925

Price. J. (1993) Joint account *Nursing times* Vol 89, No 13, pp 44-46

Price Waterhouse (1987) *Feasibility study into YTS in health and social care programmes. The final report.* Price Waterhouse, UK

Pritchard. P (1981) *Manual of primary health care* Oxford University Press,

Pritchard. P. (1984) How can we improve team working in primary care ?
The practitioner No 228, pp 1135-1139
Pritchard P. Pritchard J (1992) *Developing primary teamwork in primary health care :A practical workbook* Practical Guides for general practice No 15 Oxford Medical Publications, Oxford
Prwyes. M. (1983) The Beersheva experience : Integration of medical care and medical education. *Israel journal of medical sciences* Vol 19, pp 775-779
Purtilo. R. (1990) *Health professional and patient interaction*
W.B. Saunders Co, Philadelphia
Quataro. E.G. Hutchinson. R.R. (1976) Interdisicplinary education for community health : A case for nursing and social work collaboration. *Social work in health care* Vol 1, No 3, pp 347-356
Quinn. S.M. (1978a) Nursing -the EEC dimension (Part 1)
Nursing times Vol 74, No 1, Occasional paper pp 1-4
Quinn. S.M. (1978b) Nursing- the EEC dimension (Part 2)
Nursing times Vol 74, No 2, Occasional paper pp 5-8
Quinn. S.M. (1980a) The health professions in Europe.
1. The EEC directives. *Nursing focus* Vol 7, pp 431-432
Quinn. S.M. (1980b) The health professions in Europe
2. Nurses and midwives. *Nursing focus* Vol 8, pp 466-467
Quinn. S.M. (1980c) The health professions in Europe
3. Can we control our destiny ? *Nursing focus* Vol 9, pp 14-15
Quinn. S.M. (ed.) (1980d) *Nursing in the European Community*
Croom Helm, London
Quinn. S.M. (1989) *ICN : Past and present* Scutari Press, London
Quinn.S.M. Russell S. (eds) (1993) *Nursing : The European Dimension*
Scutari Press, London
Raisler. J. (1974) A better doctor nurse relationship *Nursing* No 4, pp 23-24
Ramos. M. Moore. G.T. (1987) *The new pathway to medical education*
Harvard Medical School, USA
Raphael. W. (1977) *Patients and their hospitals*
King Edwards Hospital Fund, London
Ratoff. L. Rose.A. Smith.C.R (1974) Social workers and G.P.'s
Social work today Vol 5, No 16, pp 497-500.
Reedy. B.L.E.C. (1981a) Discrepancies in the perceptions of a structural relationship for teamwork (No 1) *Nursing times* Vol 77, No 23, Occ. Paper
Reedy. B.L.E.C. (1981b) Discrepancies in the perceptions of a structural relationship for teamwork (No 2) *Nursing times* Vol 77, No 24, Occ. Paper
Renzulli J.S Smith L.H (1978) *Learning style inventory a measure of student preference for instructional techniques* Creative Learning Press, Connecticut

Reynolds. R.E. Bice. T.W. (1971) Attitudes of medical interns towards patients and health professionals.*Journal of health and social behavior* No 12, pp 307-311

Richards. R.Fulop. T. (1987) *Innovative schools for health personnel Report on 10 schools belonging to the NCOEIHS* WHO Offset publication No 102. Geneva

Richardson. I.M. (1977) Trainee Learning *Journal of the Royal College of General Practitioners* Vol 27, pp 666-667

Richardson. I.M. (1983) Undergraduate learning in general practice : The views of 1000 final year students *Journal of the Royal College of General Practitioners* Vol 33, pp 728-731

Ritter. S. (1989) *Manual of clinical psychiatric nursing principles and procedures* Harper Row, London

Robson. S. Foster. A. (1989) *Qualitative research in action* Hodder & Stoughton, London

Rogers. C. (1969) *Freedom to learn* Merrill Publishing Co. Ohio

Rosenaur. J.A. Fuller. D. (1973) Teaching strategies for interdisciplinary education *Nursing outlook* Vol 21, No 3, pp 159-162

Rosinski. E.F. (1965) Social classes of medical students *J.A.M.A.* No 7, pp 89

Rowbottom. R. Hey. A. (1978a) Collaboration between health and social services in Jaques. E. (ed.) *Health services, their nature organisation and the role of patients and doctors and health professions* Heinemann, London

Rowbottom. R. Hey. A. (1978b) The future of child guidance : A study in multidisciplinary teamwork. in Jaques. E. (ed.) *Health services, their nature organisation and the role of patients and doctorsand health professions* Heinemann, London

Rowbottom. R. Hey. A. (1978c) *Organisation of services for the mentally ill* BIOSS, Brunel University, Uxbridge

Royal College Of Nursing (1964) *A reform of nursing education (The Platt Report)* RCN, London

Royal College of Nursing (1974) *The state of nursing* RCN, London

Royal College of Nursing (1977) *A background to nursing in the EEC* Whitefriars Press, London

Royal College of Nursing (1985a) *The education of nurses : A new dispensation (The Judge Report)* RCN, London

Royal College of Nursing (1985b) *Annexe of research studies for the Commission on Nursing Education* RCN, London

Royal College of Nursing (1989) *Promoting professional excellence* RCN, London

Royal College of Nursing (1990) *The RMNH and the primary health care team* RCN, London

Runciman P. (1989) Health assessment of the elderly at home
Journal of advanced nursing No 14, pp 111-119
Rushmore. S. (1940) Nursing, nurses, doctors
New England journal of medicine No 222, pp 997-999
Salkind. M.R. Norell. J.S. (1980) Teaching about the primary care team :An experiment in vocational training *Journal of the Royal College of General Practitioners* Vol 30, pp 158-160
Salvage. J. (1989) The nurse practitioner in primary health care
King's Fund News Vol 12, No 3, pp 3-4
Samora. J. Saunders. L Larsen. R.F (1961) Medical vocabulary knowledge among hospital patients *Journal of health and human behaviour* No 2, pp 92
Samuel. O.V. Dodge. D. (1981) A course in collaboration for social workers and general practitioners.*Journal of Royal College of General Practitioners* Vol 31, pp 172-175
Sands. R.G. Stafford. J. McClelland. M. (1990) I beg to differ : Conflict in the interdisciplinary team *Social work in health care* Vol 14, No 3,
Satin D.G. (1987) The difficulties of interdisciplinary education : Lessons from three failures & a success *Educational gerontology* Vol 13, pp 53-69
Saunders. C.M. Caves. R.D. (1986) An empirical approach to the identification of communication skills with reference to speech therapists. *Journal of further and higher education* Vol 10, No 2, pp 29-44
Saunders. C. (1990) *Hospice and palliative care : An interdisciplinary approach* Edward Arnold, London
Schein. E.H. (1972) *Professional education : Some new directions*
McGraw Hill, New York
Schenk. F. (1979) A course on collaboration between social workers and general practitioners during their vocational training. *Medical education* Vol 13, pp 31-33
Schlotfeldt. R.M. (1965) The nurses view of the changing nurse/ physician relationship. *Journal of medical education* Vol 40, pp 772-777
Schreckenberger. P.C. (1970) Playing for the health team.
J.A.M.A. No 213, pp 279-281
Scott -Wright. M, (1976) *The relevance of multidisciplinary education in the health care team* Kings Fund Publications, London
Segall. A. Prwyes. M. Benor. D.E. Susskind. O (1978) An interim perspective in *Personnel for health care* WHO, Geneva
Seiga -Sur. J.L. Varona. Z.C (1987) Elements in the institutionalisation of the University of the Phillippines.in WHO *Innovative tracks* Geneva
Seto. W.H. (1989) The role of the alteration of patient care practices in hospital.*Journal of hospital infection* No 1 pp 29-37

Shakespeare.H. (1989) *Report of a national survey on interprofessional education in primary health care* The Institute of Community Studies, London

Sharf. B.F. Wood. B.S. Flaherty. J. (1982) Two birds with one stone : Training communication specialists while teaching medical students. *Communication education* Vol 31, pp 305-314

Sharf.B.F. Poirier. S. (1988) Exploring (un)common ground *Communication education* Vol 37, No 3, pp 224-236

Shaw. M. (1963) *Report on communications and relationships between general practitioners and hospital medical staff* King Edwards Hospital Fund, London

Shaw. M.C. (1970) *Communication processes* Penguin, London.

Shortell. S.M. (1974) Occupational prestige differences within the medical and allied health professions.*Social science and medicine* No 8, pp 1-9

Siedal. C. (1986) Part of the team *Nursing times* Vol 82, No 27, pp 64-66

Siegel. B. (1974) Organisation of the primary care team *Paediatric clinics of North America* No 21 pp 341-353

Silver. H.K. (1968) The use of new types of allied health professionals in providing care for children.*American journal of the disabled child* No 116, pp 486-490

Simon. H.A. (1961) *Administrative behavior : A study of decision making processes in administrative organisations* MacMillan, New York

Sines. D.(ed.)(1991) *Towards integration : Comprehensive services for people with mental handicaps* Lippincott Nursing Series, London

Singleton. A.F. (1981) Physician/nurse perceptions of styles of power usage. *Social science and medicine* No 15, pp 231-237

Smith M. (1993) Decubitus ulcers : A multidisciplinary view *Nursing standard* Vol 7, No 15, pp 25-28

Smith. S.J. Davis A.J. (1980) Ethical dilemmas : Conflict among rights, duties and obligations. *American journal of nursing* Vol 80, pp 1463-1466

Smith. V.M. Bass. T.A. (1982) *Communication for the health care team* Harper Row, London

Smoyak. S. (1987) Redefining roles. *Nursing times* Vol 83, No 4, pp 35-37

Snodgrass. J. (1966) Interprofessional stereotyping in the hospital *Nursing research* Vol 15, pp 350-354

Snyder. M. (1981) Preparation of nursing students for health care teams *International journal of nursing studies* Vol 18, No 2, pp 115-122

Sobral. D.T. Mejia. A. (1978) The medical school of Brasilia 1966-1976. in *Personnel for health care* WHO, Geneva

Society for Research in Higher Education (1977) *Interdisciplinarity* SRHE Ltd, University of Surrey, Guildford

Sommer. B. Sommer. R. (1991) *A practical guide to behavioral research* Oxford University Press, New York

South East Wales School of Radiography (1991) *B.Sc (Hons) Diagnostic Radiography* Document validated by the University of Wales.

South Glamorgan Health Authority (1990) *Quality Strategy* Cardiff

Spitzer. W.O. (1975) Issues for team delivery and interdisciplinary education : A Canadian perspective. *Journal of medical education* Vol 50, pp 117-121

Spruce. M.F. Snyder. F.J. (1982) An assessment of a micro counseling model for nurse training in facilitative interpersonal skills. *South African journal of psychology* Vol 12, No 3, pp 81-87

Stanfield. P.S. (1990) *Introduction to the health professions* Jones & Bartlett, Boston

Stanford. D. (1987) Nurse practitioner research : Issues in Practice and Theory. *Nurse practitioner* Vol 12, No 1, pp 64-75

Stanbrook. E. Wexler. M. (1956) The place of the behavioural sciences in the medical school. *Psychiatry* Vol 19, pp 263-269

Steel. J.E. (1981) Putting joint practice into practice *American journal of nursing* Vol 81, pp 964-967

Steele. R. (1987) *Peer learning in health science education : An alternative didactic method* WHO/EDUC/87/190 WHO, Geneva

Stein. L.I. (1967) The doctor/nurse game *Archives of general psychiatry* Vol 16, pp 699-703

Steinberg. D. (1989) *Interprofessional consultation* Blackwell Scientific, Kent

Stevenson. O. Hallet. C. (1980) *Aspects of interprofessional co-operation Child abuse : an interdisciplinary approach* Harvester Wheatsheaf, London

Stevenson O. Hallett C (1980) *Child Abuse : Aspects of interprofessional cooperation* Allen & Unwin, London

Stimson. G.V. Webb. B. (1975) *Going to see the doctor* Routledge, Kegan & Paul, London

Stotts. M.L. (1986) Teaching geriatrics away form the medical model *Education gerontology* Vol 12, No 1, pp 3-12

Strang. J.R. Caine. N. Acheson. R.M. (1983) Team care of elderly patients in general practice *British medical journal* Vol 4, No 286, pp 851-854

Streiner. D.L. Norman. G.R. (1991) *Health measurement scales* Oxford Medical. Oxford

Stroller. R.J. Geertsma. R.M. (1958) Measurement of medical students acceptance of emotionally ill patients. *Journal of medical education* Vol 33, pp 585-590

Styles. M. Gottdauk. M. (1978) Nursings vulnerability *American journal of nursing* Vol 12, pp 1978-1980

Sundstrom E De Meuse K P. Futrell D (1990) Work teams : Application & effectiveness *American Psychologist* Vol 45, pp 120-133

Susman. G. Evered. R. (1978) An assessment of the scientific merit of action research *Administrative science quarterly* Vol 23, pp 582-603

Swift. G. MacDougall. I.A. (1964) The family doctor and the family nurse. *British medical journal* Vol 1, No 5399, pp 1697-1699

Szasz. G. (1970) Education for the health team. *Canadian journal of public health* Vol 61, No 5, pp 386-390

Szasz. T.S. Hollander. M. (1956) A contribution to the philosophy of medicine : The basic models of the doctor/patient relationship. *American Medical Association Archives of Internal Medicine* No 97, pp 585

Tanner. L. Linn. M.W. Carmichael. L.P. (1972) An interdisciplinary student health team project in comprehensive family health care. *Journal of medical education* Vol 47, pp 656-661

Tanner. L.A. Soulary. E.J. (1972) Interprofessional student health teams. *Nursing outlook* Vol 20, No 2, pp 111-115

Tanner. O. (1991) Interdisciplinary pain management. *Nursing standard* Vol 5, No 52, pp 33-36

Taylor. C. (ed.) (1964) *Creativity : Progress and potential* McGraw Hill, New York

Temkin-Greener. H. (1983) Interprofessional perspectives on teamwork in health care. *Milbank Memorial Fund Quarterly* Vol 61, No 4, pp 641-658

Tesch. R. (1990) *Qualitative research* Falmer Press : London

Thompson. D.F. (1988) Attitudes of pharmacologists and nurses towards interprofessional relations and decentralised pharmaceutical services. *American journal of hospital pharmacists* Vol 45, No 2, pp 345-351

Thompson. R.F. (1988) Using an interdisciplinary team for geriatric education in a nursing home. *Journal of medical education* Vol 63, No 10, pp 796-798

Tigyi. J. (1978) A community oriented medical education programme at the Medical University of Pecs, Hungary in *Personnel for health care* WHO, Geneva

Tolliday. H. (1978) *Clinical Autonomy* Heinemann, London

Towle.A. (1991) *Critical thinking : The future of undergraduate medical education* King Edwards Hospital Fund, London

Treece.E.W. Treece.J.W. (1986) *Elements of research in nursing (4th Ed)* C.V. Mosby, Missouri

Trotter. B. (1992) Team spirit *Nursing times* Vol 88, No 28, pp 33-35

Trowell. J. (1992) Does interprofessional care matter in child protection? *Journal of interprofessional studies* Vol 6, No 2, pp 103-109

Turnbull. E.N. (1981) Health care issues as an interdisciplinary course *Nursing outlook* No 1, pp 42-45

Turnbull. E.N. (1982) Interdisciplinarism : problems and promises. *Journal of nursing education* Vol 21, No,2, pp 24-31

Turner. B.S. (1990) The interdisciplinary curriculum from social medicine to post modernism. *Sociology of health and illness* Vol 12, No 1, pp 1-23

Turrell. E.A. (1986) *Change and innovation : A challenge for the NHS* Institute of Health Services Management, London

Uhlemann. M.R. Stone. G.L. Evans. D.R. (1982) Evaluation of microtraining modifications: implications for paraprofessional trainining within community counselling agencies.*Canadian counsellor* Vol 16, No 2, pp 115-121

Ulin. P.R. (1989) Global collaboration in primary health care *Nursing outlook* Vol 37, No 3, pp 134-137

United Kingdom Central Council for Nursing, Midwifery and Health Visiting (1992) *Code of professional conduct for the nurse, midwife and health visitor (3rd edition)* UKCC, London

UKCC (1987) *Confidentiality : An elaboration of Clause 9* UKCC, London

UKCC (1992) *Personal communication*

Vachon. M.L.S. Lyall. W.A.L. Freeman. S.J.T (1978) Measurement and management of stress in health professionals working with cancer patients. *Death education* Vol 1, No 4, pp 365-375

Vachon. M.L.S. (1978) Motivation and stress experienced by staff working with the terminally ill. *Death education* Vol 2, No 1, pp 113-122

Valle. F.C. Siordia. E.V. Wood. H.G. Carnicer. J.V De La Vega. A.R. Garcia. L.C Durazo. A.L. Silva. P.M. (1987) The general integrated medical program. National Autonomous University of Mexico. in *Innovative tracks for health personnel* WHO, Geneva

Van Dalen. J. (1989) The curriculum of communication skills teaching at Maastricht medical school.*Medical education* Vol 1, pp 55-61

Van Der Merwe. N. (1989) Teaching effective communication on ward rounds *South African medical journal* Vol 76, No 2, p 4-7

Vaughan. Morrow. (1989) *Manual of epidemiology for district health management*

Verby. J. Holden. P Davis. R.H.. (1979) Peer review of consultations in primary care : The use of audio visual recordings. *British medical journal* Vol 2, No 72, pp 1686-1688

Verma. D.K. (1988) Multi-disciplinary, problem based self directed learning in occupational health. *Journal of the society of occupational medicine* Vol 38, No 4, pp 101-104

Von Schilling. K. (1982) The consultant role in multi-disciplinary team development. *International nursing review* Vol 29, No 3, pp 73-75, 96

Wallace. L. (1966) Educational functions of occupational therapy in a multi-disciplinary university based home care program. *American journal of occupational therapy* Vol 20, No 6, pp 286-287

Walsh. W.J. (1978) Developing problem solving abilities : The McMaster programme of medical education, Hamilton, Ontario. in *Personnel for health care* WHO, Geneva

Ward. A.W.M. (1974) Telling the patient. *Journal of the Royal College of General Practitioners* Vol 24, pp 465-468

Ward. C.G. (1979) Burn care : A multi-disciplinary speciality *Quality review bulletin* No 5, pp 2-3

Ward. N.G. Stein. L. (1975) Reducing emotional distance : A new method to teach interviewing skills. *Journal of medical education_* No 50, pp 605

Waters. W.H.R. Sandeman. J.M Lunn. J.E. (1980) A four year prospective study of the work of the practice nurse in the treatment room of a South Yorkshire practice *British medical journal* Vol 2, No 80, pp 87-89

Watts. M. (1988) *Shared Learning* Royal College of Nursing, Research Series, Scutari Press, London

Watts. P.R. (1977) Evaluation of a death attitude change resulting from a death education instructional unit. *Death education* Vol 1, No 2, pp 187-193

Webster. D. (1985) Medical students views of the role of the nurse *Nursing research* No 34, pp 313-317

Webster. D. (1988) Medical students and nurses. *Nursing outlook* Vol 36, No 3, pp 130-135

Webster. T.G. (1967) Psychiatry and behavioral science curriculum time in US schools of medicine and osteopathy. *Journal of medical education* Vol 42, No 6, pp 687-696

Weil. T.P. Parrish. H.M. (1967) Development of a co-ordinated approach for the training of health personnel. *Journal of medical education* Vol 42, No 6, pp 651-659

Weinberger. L.E. Millham. J. (1975) A multidimensional, multiple method analysis of attitudes towards the elderly *Journal of gerontology* Vol 75, No 30, pp 343-348

Weiss. C.H. (1975) *Interviewing in evaluation research* Sage Publications, Beverly Hills

Welsh Office (1983) *All Wales Strategy for the development of services for mentally handicapped people* Welsh Office, Cardiff

Welsh Office (1987) *Nursing in the community : A team approach for Wales.* Welsh Office, Cardiff

Welsh Office (1988) *The corporate management programme for the health service in Wales. Development and change 1988-1993* Welsh Office, Cardiff

Welsh Office (1989a) *Caring for People : Community care in the next decade and beyond. The proposals for Wales* Welsh Office, Cardiff

Welsh Office (1989b) *Strategic intent and direction for the NHS in Wales* Welsh Health Planning Forum, Welsh Office, Cardiff

Welsh Office (1989c) *Local strategies for health : A new approach to strategic planning.* Welsh Health Planning Forum, Welsh Office, Cardiff

Welsh Office (1989d) *The health service in Wales : Towards 2000 Manpower planning, education and training* Welsh Office, Cardiff

Welsh Office (1990a) *A quality health service for Wales* Welsh Office, Cardiff

Welsh Office (1990b) *Protocol for investment in health gain : Cancers* Welsh Health Planning Forum, Welsh Office, Cardiff

Welsh Office (1990c) *Guidance on social care plans* Doc/SHM/3-18-6. Welsh Office, Cardiff

Welsh Office (1991a) *NHS Wales : Agenda for Action 1991-1993* Welsh Office, Cardiff

Welsh Office (1991b) *Managing care : Guidance on assessment and the provision of social and community care* Welsh Office, Cardiff

Welsh Office (1991c) *People : Personnel principles for NHS Wales* Welsh Office, Cardiff

Wessell. M.A. (1981) Learning about interdisciplinary collaboration *Journal of nursing education* Vol 20, No 3, pp 39-44

Wessen. A.F (1966) Hospital ideology and communication between ward personnel. *Medical care* pp 458-475

Westbrook. M. (1978) Professional stereotypes : How occupational therapists and nurses perceive themselves and each other. *Australian occupational therapists journal* Vol 25, No 12, pp 613-619

Whitehouse. C.R. (1986) Conflict and co-operation between doctors and nurses in primary health care.*Nurse Practitioner* Vol 1, No 4, pp 242-245

Willcocks. A. (1979) Weakness of consultation *Health and social services journal* Vol LXXXIX No 4639, pp 481

Willer. B. Ross. M Intagliata. J. (1980) Medical school education in mental retardation *Journal of medical education* Vol 55, No 7 pp 589-594

Williams. C.C. Bracht. N.F. Williams. R.A. (1978) Social work and nursing in hospital settings : A study of interprofessional experiences *Social work health care_* No 3, pp 311-322

Williams. P Clare. A. (1982) Social workers in primary health care : The general practitioners viewpoint. *Social work and primary health care* London

Williams. R.A. Williams. C. (1982) Hospital social workers and nurses : Interprofessional perceptions and experiences. *Journal of nursing education* Vol 21, No 5, pp 16-21

Wilson. C. (1982) Patient oriented management *Health management forum* No 3, pp 40-57

Wise. H. (1974) Making health teams work *American journal of the disabled child* No 537, pp 1974-1977

Wise. H.Beckhard. R. Rubin. I. Kyte. A. (1974) *Making health teams work* Ballinger, Cambridge, USA

Wiseman. J.P. Aron. M.S. (1972) *Field projects in sociology* Transworld Student Library, Massachusetts

Woodruff. D. Birren. V. (1975) *Ageing : Social Perspectives and social issues* Van Nostrand, New York

World Health Organisation (1973a) *Continuing education for physicians* Technical Report Series No 534 WHO, Geneva

WHO (1973b) *Training and preparation of teachers for schools of medicine and allied health sciences* Technical Report Series, No 521 WHO, Geneva

WHO (1976) *Health manpower development* Doc/ A29/15 (unpublished) Presented at 29th World Health Assembly

WHO (1977) *Criteria for the evaluation of learning objectives in the education of health personnel* Technical Report Series, No 608 WHO, Geneva

WHO (1978a) *Primary Health Care. Report of the International Conference on primary health care The Alma Ata Declaration* Health for All Series No 1, WHO, Geneva

WHO (1978b) *Guidelines for evaluating a training programme for health personnel* WHO, Geneva

WHO (1978c) *Personnel for health care : Case studies of educational programmes* Public Health Paper Vol 1, No 70 WHO, Geneva

WHO (1979a) *Continuing education of health personnel and its evaluation* WHO, Geneva

WHO (1979b) *Primary health care in Europe* Euro. Report No 14, WHO, Geneva

WHO (1979c) *Training and utilisation of auxillary personnel for rural health teams in developing countries* Technical Report Series, No 633 WHO, Geneva

WHO (1981a) *Global strategy for health for all by the year 2000* Health for All - Series No 3 WHO, Geneva

WHO (1981b) *Teamwork for primary health care* Doc/SEA/HSD/20 WHO, New Delhi

WHO (1983) *Primary health care in undergraduate medical education* WHO, Copenhagen

WHO (1983) *Graduate medical education in the European Region* Euro. Reports and Studies, No 77 WHO, Geneva

WHO (1984a) *The role of Universities in the strategies for health for all* Technical discussions 11-12 May 1984 Doc. A/37/ Tec. Discussion/3 WHO, Geneva

WHO (1984b) *Nurses and physicians of tomorrow : A world wide survey on professional roles and their use as a basis for educational programmes* Unpublished Doc. WHO/EDUC/84.183 WHO, Geneva
WHO (1984c) *Multidisciplinary undergraduate education for the professions. Some aspects of how and why* Report ICP/HMD 103 MO2/6 4323E WHO, Copenhagen
WHO (1985a) *Targets for health for all* WHO, Copenhagen
WHO (1985b) *Training for primary health care* Report on Tech. Discussions EUR/RC34 WHO, Geneva
WHO (1985c) *Contribution of psychology to programme development in the WHO* ICP/PSF 199m04 WHO, Geneva
WHO (1986a) *Leadership for health for all : The challenge to nursing A strategy for action* WHO/HMD/NUR/86.1WHO, Geneva
WHO (1986b) *Targets for health for all : Implications for nursing/ midwifery* Nursing/Euro 86.1. 80171 WHO, Geneva
WHO (1986c) *Multiprofessional education of health personnel in th European Region* Unpublished Doc. EURO/KP/HMD/136 (S) WHO, Copenhagen
WHO (1986d) *Intersectoral action for health : The role of international co-operation in national strategies for health for all* WHO, Geneva
WHO (1987a) *Peer learning in health science education : An alternative didactic method* WHO/EDUC/87/190
WHO (1987b) *Innovative schools for health personnel. Report on 10 schools belonging to the NCOEIHS* WHO Offset Publication No 102, Geneva
WHO (1987c) *Innovative tracks at established institutions for the education of health personnel :An experimental approach to change relevant health needs.* WHO Offset Publication No 101 WHO, Geneva
WHO (1987d) *The role of intersectoral co-operation in combating inequities in health in national strategies for health for all* ICP/HSR/816 WHO, Geneva
WHO (1987e) *Community based education of health personnel* WHO Technical Report Series No 746 WHO, Geneva
WHO (1987f) *The community health worker : Working guide, guidelines for training, guidelines for adaptation* WHO, Geneva
WHO (1987g) *Education handbook for health personnel (revised edition)* WHO Offset Publication, No 35 WHO, Geneva
WHO (1987h) *Information exchange and collaboration in health related activities in Europe* ICP/COR/112, WHO, Geneva
WHO (1988a) *The role of nursing and midwifery personnel in the strategy for health for all* EB83/6 WHO, Geneva
WHO (1988b) *Learning together to work together for health* Technical Report Series No 769, WHO, Geneva

WHO (1988c) *Review of the need for a college of health sciences* Assignment Report -Project No 1, CXP/4 MD/003 WHO, Geneva
WHO (1988d) *European nursing : A major force for change* ICP/HSR 329/5 1530V WHO, Geneva
WHO (1988e) *European Conference on Nursing* EUR/ICP/HSR 329(S) 6694. N.WHO, Geneva
WHO (1988f) *Study group on multiprofessional education Learning to work together for health : The team approach* WHO Technical Report Series, No 769 WHO, Geneva
WHO (1988g) *Megatrends affecting the reorientation of nursing in Europe* ICP/HSR 329/8 WHO, Geneva
WHO (1988h) *Interaction between health and social services and the public in the provision of health care* EUR/ICP/PHC 330, WHO, Geneva
WHO (1988i) *Multiprofessional of health personnel in the European Region* EUR/ICP/HMD 136, WHO, Geneva
WHO (1989a) *Nursing in primary health care : Ten years after Alm Ata and perspectives for the future* HMD/NUR/ 89.1, WHO Geneva
WHO (1989b) *Summary Report : First meeting of Government Chief Nursing Officers and WHO Collaborating Centres on the implications of health for all targets for nursing and midwifery* EUR/ICP/HSR 334 (S) 3639R WHO, Geneva
WHO (1989c) *Specialised medical education in the European Region* Euro. Reports and Studies, No 112, WHO, Geneva
WHO (1989d) *Intersectoral action : Practical augumentation and mechanisms* EUR/ICP/MPN 016 WHO, Geneva
WHO (1989e) *Psychosocial interventions in primary health care settings in Europe* EUR/ICP/PSF 020 WHO, Copenhagen
WHO (1991a) *Health for all : The nursing mandate* Health for all nursing series No1, WHO, Copenhagen
WHO (1991b) *Missions and functions of the nurse* Health for all nursing series No 2, WHO, Copenhagen
WHO (1991c) *The nursing in action project* Health for all nursing series No 3, WHO, Copenhagen
Wright. S. (1985) New nurses : New boundaries *Nursing practice* No 1, pp 32-39
Xue-Min. L Yi. Fei. W. (1987) The problem oriented basic medical science curriculum track, Shanghai University, China in WHO (1987) *Innovative tracks for health personnel*, WHO, Geneva
Yalof. I. (1979) The multidisciplinary team : An effective approach to the management of cardiac surgery patients. *Heart and Lung* Vol 8, pp 699-705
Yeaworth. R. Fern. M. (1973) Interdisciplinary education as an influence system *Nursing outlook* Vol 21, No 11, pp 696-699

Young. G.L. (1993) Evolution not revolution *Nursing standard* Vol 7, No 28 pp 20-21

Youngman. M.B. (1978) *Designing and analysing questionnaires* Rediguide 12, School of Education,University of Nottingham, UK

Youngman. M.B. (1979) *Analysing social and educational research data* McGraw Hill, London

Youngman. M.B. (1982) *Presenting research results* Rediguide 25, School of Education University of Nottingham, UK

Youngman. M.B. (1986) *Analysing questionnaires* School of Education, University of Nottingham, UK

Youngman. M.B.(ed.) (undated) *Chi squared and contingency tables* Rediguide 31, School of Education University of Nottingham, UK

Zangwill. H. (1980) *Behaviour modification : Report of the Joint Working Party Appendix IX, Legal Responsibility* Royal College of Physicians, Royal College of Nursing and the British Psychological Society

Bibliography

Acheson. D. (1972) Southampton - Some first year experiences. *British medical journal* No 2, pp 166-170

Agich. G. (1982) *Responsibility in health care* Reidel Boston, New York

Akinsanya. J.A.(1990) Nursing links with higher education :A prescription for change in the 21st Century. *Journal of advanced nursing* Vol 15, pp 744-754

Alaszewski. A.(1977) Occupational therapy - Case study of a professional strategy. *Health and social services journal* Vol CLXXXVIII, No 4562, pp B5-B8

Allport. G.(1954) *The nature of prejudice* Addison-Wesley, Massechussets.

Anderson. O.J. Finn. M.C.(1983) Collaborative practice: Developing a structure that works. *Nursing administration quarterly* Vol 8, No 3, pp 19-25

Ansell. P. (1992) *Shared learning in health visitor education.* Unpublished Ph.D. Thesis University of Manchester

Anson. E. Lynch. J. Fawcett-Henesy. A. (1988) From the other side of the fence. *Community care* 28/4/88 pp 20-21

Archer. S.E. Kelly. C.D. Bisch. S.A. (1984) *Implementing change in communities: A collaborative process* C.V. Mosby, St Louis.

Argyle. M. (ed.) (1981) *Social skills and health.* Methuen, London

Armstrong. D. (1976)The decline of medical hegemony :A review of Government reports during the NHS. *Social science and medicine* Vol 10, pp 157-163

Bach. C.A. (1979) Who teaches foundations in an integrated curriculum ? *Nursing outlook,* Vol 27, pp 112-115

Baric. L.(1990) The new approach to community participation. *Journal of the Institute of Health Education* Vol 28, No 2, pp 41-52

Barrows. H.S. Tamblyn R.M.(1976a) An evaluation of problem based learning in small groups utilising a simulated patient. *Journal of medical education.* Vol 51, No 1, pp 52-54.

Barrows. H.S. Tamblyn. R.M. (1976b) Self assessment units *Journal of medical education* Vol 51, No 4, pp 334-336

Barrows. H.S. Tamblyn. R.M (1980) *Problem based learning : An approach to medical education* Springer, New York.

Bassoff. B.Z.(1983) Interdisciplinary education as a facet of health education policy : The impact of attitudinal research. *Journal of Allied Health.* No 12, pp 280-286

Berger. A. Schaffer. S. (1986) An interdisciplinary continuity of care experience for pre clinical medical students. *Journal of medical education* Vol 61, No 9, pp 771-773Bergman. R. Stockler. R Gilad. Z. (1971) Opinion on nursing. *International nursing review* Vol 18, No 3, pp 195-230

Billups. J.O. (1987) Interprofessional team process *Theory into practice* Vol 26, No 2, pp 146-152

Brandt. P.A.(1989) Preparation of clinical nurse specialists *Infants and young children* Vol 3, No 1, pp 51-62

Brooke. R.I. Fischman. D.M. Drinnan. A.J. (1972) An integrated course in human disease *The New York State dental journal* Vol 38, No 4, pp 203-206

Brown. C.A. (1973) The division of labourers : The allied health professions. *International journal of health services.* Vol 3, No 3, pp 435-444

Bucher. R. Strauss. A.L. (1961) Professions in practice *American journal of sociology* Vol 66, pp 325-334

Burnard. P.(1986) Integrated self awareness training A holistic model. *Nurse education today* Vol 6, No 5, pp 219-222

Burrows. S. (1989) A strategy for curriculum integration of information skills instruction. *Bulletin of Medical Libraries Association* Vol 77, No 3, pp 89

Butterworth. A. (1984) The future training of psychiatric and general nurses. *Nursing times* Vol 80, No 30, pp 65-66

Cassidy. R.C.(1983) Teaching biopsychoethical medicine in a family practice clerkship *Journal of medical education* Vol 58, No 10, p 778-783

Chacko. T. I. Wong. J.K. (1984) Correlates of role conflict between physicians and nurse practitioners. *Psychological reports* Vol 54, No 3, pp 783-789

Chant. A. (1989) *The stem doctor* Western Printing Co. Southampton

Charmaz. K. (1986) Social science in health studies : An interdisciplinary approach. *Sociology of health and illness* Vol 8, No 3,

Chartier. L.(1984) Une experience de formation a interdisciplinarite. *L'Infirmiere Canadienne* Vol 81, No 7, pp 10-15

Chester. T.E. (1975) European health and hospital care *International series No 12* Ravenswood Publications, Kent.

Christopherson. A. Pretty. J (1986) Learning to communicate *Senior nurse* Vol 4, No 6, pp 20-22

Clearage. D.K. (1984) An integrated curriculum : Idealism or pragmatism ? *Journal of nurse education* No 7, pp 308-310

Clegg. F. (1982) *Simple statistics : A course book for the social sciences* Cambridge University Press, Cambridge.

Colby. K.K. (1986) Problem based learning of social sciences and humanities by fourth year medical students. *Journal of medical education* Vol 61, No 5, pp 413-415

Coombes. R.B. Rana. S.C (1981) An integrated SRN/RMN course : A future for nurse training. *Nursing times* Vol 77, No 12, Occasional paper pp 45-48

Coombes. R.B. Rana. S.C. (1981) An integrated SRN/RMN course A survey : What happens to integrated nurses? *Nursing times* Vol 77, No 13, Occasional paper.

Connelly. T. (1978) Basic organisational considerations for interdisciplinary education development in the health sciences . *Journal of allied health* Vol 4, pp 274-280

Critchley. B Casey. D. (1984) Second thoughts on team building. *Management, education and development* Vol 15, No 2, pp 163-175

Croen. L.G. Hamerman.D (1984) Interdisciplinary training for medical and nursing students : Learning to collaborate in the care of geriatric patients. *Journal of the American Geriatrics Society.* Vol 32, No 1, pp 56-61.

Davis. B.D. (1983) *Perceptions by nurses, doctors, physiotherapists of pre-operative information giving.* Nursing Research Unit, Univ. of Edinburgh

Davis. B.D. (1984a) *Pre-operative information giving and patients post operative outcomes : An implementation study* Nursing Research Unit, Univ.of Edinburgh

Davis. B.D. (1984b) *Study of patients fears and worries* Nursing Research Unit, Univ. of Edinburgh

Davis. F. (1964) Baccalaureate students images of nursing *Nursing research* Vol 13, pp 8-15

Davis. L.L (1986) The politics of interdisciplinary collaborationin professonal practice. *Journal of professional nursing* Vol 2, No 4, pp 206, 266.

Dodge. J.S. (1969) Factors relating to patients perceptions of their cognitive needs. *Nursing research,* Vol 18, No 6, pp 31-35

Dowie. R. (1987) *Postgraduate medical education and training : The system in England and Wales* King Edwards Hospital Fund, London

Downie. N.M. Heath. R.W.(1974) *Basic statistical methods* Harper International, London

Draper. J. Farmer. S. Field. S. (1984a) The working relationship between the health visitor and the community midwife. *Health visitor* Vol 57, pp 366-368

Draper. J. Farmer. S. Field. S. (1984b) The working relationship between the general practitioner and the health visitor. *Journal of the Royal College of General Practitioners* Vol 34, pp 264-268

Drinkwater. C.K. (1972) Vocational training for general practice :A comparison of the views of trainees and teachers. *British medical journal* No 4 pp 96-98

Dunkin. E.N. (1982) *Psychology for physiotherapists* Macmillan, London

Dyer. W.G. (1977) *Team building : Issues and Alternatives* Addison Wesley, Mass.

Earl. F.A. (1980) Working group A Multidisciplinary health care and education .*Journal of medical education* Vol 55, No 14, pp 68

Edwards. J. Gastrell. P. (1991) A common core. *Primary health care* No 2, pp 28-29

Ellis. R. (ed.) (1988) *Professional competence and quality assurance in the caring professions.* Croom Helm, London.

England. H. (ed.) (1980) Education for co-operation in health and social work. *Journal of the Royal College of General Practitioners.* Occasional Paper 14.

England. H. (1984) Working relationships : A workshop for increasing mutual understanding in socialwork, general practice and health visiting *Trainee* September 1984, pp 100-104

Evans. R.L .(1984) The resource manager in physical rehabilitation. *Rehabilitation literature* Vol 45, No 1, pp 2.

Flood. A.B. Scott. W.R. (1978) Professional powers and professional effectiveness :The power of the surgical staff and quality of surgical care in hospital . *Journal of health and social behavior* Vol 19, pp 240-254

Foss. B. (ed.) (1966) *New horizons in psychology* Penguin, Harmondsworth.

Fransella. F. (1982) *Psychology for occupational therapists* Macmillan, London

Freidson. E. (1970) *Profession of medicine* Dodd, Mead & Co. New York.

Fox. R. (1981) The sting of death in American society. *Social service review* pp 42-59

Fuller. D.S. Quesada. G.M.(1973) Communication in medical therapeutics. *Journal of communication* Vol 23, No 12, pp 361-370

Garrett. G. (1988)Teamwork : An equal partnership ? *The professional nurse* Vol 4, pp 259-262

Gay. L. (1976) *Educational research:Competencies for analysis and application* C. E. Merrill, Columbus.

Gearing. B. Johnson. M. Heller. J. (eds) (1988) *Mental health problems in old age* Wiley, Chichester.
Gellhorn. A. Schever. R. (1978) The experiment in medical education at the City College of New York *Journal of medical education* Vol 53, No 7, pp 574-582
Gilhespy. N. (1991) Part of the team or some sort of threat ? *Nursing times* Vol 87, No 12, pp 31-32
Gillis. C.L. (1983) Collaborative practice in the hospital : Whats in it for nursing? *Nursing Administration* Summer 1983
Golden. A.S. Carlson. D.G. Harris. B. (1973) Non physician health teams for health maintenance organisations. *American journal of public health* No 63, pp 732
Grady. C.(1984) In defence of the integrated curriculum. *Journal of nursing education* Vol 23, No 7, pp 322-323
Grau. L. (1986) Britains community psychiatric nursing teams *Geriatric nursing* Vol 3, pp 143-146
Green. M. (1988) Planning for change in education. *British journal of occupational therapy* Vol 51, No 3, pp 88
Greenfield. H.L. Brown. C.A (1969 *) Allied health manpower:Trends and prospects* Columbia Univ. Press, New York
Griffiths. D. (1981) *Psychology and medicine* British psychological society, Leicester
Grove. E. (1988) Working together *British journal of occupational therapy* Vol 51, No 5, pp 150-156
Hall. J. (1982) *Psychology for nurses and health visitors* Macmillan, London
Hall. M. (1980) An account of two in service courses *Journal of Royal College of General Practitioners* Occasional paper 14, pp 21-23
Hall . T. (1965) Experiment in co-operation *The Lancet* Vol 1, No 7399, p 1325-1327
Halmos. P. (1965) *The faith of the counsellors* Constable, London
Hamer. S. (1992) Nursing in Europe : What 1992 has to offer. *British journal of nursing* Vol 1, No 1, pp 32-35
Hammersley. R. Don Read. J. (1986) What is integration ? Remembering a story and remembering false implications about the story. *British journal of psychology* Vol 77, pp 329-341
Harbaugh.G.L. Casto. R.M. Burgess-Ellison. J.A. (1987) Becoming a professional : How interprofessional training helps *Theory into practice* Vol 26, No 2, pp 141-145
Harris. J.L. Saunders. D.N. Zasorin- Connors. J. (1976) A training programme for interprofessional healthcare teams. *Health and social work* Vol 3, pp 35-53
Harris. J.L. (1978) Interdisciplinary health education : A case study of fact and fancy. *Journal of community health* Vol 3, No 4, pp 357-368

Heaney. R.P. (1975) Integration of health professions education *American journal of pharmaceutical education* Vol 39, No 4, pp 440-445

Hertz. C.G. Williams. H. Hutchins. E.B. (1976) Clinical curriculum setting *Journal of medical education* Vol 51, No 3, pp 22-25

Hipps. O.S. (1981) The integrated curriculum : The emperor is naked *Amercian journal of nursing* Vol 81, No 5, pp 976-980

Holm. K. Llewellyn. J.G. (1986) *Nursing research for nursing practice* W B Saunders, Philadelphia

Hollm.C. Trower.P (eds) (1986) *Social skills training for health professionals* Pergamon, Oxford

Horwitz. J. (1970) *Team practice and the specialist* Charles Thomas, Springfield.

Hubbard. R .(1989) Medical career destroyed by the Hippocratic curse *Sunday Times* Section F3 18/6/1989

Humphries. D. (1988) Team working : Breaking down the barriers *Nursing* Vol 3, No 27, pp 999-1001

Hunt. J. Macleod Clark. J. (1981) *Communication in patient care* King Edwards Hospital Fund, London

Hunt. S. (1990) Building alliances : professional and political issues in community participation. Examples from a health and community development project. *Health promotion international* Vol 5, No 3, pp 179-185

Ingmire. A.E. Blansfield. M.G.(1967) A development programme for the hospital team *Nursing forum* Vol 6, No 4, pp 382-398

Irwin. W.G.(1988) Multidisciplinary teaching in a formal medical ethics course for clinical students. *Journal of medical ethics* Vol 14, No 3, pp 125-128

Irwin. W.G. (1989) Communication skills training for medical students : An integrated approach. *Medical education* Vol 23, No 4, pp 387-394

Jacobsen-Webb. M.L. (1985) Increasing team skills : An evaluation of programme effectiveness. *Journal of allied health* Vol 14, No 4, pp 387- 394.

Jessett. D.F. (1976) *Chiropody training and the concept of the College of Health* Unpublished M.Ed Dissertation, University of Bristol

Johnson. T. (1972) *Professions and power* Macmillan, London

Kappeli. S. (1991) Good nursing care : Under what conditions and at what price? *Hoitotiede* Vol 3, No 5, pp 189-199

Kerr. J.F. (1968) *Changing the curriculum* University of London Press, London

Keyzer. D. (1986) Two's company *Nursing times* Vol 82, No 36, pp 57-59

King. D. (1990) Teamwork in primary care *Nursing* Vol 8, No 6, pp 36-37

Klinger. M. (1980) An account of two experiments for students in training *Journal of the Royal College of General Practitioners* Occasional Paper 14, pp 19-21

Knopke. H.J. Diekelmann. N.L. (1978) *Approaches to teaching in the health sciences* Addison Wesley, London

Korsch. B. Negreti. V.F. (1972) Doctor patient communication *Scientific American* No 227, pp 66-75

Krevans. J.R. Condliffe. B. (1970) *Reform of medical education* Macmillan, London

Kronus. C.L. (1976) The evolution of occupational power *Sociology of work and occupations* Vol 3, No 1, pp 3-37

Kuhn. A. Wolpe. A.M. (1978) *Feminism and materialism : Women and modes of production* Routledge, Kegan & Paul, London

Laquillo. E. (1988) Home care services as teaching sites for geriatrics in family medicine residencies. *Journal of medical education* Vol 63, No 9, pp 667- 674 *Nursing* Vol 4, No 33, pp13-15

Lenburg.C.B. (1975) *Openess and mobility in nursing education* C.V. Mosby, St Louis

Levitt. R. (1975) Attitudes of hospital patients. *Nursing times* Vol 71, No 41, pp 497-499

Lewis. P. (1984) *Multidisciplinary teams : A discussion paper* (unpublished). North Western Regional Health Authority.

Lichter. I. (1987) *Communication in cancer care* Churchill Livingstone, Edinburgh

Liftshitz. M. (1974) Quality professionals -does training make a difference? *British journal of social and clinical psychology* No 13, pp 183-189

Lloyd. G. Borland. M. Thwaites. M. Waddicor. P. (1973) An interdisciplinary workshop *Journal of the Royal College of General Practitioners* Vol 23, No 11, pp 463-473

Lorensen.M.(1984) *Studies on communication and collaboration between health professionals* Paper given at a conference - Nursing research, does it make a difference ? 13th April 1984, London

Loxley. A. (1980) A multidisicplinary in - service training in the interests of health care *Social work service* No 24, pp 35-52

Lyne. P. (1990) Talent waiting to be tapped. *The health service journal* Vol 4, No 12, pp 31

Lysaught. J.P.(ed.) (1970) National commission for the study of nursing and nursing education Report *American journal of nursing* Vol 70, No 6, pp 553-561

McClymont. A. (1984) *Teaching for reality* English National Board for Nursing, Midwifery and Health Visiting, London

McGuire. C.H.(ed.) (1983) *Handbook on health professions education* Jossey Bass, San Francisco

McMahon. B. (1989) Teamwork- A complete service with specialist *The professional nurse* Vol 11, No 6, pp 433-435

MacDonald. G. (1964)Baccalaureate education for graduates of diploma and associated degree programmes *Nursing outlook* Vol 12, No 6, pp 52-56

Madsen. M.K. (1988) An interdisciplinary clinic *Journal of allied health* Vol 17, No 2, pp 135-141

Malin. N. (ed.) (1987) *Reassessing community care* Routledge, London

Mann. C.J.H. (1966) *An experiment in communication between G.Ps and hospital staff* Oxford University Press

Marshall. C. (1985) Appropriate criteria for trustworthiness and goodness for qualitative research on education organisations *Quality and Quantity* No 19, pp 353-373

Marshall. M. Preston-Shoot. M. Winicott. E.(1979) *Teamwork : For and against* BASW publications, Birmingham

Mason. S.A. (1979) The multi hospital movement defined *Public health reports* No 94, pp 446-453

Matteson. M.T. Smith. S.V. (1977) Selection of medical specialities, preferences versus choices. *Journal of medical education* Vol 52, No 8, pp 548-554

Metcalfe. D. (1980) An education for practice. *Journal of the Royal College of GeneralPractitioners* Occasional Paper 14, pp 15-19

Miller. G.E. (1962) *Teaching and learning in medical school* Harvard University Press, Cambridge, Mass.

Moores. B. Thompson. AGH (1986) What 1357 hospital patients think about aspects of their stay in British acute hospitals. *Journal of advanced nursing* Vol 11, No 1, pp 87-102

Morgan. W.L. Engel. G.L. (1969) *The clinical approach to the patient* WB Saunders, Philadelphia.

Morrill. R.G. (1972) A new mental health services model for the comprehensive neighborhood health center *American journal of public health* No 68, pp1108

Mortimer.E. (1980) Interdisciplinary learning at the qualifying and post qualifying stages. *Journal of the Royal College of GeneralPractitioners* Occasional Paper 14, pp 15-17

Mullen P.D. (1988) Selected allied health professionals self confidence *Journal of allied health* Vol 17, No 2, pp 123-133

Murdock. J.E. (1978) Regrouping for an allied curriculum *Nursing outlook* Vol 26, No 8, pp 514-519

NHS Management Executive (1990) *Nursing in the community* Report of the working group

Nicholls. A. (1983) *Managing educational innovations* Unwin, London

Noack. H.(ed.) (1980) *Medical education and primary health care* Croom Helm, London

Oaker. G. Brown. R. (1986) Intergroup relations in a hospital setting : A further test of identity theory. *Human relations* Vol 39, No 8, pp 767-778

Palmore. E. (1979) Predictors of successful aging *The gerentologist* Vol 19, pp 427-431

Parkin. D.M. (1976) Survey of the success of communication between hospital staff and patients *Public health* No 90, pp 203-209

Patterson. M. Hayes. S.O. (1977) Verbal communication between students in multidisciplinary teams *Journal of medical education* Vol 52, No 3, pp 205-210

Payne. S. (1972) Atlas of a health team *Health visitor* Vol 45, No 3, pp 69

Pfeifle. W.G. Lacefield. W.E. Cole. H.P. (1981) Motivational factors in the careers of health care educators *Journal of allied health* 10, No 2, pp 73-90

Pine. G.J. Horne. P.J (1969) *Principles and conditions for learning in adult education* October 1969, pp 108-134

Poole. D.L. Wilson. F. (1975) Integrated teach-ins *Nursing times* Vol 71, No 33, pp 1310-1311

Poulton. B. (1991) Does your team really work? *Primary health care* Vol 11, No 2, pp 11-14

Porrit. L. (1990) *Interaction strategies : An introduction for health professionals* Churchill Livingstone, London

Prospect Centre (1989) *A first degree in health care in the National Health Service* Prospect Centre, London

Purser. H. (1982) *Psychology for speech therapists* Macmillan, London

Purtillo. R.B. Cassel. C.K.(1981) *Ethical dimensions in the health professions* WB Saunders, Philadelphia.

Quinn. C.A. Smith. M.D. (1987) *The professional commitment* WB Saunders, Philadelphia

Redman. B.K. (1978) On problems with integrated curricula in nursing *Journal of nursing education* Vol 17, No 6, pp 26-29

Rees. C.B. (1984) *Developments in professional education : The case of the remedial professions* Paper given at the RCN Research Society 4/2/1984, London

Regan Smith. M.G. (1988) Teaching communication and interviewing skills to medical students. *Journal of medical education* Vol 63, No 10, pp 801- 803

Revans. R.W. (1964) *Standards for morale : Cause and effects in hospitals* Oxford University Press, Oxford

Riccardi. V.M. Kurtz. S.M. (1983) *Communication and counselling in health care* Charles C Thomas, Illinois

Ritchie. R.T. (1979) Multidisciplinary teams *British medical journal* No2, p 1590

Robinson. K.M. (1988) A social skills training program for adult care givers *Advances in nursing science* Vol 10, No 2, pp 59-72

Roehampton Institute (1991) *B.Sc Degree(Hons) in health studies* Roehampton Institute, London

Rogers. M.E. (1961) *Educational revolution in nursing* Macmillan, New York

Rose. A.M. Peterson. W.A (1965) *Older people and their social worlds* F.A. Davis, Philadelphia

Routledge. J. Wilson. M. (1992) Joint does not mean generic *Therapy weekly* 5 November, p 6.

Rowe. A. (1977) *Collaboration and co-operation between the professions in the EEC* Royal College of Nursing, London

Rubin. I.M. Plovnick. M. Fry.R.E. (1978) *Task oreintated team development* McGraw Hill, New York

Rusnack. B. (1977) Planned change : Interdisciplinary education for health care. *Journal of education for social work* Vol 13, No 1, pp 104-111

Ryden. M.B. Duckett. L. Crisham.P. Caplan. A.Schmitz.K. (1989) Multi course sequential learning as a model for integration : Ethics as a prototype *Journal of nursing education* Vol 28, No 3, pp 102-105

Ryland. R. Moysey. J. (1983) Collaboration for a more productive future *Nursing times* Vol 79, No 41, pp 51-53

Sakalys. J.A. Watson. J. (1986) Professional education : Post baccalaureate education for professional nursing *Journal of professional nursing* Vol 2, No 2, pp 37-39

Salmon. M. Talashek. M. Tichy. A. (1988) Health for all : A transnational model for nursing *International nursing review* Vol 35, No 4, pp 104-109

Sanson-Fisher. R. Poole.A. (1979) Teaching medical students communication skills *Research in psychology and medicine* Academic Press, London

Scammell. B. (1983) The evaluation of nursing education today *Nursing times* Vol 79, No 32, pp 42-46

Schmidt. H.G. De Volder M.L. (1984) *Tutorials in problem based learning: New directions in training for the health professions* Van Gorcum Assen, Maastricht

Schwab. J.J. (1969)The practical : A language for the curriculum *School review* No 78, pp 1-24

Shepard. K.F. Yeo. G. (1985) Successful components of interdisciplinary education *Journal of allied health* Vol 14, pp 297-302

Shortliffe. E.H. Fagan. L.M.(1989) Research training in medical informatics : The Stanford experience *Academic medicine* No 10.

Siegal. S. (1956) *Nonparametric statistics for the behavioral sciences* McGraw Hill, Tokyo

Simons. W. (1984) Towards integration *Senior nurse* Vol 11, No 28, pp 14-16

Sims. D. (1986a) Interorganisations : Some problems of multiorganisational teams *Personnel review* Vol 15, No 4, pp 27-31

Sinson. J. (1983) Training for the team *The health services journal* Vol 7, No 10, p 14

Skeet. M. Elliot. K. (1978) *Health auxilliaries and the health team* Croom Helm, London

Smail. S. (1980) A model for use in shared teaching *Journal of Royal College of General Practitioners* Occasional Paper 14, pp 17-19

Smith. E.C. (1981) The integrated curriculum from a developmental curriculum *Nursing outlook* Vol 10, pp 577-578

Smith. L. (1992) Ethical issues in interviewing *Journal of advanced nursing* Vol 17, No 1, pp 98-103

Smith. M. Beck. J. Cooper. C.L. (1982) *Introducing organisational behaviour* Macmillan, London

Smith. P.B. (ed.) (1970) *Modern psychology readings* Penguin, London

Snow. C.P. (1964) *The two cultures and a second look* Cambridge University Press, Cambridge

Snyder. R.C. (1987) A societal backdrop for interprofessional education and practice *Theory into practice* Vol 26, No 2, pp 94-98

Stacey. M. Reid. M Heath. C. Dingwall. R. (eds) (1977) *Health and the division of labour* Croom Helm, London

Stevenson. O. (1985) Education for community care *British medical journal* Vol 290, pp 1966-1968

Stott. N.C.H. Davies. R.H. (1979) The exceptional potential in each primary care consultation *Journal of the Royal College of General Practitioners* Vol 29, pp 201-205

Straus. R. (1959) A department of behavioural science *Journal of medical education* No 34, pp 662-666

Styles. M.M. (1986) In the name of integration *Nursing outlook* Vol 12, No 24, pp 738-744

Tansley. P. (1989) *Course teams. The way forward in F.E. ?* NFER/Nelson,. London

Thomas. L.F. Harri-Augstein. E.S. (1984) Education and the negotiation of personal meaning *Education section review* Vol 8, No 1, pp 7-36

Thomstad. B. (1975) Changing the rules of the doctor-nurse game *Nursing outlook* Vol 23, No 7, pp 422-427

Tichy. M.K. (1974) *Health care teams : An annotated bibliography* Prager, New York

Titmuss. R.M.(ed.) (1969) Colleagues or competitors *Occasional papers on social administration* No 31, Bell & Son, London

Todd. F. (ed.) (1987) *Planning continual professional development* Croom Helm, USA

Tomich. J. (1966) Home care : A technique for professional identity *Journal of medical education* No 41, pp 202-208

Turner.B.S. (1990) The interdisciplinary curriculum : From social medicine to post modernism *Sociology of health and illness* Vol 12, No 1, pp 1-23

Vineberg. U. Willems.P (1971) Observation and analysis of patient behavior in the rehabilitation hospital. *Archives of physical medicine Rehabilitation* January 8-13.

Waddington. I. (1973) The role of the hospital in the development of modern medicine : A sociological analysis. *Sociology* No 7, pp 43-49
Wagner. V. (1990) Joining the team *Nursing standard* Vol 4, No 21, p 5.
Walton. H.J. Drewery. J. Phillip. A.E. (1964) Typical medical students *British journal of medicine* Vol 2, No 9, pp 744-748
Watkin. B. (1975) *Documents on health and social services* Methuen, London
Weir. M. (1991) Towards a holistic understanding of health and illness *Health visitor* Vol 64, No 3, pp 77-79
White. K.L. (1973) Life and death medicine *Scientific American* Vol 229, No 3, pp 22-33
Williams. C.A. (1989) Empathy and burnout in male and female helping professionals *Residential nurse health* Vol 12, No 3, pp 169-178
Williams. P. (1990) Creating common purpose *The health service journal* Vol 10, No 11, pp 1700
Williams. J.W. Alexander.M. Miller G.E. (1967) Continuing education and patient care research *J.A.M.A* No 201, pp 118-122
Wilson .P. MacMurray. V.D. (1974) Interdisciplinary education : Lowering the barriers to effective learning *Educational research* No 17, pp 27-33
Winefield. H.R. (1982) Subjective and objective outcomes of communication skills training in the first year *Medical education* Vol 16, No 4, pp 192
World Health Organisation (1966) *WHO expert committe on nursing 5th report* Technical report series No 347, Geneva
World Health Organisation (1983) *Education in primary health care.* Report on WHO meeting held in Exeter Copenhagen
World Health Organisation (1980) *Assessing health workers performance : A manual for training and supervision* Public health papers, No 72.
Young. R. Freiberg. E. Stringham.P. (1981) The home visit in the multidisciplinary teaching of primary care physicians *Journal of medical education* Vol 56, No 4, pp 341-346
Young. L.D. (1986) Use of external examinations to involve faculty in curriculum content evaluation *Evaluation and the health professions* Vol 9, No 3, pp 325-338
Young. P. (1986) Linked for success *Nursing times educational supplement* Vol 6, No 4, pp 55-57

Index to the appendices

Appendix 1.1 Examples of topics suggested as suitable for interdisciplinary learning

Topics	References
Communication skills	Sharf et al (1982), Sharf & Poirier (1988), Owen (1988)
Teamwork	Seidel (1986), Adair (1987), Abbatt & McMahon (1985), Adcock et al (1977), Allen (1992), Bligh (1980), Broad (1985), Brooks et al (1981), Bryar (1991), Allibone (1981), Barber & Kratz (1980), Bassett (1989), Boss (1983), Given & Simmons ((1979), Grove (1988), Haggard (1990), Harris et al (1976), Owen (1982)
The patient in pain	Marcer & Deighton (1988), Saunders (1990), Guck et al (1985), Llewellyn (1990)
Family Planning, sexuality	Fairweather & Law (1978) Yeaworth & Fern (1973)
Research Methods	Shortell & Fagan (1989), Salvage (1989) Lorenz (1986)
Maternity Care	Iles & Auluck (1990), Donnison (1977), Opoku (1992)
Mental Health	Nodder (1980), Nitsuri et al (1981), Gelder et al (1985), Gomez (1986), Steinberg (1989), Crews (1990), Gearing et al (1988)
Learning disabilities	Sines (1991), Hudson (1991), Ovretveit (1986), Williams (1980), Willer et al (1980)
Child Abuse	Goble (1991), Trowell (1992), Stevenson & Hallett (1980)
Care of the elderly	Runciman (1989), Thompson et al (1988), Stotts (1986) Croen (1984), Dartington (1986), Weinberger & Millham (1975), Beynon (1978), Hutt (1980) Woodruff (1975), Fielding (1987), Hooyman (1982) Kosberg (1983)
Occupational Health	Verma (1988)
Death Education	Agatstein (1980), Watts (1977), Lewis (1966), Nash (1984), Barbou (1975), Hockey (1990) Saunders (1990) Bakemeier (1984) Cramond (1973)
Paediatrics	Ulin (1989), Court (1972), Dingwall et al (1983), Wise (1974), Burkinshaw et al (1991)
Burns & Plastics	Ward (1959)
Cardiac surgery	Yaloff (1979)
Ethical Issues	McElhinney (1981) Smith & Davis (1980), Purtillo (1990), Moore (1989)
Legal Issues	Moore (1989)
Substance abuse	Iles & Auluck (1990) Ulin (1989) Kingdon (1992)
Primary health care	Eichenberger et al (1969), Balasonne (1981), Tanner & Soulary (1972), Fenwick (1979), Fried & Leatt (1986), Evans (1984) Turnbull (1981), Weil & Parrish (1967), Polgar (1961), Owen (1982)
Management	Weil & Parrish (1967) Owen (1982)

Appendix 2.1

Suggestions for designing & launching an interdisciplinary programme

Learning together to work together for health (WHO 1988)	Community based education of health personnel (WHO 1987)
1. Justify the decision to carry out multiprofessional education in a given institution	1. Justify the proposal to start a community based educational programme at a given institution
2. Collect information on how to carry out multiprofessional education and adapt it to local conditions	2. Obtain information on how to realise a community based educational programme & adapt it to the local situation
3. Form a nucleus of colleagues to launch a programme	3. Obtain political commitment & the authority of supervisors to proceed
4. Promote political support for multiprofessional education & obtain clearance from supervisory levels	Ask a number of colleagues to serve as members of a core group for the initiation & implementation of the programme
5. Obtain support from participating schools	5. Review the recommendations presented here to seek out the obstacles that might impede progress, taking local circumstances into consideration
6. Set up a continuous teacher training programme	6. Establish a continuing teacher training programme
7. Improve the administration of the Institution	7. Improve the administration of the educational institution
8. Select priority health problems in the communities to be served	8. Compile professional profiles of the types of health personnel the institution expects to train
9. Determine health service activities that require a team approach for solving community health problems	9. Construct instruments for assessing the performance of the students
10. Determine the professional categories needed for the selected service activities	10. Set up a mechanism for selecting students suitable for community based education
11. Draw up the professional profiles of the types of health personnel that the institute expects to educate together.	11. Select the sites for community based learning activities
12. Select learning activities for student teams	12. Approach the communities selected as sites for community based learning activities
13. Organise the resources needed	13. Introduce improvements at the sites for community based learning activities
14. Determine the other categories of student health personnel that might benefit from joint training	14. Train the students to make the best use of community based education

Continued next page

Appendix 2.1 (Continued)

Learning together to work together for health (Continued) (WHO 1988)	Community based education for health personnel (Continued) (WHO 1987)
15. Approach the communities selected as settings for multiprofessional education activities	15. Ascertain which categories of students other than those studying the health sciences will benefit from joint training.
16. Select settings for multiprofessional learning activities	16. Plan the sequence of community based learning activities
17. Prepare the students to make the best use of multiprofessional education	17. Ensure that there is a built in programme evaluation mechanism
18. Plan the sequence of multiprofessional activities	
19. Devise instruments for assessing student performance	
20. Incorporate a means of programme evaluation	
21. Review the planning steps presented here & single out obstacles to their implementation with due regard for local circumstances	
22. Use an efficient strategy to introduce change	

Appendix 2.2

How the European Community Works

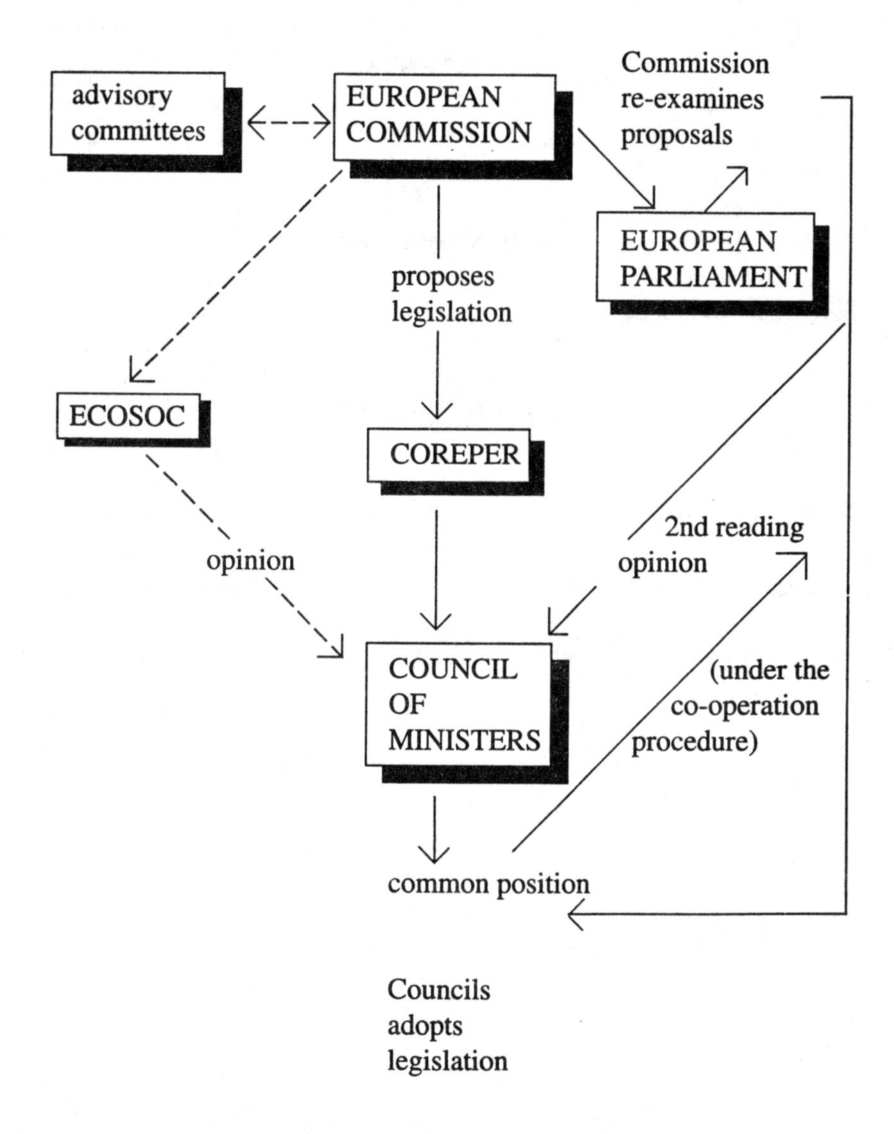

Appendix 2.3

The change from primary medical to primary health care (WHO 1984. EUR/RC 34)

FROM		TO
	FOCUS	
Illness	⇒	Health
Cure	⇒	Prevention & Cure
	CONTENTS	
Treatment	⇒	Health promotion
Episodic care	⇒	Continuous care
Attention to specific problems	⇒	Comprehensive care
	ORGANISATION	
Physicians	⇒	Other personnel groups
Single handed practices	⇒	Multiprofessional teamwork General practitioners
	RESPONSIBILITY	
Health sector alone	⇒	Intersectoral collaboration
Professional dominance	⇒	Community participation
Passive reception	⇒	Self resposibility

Appendix 2.4

UKCC : CODE OF PROFESSIONAL PRACTICE (1992)

Each registered nurse, midwife and health visitor shall act, at all times, in such a way as to:

- **safeguard and promote the interests of individual patients and clients;**
- **serve the interests of society**
- **justify public trust and confidence and**
- **uphold and enhance the good standing and reputation of the professions.**

As a registered nurse, midwife, or health visitor, you are personally accountable for your practice and, in the exercise of your professional accountability, must:

1. act always in such a manner as to promote and safeguard the interests and well-being of patients and clients;
2. ensure that no action or omission on your part, or within your sphere of responsibility, is detrimental to the interests, conditions or safety of patients an clients;
3. maintain and improve your professional knowledge and competence;
4. acknowledge any limitations in your knowledge and competence and decline any duties or responsibilities unless able to perform them in a safe and skilled manner;
5. work in an open and co-operative manner with all patients, clients and their families, foster their independence and recognise and respect their involvement in the planning and delivery of care;
6. work in a collaborative and co-operative manner with health care professionals and others involved in providing care, and recognise their particular contributions within the health care team;
7. recognise and respect the uniqueness and dignity of each patient and client, and respond to their need for care irrespective of their ethnic origin, religious beliefs, personal attributes, the nature of their health problems or any other factor;
8. report to an appropriate person or authority, at the earliest time, any conscientious objection which may be relevant to your professional practice;

9. avoid any abuse of your privileged relationship with patients and clients and of the privileged access allowed to their person, property, residence or workplace;
10. protect all confidential information concerning patients and clients obtained in the course of professional practice and make disclosures only with consent, where required by the order of the court or where you can justify disclosure in the wider public interest;
11. report to an appropriate person or authority, having regard to the physical, psychological and social effects on patients and clients, any circumstances in the environment of care which could jeopardise standards of practice;
12. report to an appropriate person or authority any circumstances in which safe and appropriate care for patients and clients cannot be provided;
13. report to an appropriate person or authority where it appears that the health or safety of colleagues is at risk, as such circumstances may compromise standards of practice and care;
14. assist professional colleagues, in the context of your own knowledge, experience and sphere of responsibility, to develop their professional competence, and assist others in the care team, including informal carers, to contribute safely and to a degree appropriate to their roles;
15. refuse any gift, favour or hospitality from patients or clients currently in your care which may be interpreted as seeking to exert influence to obtain preferential consideration;
16. ensure that your registration status is not used in the promotion of commercial products or services, declare any financial or other interests in relevant organisations providing such goods or services and ensure that your professional judgement is not influenced by any commercial considerations.

Appendix 4.1

Interview schedule : Overseas Teachers

Date............................

Time Commenced.......................

Introduction : Purpose of research ie why the interview is being conducted.

1. Confirm profession.

medicine
dentistry
nursing
radiography
physiotherapy
occ. therapy
O.D.A
speech therapy
podiatry
dental tech.
nutrition and diet.
soc. work
DSA/Den. Hyg.

2. Since you qualified how many years in clinical practice?

3. How many years teaching ? Full time/part time

4. Areas of teaching specialisation ? (Give examples)

5. Which of the above professions do you teach..........................List

6. In which year of training are the students?

7. What do you teach them?

8. How many hours do the students spend together on these subjects?

9. Is it a joint curriculum? YES NO

10. If "Yes", which other disciplines were involved in the curriculum planning?

11. Which teaching methods are used? Lectures, tutorials, seminars, debates, contract learning, practicals, others..

12. What do you think are the advantages of interdisciplinary learning?

13. What are the disadvantages?

14. What preparation did the staff need before commencing interdisciplinary learning?

15. Have you noticed any partciular problems of integration between either the staff or the students of any of the professions in particular? YES NO

16. If "Yes", which ones and why do you think this is?

17. If "Yes", what are these? Why are these a problem?

18. Do you think that there could be any specific problems in shared learning with any of the above groups. YES NO
    If "Yes", which ones in particular :-

19. Do you personally have any reservations about shared learning?

20. Are there any further developments planned in interdisciplinary learning in your Faculty?

(Thank respondent, enquire if they wish to ask any questions, promise results will be sent to the Faculty as soon as the study is completed)

Time completed ....

Appendix 4.2

Main interview schedule : Teachers

Date............................

Time Commenced.......................

Introduction : Purpose of research ie why the interview is being conducted.

1. Confirm profession.

medicine
dentistry
nursing
radiography
physiotherapy
occ. therapy
O.D.A
speech therapy
podiatry
dental tech.
nutrition and diet.
soc. work
DSA/Den. Hyg.

2. Since you qualified how many years were you in clinical practice before you started teaching ?

3. How many years teaching ? Full time/part time

4. Areas of teaching specialisation ? (Give examples)

5. Have you had the opportunity to teach other disciplines ? Yes No
(if yes details)

6. Have you ever experienced shared learning with other professions?
(if yes details) Yes No

7. Which subject areas would you include in the behavioural sciences ? From answer clearly define.

8. Do you agree/disagree that a knowledge of the behavioural sciences are essential to the health and social care professions ? Agree Disagree
If agree proceed to Q 10. If disagree proceed to Q 9.

9. Why don't you feel they are essential ? (Encourage short discussion on reasons why. Do not try to change point of view. If very strong objections offer to terminate interview at this point.)

10. As you feel that the behavioural sciences are essential to all health and social professions, do you feel that there would be any advantage in learning these together ? Yes No
If yes what would these advantages be ?

Either response - What would the disadvantages be ?

11. As an individual do you feel that you personally would have reservations about teaching other professions ? Yes No
If yes what are these ?

12. Which word do you use to describe these activities ?
(ie multi-disciplinary, interdisciplinary etc)

13. What do you understand by the word you have chosen ?

(Give description of the differences between the words. Explain rationale for using the word "interdisciplinary")

14. Given the opportunity (not with standing your reservations) how interested would you be in participating in some interdisciplinary teaching ?

15. Do you feel that teacher participants would need special preparation ? Yes No
If yes, what type of preparation would be needed ?

16. Are there any topics apart from specialist practitioner areas which you would reject as being unsuitable for interdisciplinary learning ? Yes No
If yes what are these ?

17. Which of the following disciplines do you feel could be included in some interdisciplinary learning initiatives with your own profession.

medicine	Yes/No
dentistry	Yes/No
nursing	Yes/No
radiography	Yes/No
physiotherapy	Yes/No
occ.therapy	Yes/No
ODA'S	Yes/No
speech therapy	Yes/No
podiatrists	Yes/No
nutrition and diet.	Yes/No
dental tech.	Yes/No
social work	Yes/No
DSA/Den. Hyg.	Yes/No

18. Do you think that there could be any specific problems in shared learning with any of the above groups. Yes No

If yes which ones in particular :-

19. At which stage do you think interdisciplinary learning should be introduced?

At the beginning of training ?	Yes/No
In the middle of training?	Yes/No
At the end of training ?	Yes/No
Following qualification ?	Yes/No
Any other response ?	

Please give the reasons why you have chosen this option.

20. Which teaching methods do you think would be the most appropriate ones to adopt ?

Thank you very much for your participation. Are there any questions you wish to ask me ?

Time completed ....

Appendix 4.3

Main interview schedule : Students

Date............................

Time Commenced.......................

Introduction : Purpose of research i.e. why the interview is being conducted.

1. Confirm profession.

medicine
dentistry
nursing
radiography
physiotherapy
occ. therapy
O.D.A
speech therapy
podiatry
dental tech.
nutrition and diet.
soc. work
DSA/DH

2. Which year of training are you in ?

3. Have you ever experienced shared learning with other professions ? Yes No
   (if yes details)

4. What does the term behavioural sciences mean to you? From answer clearly define.

5. Do you agree/disagree that the behavioural sciences are basic to the health and social care professions ? Agree Disagree
   If agree proceed to Q 7. If disagree proceed to Q 6.

6. Why don't you feel they are essential? Encourage short discussion on reasons why. Do not try to change point of view. If very strong objections terminate interview at this point.

7. If you feel that the behavioural sciences are essential to all health and social professions, do you feel that there would be any advantage in learning these together ? Yes No
   If yes what would these advantages be ?

   Either response - What would the disadvantages be ?

8. As an individual do you feel that you personally would have reservations about learning with other professions ? Yes No
   If yes what are these ?

9. Which word would you use to describe learning together with other professions ? (ie multi-disciplinary, interdisciplinary)

10. What do you understand by the word you have chosen ?

11. Given the opportunity (not withstanding your reservations) how interested would you be in having the opportunity to participate in interdisciplinary learning ?

12. Do you feel that the teachers participating would need special preparation ?
    If yes, what type of preparation would be needed ? Yes No

13. Are there any topics apart from specialist practitioner areas which you would reject as being unsuitable for interdisciplinary learning ? Yes No
    If yes what are these ?

14. Which of the following disciplines do you feel could be included in some interdisciplinary learning initiatives with your own profession.

medicine	Yes/No
dentistry	Yes/No
nursing	Yes/No
radiography	Yes/No
physiotherapy	Yes/No
occ.therapy	Yes/No
ODA'S	Yes/No
speech therapy	Yes/No
podiatrists	Yes/No
nutrition and diet.	Yes/No
dental tech.	Yes/No
social work	Yes/No

15. Do you think that there could be any specific problems in shared learning with any of the above groups. Yes No
    If yes which ones in particular :-

16. At which stage do you think interdisciplinary learning should be introduced ?

    At the beginning of training ? Yes/No
    In the middle of training? Yes/No
    At the end of training ? Yes/No
    Following qualification ? Yes/No
    Any other response ?

    Please give the reasons why you have chosen this option.

17. How would you like to see the whole concept of interdisciplinary learning put into action ? (workshops, conferences, meetings etc.)

18. Which learning methods do you think would be the most appropriate ones to adopt ?

Thank you very much for your participation. Are there any questions you wish to ask me ?

Time completed ....

Appendix 4.4

SHARED LEARNING IN THE HEALTH & SOCIAL CARE PROFESSIONS

MAIN STUDY : TEACHER QUESTIONNAIRE

The purpose of this questionnaire is to elicit your opinions of the feasibility and desirability of common learning experiences between the health and social care professions. Please answer all questions as accurately as possible to reflect your honest opinions. You will not be identified in any way either during or following completion of this study. THANK YOU. Rosemary Tope.

PART A BIOGRAPHIC DATA

Please circle the number opposite to your answer in COLUMN "A" **Please DO NOT use "B" or "C".**

Question	Answer	A	B	C
1. To which profession do you belong ?	Dental Surgeon	1	1	
	DSA/ Dental Hygienist	2	2	
	Dental Technician	3	3	
	Medicine	4	4	
	Nursing	5	5	
	Nutrition and Dietetics	6	6	
	Occupational Therapy	7	7	
	Operating Department Practitioner	8	8	
	Physiotherapy	9	9	
	Podiatry (chiropody)	10	10	
	Radiography	11	11	
	Social Work	12	12	
	Speech Therapy	13	13	
2. Your gender	Male	1	14	
	Female	2	15	
3. Your age group	Under 25 years	1	16	
	25 - 30	2	17	
	31 - 35	3	18	
	36 - 40	4	19	
	41 - 45	5	20	
	46 - 50	6	21	
	51 - 55	7	22	
	56 - 60	8	23	
	Over 60 years	9	24	
4. After qualifying, how many years were you in practice before you commenced teaching ? (Please INCLUDE any post-graduate training periods)	Less than 1 year	1	25	
	1 - 5 years	2	26	
	6 - 10	3	27	
	11 - 15	4	28	
	16 - 20	5	29	
	21 - 25	6	30	
	Over 25 years	7	31	
5. How many years have you had a **designated** teaching post ? (Either full-time or part-time in an educational institution and/or within clinical areas as part of a clinical post.)	Less than 1 year	1	32	
	1 - 5 years	2	33	
	6 - 10	3	34	
	11 - 15	4	35	
	16 - 20	5	36	
	21 - 25	6	37	
	Over 25 years	7	38	

		A	B	C
6.a. EXCLUDING subjects specific to your own profession, do you have any other RELATED areas of knowledge that you can teach?	YES	1	39	
	NO	2	40	

b. If "Yes", Please give details..

....

....

(Please use the reverse of this page if there is insufficient room for your answer above)

		A	B
7a. Within your personal teaching experience, have you had the the opportunity to teach other professional groups ?	YES	1	41
	NO	2	42
b. If "Yes", Please identify which profession(s).	Dental Surgeon	1	43
	DSA/Dental Hygienist	2	44
	Dental Technician	3	45
	Medicine	4	46
	Nursing	5	47
	Nutrition and Dietetics	6	48
	Occupational Therapy	7	49
	Operating Department Practitioner	8	50
	Physiotherapy	9	51
	Podiatry (Chiropody)	10	52
	Radiography	11	53
	Social Work	12	54
	Speech Therapy	13	55
	Other profession	14	56

c. If "Other Profession",Please give details..

....

....

(Please use the reverse of this page if there is insufficient room for your answer above)

		A	B
8. Have you ever participated in learning with any other profession ?	YES	1	57
	NO	2	58

<u>If "YES", please answer questions 9 and 10 below. If "NO", please go direct to Question 11 on the NEXT page</u>

		A	B
9. Was your shared learning experience Before or After you obtained your MAIN professional qualification ?	BEFORE	1	59
	AFTER	2	60
10a With which other professions did you share learning ?	Dental Surgeons	1	61
	DSA/Dental Hygienist	2	62
	Dental Technician	3	63
	Medicine	4	64
	Nursing	5	65
	Nutrition and Dietetics	6	66
	Occupational Therapy	7	67
	Operating Department Practitioner	8	68
	Physiotherapy	9	69
	Podiatry (Chiropody)	10	70

PLEASE CONTINUE ON THE NEXT PAGE

Question 10 continued

	A	B	C
Radiography	11	71	
Social Work	12	72	
Speech Therapy	13	73	
Other Profession(s)	14	74	

b. If "Other Profession(s)", please give details..

....

PART B OPINIONS

This part of the questionnaire is concerned with your opinions regarding the concept of introducing some shared learning of the behavioural sciences in the education and training of the health and social care professions. Please continue to circle the number in Column "A"opposite to your response.

Please circle the number opposite your answer in column "A" Please DO NOT use "B" or "C"

		A	B	C
11a. Which term do you generally use when referring to Shared Learning ?	Do not use any specific term	1	75	
	Multidisciplinary	2	76	
	Interdisciplinary	3	77	
	Multiprofessional	4	78	
	Interprofessional	5	79	
	Pluridisciplinary	6	80	
	Other	7	81	

b. If "Other", please specify..

		A	B
12a. Do you believe that there should be SOME shared learning of the behavioural sciences between the health and social care professions ?	YES	1	82
	NO	2	83
	UNDECIDED	3	84
b. Do you believe that Advantages could result from shared learning ?			
	YES	1	85
	NO	2	86
	UNDECIDED	3	87

c. Please List/State any ADVANTAGES that you consider could result from shared learning.

.... **88**

....

(Please use the reverse of this page if there is insufficient room for your answer above)

d. Please List/State any DISADVANTAGES that you consider could result from shared learning.

.... **89**

....

(Please use the reverse of this page if there is insufficient room for your answer above)

		A	B	C
13a. IN CONJUNCTION WITH your own profession, which of the following do you feel could be included in a possible shared learning initiative ?				
	Dental Surgeon	1	90	
	DSA/Dental Hygienist	2	91	
	Dental Technician	3	92	
	Medicine	4	93	
	Nursing	5	94	
	Nutrition and Dietetics	6	95	
	Occupational Therapy	7	96	
	Operating Department Practitioner	8	97	
	Physiotherapist	9	98	
	Podiatry(Chiropody)	10	99	
	Radiography	11	100	
	Social Work	12	101	
	Speech Therapy	13	102	
b. Do you believe that there could be any problems in shared learning between your profession and any of the above groups ?	YES	1	103	
	NO	2	104	
	UNDECIDED	3	105	

c. If "Yes", please state the nature of these problems..

....

....

....

14a. At which stage of Professional education and training do you feel that shared learning could take place ?	BEGINNING	1	106	
	MIDDLE	2	107	
	END	3	108	
	THROUGHOUT	4	109	
	AFTER QUALIFYING	5	110	

b. Please briefly state the reason(s) for making this choice.

....

....

....

(Please use the reverse of this page if there is insufficient room for your answer above)

15a. Are there any TOPICS apart from SPECIALIST PRACTITIONER AREAS which you would REJECT as being unsuitable for shared learning ?	YES	1	111	
	NO	2	112	

b. If "Yes", please list these topics...

....

....

(Please use the reverse of this page if there is insufficient room for your answer above)

		A	B	C
16. Given the opportunity, how interested would you be in participating as a TEACHER in a shared learning initiative ?	VERY INTERESTED	1	113	
	INTERESTED	2	114	
	NEITHER INTERESTED NOR UNINTERESTED	3	115	
	UNINTERESTED	4	116	
	TOTALLY UNINTERESTED	5	117	

17a. Do you feel that teachers would benefit from receiving special preparation if they participated in a shared learning initiative ?

YES	1	118
NO	2	119
UNCERTAIN	3	120

b. If "Yes", what do you feel should be included in the preparation ?

....

....

....

(Please use the reverse of this page if there is insufficient room for your answer above)

18. Below is a list of Subjects/Topics to be found in current health and social care curricula and as such are required teaching/learning. Please give your opinion on their SUITABILITY for SOME shared learning BETWEEN the professions.

Subject/Topic			
A/. PSYCHOLOGY	SUITABLE	1	121
	UNSUITABLE	2	122
B/. SOCIOLOGY	SUITABLE	1	123
	UNSUITABLE	2	124
C/. ETHICS	SUITABLE	1	125
	UNSUITABLE	2	126
D/. LAW & PRACTICE	SUITABLE	1	127
	UNSUITABLE	2	128
E/. BEHAVIOURAL RESEARCH METHODS	SUITABLE	1	129
	UNSUITABLE	2	130
F/. MANAGEMENT	SUITABLE	1	131
	UNSUITABLE	2	132
G/. ECONOMICS OF HEALTH CARE	SUITABLE	1	133
	UNSUITABLE	2	134
H/. HEALTH PROMOTION/ EDUCATION	SUITABLE	1	135
	UNSUITABLE	2	136

PLEASE CONTINUE ON FINAL PAGE

		A	B	C
I/. STUDY SKILLS	SUITABLE	1	137	
	UNSUITABLE	2	138	
J/. QUALITY IN HEALTH & SOCIAL CARE	SUITABLE	1	139	
	UNSUITABLE	2	140	
K/. STRUCTURAL ORGANISATION IN HEALTH & SOCIAL CARE	SUITABLE	1	141	
	UNSUITABLE	2	142	
L/ COMPUTING SKILLS	SUITABLE	1	143	
	UNSUITABLE	2	144	

THANK YOU for taking the time to complete this questionnaire. When this study has been completed the results will be made widely available. If you have any queries please do not hesitate to contact me at the address on the enclosed envelope.

Appendix 4.5

SHARED LEARNING IN THE HEALTH & SOCIAL CARE PROFESSIONS

MAIN STUDY : STUDENT QUESTIONNAIRE

The purpose of this questionnaire is to elicit your opinions of the feasibility and desirability of shared learning experiences between the health and social care professions. Please answer all questions as accurately as possible to reflect your honest opinions. You will not be identified in any way either during or following completion of this study. THANK YOU. Rosemary Tope.

PART A BIOGRAPHIC DATA

Please circle the number opposite to your answer in COLUMN "A" **Please DO NOT use "B" or "C".**

Question	Answer	A	B	C
1. For which profession are you training ?	Dental Surgeon	1	1	
	DSA/ Dental Hygienist	2	2	
	Dental Technician	3	3	
	Medicine	4	4	
	Nursing	5	5	
	Nutrition and Dietetics	6	6	
	Occupational Therapy	7	7	
	Operating Department Practitioner	8	8	
	Physiotherapy	9	9	
	Podiatry (Chiropody)	10	10	
	Radiography	11	11	
	Social Work	12	12	
	Speech Therapy	13	13	
2. In which year of training are you ?	Year 1	1	14	
	Year 2	2	15	
	Year 3	3	16	
	Year 4	4	17	
	Year 5	5	18	
	Other	6	19	
3. Your gender	Male	1	20	
	Female	2	21	
4. Your age group	20 years or less	1	22	
	21 - 25	2	23	
	26 - 30	3	24	
	31 - 35	4	25	
	36 - 40	5	26	
	41 - 45	6	27	
	46 - 50	7	28	
	51 - 55	8	29	
	Over 55 years	9	30	
5. Have you PREVIOUSLY undertaken any courses which you consider RELEVANT to your current training ? (EXCLUDE SCHOOL QUALIFICATIONS)	Yes	1	31	
	No	2	32	

If "YES" please give details...

....

PLEASE CONTINUE ON THE NEXT PAGE

		A	B	C

6. Have you PREVIOUSLY had any work experience which you consider RELEVANT to health or social care ?

	A	B	C
Yes	1	33	
No	2	34	

If "YES" please give details..

....

---

7. (EXCLUDING THE CLINICAL AREAS) Have you experienced any shared learning with other health and social care professions ?

	A	B	C
Yes	1	35	
No	2	36	

If "YES" please identify which profession(s)

	A	B	C
Dental Surgeons	1	37	
DSA/Dental Hygienist	2	38	
Dental Technician	3	39	
Medicine	4	40	
Nursing	5	41	
Nutrition & Dietetics	6	42	
Occupational Therapy	7	43	
Operating Department Practitioner	8	44	
Physiotherapy	9	45	
Podiatry (Chiropody)	10	46	
Radiography	11	47	
Social Work	12	48	
Speech Therapy	13	49	
Other profession	14	50	

If "Other Profession" please give details..

....

PART B OPINIONS.

This part of the questionnaire is concerned with your opinions regarding the concept of introducing some shared learning of the behavioural sciences in the education and training of the health and social professions. Please continue to circle the number in Column "A" opposite to your response.

8. Which of the following subjects would you include in the term "behavioural sciences" ?

		A	B	C
Psychology	Yes	1	51	
	No	2	52	
	Undecided	3	53	
Sociology	Yes	4	54	
	No	5	55	
	Undecided	6	56	
Ethics	Yes	7	57	
	No	8	58	
	Undecided	9	59	

PLEASE CONTINUE ON THE NEXT PAGE

		A	B	C
Law & Practice	Yes	10	60	
	No	11	61	
	Undecided	12	62	
Management	Yes	13	63	
	No	14	64	
	Undecided	15	65	
Health Promotion	Yes	16	66	
	No	17	67	
	Undecided	18	68	
Study Skills	Yes	19	69	
	No	20	70	
	Undecided	21	71	
Quality Issues	Yes	22	72	
	No	23	73	
	Undecided	24	74	

---

9. Do you believe that there should be SOME shared learning of the behavioural sciences between the health and social care professions ?

Yes	1	75
No	2	76
Undecided	3	77

10a. Do you believe that any advantages could result from shared learning ?

Yes	1	78
No	2	79
Undecided	3	80

b. Please list/state any ADVANTAGES which you consider could result from shared learning.

....

....

c. Please list/state any DISADVANTAGES which you consider could result from shared learning.

....

....

11a. IN CONJUNCTION WITH your own profession, which of the following do you feel could be included in SOME shared learning initiatives ?

Dental Surgeon	1	81
DSA/Dental Hygienist	2	82
Dental Technician	3	83
Medicine	4	84
Nursing	5	85
Nutrition & Dietetics	6	86
Occupational Therapy	7	87

PLEASE CONTINUE ON THE NEXT PAGE

	A	B	C
Operating Department Practitioners	8	88	
Physiotherapy	9	89	
Podiatry (Chiropody)	10	90	
Radiography	11	91	
Social Work	12	92	
Speech Therapy	13	93	

b. Do you believe that there could be any problems in shared learning between your profession and any of the above groups ?

Yes	1	94
No	2	95
Undecided	3	96

c. If "Yes" please state the nature of these problems.

....

....

....

12a. At which stage of training do you feel that shared learning could take place ?

At the beginning	1	97
Middle of training	2	98
End of Training	3	99
Throughout	4	100
After Qualifying	5	101

b. Please briefly state the reasons for making this choice.

....

....

13a. APART FROM KNOWLEDGE YOU CONSIDER SPECIFIC TO YOUR OWN PROFESSION are there any topics which you would REJECT as being unsuitable for shared learning ?

Yes	1	102
No	2	103

b. If "YES" please list these topics..

....

....

---

14. Given the opportunity how interested would you be in participating as a STUDENT in SOME shared learning with the other health and social care professions ?

Very Interested	1	104
Interested	2	105
Neither Interested Nor Uninterested	3	106
Uninterested	4	107
Totally uninterested	5	108

PLEASE CONTINUE ON THE NEXT PAGE

15. Which learning methods do you feel would be appropriate for any shared learning initiatives ?

		A	B	C
Mixed Tutorials	Yes	1	109	
	No	2	110	
	Undecided	3	111	
Workshops	Yes	1	112	
	No	2	113	
	Undecided	3	114	
Case Studies	Yes	1	115	
	No	2	116	
	Undecided	3	117	
Seminars	Yes	1	118	
	No	2	119	
	Undecided	3	120	
Problem Based Learning	Yes	1	121	
	No	2	122	
	Undecided	3	123	
Role Play	Yes	1	124	
	No	2	125	
	Undecided	3	126	
Lectures	Yes	1	127	
	No	2	128	
	Undecided	3	129	
Visits to clinical areas	Yes	1	130	
	No	2	131	
	Undecided	3	132	

16. Below is a list of subjects/topics found in the curriculum of the health and social care professions. Please give your opinion on their suitability for SOME shared learning.

Psychology	Yes	1	133
	No	2	134
Sociology	Yes	1	135
	No	2	136
Ethics	Yes	1	137
	No	2	138
Law & Practice	Yes	1	139
	No	2	140
Research Methods	Yes	1	141
	No	2	142
Management	Yes	1	143
	No	2	144
Economics of Health Care	Yes	1	145
	No	2	146

PLEASE CONTINUE ON FINAL PAGE

		A	B	C
Health Education/ Promotion	Yes	1	147	
	No	2	148	
Study Skills	Yes	1	149	
	No	2	150	
Quality Issues	Yes	1	151	
	No	2	152	
Structural Organisation in health & social care.	Yes	1	153	
	No	2	154.	
Computing skills	Yes	1	155	
	No	2	156	

Thank you for taking the time to complete this questionnaire. When this study has been completed the results will be made widely available.

Appendix 5.1

Biographic details of teacher respondents in structured interviews

Respondent	Profession	Years in Practice	Years in Teaching
1	Dentist	16	10
2	Dentist	5	26
3	DSA/DH	6	15
4	DSA/DH	9.5	2.5
5	Dental Tech.	4	18
6	Dental Tech.	2	11
7	Medicine	6	20
8	Medicine	5	6
9	Nursing	11	2
10	Nursing	2.5	6.5
11	Nursing	5	7
12	Nursing	7	21
13	Nursing	12	8
14	Nutrit. & Diet.	4	11
15	Nutrit. & Diet.	0	27
16	Occ. Therapy	8	16
17	Occ. Therapy	6	4
18	Op. Dept. Pract.	3.5	2
19	Op. Dept. Pract.	2	7
20	Physiotherapy	20	3
21	Physiotherapy	3	19
22	Podiatry	6	22
23	Podiatry	6	35
24	Radiography	8	7
25	Radiography	7	19
26	Social Work	14	0.25
27	Social Work	3.5	10
28	Speech Therapy	12	17
29	Speech Therapy	17	11

Appendix 5.2

Topics additional to profession specific subjects

Respondent	Additional topics identified
1	Behavioural sciences.
2	Nil.
3	Health education, health promotion.
4.	Nil.
5.	Nil.
6.	Computing skills, behavioural sciences.
7.	Health education, health promotion, community health.
8.	Nil.
9.	Nil.
10.	Psychology.
11.	Philosophy, ethics, social policy.
12.	Management, behavioural sciences.
13.	Research methods, counselling, management.
14.	Education methods, research methods.
15.	Research methods.
16.	Nil.
17.	Teaching and supervision skills.
18.	Nil.
19.	Nil.
20.	Nil.
21.	Anatomy.
22.	Skills analysis, teaching methods.
23.	Nil.
24.	Nil.
25.	Philosophy, professional studies, study skills.
26.	Social policy, mental health, disability.
27.	Communication skills, staff development, management.
28.	Counselling, developmental studies.
29.	Nil.

Appendix 5.3

Teacher's experiences of learning with other disciplines

Res. No.	Stage	Experience
1	Post Qual	Conferences, short courses
2	Post Qual	Conferences, study days.
3	Post Qual	Conferences, study days.
4	Post Qual	FETC.
5	Post Qual	Conferences & workshops.
6	Post Qual	Conferences.
7	Post Qual	Conferences...... "I elect to go"
8	Post Qual	Study days...... "I choose to go"
9	Post Qual	FETC,PGCE.
10	**Pre Qual**	Lectures "Psychology with arts and science students"
11	Post Qual	MA Philosophy of Health Care.
12	Post Qual	NHS Management Course
13	Post Qual	Management Course, Cert. Ed. M.Sc Research.
14	**Pre Qual**	"With food science courses" + Post Qual. Management
15	Post Qual	"Odd lectures"
16	Post Qual	"Sat in the same lecture room as physios, radiographers, orthoptists on conferences/study days if that is what you mean"
17	Post Qual	MSc Management in Community Care
18	Post Qual	NHS Management Course, Cert. Ed.
19	Post Qual	Cert. Ed. Diploma in Management Studies, Cert.Ed.
20	Post Qual	Cert.Ed. M.Ed. "odd conferences"
21	Post Qual	MSc (not specified)
22	Post Qual	Conferences
23	Post Qual	Cert.Ed. M.Ed, "Odd study days"
24	Post Qual	MSc Interprofessional Health Studies
25	Post Qual	FETC,Cert.Ed. B.Ed. MSc Research, Management.
26	Post Qual	Conferences
27	Post Qual	Induction course for new staff, MBA
28	Post Qual	Conferences.
29	Post Qual	Conferences.

Appendix 5.4

Subject areas which teachers include in the behavioural sciences

All 29 respondents identified psychology and sociology as being core subjects in the behavioural sciences. Additional inclusions are presented below.

Respondent Number	Additional Subjects/Comments
1	Nil
2	"It seems that everything is lumped in these days"
3	"Life skills, communication, the environment"
4	Nil
5	Anthropology
6	Anthroplogy, philosophy, ethics, law, organisation, management.
7	Ethics, legal practice, communication, "anything and everything that cannot be described as a life science."
8	"It cant' be isolated from communication, ethics, philosophy"
9	Social policy
10	Economics, law, ethics, social policy.
11	Social policy, health
12	"The individual & society, economics, law, ethics."
13	Ethics, law.
14	Management, organisation.
15	Research methods, education, management, organsiation.
16	Management, philosophy, ethics, law
17	Education
18	Nil
19	Ethics, law, equal opportunities.
20	Ethics, law, management.
21	Research methods, ethics, law.
22	Nil
23	Ethics, professional issues
24	Law, ethics, management.
25	Health studies, ethics, law, economics, management.
26	Occupations
27	"Unhappy with the term behavioural, it has a negative connotation and is a limiting concept."
28	Nil
29	Nil

Appendix 5.5

Additional comments regarding participation in interdisciplinary teaching

Respondent Number	Additional Comments
4	"I think it would be fantastic.....we could learn such a lot from each other"
5	"I would probably find it a challenge and very interesting"
7	"I already do it whenever I get the opportunity"
9	"Given the right situation & topics it would be an interesting experience"
10	"It would depend on my teaching load"
12	"The only thing to stop me would be the time commitment"
13	"It's my ultimate goal. Thats one of the reasons I'm doing the degree that I'm doing."
14	"Yes, it would be quite interesting"
16	"As an individual I would prefer to participate later in the course"
19	"Yes I would, I want to see us all move forward"
20	"It's a very interesting idea....it would make you really analyse everything"
23	"I should reall enjoy it"
24	"I would be dead chuffed"
26	"Yes, lets experiment I would really like to do that"
27	"Yes I am, because I think it is the only way forward & political influences regardless of agreement or not, will suggest we must"

Appendix 5.6

Where there any topics unsuitable for interdisciplinary learning ?
Individual responses YES = 3 (N=29)

Res. No.	Profession	Individual Comments
11	Nursing	"Life sciences would be difficult because of the different levels of knowledge needed."
16	Occ. Therapy	"The basic life sciences from our point of view."
25	Radiography	"Yes the biological sciences."

NO =26 (N=29)

Resp. No.	Profession	Individual Comments.
1	Dentist	"No providing profession specific competence stays."
2	Dentist	"No I dont think so although some professions may need greater depth and emphasis."
3	DH/DSA	"I cant think of anything."
4	DH/DSA	"None at all, at the end of the day we should all be doing the same thing - caring for people."
5	Den. Tec.	"I dont think anything unsuitable although maybe irrelevant in some cases."
6	Den. Tec.	"No not really, my personal view is that education ought to be broad. People should be more open minded."
7	Medicine	"None at all, although different levels of knowledge would be needed."
8	Medicine	"No the behavioural sciences would be particularly relevant."
9	Nursing	"No I dont think so"
10	Nursing	"All the supportive 'ologies'. Anything & everything could be taught."
12	Nursing	"No, I dont think hand on heart there is anything."
13	Nursing	"No providing profession specific tutorials were also given."
14	Nut. & Diet.	"No as long as there was provision for profession specific things."
15	Nut. & Diet.	"No I dont think so."
17	Occ. Therapy.	"I wouldnt have thought so."
18	ODP	"It is difficult to think of anything immediately."
19	ODP	"None immediately come to mind."
20	Physiotherapy	"Not if in conjunction with specialist tutorials."

Appendix 5.6 continued next page

Appendix 5.6 Continued

Resp. No.	Profession	Individual Comments
21	Physiotherapy	"No we are too narrow on our course. We could easily develop the behavioural sciences."
22	Podiatry	"No I cant bring anything to mind."
23	Podiatry	"No I wouldnt think so."
24	Radiography	"I cant think of anything off hand."
26	Social Work	"All the behavioural sciences would be relevant to us."
27	Social Work	"If you mean the behavioural sciences it would be OK."
28	Speech Therapy	"It would be fine at an introductory level."
29	Speech Therapy	"No, I guess overall the principles would be applicable to all disciplines & then target specific knowledge."

Appendix 5.7

Additional individual responses regarding teacher's own professions learning with other professions

Resp. No.	Profession	Individual Comments
1	Dentist	"I'm not so sure about ODP's, I'm sure that there are good reasons"
2	Dentist	"I don't know about podiatrists"
3	DH/DSA	"I would like to rank these"
4	DH/DSA	"ODP who are they?" Explanation offered..... Decision made "Oh Yes"
5	Den. Tec.	"Tenuous links only with social work"
6	Den.Tec.	"Maybe ODP's I dont know enough about them"
10	Nursing	"I dont know anything about ODP's"
14	Nut. & Diet.	"Radiography & Physiotherapy possibly"
17	Occ. Therapy	"ODP's I dont know anything about them"
18	ODP	"Occ. Therapists. I dont' understand their role."
24	Radiography	"Speech therapy & dental technology with reservations as I am not really sure what they do"
25	Radiography	"Regarding social workers I've got a gut feeling 'yes' but I dont really know enough about them".
27	Social work	"Dentists.. I am not sure...maybe on something like crisis intervention"
29	Speech therapy	"If behavioural sciences are being taught then all of them otherwise I'm not so sure"

Appendix 5.8

At which stage of training should interdisciplinary learning commence ?
Individual teachers responses

Resp. No. (N=23)	Rationale for the beginning of training.
1	"It should be throughout training"
2	"it should be straight through at appropriate times"
3	"At the beginning at then at appropriate times"
4	"It is important to link right at the beginning & then maintain these links throughout"
7	"Right through & then throughout to post graduate level"
8	"Throughout I should think so that we get used to each other"
10	"Basic learning is best at the beginning.. it should be an evolutionary process"
11	"It should go right through"
12	"There should be a core model like there is in the Common Foundation Programme"
13	"Right at the beginning.. if they learn separately & then they are brought together it ties in with professional isolation. They should be socialised to grow up together... joint knowledge is power"
14	"All the way through, at different times & at different levels"
15	"At various stages throughout"
18	"When it is needed... probably at the beginning"
19	"There should be a base foundation"
20	"The earlier the better, student will find their own roles"
21	"Theory at the beginning , application at the end, therefore throughout"
22	"It is as important to know who they are as who you are"
23	"As early as possible & then straight through"
24	"It needs to be reinforced throughout"
25	"I mainly see it at the beginning & then at the end....an introduction & consolidation"
26	"It must not be bolted on but integrated"
27	"As early as possible it should be integral to the whole culture"
28	"A core module... some might be better after qualification but by then they have channelled"

Appendix 5.8 (Continued)

Resp. No. (N=3)	Rationale for the middle of training.
9	"Once they settle down but before they develop concrete thoughts"
17	"They should concentrate at the beginning on defining their own role & specific job"
29	"Students will have an understanding of their own identity & may be prepared to try & understand others roles"

Resp.No. (N=3)	Rationale for the end of training.
5	"Towards the end of training as the first years would see it as irrelevant"
6	"When starting they need a good introduction into their own field then they can look at other aspects from their own foundation"
16	"I feel it is important for students to be comfortable with their own professional identity & find their feet"

Appendix 5.9

How would teachers put interdisciplinary learning into action. Individual responses

Resp. No. (N=29)	Recommended teaching strategies
1	"Workshops, small groups, interactive"
2	"Workshops"
3	"Must be interactive in small groups"
4	"Need a lot of interaction, workshops, case studies, problem based."
5	"Lots of planning meetings, then workshops"
6	"Tutorials, workshops, seminars"
7	"All sorts, mixed tutorials would be excellent after lectures"
8	"Tutorials, case studies, role playing"
9	"Workshops, tutorials, lectures, interaction & dialogue"
10	"Small mixed groups, case studies, problem based learning"
11	"A wide range, lectures, seminars tutorials."
12	"Student led, lectures, workshops, seminars, case studies, anything"
13	"Lectures, tutorial groups, case studies, clinical visits"
14	"Lectures, followed by tutorials, case studies, problem based learning"
15	"Workshops, seminars, case studies"
16	"Case studies, workshops, student led seminars"
17	"A case study approach, tutorials, discussion groups"
18	"Subject related tutorials, role play, must be an integrated approach"
19	"Case studies would make an excellent approach"
20	"Workshops, lectures when appropriate, role play, tutorials"
21	"Small mixed groups with facilitator, case studies"
22	"Lead lecture, profession specific tutorial, mixed tutorial"
23	"Lecture followed by interdisciplinary tutorial, case studies"
24	"Lectures, tutorials, case studies, role play, problem solving"
25	"Mixed tutorials, workshops, case studies"
26	"Joint project work, role play, problem solving, interaction"
27	"Small mixed groups, interaction using a process model"
28	"Student centred, seminars, case studies, joint project work"
29	"Workshops, case studies using a problem solving approach, interaction"

Appendix 5.10

Subject areas which students would include in the behavioural sciences

Respondent Number	Subject Areas
1	Sociology, psychology
2	The way people act
3	Sociology, psychology
4	Psychology, sociology, ethics.
5	Psychology, sociology
6	Psychology, sociology, interpersonal skills
7	Sociology, psychology, anthroplogy, philosophy
8	Psychology, sociology
9	Psychology, sociology
10	Psychology, sociology
11	Psychology, physiology
12	Sociology, psychology, psychiatry
13	Teamwork. I dont know I've never heard the term.
14	Patient ethics, patient safety
15	Psychology, sociology
16	Psychology, sociology
17	Health care, social services, anything
18	Social behaviour, the mind
19	Psychology, care of patients
20	Psychology, communication, teaching, legal and ethical issues
21	"People sciences, the way people behave and why they behave in the way they do... the environment and community in which an individual lives and the effect that has on their behaviour."
22	Psychology, sociology

Appendix 5.11 Teacher questionnaire results

VARIABLES		DENTISTS	DSA/DH	DEN. TEC.	MEDICINE	NURSING	NUT. & DIET.	OCC. THERAPY	ODP.	PHYSIOTHERAPY	PODIATRY	RADIOGRAPHY	SOCIAL WORK	SPEECH THERAPY	TOTAL
PART A BIOGRAPHIC DATA		**1**	**2**	**3**	**4**	**5**	**6**	**7**	**8**	**9**	**10**	**11**	**12**	**13**	
1. Profession															
Dental Surgeon	**1**	40	0	0	0	0	0	0	0	0	0	0	0	0	**40**
DSA/Dental Hygienist	**2**	0	4	0	0	0	0	0	0	0	0	0	0	0	**4**
Dental Technician	**3**	0	0	6	0	0	0	0	0	0	0	0	0	0	**6**
Medicine	**4**	1	0	0	107	0	0	0	0	0	0	0	0	0	**108**
Nursing	**5**	0	0	0	0	97	0	0	0	0	0	0	0	0	**97**
Nutrition & Dietetics	**6**	0	0	0	0	0	4	0	0	0	0	0	0	0	**4**
Occupational Therapy	**7**	0	0	0	0	0	0	7	0	0	0	0	0	0	**7**
Operating Department Practitioner	**8**	0	0	0	0	0	0	0	2	0	0	0	0	0	**2**
Physiotherapy	**9**	0	0	0	0	0	0	0	0	10	0	0	0	0	**10**
Podiatry (Chiropody)	**10**	0	0	0	0	0	0	0	0	0	8	0	0	0	**8**
Radiography	**11**	0	0	0	0	0	0	0	0	0	0	6	0	0	**6**
Social Work	**12**	0	0	0	0	0	0	0	0	0	0	0	7	0	**7**
Speech Therapy	**13**	0	0	0	0	0	0	0	0	0	0	0	0	2	**2**
2. Gender															
Male	**14**	29	0	5	80	29	0	2	2	3	4	3	3	0	**160**
Female	**15**	11	4	1	26	67	4	5	0	6	4	3	4	2	**137**
3. Age Group															
Under 25	**16**	0	0	0	0	0	0	0	1	0	0	0	0	0	**1**
25 - 30	**17**	2	0	2	0	0	0	1	0	1	0	0	2	0	**8**
31 - 35	**18**	4	2	1	11	16	0	2	0	0	0	2	0	0	**38**
36 - 40	**19**	9	0	0	21	23	1	0	0	3	0	2	1	0	**60**
41 - 45	**20**	12	0	2	18	27	1	3	1	4	5	0	3	1	**77**
46 - 50	**21**	8	0	0	20	13	2	1	0	1	2	1	1	0	**49**
51 - 55	**22**	0	0	0	19	5	0	0	0	0	0	1	0	1	**26**
56 - 60	**23**	1	1	1	12	6	0	0	0	0	0	0	0	0	**21**
Over 60	**24**	3	0	0	4	0	0	0	0	1	1	0	0	0	**9**
4. Practice before teaching															
Less then one year	**25**	4	0	0	25	0	1	0	0	0	1	0	1	0	**32**
1 - 5 yrs	**26**	20	3	1	55	26	2	0	2	4	3	1	1	1	**119**
6 - 10 yrs	**27**	8	0	4	23	42	1	3	0	0	4	4	1	0	**90**
11 - 15 yrs	**28**	4	1	1	2	18	0	4	0	4	0	1	4	1	**40**
16 - 20 yrs	**29**	3	0	0	0	10	0	0	0	2	0	0	0	0	**15**
21 - 25 yrs	**30**	0	0	0	0	0	0	0	0	0	0	0	0	0	**0**
Over 25 yrs	**31**	0	0	0	1	0	0	0	0	0	0	0	0	0	**1**
5. Years in teaching post															
Less than one year	**32**	0	0	0	1	2	0	0	0	2	0	0	3	0	**8**
1 - 5 yrs	**33**	9	1	3	20	27	0	4	1	2	0	3	2	0	**72**
6 - 10 yrs	**34**	12	2	0	23	23	0	2	0	3	1	1	2	0	**69**
11 - 15 yrs	**35**	10	0	2	18	28	1	0	0	1	1	0	0	1	**62**
16 - 20 yrs	**36**	3	1	0	18	10	1	1	0	0	3	1	0	0	**38**
21 - 25 yrs	**37**	1	0	0	17	4	1	0	1	2	2	1	0	1	**30**
Over 25 yrs	**38**	5	0	1	9	2	1	0	0	0	1	0	0	0	**19**
6a. Additional related areas can teach															
YES	**39**	9	0	1	34	59	3	5	2	5	4	2	5	1	**130**
NO	**40**	31	4	5	70	37	1	2	0	5	4	4	2	1	**166**
6b. If YES gave details															
YES		9	0	1	34	58	3	5	2	5	4	2	5	1	**129**
NO		30	4	5	70	38	1	2	0	5	4	4	2	1	**166**

		1	2	3	4	5	6	7	8	9	10	11	12	13	
7a. Opportunity teach other prof.															
YES	**41**	30	3	4	96	60	4	7	2	9	3	5	7	2	**232**
NO	**42**	9	1	2	10	35	0	0	0	0	5	1	0	0	**63**
7b. If YES which professions?															
Dental Surgeons	**43**	3	0	4	37	0	0	0	0	0	0	1	0	1	**46**
DSA/Dental Hygienist	**44**	27	1	0	2	1	0	0	0	0	0	1	0	0	**32**
Dental Technician	**45**	12	1	1	3	2	0	0	0	0	0	0	0	0	**19**
Medicine	**46**	8	0	0	33	18	1	3	0	1	2	2	0	1	**69**
Nursing	**47**	13	3	0	90	6	3	3	2	7	1	1	3	1	**133**
Nutrition & Dietetics	**48**	3	0	0	25	7	0	3	0	0	0	0	2	0	**40**
Occupational Therapy	**49**	1	1	0	22	17	0	2	0	3	1	0	1	1	**49**
Operating Dept. Practitioner	**50**	2	0	0	12	11	0	0	1	1	0	2	0	0	**29**
Physiotherapy	**51**	0	1	0	37	26	0	4	0	2	2	2	0	1	**75**
Podiatry	**52**	1	0	0	18	1	0	0	0	0	0	1	0	0	**21**
Radiography	**53**	1	0	0	17	10	0	3	0	5	0	1	0	0	**37**
Social Work	**54**	1	0	0	22	17	1	2	0	0	0	0	0	2	**45**
Speech Therapy	**55**	6	0	0	11	2	1	2	0	0	0	0	0	0	**22**
Other professions	**56**	11	0	1	35	22	2	3	1	3	1	1	3	2	**85**
7c. If other professions gave details															
YES		12	0	1	40	29	2	4	1	4	2	1	4	2	**102**
NO		28	4	5	67	67	2	3	1	6	6	5	3	0	**197**
8. Learning partic. with other prof.															
YES	**57**	24	4	3	54	70	2	7	2	7	3	5	3	2	**186**
NO	**58**	16	0	3	52	26	2	0	0	3	5	1	4	0	**112**
If YES answer 9 & 10 if NO go to 11)															
9. Shared learning before/after															
BEFORE	**59**	11	2	2	17	6	1	2	1	2	0	1	1	0	**46**
AFTER	**60**	12	2	2	62	64	1	7	1	7	3	5	3	2	**171**
10a. Which other prof shared learning ?															
Dental Surgeon	**61**	0	0	2	8	4	1	0	0	0	0	1	0	0	**16**
DSA/DH	**62**	6	0	0	2	1	0	1	1	0	0	2	0	0	**13**
Dental Technicians	**63**	5	0	0	1	2	1	0	0	0	0	1	0	0	**10**
Medicine	**64**	24	0	0	8	26	1	1	0	2	0	0	2	2	**66**
Nursing	**65**	5	2	1	27	5	1	4	2	5	2	3	1	0	**58**
Nutrition & Dietetics	**66**	2	0	0	8	19	0	1	1	1	0	1	0	0	**33**
Occupational Therapy	**67**	1	1	0	6	20	0	0	0	6	2	4	1	1	**42**
Operating Dept. Pract.	**68**	1	2	0	4	2	0	0	1	0	0	0	0	0	**10**
Physiotherapy	**69**	1	1	0	8	21	0	5	0	1	2	4	0	1	**44**
Podiatry	**70**	0	0	1	3	7	1	1	0	2	0	2	0	0	**17**
Radiography	**71**	2	1	0	9	15	0	2	0	3	0	0	0	0	**32**
Social Work	**72**	1	1	1	18	31	1	2	0	3	0	1	0	1	**60**
Speech Therapy	**73**	2	0	0	5	7	1	0	0	3	0	1	0	0	**19**
Other Professions	**74**	1	0	2	19	39	1	5	0	4	0	0	0	2	**73**
10b. If other professions gave details															
YES		1	0	2	23	43	1	5	0	4	0	0	1	2	**82**
NO		39	4	1	29	26	1	2	2	6	3	5	2	0	**120**
PART B OPINIONS															
11a. Terminology for shared learning															
None specific	**75**	12	1	5	39	21	3	1	2	3	1	2	3	1	**94**
Multidisciplinary	**76**	16	1	0	51	58	0	3	0	3	4	3	4	1	**144**
Interdisciplinary	**77**	7	1	0	12	8	1	4	0	2	1	2	0	0	**38**
Multiprofessional	**78**	3	1	0	4	8	0	1	0	1	0	0	0	0	**18**
Interprofessional	**79**	2	0	1	3	2	0	1	0	1	1	1	0	0	**12**
Pluridisciplinary	**80**	0	0	0	0	1	0	0	0	0	0	0	0	0	**1**
Other	**81**	0	0	0	2	6	0	0	0	0	1	0	0	0	**9**

		1	2	3	4	5	6	7	8	9	10	11	12	13	
11b. If other gave details															
YES		0	0	0	4	9	0	0	0	0	1	0	0	0	**14**
NO		40	4	6	103	87	4	7	2	10	7	6	7	2	**285**
12a. Belief in some shared learning															
YES	**82**	36	4	5	83	83	4	5	1	6	7	4	7	2	**247**
NO	**83**	1	0	0	5	5	0	0	0	0	1	0	0	0	**12**
UNDECIDED	**84**	3	0	1	19	8	0	2	1	4	0	2	0	0	**40**
12b. Belief in advantages															
YES	**85**	36	4	4	84	84	4	5	2	4	7	5	7	2	**248**
NO	**86**	1	0	0	4	3	0	0	0	0	1	0	0	0	**9**
UNDECIDED	**87**	3	0	2	18	8	0	2	0	6	0	1	0	0	**40**
12c. Listed advantages	**88**														
YES		30	2	5	65	80	4	6	2	9	7	5	6	2	**223**
NO		10	2	1	42	16	0	1	0	1	1	1	1	0	**76**
12d. Listed disadvantages	**89**														
YES		16	0	2	51	62	4	6	1	8	7	5	5	2	**169**
NO		24	4	4	56	34	0	1	1	2	1	1	2	0	**130**
13a. With own prof. poss. share learn															
Dental Surgeons	**90**	0	2	6	52	31	0	0	1	1	3	5	2	0	**103**
DSA/Dental Hyg.	**91**	30	0	3	22	28	0	1	0	1	1	3	2	0	**91**
Dental Tec.	**92**	27	2	3	18	21	0	0	0	0	1	1	1	0	**74**
Medicne	**93**	30	1	0	0	80	2	3	1	8	7	6	7	2	**147**
Nursing	**94**	29	4	1	87	0	4	5	2	7	6	5	7	1	**158**
Nutrition & Dietetics	**95**	30	3	0	55	66	0	4	0	2	2	3	4	1	**170**
Occupational Therapy	**96**	7	2	0	57	75	3	1	1	8	4	3	7	2	**170**
Operating Depart. Prac.	**97**	6	2	0	33	34	0	0	2	1	2	2	1	0	**83**
Physiotherapy	**98**	7	1	0	67	80	2	4	2	0	5	5	3	2	**178**
Podiatry	**99**	6	1	1	32	43	1	1	0	4	0	4	2	0	**95**
Radiography	**100**	20	3	1	53	39	1	0	2	4	6	0	2	1	**132**
Social Work	**101**	17	1	0	72	81	3	7	0	6	3	3	0	2	**195**
Speech Therapy	**102**	22	1	2	46	60	4	3	0	6	3	4	6	0	**157**
13b. Belief in problems in shared learn															
YES	**103**	14	0	1	39	56	3	5	0	8	6	3	3	1	**139**
NO	**104**	21	2	2	53	29	1	1	1	0	1	1	3	0	**115**
UNDECIDED	**105**	5	2	3	15	11	0	1	0	2	1	2	1	1	**44**
13c. If YES listed problems															
YES		13	0	1	40	61	3	5	0	8	7	3	3	1	**145**
NO		26	3	5	67	35	1	2	1	2	1	3	4	1	**151**
14a. Stage should take place															
Beginning	**106**	4	2	0	21	22	0	0	0	0	3	3	2	0	**57**
Middle	**107**	3	0	0	12	2	1	1	1	0	1	0	0	0	**21**
End	**108**	2	0	0	2	4	0	2	0	4	1	0	1	0	**16**
Throughout	**109**	30	2	6	70	69	3	3	1	4	2	4	5	2	**201**
After Qualifying	**110**	7	1	0	10	16	2	2	0	5	2	1	1	0	**47**
14b Gave reasons for choice															
YES		27	3	4	61	82	4	7	1	9	8	5	5	2	**218**
NO		13	1	2	45	13	0	0	1	1	0	1	2	0	**79**
15a. Any topics rejected															
YES	**111**	3	1	0	13	20	2	1	0	6	1	1	1	1	**50**
NO	**112**	37	2	6	90	70	2	5	2	3	7	5	6	1	**236**
15.b If YES listed topics															
YES		4	1	0	12	22	2	2	0	6	2	1	1	1	**54**
NO		36	3	6	93	69	2	4	2	3	6	5	6	1	**236**

		1	2	3	4	5	6	7	8	9	10	11	12	13	
16. Level of interest teaching others															
VERY INTERESTED	**113**	9	0	0	23	41	0	2	0	1	2	3	5	1	**87**
INTERESTED	**114**	22	3	6	46	41	4	4	1	3	6	1	2	0	**139**
NEITHER	**115**	7	1	0	29	8	0	1	1	4	0	2	0	1	**54**
UNINTERESTED	**116**	0	0	0	5	3	0	0	0	2	0	0	0	0	**10**
TOTALLY UNINTERESTED	**117**	2	0	0	5	2	0	0	0	0	0	0	0	0	**9**
17a. Benefit from special preparation															
YES	**118**	28	3	2	60	73	3	5	2	5	7	4	7	2	**201**
NO	**119**	4	1	1	13	5	0	0	0	0	0	0	0	0	**24**
UNDECIDED	**120**	8	0	3	25	18	1	2	0	5	1	1	0	0	**64**
17b. If YES gave details															
YES		20	2	2	41	64	3	5	1	5	5	3	6	2	**159**
NO		20	2	4	65	32	1	2	1	5	3	2	1	0	**138**
18. List of topics suitable/unsuitable															
Psychology															
SUITABLE	**121**	40	3	6	97	91	4	4	1	10	7	5	7	2	**277**
UNSUITABLE	**122**	0	1	0	7	3	0	2	1	0	0	1	0	0	**15**
Sociology															
SUITABLE	**123**	36	4	4	90	92	4	4	1	9	7	5	7	2	**265**
UNSUITABLE	**124**	4	0	2	15	2	0	2	1	1	0	1	0	0	**28**
Ethics															
SUITABLE	**125**	37	3	6	103	89	4	6	2	10	7	6	6	2	**281**
UNSUITABLE	**126**	3	1	0	4	5	0	0	0	0	0	0	1	0	**14**
Law & Practice															
SUITABLE	**127**	34	3	6	98	85	3	6	2	9	7	6	5	2	**266**
UNSUITABLE	**128**	6	1	0	9	9	1	0	0	1	0	0	2	0	**29**
Research Methods															
SUITABLE	**129**	34	2	5	80	86	4	6	2	7	6	4	6	2	**244**
UNSUITABLE	**130**	6	2	1	26	8	0	0	0	3	1	2	1	0	**50**
Management															
SUITABLE	**131**	33	3	6	100	81	4	6	1	7	6	6	4	2	**259**
UNSUITABLE	**132**	7	1	0	6	13	0	0	1	3	1	0	2	0	**34**
Economics of health care															
SUITABLE	**133**	31	2	5	99	88	4	6	1	7	6	6	4	2	**261**
UNSUITABLE	**134**	9	2	1	8	6	0	0	1	3	1	0	2	0	**33**
Health Promotion/Education															
SUITABLE	**135**	37	4	5	101	92	4	5	2	9	7	6	3	2	**277**
UNSUITABLE	**136**	3	0	1	5	2	0	1	0	1	0	0	3	0	**16**
Study Skills															
SUITABLE	**137**	32	4	6	86	90	4	5	2	9	7	6	7	2	**260**
UNSUITABLE	**138**	8	0	0	20	4	0	1	0	1	0	0	0	0	**34**
Quality in Health/Social Care															
SUITABLE	**139**	31	4	6	94	88	4	6	2	9	7	5	6	2	**264**
UNSUITABLE	**140**	9	0	0	12	6	0	0	0	1	0	1	1	0	**30**
Organisation in health/social care															
SUITABLE	**141**	34	4	6	94	91	4	6	2	8	7	6	6	2	**270**
UNSUITABLE	**142**	6	0	0	13	3	0	0	0	2	0	0	1	0	**25**
Computing Skills															
SUITABLE	**143**	36	3	6	95	91	4	6	2	10	7	6	6	2	**274**
UNSUITABLE	**144**	4	1	0	12	3	0	0	0	0	0	0	1	0	**21**

Appendix 5.12		**Student questionnaire results**													
VARIABLES		**DENTISTS**	**DSA/DH**	**DEN.TEC.**	**MEDICINE**	**NURSING**	**NUT. & DIET.**	**OCC. THERAPY**	**ODP**	**PHYSIOTHERAPY**	**PODIATRY**	**RADIOGRAPHY**	**SOCIAL WORK**	**SPEECH THERAP**	**TOTAL**
PART A BIOGRAPHIC DATA		**1**	**2**	**3**	**4**	**5**	**6**	**7**	**8**	**9**	**10**	**11**	**12**	**13**	**14**
1. Profession															
Dental Surgeon	**1**	93	0	0	0	0	0	0	0	0	0	0	0	0	**93**
DSA/Dental Hygienist	**2**	0	36	0	0	0	0	0	0	0	0	0	0	0	**36**
Dental Technician	**3**	0	0	30	0	0	0	0	0	0	0	0	0	0	**30**
Medicine	**4**	0	0	0	269	0	0	0	0	0	0	0	0	0	**269**
Nursing	**5**	0	0	0	0	396	0	0	0	0	0	0	0	0	**396**
Nutrition & Dietetics	**6**	0	0	0	0	0	45	0	0	0	0	0	0	0	**45**
Occupational Therapy	**7**	0	0	0	0	0	0	89	0	0	0	0	0	0	**89**
Operating Department Practitioner	**8**	0	0	0	0	0	0	0	25	0	0	0	0	0	**25**
Physiotherapy	**9**	0	0	0	0	0	0	0	0	101	0	0	0	0	**101**
Podiatry (Chiropody)	**10**	0	0	0	0	0	0	0	0	0	63	0	0	0	**63**
Radiography	**11**	0	0	0	0	0	0	0	0	0	0	52	0	0	**52**
Social Work	**12**	0	0	0	0	0	0	0	0	0	0	0	130	0	**130**
Speech Therapy	**13**	0	0	0	0	0	0	0	0	0	0	0	0	54	**54**
2. Year of Training															
Year 1	**14**	0	29	13	0	234	15	30	11	38	31	20	78	18	**517**
Year 2	**15**	0	7	8	0	125	5	26	14	29	16	18	51	12	**311**
Year 3	**16**	18	0	0	78	22	10	33	0	33	16	14	0	16	**240**
Year 4	**17**	33	0	3	119	8	15	0	0	0	0	0	0	8	**186**
Year 5	**18**	42	0	4	65	0	0	0	0	0	0	0	0	0	**111**
Other	**19**	0	0	1	7	2	0	0	0	0	0	0	0	0	**10**
3. Gender															
Male	**20**	53	0	18	120	63	4	9	16	23	15	10	35	1	**367**
Female	**21**	40	36	10	147	328	41	80	9	77	47	42	92	53	**1002**
4. Age Group															
20 Years or Under	**22**	23	16	10	5	159	11	21	0	42	19	29	0	17	**352**
21 - 25	**23**	62	15	11	239	128	27	36	14	29	18	16	13	22	**630**
26 - 30	**24**	6	2	4	16	40	3	13	8	18	9	5	35	1	**160**
31 - 35	**25**	1	3	3	7	31	1	6	2	6	7	1	34	4	**106**
36 - 40	**26**	0	0	0	0	24	1	2	1	4	6	1	17	2	**58**
41 - 45	**27**	0	0	1	0	6	1	7	0	0	3	0	20	4	**42**
46 - 50	**28**	0	0	0	0	2	0	3	0	1	1	0	8	3	**18**
51 - 55	**29**	0	0	0	0	0	0	0	0	0	0	0	2	0	**2**
Over 55 years	**30**	0	0	0	0	0	0	0	0	0	0	0	0	0	**0**
Previous relevant courses															
YES	**31**	9	17	10	46	119	5	21	7	22	20	9	77	10	**372**
NO	**32**	84	19	19	221	272	40	68	18	78	43	43	52	44	**1001**
5b. If YES gave details															
YES		9	16	10	46	121	4	21	6	22	19	9	75	9	**367**
NO		84	20	19	221	270	41	68	19	78	44	43	54	45	**1006**

		1	2	3	4	5	6	7	8	9	10	11	12	13	
Previous relevant work experience															
YES	**33**	25	25	11	122	256	27	62	20	60	38	17	113	34	**810**
NO	**34**	68	11	18	145	135	18	27	5	40	25	35	16	20	**563**
6b. If YES gave details															
YES		24	24	11	118	257	27	63	20	59	37	17	109	34	**800**
NO		69	12	18	148	134	18	26	5	41	26	35	20	20	**572**
7a. Experienced shared learning															
YES	**35**	68	16	11	62	79	3	8	6	7	12	9	61	15	**357**
NO	**36**	25	20	18	205	312	42	81	19	93	51	43	68	39	**1016**
7b. If YES which professions?															
Dental Surgeons	**37**	0	7	10	46	7	0	0	0	2	0	0	0	0	**72**
DSA/Dental Hygienist	**38**	0	0	5	0	8	0	0	0	0	2	0	3	0	**18**
Dental Technician	**39**	6	0	0	0	3	0	0	0	0	0	0	2	0	**11**
Medicine	**40**	58	0	1	0	25	0	1	0	3	5	0	15	2	**110**
Nursing	**41**	1	3	0	4	0	1	3	4	3	7	4	41	1	**72**
Nutrition & Dietetics	**42**	1	0	0	3	16	0	0	0	0	1	0	9	1	**31**
Occupational Therapy	**43**	0	0	0	7	25	0	0	0	2	3	6	34	1	**78**
Operating Dept. Practitioner	**44**	0	0	1	1	4	0	1	1	0	0	0	1	0	**9**
Physiotherapy	**45**	0	0	0	11	29	1	4	0	2	6	7	10	1	**71**
Podiatry	**46**	0	0	0	0	4	0	0	0	0	1	0	1	0	**6**
Radiography	**47**	1	0	0	6	8	0	0	0	0	1	0	1	0	**17**
Social Work	**48**	0	2	1	5	21	0	4	0	2	1	0	0	1	**37**
Speech Therapy	**49**	0	1	0	5	12	0	1	0	1	2	0	13	0	**35**
Other professions	**50**	4	2	2	9	15	1	3	2	0	1	5	24	11	**79**
7c. If other professions gave details															
YES		4	2	2	12	19	1	4	3	0	1	5	27	11	**91**
NO		89	34	27	254	372	44	85	22	99	62	47	102	43	**1280**
PART B OPINIONS															
8. Subjects to include under Behav.Sc.															
Psychology															
YES	**51**	91	35	27	262	381	45	88	20	98	61	51	128	54	**1341**
NO	**52**	1	0	1	2	3	0	0	1	0	0	0	0	0	**8**
Undecided	**53**	1	1	1	2	7	0	1	4	2	2	1	1	0	**23**
Sociology															
YES	**54**	83	33	24	241	357	43	79	20	99	55	45	114	45	**1238**
NO	**55**	2	1	0	13	13	0	4	1	0	2	5	4	2	**47**
Undecided	**56**	8	2	5	12	21	2	6	4	1	6	2	11	7	**87**
Ethics															
YES	**57**	62	17	14	147	176	24	46	16	82	33	30	78	33	**758**
NO	**58**	20	4	7	56	91	2	13	5	8	13	8	5	5	**237**
Undecided	**59**	11	15	8	63	124	19	30	4	10	17	14	46	16	**377**
		1	2	3	4	5	6	7	8	9	10	11	12	13	
Law & Practice															
YES	**60**	35	15	12	72	131	6	24	15	47	23	23	64	13	**480**
NO	**61**	41	10	5	136	174	19	39	3	38	21	23	37	26	**572**
Undecided	**62**	17	11	12	58	86	20	26	7	15	19	6	28	16	**321**

		1	2	3	4	5	6	7	8	9	10	11	12	13	
Management															
YES	**63**	45	16	14	71	121	12	27	12	48	30	17	78	27	**518**
NO	**64**	34	13	9	149	166	16	40	6	33	19	25	21	14	**545**
Undecided	**65**	14	7	6	46	92	17	22	7	19	14	10	30	14	**298**
Health Promotion															
YES	**66**	73	27	22	200	234	35	44	18	64	51	36	79	35	**918**
NO	**67**	14	0	4	36	86	4	16	2	22	2	13	22	9	**230**
Undecided	**68**	6	9	3	30	68	6	29	5	14	10	3	28	10	**221**
Study Skills															
YES	**69**	34	16	16	84	139	19	29	19	53	28	15	59	27	**538**
NO	**70**	43	6	5	134	163	11	29	4	32	21	29	33	12	**522**
Undecided	**71**	16	14	8	48	89	15	31	2	15	13	8	37	15	**311**
Quality Issues															
YES	**72**	27	12	8	60	113	12	25	13	45	17	18	67	14	**431**
NO	**73**	22	8	8	110	108	12	24	3	25	19	19	26	13	**397**
Undecided	**74**	44	16	13	96	170	21	40	9	30	27	15	36	27	**544**
9. Belief in some shared learning															
YES	**75**	71	29	26	177	324	42	84	21	71	60	45	124	47	**1121**
NO	**76**	11	2	0	42	9	1	0	1	5	1	5	1	0	**78**
Undecided	**77**	11	6	3	47	58	2	5	3	24	2	2	5	7	**175**
10a. Believe any advantages result															
YES	**78**	65	27	25	151	314	41	86	20	86	59	42	122	51	**1089**
NO	**79**	8	1	1	36	10	0	0	1	4	1	5	1	0	**68**
Undecided	**80**	20	8	3	79	67	4	3	4	10	2	5	6	3	**214**
10b. Listed ADVANTAGES															
YES		47	28	24	131	293	44	83	17	96	60	43	113	50	**1029**
NO		46	8	5	135	98	1	6	8	4	3	9	13	4	**340**
10c. Listed DISADVANTAGES															
YES		23	13	14	100	134	31	50	11	66	29	32	44	38	**585**
NO		70	23	15	166	257	14	39	14	34	34	20	85	16	**787**
11a.With own prof.shared learning?															
Dental Surgeons	**81**	0	28	28	93	72	24	5	3	8	6	16	5	28	**316**
DSA/Dental Hyg.	**82**	82	0	25	15	164	16	5	1	4	1	4	13	11	**341**
Dental Tec.	**83**	61	12	0	4	51	4	3	4	3	0	4	3	15	**164**
Medicine	**84**	85	12	0	0	309	41	70	20	88	61	41	97	42	**866**
Nursing	**85**	37	22	4	171	0	45	85	23	80	51	48	114	45	**725**
Nutrition & Dietetics	**86**	62	20	10	148	340	0	59	3	45	33	9	77	20	**826**
Occupational Therapy	**87**	21	9	6	157	328	30	0	5	93	46	16	121	46	**878**
Operating Depart. Prac.	**88**	13	7	4	43	178	8	11	0	18	38	17	19	5	**361**
Physiotherapy	**89**	17	2	3	175	317	27	86	10	0	59	33	79	44	**852**
Podiatry	**90**	4	0	1	35	149	12	20	1	39	0	4	19	3	**287**
Radiography	**91**	59	14	8	150	137	20	11	11	50	45	0	9	12	**526**
Social Work	**92**	40	13	4	139	317	37	86	5	71	38	21	0	46	**817**
Speech Therapy	**93**	45	5	18	91	254	30	74	4	69	9	11	102	0	**712**
		1	2	3	4	5	6	7	8	9	10	11	12	13	
11b. Believe problems own prof/others															
YES	**94**	20	11	11	108	119	15	45	10	49	20	18	43	23	**492**
NO	**95**	51	9	12	75	129	16	16	7	22	29	17	54	10	**447**
Undecided	**96**	22	16	6	83	142	14	28	8	29	14	17	4	21	**404**
YES		18	11	12	90	111	15	43	10	45	20	20	41	26	**462**
NO		75	25	17	176	279	30	46	15	55	43	32	88	28	**909**

		1	2	3	4	5	6	7	8	9	10	11	12	13	
12a. Stage Share. Learn. take place															
Beginning	**97**	5	9	2	37	51	7	17	7	19	8	19	17	3	**201**
Middle	**98**	16	9	9	69	81	6	5	5	20	18	7	20	11	**276**
End	**99**	7	2	4	33	23	8	2	2	5	5	5	7	5	**108**
Throughout	**100**	61	15	15	119	239	27	59	7	49	35	20	85	33	**764**
After Qualifying	**101**	4	4	1	28	107	2	8	4	12	6	4	7	7	**194**
12b. Gave reasons for choice															
YES		60	28	24	125	282	41	77	19	89	54	45	95	51	**990**
NO		33	8	5	139	107	4	12	6	11	9	7	34	3	**378**
13a. Any topics rejected															
YES	**102**	7	3	5	50	31	12	14	1	27	14	9	18	10	**201**
NO	**103**	86	33	24	214	359	33	75	24	73	49	43	111	44	**1168**
13b. If YES listed topics															
YES		5	3	5	35	28	13	16	1	29	15	9	15	10	**184**
NO		88	33	24	229	362	32	73	24	71	48	43	114	44	**1185**
14 . Interest in participating in sh.learn															
VERY INTERESTED	**104**	15	9	8	25	117	25	37	7	20	33	15	78	28	**417**
INTERESTED	**105**	53	17	16	118	201	18	49	13	54	23	25	47	20	**654**
NEITHER	**106**	19	7	3	82	56	1	3	5	17	6	9	2	3	**213**
UNINTERESTED	**107**	4	1	1	18	5	1	0	0	7	1	2	1	3	**44**
TOTALLY UNINTERESTED	**108**	2	2	1	18	5	0	0	0	2	0	1	1	0	**32**
15. Which sh.learn. methods approp.															
Mixed Tutorials															
YES	**109**	73	23	19	154	242	36	60	17	66	44	41	75	38	**888**
NO	**110**	10	3	5	67	57	5	11	5	19	5	8	13	6	**214**
Undecided	**111**	10	10	5	35	87	4	18	3	14	14	3	41	9	**253**
Workshops															
YES	**112**	49	13	18	123	281	32	74	22	60	43	32	119	45	**911**
NO	**113**	18	6	4	75	44	1	7	1	21	5	8	2	3	**195**
Undecided	**114**	26	17	7	58	47	12	8	2	19	15	12	8	5	**236**
Case Studies															
YES	**115**	76	20	21	119	256	33	63	12	58	38	39	112	44	**891**
NO	**116**	8	3	22	86	39	3	12	8	20	10	5	3	3	**222**
Undecided	**117**	9	13	6	50	91	9	14	5	22	15	8	14	6	**262**
Seminars															
YES	**118**	68	22	10	161	211	25	47	18	52	33	30	96	28	**801**
NO	**119**	10	3	8	57	56	7	17	4	27	12	7	12	11	**231**
Undecided	**120**	15	11	11	37	106	13	25	3	9	18	15	21	14	**298**
Problem Based Learning															
YES	**121**	47	15	15	132	244	27	51	13	61	38	28	100	24	**795**
NO	**122**	20	3	4	57	35	2	16	6	22	7	7	6	7	**192**
Undecided	**123**	26	18	10	66	108	16	22	6	17	18	17	23	23	**370**
Role Play															
YES	**124**	38	11	8	81	116	5	36	10	20	19	16	81	15	**456**
NO	**125**	38	14	13	120	171	19	34	12	54	19	20	18	28	**560**
Undecided	**126**	17	11	8	51	99	21	19	3	26	25	16	30	11	**337**

			1	2	3	4	5	6	7	8	9	10	11	12	13	
Lectures																
YES	**127**		46	20	15	90	200	26	64	21	56	40	34	73	27	**712**
NO	**128**		29	9	8	120	82	13	12	1	25	6	8	20	13	**346**
Undecided	**129**		18	7	6	45	104	6	13	3	19	17	10	36	13	**297**
Visits to Clinical Areas																
YES	**130**		78	25	27	182	297	35	66	19	73	58	44	98	43	**1045**
NO	**131**		7	4	0	38	37	2	11	4	16	1	4	7	3	**134**
Undecided	**132**		8	7	2	35	52	8	12	2	11	4	4	24	7	**176**
16. Opinion on topic suitable sh.learn.																
Psychology																
YES	**133**		83	34	22	185	342	40	83	17	93	54	44	125	51	**1173**
NO	**134**		10	2	7	67	36	5	6	8	7	9	8	3	2	**170**
Sociology																
YES	**135**		77	28	16	155	339	43	87	13	89	50	41	119	41	**1098**
NO	**136**		16	8	13	97	35	2	2	12	11	13	11	9	12	**241**
Ethics																
YES	**137**		67	16	17	192	324	36	79	23	83	46	42	114	48	**1087**
NO	**138**		26	20	12	60	55	9	10	2	17	17	10	14	5	**257**
Law & Practice																
YES	**139**		60	16	14	144	239	15	58	14	64	40	27	115	25	**831**
NO	**140**		33	20	15	108	145	30	31	11	36	23	25	13	28	**518**
Research Methods																
YES	**141**		44	11	21	95	246	33	63	16	40	42	36	96	35	**778**
NO	**142**		49	25	8	157	138	12	26	9	60	21	16	32	18	**571**
Management																
YES	**143**		62	14	16	129	223	22	58	16	48	36	23	97	30	**774**
NO	**144**		31	22	13	123	161	23	31	9	52	27	29	31	23	**575**
Economics of health care																
YES	**145**		72	22	19	136	299	31	64	16	77	46	28	99	39	**948**
NO	**146**		21	14	10	116	85	14	25	9	23	17	24	29	14	**401**
Health Promotion/Education																
YES	**147**		84	31	26	205	251	39	76	21	75	55	39	108	44	**1054**
NO	**148**		9	5	3	47	33	6	13	4	25	8	13	20	9	**195**
Study Skills																
YES	**149**		47	16	18	104	240	28	58	22	58	39	32	87	34	**783**
NO	**150**		46	20	11	148	144	17	31	3	42	24	20	41	19	**566**
Quality in Health/Social Care																
YES	**151**		49	12	13	98	238	27	64	15	63	32	32	104	29	**776**
NO	**152**		44	24	16	154	146	18	25	10	37	31	20	24	24	**573**
Organisation in health/social care																
YES	**153**		71	20	23	164	303	34	80	13	87	53	43	111	45	**1047**
NO	**154**		22	16	6	88	81	11	9	11	13	10	9	17	8	**301**

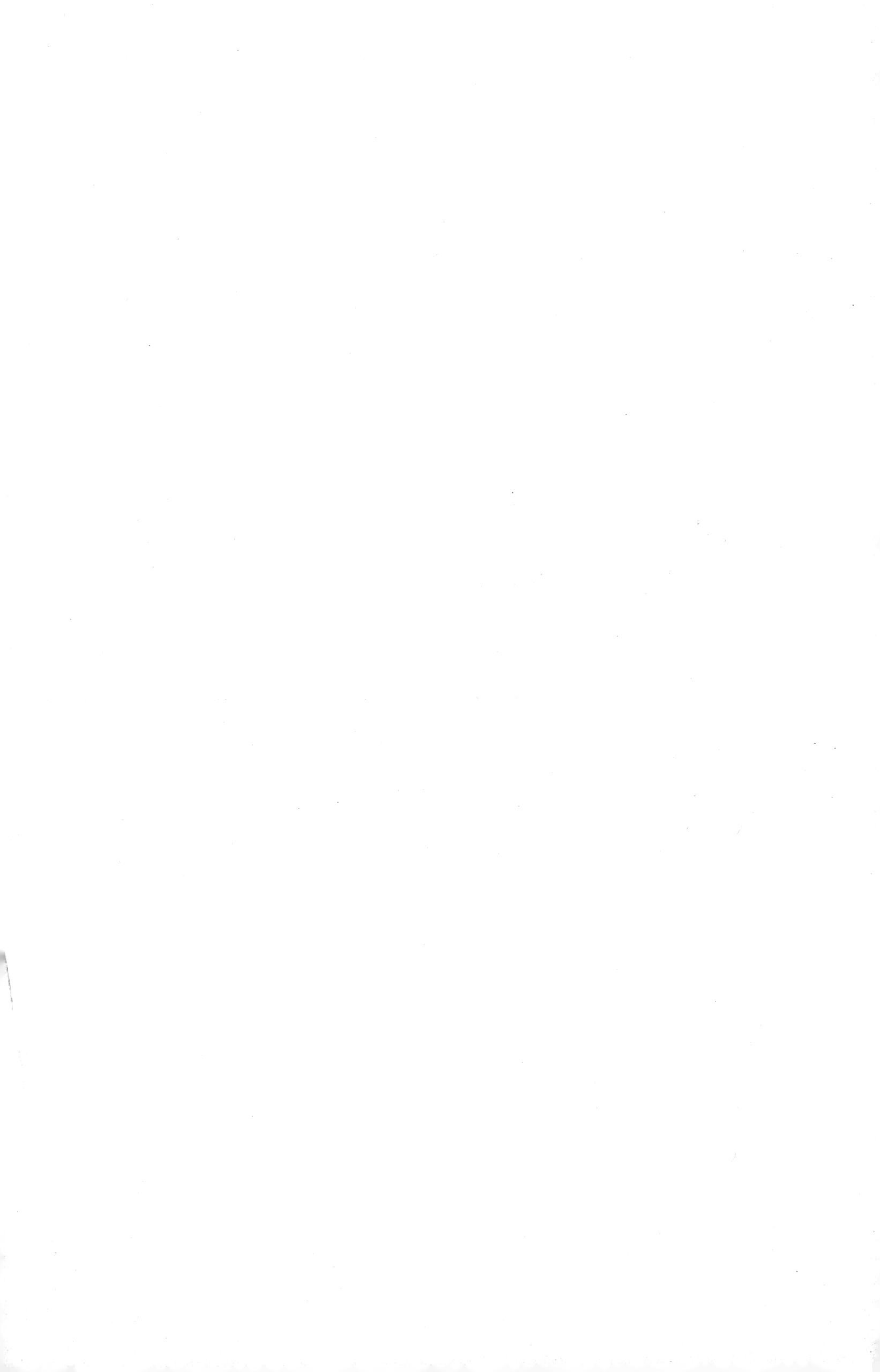